W0051018

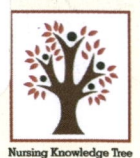

Nursing Knowledge Tree
An Initiative by CBS Nursing Division

Textbook of
# Midwifery and Gynecological Nursing
## for GNM Nursing Students

*(As per the Syllabus of Indian Nursing Council)*

Textbook of
# Midwifery and Gynecological Nursing

## for GNM Nursing Students

*(As per the Syllabus of Indian Nursing Council)*

**Second Edition**

**Sandeep Kaur**

MSc, PhD(N) (Obstetrics and Gynecological Nursing)

*Professor cum HOD*
Khalsa College of Nursing
Amritsar, Punjab

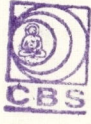

## CBS Publishers & Distributors Pvt Ltd

• New Delhi • Bengaluru • Chennai • Kochi • Kolkata • Lucknow • Mumbai
• Hyderabad • Jharkhand • Nagpur • Patna • Pune • Uttarakhand

Textbook of
## Midwifery and Gynecological Nursing
for GNM Nursing Students
*(As per the Syllabus of Indian Nursing Council)*

ISBN: 978-93-90619-18-4

**Reprint: 2025**

**Second Edition: 2022**

**First Edition: 2019**

Published by **Satish Kumar Jain** and produced by **Varun Jain** for

**CBS Publishers & Distributors Pvt Ltd**
4819/XI Prahlad Street, 24 Ansari Road, Daryaganj, New Delhi 110 002, India.
Ph: +91-11-23289259, 23266861, 23266867        Website: www.cbspd.com
Fax: 011-23243014
e-mail: delhi@cbspd.com; cbspubs@airtelmail.in.

*Corporate Office:* 204 FIE, Industrial Area, Patparganj, Delhi 110 092
Ph: +91-11-4934 4934        Fax: 4934 4935
e-mail: feedback@cbspd.com; bhupesharora@cbspd.com

*Branches*

- **Bengaluru:** Seema House 2975, 17th Cross, K.R. Road, Banasankari 2nd Stage, Bengaluru-560 070, Karnataka
  Ph: +91-80-26771678/79              Fax: +91-80-26771680              e-mail: bangalore@cbspd.com
- **Chennai:** 7, Subbaraya Street, Shenoy Nagar, Chennai-600 030, Tamil Nadu
  Ph: +91-44-26680620, 26681266       Fax: +91-44-42032115              e-mail: chennai@cbspd.com
- **Kochi:** 68/1534, 35, 36-Power House Road, Opp. KSEB, Cochin-682018, Kochi, Kerala
  Ph: +91-484-4059061-65              Fax: +91-484-4059065             e-mail: kochi@cbspd.com
- **Kolkata:** Hind Ceramics Compound, 1st Floor, 147, Nilganj Road, Belghoria, Kolkata-700056, West Bengal
  Ph: +033-2563-3055/56                                                e-mail: kolkata@cbspd.com
- **Lucknow:** Basement, Khushnuma Complex, 7-Meerabai Marg (Behind Jawahar Bhawan), Lucknow-226001, Uttar Pradesh
  Ph: +0522-4000032                                                    e-mail: tiwari.lucknow@cbspd.com
- **Mumbai:** PWD Shed, Gala No. 25/26, Ramchandra Bhatt Marg, Next to J.J. Hospital Gate No. 2, Opp. Union Bank of India, Noor Baug, Mumbai-400009, Maharashtra
  Ph: +91-22-66661880/89              Fax: +91-22-24902342             e-mail: mumbai@cbspd.com

*Representatives*

| | | |
|---|---|---|
| **Hyderabad** +91-9885175004 | **Jharkhand** +91-9811541605 | **Nagpur** +91-9421945513 |
| **Patna** +91-9334159340 | **Pune** +91-9623451994 | **Uttarakhand** +91-9716462459 |

Printed at : Goyal Offset Works Pvt. Ltd. Haryana

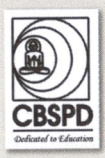

## CBS Nursing Knowledge Tree

## Extends its Tribute to

# *Florence Nightingale*

"

*For glorifying the role of women as nurses,
For holding the title of " The Lady with the Lamp,"
For working tirelessly for humanity—
Florence Nightingale will always be
remembered for her
selfless and memorable services to the
human race.*

"

**Florence Nightingale
(May 1820 – August 1910)**

# Dedicated to

My parents, husband and teachers
who blessed my life with their tireless support and
encouragements

# Preface to the Second Edition

It gives me immense pleasure and satisfaction to present the 2nd edition of *Textbook of Midwifery and Gynecological Nursing* for GNM Nursing Students.

Midwifery is the oldest art that requires in-depth professional knowledge. Present era of evidence-based nursing practices has imposed increasing demand on nurses to generate sound evidence-based knowledge to improve nursing practice, shape health policy and protect the health of people.

This edition has come out with an international standard to meet the overwhelming demand of a quality book in many parts of the world. The new edition of this book offers a unique opportunity to students as well as teachers, to assimilate the ever-growing body of scientific knowledge and to develop the technical and analytical skills necessary to apply the same into practice.

This book has been organized into two sections. Section I (Midwifery) that includes 14 Chapters and Section II (Gynecological Nursing) that contains 7 Chapters which are strictly based on revised GNM curriculum by INC. At the end of the book, Midwifery Procedures and Instruments, commonly used in obstetrics and gynecological procedures are included.

Each chapter of this book starts with learning objectives, chapter outline and ends with frequently asked questions in exams and multiple choice questions. Special care has been taken to develop the content by avoiding the unnecessary details and keeping the text according to the requirement and structure of the recent trends of the paper.

The feedback that I received from the teachers and students was invaluable. Many of these suggestions have been addressed in this edition. I hope, this comprehensive textbook will continue to be of immense educational resource to the readers as ever.

**Sandeep Kaur**

# Preface to the First Edition

Midwifery is recognized as a responsible and accountable profession. A midwife works in association with women to give the necessary support, care and advice during pregnancy, labor and postpartum period and to conduct births. The midwives are also responsible to provide care to the newborn and infants. The care includes preventive measures, the promotion of normal birth, the detection of complications in mother and child, providing access to medical care or other appropriate assistance and then carrying out emergency measures.

Being constantly insisted by my beloved students, I have attempted to write a compact, comprehensive and practically oriented textbook on midwifery and gynecology. It is an effort to provide the students comprehensive and easy techniques of obstetrics with an aim to emphasize the text in a simple rather than in complex way.

"Textbook of Midwifery and Gynecological Nursing for GNM Students" offers a unique opportunity to students as well as teachers, to assimilate the ever-growing body of scientific knowledge and to develop the technical and analytical skills necessary to apply the same into practice. This book is organized into two sections. Section I (Midwifery) that includes 14 chapters and Section II (Gynecological Nursing) that contains 7 chapters which are strictly based on revised GNM curriculum by INC. Thorough and updated text matter has been presented in a concise and lucid language, which will make this textbook reader-friendly.

The book has flavor of its own, both in scope and content distinctly different from a number of existing textbooks. It is an attempt to encourage the students to learn midwifery in a comparatively easy way. Each chapter starts with learning objectives, chapter outline and ends with frequently asked questions in exams and multiple choice questions. Special care has been taken to develop the content by avoiding the unnecessary details and keeping the text according to the requirement and structure of the recent trends of the paper.

The critical evaluation and feedback of the readers regarding the content are welcome.

**Sandeep Kaur**

# Acknowledgments

First and foremost, I would like to thank the Almighty for all His blessings to me. Thank you God for the strength you have bestowed upon me and also for keeping your protective hands on me.

No endeavors are complete in isolation and likewise this book too is a product of efforts and blessings of many noble people around me. I am very fortunate to have the valuable guidance, help and support of all those who have been my advisors, Dr Darshan Soni, Dr Monika Dogra and Dr Neelam Hans, friends, well-wishers and family members. I convey my heartfelt thanks to all those who have been associated with this book and have contributed to it in one way or the other.

I would like to thank **Mr Satish Kumar Jain** (Chairman) and **Mr Varun Jain** (Managing Director), M/s CBS Publishers and Distributors Pvt Ltd for providing me the platform in bringing out the book. I have no words to describe the role, efforts, inputs and initiatives undertaken by **Mr Bhupesh Aarora**, Sr. Vice President – Publishing and Marketing (Health Sciences Division) for helping and motivating me.

Last but not least, I sincerely thank the entire CBS team for bringing out the book with utmost care and attractive presentation. I would like to thank Ms Nitasha Arora (Publishing Head and Content Strategist – Medical and Nursing), Ms Daljeet Kaur (Assistant Publishing Manager) and Dr Anju Dhir (Product Manager and Medical Development Editor) for their editorial support. I would also extend my thanks to Mr Shivendu Bhushan Pandey (Sr. Manager and Team Lead), Mr Ashutosh Pathak (Sr. Proofreader cum Team Coordinator) and all the production team members for devoting laborious hours in designing and typesetting the book.

All the suggestions and critical evaluation by readers and academicians are highly appreciated.

# Reviewers

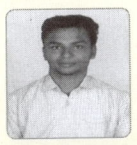

**Ashish Pandya**
BSc(N)
*Nursing Tutor*
Chitrini Nursing College
Prantij, Gujarat

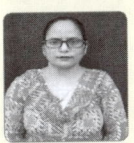

**Bhupinder Kaur**
MSc (OBG)
*Professor*
University College of Nursing
Faridkot, Punjab

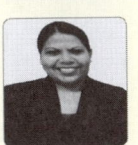

**Cristina Francis**
*Professor and Principal*
Mata Saraswati Institute of Nursing
Ludhiana, Punjab

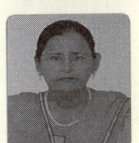

**Darshan Sohi**
PhD, MSc(N)
*Professor and Principal*
Chief Khalsa Diwan College of
Nursing
Amritsar, Punjab

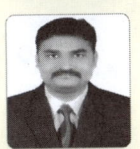

**Jeenath Justin Doss K**
MSc(N) PhD Scholar
*Principal*
Shri Anand Institute of Nursing
Anand, Gujarat

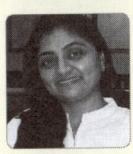

**Mallika Vhora**
MSc(N), PhD Scholar
*I/C Principal*
Knowledge Institute of Nursing
Anand, Gujarat

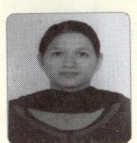

**Monika Dogra**
PhD, MSc(N)
*Associate Professor*
Khalsa College of Nursing
Amritsar, Punjab

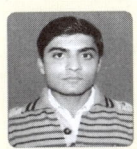

**Narendra Kumar Sharma**
MSc(N)
*Principal*
Chitrini Nursing College
Prantij, Gujarat

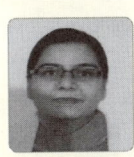

**Neelam Hans**
PhD, MSc(N)
*Professor and Principal*
Khalsa College of Nursing
Amritsar, Punjab

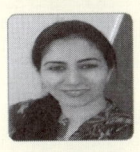

**Nidhi Sagar**
MSc(N)
*Professor and Vice-Principal*
Dayanand Medical College and
Hospital
Ludhiana, Punjab

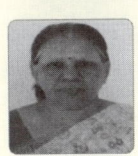

**Pratima Mali**
MSc(N)
*Principal*
SKUM College of Nursing
Ahmedabad, Gujarat

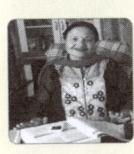

**Ramesh Kumari**
PhD, MSc(N)
*Professor and Principal*
Mai Bhago College of Nursing
Tarn Taran, Punjab

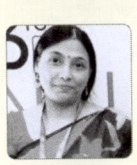

**Saonli Jha**
MSc(N) (OBG)
*Professor*
Woodlands College of Nursing
Alipore Road, Kolkata

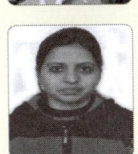

**Timsy**
MSc(N) (OBG)
*Associate Professor*
Desh Bhagat University Mandi
Gobindgarh, Punjab

*The name of the reviewers are arranged in alphabetical order*

# From Publisher's Desk

*Dear Reader,*

Nursing Education has a rich history, often characterized by traditional teaching techniques that have evolved over time. Primarily, teaching took place within classroom settings. Lectures, textbooks, and clinical rotations were the core teaching tools; and students majorly relied on textbooks by local or foreign publishers for quality education. However, today, technology has completely transformed the field of nursing education, making it an integral part of the curriculum. It has evolved to include a range of technological tools that enhance the learning experience and better prepare students for clinical practice.

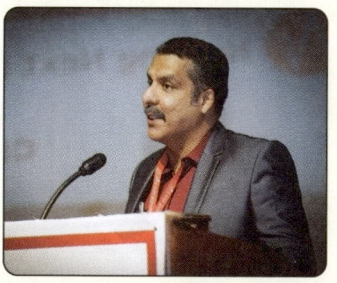

As publishers, we've been contributing to the field of Medical Science, Nursing and Allied Sciences and earned the trust of many. By supporting **Indian authors**, coupled with **nursing webinars and conferences**, we have paved an easier path for aspiring nurses, empowering them to excel in national and state level exams. With this, we're not only enhancing the quality of patient care but also enabling future nurses to adapt to new challenges and innovations in the rapidly evolving world of healthcare. Following the ideology of **Bringing learning to people instead of people going for learning**, so far, we've been doing our part by:

- Developing quality content by qualified and well-versed authors
- Building a strong community of faculty and students
- Introducing a smart approach with Digital/Hybrid Books, and
- Offering simulation Nursing Procedures, etc.

Innovative teaching methodologies, such as modern-age Phygital Books, have sparked the interest of the Next-Gen students in pursuing advanced education. The enhancement of educational standards through **Omnipresent Knowledge Sharing Platforms** has further facilitated learning, bridging the gap between doctors and nurses.

At Nursing Next Live, a sister concern of CBS Publishers & Distributors, we have long recognized the immense potential within the nursing field. Our journey in innovating nursing education has allowed us to make substantial and meaningful contributions. With the vision of strengthening learning at every stage, we have introduced several plans that cater to the specific needs of the students, including but not limited to **Plan UG** for undergraduates, **Plan MSc** for postgraduate aspirants, **Plan FDP** for upskilling faculties, **SDL** for integrated learning and **Plan NP** for bridging the gap between theoretical & practical learning. Additionally, we have successfully completed seven series of our **Target High** Book in a very short period, setting a milestone in the education industry. We have been able to achieve all this just with the sole vision of laying the foundation of diversified knowledge for all. With the rise of a new generation of educated, tech-savvy individuals, we anticipate even more remarkable advancements in the coming years.

We take immense pride in our achievements and eagerly look forward to the future, brimming with new opportunities for innovation, growth and collaborations with experienced minds such as yourself who can contribute to our mission as Authors, Reviewers and/or Faculties. Together, let's foster a generation of nurses who are confident, competent, and prepared to succeed in a technology-driven healthcare system.

**Mr Bhupesh Aarora**
(Sr Vice President – Publishing & Marketing)
bhupeshaarora@cbspd.com| +91 95553 53330

# Special Features of the Book

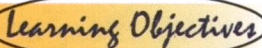
**Learning Objectives**

Learning Objectives given in all the chapters focus on the areas that a student shall comprehend after completing the chapter

**Upon completing this chapter, the learner will be able to:**
- Define midwifery and obstetrical nursing
- Describe the scope of midwifery
- Enlist the basic competencies of a midwife

Every chapter starts with a chapter outline that gives the glimpse of the content covered in the chapter

**Chapter Outline**

- Maternity Care: Key Terms and Concepts
- Scope of Midwifery
- History of Midwifery
- History of Midwifery in India
- Trends of Maternity Services in India
- Vital Statistics
- Basic Competencies of Nurse Midwives

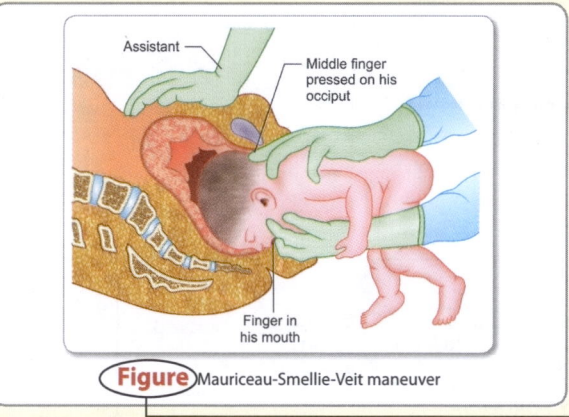
**Figure** Mauriceau-Smellie-Veit maneuver

Several images and diagrams have been used at relevant places to simplify the concepts for the students

Numerous tables are used in text to provide necessary data and information to supplement the text

**TABLE 1:** Malpositions in vertex presentation

| Malposition | Occiput points towards | Sagittal suture of fetus in mother's pelvis |
| --- | --- | --- |
| Left occipitolateral position (LOL) | Left iliopectineal line (midway between iliopectineal eminence and ileosacral joint) | Transverse diameter |
| Right occipitolateral position (ROL) | Right iliopectineal line (midway between iliopectineal eminence and ileosacral joint) | Transverse diameter |
| Left occipitoposterior position (LOP) | Left sacroiliac joint | Left oblique diameter |
| Right occipitoposterior position (ROP) | Right sacroiliac joint | Right oblique diameter |
| Occipitoanterior position | Symphysis pubis | Anteroposterior diameter |
| Occipitoposterior position | Sacrum | Anteroposterior diameter |

Numerous flow diagrams are used to enhance your learning experience

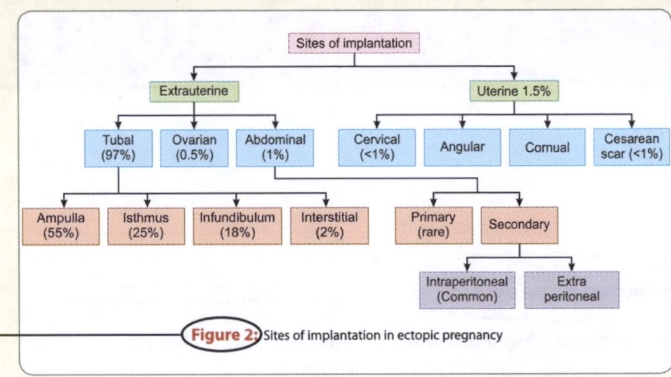

**Figure 2:** Sites of implantation in ectopic pregnancy

At the end of every chapter, *Assess yourself* section which contains frequently asked questions in exams and multiple choice questions, helps you to attain mastery over the subject

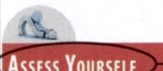

## ASSESS YOURSELF

**FREQUENTLY ASKED QUESTIONS IN EXAMS**

1. Define breech presentation, its types and complication of breech. Explain the nursing responsibility during breech delivery.
2. Define postpartum hemorrhage. Explain the types of PPH, its causes and diagnostic evaluation.
3. Describe the management of true PPH.
4. Differentiate between contraction ring and retraction ring.
5. What do you mean by prolonged labor? What are the causes and complication of prolonged labor?
6. How can you manage a case of prolonged labor?
7. Write short notes on:
   1. Precipitate labor
   2. Contracted pelvis
   3. Cord prolapse
   4. Management of retained placenta
   5. Obstetrical shock

**MULTIPLE CHOICE QUESTIONS**

1. Contracted pelvis may be caused by the deficiency of which vitamin during early childhood:
   a. Vitamin $B_{12}$
   b. Vitamin C
   c. Vitamin D
   d. Vitamin A
2. When the ALAE of both sides are absent and the sacrum directly fused with the innominate bones, the pelvis is known as:
   a. Robert pelvis
   b. Naegele pelvis
   c. Android pelvis
   d. Anthropoid pelvis

## Appendices

### 1

### ANTENATAL EXAMINATION

**Definition:** It is systematic examination of the pregnant woman externally to know about the pregnant uterus and condition of fetus.

#### Purposes

- To detect the high risk conditions of mother and fetus.
- To promote and maintain physical health.
- To ensure continued medical surveillance and prophylaxis.

## Instruments used in Obstetrics and Gynecological Procedures

### ARTERY FORCEPS

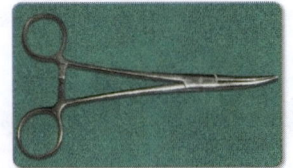

#### Purposes

- To clamp bleeding vessels during hemorrhage.
- To grasp tissue at the time of operation.
- To hold stay sutures.

Appendices are added at the end which include Midwifery procedures & Instruments used in obstetrics & gynecological procedures to improve clinical nursing skills.

# Syllabus

## Midwifery and Gynecological Nursing

**Placement: Third Year**

**Total Hours: 140**

Midwifery: 120 hours
Gynecological Nursing: 20 hours

## MIDWIFERY

### Course Description

This course is designed to help students acquire knowledge and gain skills to meet the needs of women during pregnancy, labor and puerperium and care for the newborn.

**Total Hours: 120**

| Unit No. | Learning objectives | Contents | Hrs | Teaching learning activities | Assessment methods |
|---|---|---|---|---|---|
| I | Describe the scope and trends in midwifery | **Introduction:**<br>• Definition of midwifery and obstetrical nursing<br>• Scope of midwifery<br>• Basic competencies of a midwife<br>• History of midwifery<br>• Trends of maternity services in India<br>• Vital statistics related to maternal health in India. | 4 | • Lecture cum discussions<br>• Videos | • Short answers<br>• Objective type<br>• Essay type |
| II | Describe the anatomy and physiology of female reproductive system | **Reproductive system**<br>• Review of structure and function of female reproductive system<br>• Female pelvis—structure, types and diameters | 5 | • Lecture cum discussions<br>• Demonstrations<br>• Charts, specimen models and objects | • Short answers<br>• Objective type<br>• Essay type<br>Viva |
| III | Describe the stages of embryological and fetal development | **Embryology and fetal development**<br>• Oogenesis, spermatogenesis, fertilization and implantation.<br>• Embryology and fetal development<br>• Placenta and membranes:<br>  ▪ Structure<br>  ▪ Functions<br>  ▪ Abnormalities<br>  ▪ Liquor amni<br>  ▪ Umbilical cord | 8 | • Lecture cum discussions<br>• Charts<br>• Models and objects<br>• Specimens | • Short answers<br>• Objective type<br>• Essay type<br>• Oral presentation |

*Contd...*

| Unit No. | Learning objectives | Contents | Hrs | Teaching learning activities | Assessment methods |
|---|---|---|---|---|---|
| | | • Fetal skull:<br>  ▪ Structure<br>  ▪ Diameters<br>  ▪ Fontanels and sutures<br>• Fetal circulation | | | |
| IV | • Describe the physiological changes in pregnancy and the management of normal pregnancy<br>• Demonstrate skill in caring for pregnant women | **Normal pregnancy and its management**<br>• Pre-conception care<br>• Genetic counseling<br>• Physiological changes in pregnancy<br>• Diagnosis of pregnancy<br>  ▪ History<br>  ▪ Signs and symptoms<br>• Antenatal care:<br>  ▪ History taking<br>  ▪ Calculation of expected date of delivery,<br>  ▪ Examination and investigations<br>  ▪ Health education and counselling<br>  ▪ Drugs and immunizations<br>• Minor disorders and their management | 12 | • Lecture cum discussions<br>• Demonstration<br>• Clinical teaching Simulation<br>• Charts and videos<br>• SBA module of government of India, handbook for staff nurses (Government of India) | • Short answers<br>• Objective type<br>• Essay type<br>• Assessment of skill using checklist |
| V | • Describe the various stages of labor and the role of the midwife in caring for a woman in labor<br>• Demonstrate skill in conducting the normal delivery | **Normal labor and its management**<br>• Definition and stages<br>• Causes and signs of onset of labor<br>• True and false labor<br>• First stage of labor:<br>  ▪ Physiology<br>  ▪ Monitoring using partograph and its interpretation<br>  ▪ Care of mother: physical and psychological<br>  ▪ Pain management<br>  ▪ Setting up of the labor room including newborn corner<br>• Second stage:<br>  ▪ Physiology and mechanism<br>  ▪ Monitoring<br>  ▪ Conduction of normal delivery<br>  ▪ Episiotomy<br>  ▪ Essential newborn care<br>• Third stage:<br>  ▪ Physiology and signs<br>  ▪ Active management of third stage<br>  ▪ Examination of the placenta<br>  ▪ Episiotomy suturing<br>• Fourth stage:<br>  ▪ Physiology<br>  ▪ Care of the mother and baby<br>  ▪ Postpartum family planning | 18 | • Lecture cum discussions<br>• Demonstrations<br>• Case studies<br>• Simulation<br>• Videos exercises<br>• SBA module of government of India, handbook for staff nurses (Government of India) | • Short answers<br>• Objective type<br>• Essay type<br>• Assessment of skill using checklist |

*Textbook of Midwifery and Gynecological Nursing*

*Contd...*

| Unit No. | Learning objectives | Contents | Hrs | Teaching learning activities | Assessment methods |
|---|---|---|---|---|---|
| VI | • Describe the management of normal newborn<br>• Development of skill in caring for the normal newborn | **Management of newborn**<br>• Assessment<br>• Physiological adaptation<br>• Apgar scoring<br>• Examination for defects<br>• Breastfeeding- BFHI<br>• Care of newborn—Skin, eyes, buttocks, etc.<br>• Bonding and rooming in<br>• Minor disorders of new born:<br>  ▪ Birth marks, rashes, skin<br>  ▪ Infections, sore buttocks,<br>  ▪ Infection of eyes. | 14 | • Lecture cum discussion<br>• Demonstrations<br>• Clinical teaching<br>• Chart<br>• Videos<br>• SBA module, ENBC, NSSK, PPIUCD module, handbook for staff nurses of Government of India | • Short answers<br>• Objective type<br>• Essay type<br>• Assessment of skill using checklist |
| VII | Describe normal pureperium and the role of midwife in the caring for woman in puerperium | **Management of normal puerperium**<br>• Definition and objectives of care<br>• Physiological changes<br>• Postnatal counseling<br>• Lactation and feeding<br>• Care during puerperium—breast and perineal care, postnatal exercise, postnatal examination, follow up, family welfare<br>• Minor ailments and management<br>• Family planning | 10 | • Lecture cum discussion<br>• Demonstration<br>• Simulation role play SBA module, PPIUCD module, handbook for staff nurses of Government of India | • Short answers<br>• Objective type<br>• Essay type<br>• Assessment of skill using checklist |
| VIII | • Describe the complications of pregnancy<br>• Demonstrate skills in providing care for women with complicated pregnancy | **Management of complications during pregnancy**<br>• Bleeding in pregnancy<br>  ▪ Early and late<br>  ▪ Ectopic pregnancy<br>  ▪ Abortion<br>  ▪ Antepartum hemorrhage<br>  ▪ Vesicular mole<br>• Hyperemesis gravidarum<br>• Gestational diabetes mellitus<br>• Pregnancy induced hypertension<br>  ▪ Preeclampsia<br>  ▪ Eclampsia<br>• Hydromnios—poly and oligo<br>• Pelvic inflammatory diseases<br>• Intrauterine growth retardation<br>• Post maturity<br>• Intrauterine death<br>  ▪ High-risk pregnancy<br>  ▪ Monitoring—NST, USG<br>  ▪ Anemia<br>  ▪ Jaundice<br>  ▪ Viral<br>  ▪ Urinary tract infections<br>  ▪ Hearts diseases<br>  ▪ Diabetes | 12 | • Lecture cum discussions<br>• Case presentation<br>• Clinical teaching<br>• Videos simulation<br>• Case studies and exercises SBA module | • Short answers<br>• Essay type<br>• Objective type<br>• Assessment of skill using checklist |

*Contd...*

| Unit No. | Learning objectives | Contents | Hrs | Teaching learning activities | Assessment methods |
|---|---|---|---|---|---|
| | | • AIDS and STD's<br>• Osteomalacia<br>• Teenage pregnancy<br>• Elderly primigravida<br>• Multipara<br>• Multiple pregnancy | | | |
| IX | • Describe the management high-risk labor<br>• Demonstrate skills in early detection and prompt management of high-risk labor | **Management of high-risk labor**<br>• Malposition, malpresentations<br>• Contracted pelvis<br>• Abnormal uterine actions<br>• Cervical Dystocia<br>• Premature rupture of membranes, precipitate and prolonged labor, induction of labor obstructed labor,<br>• Obstetrics Emergencies-Cord prolapse, cord presentation, amniotic fluid embolism, obstetric shock, rupture of uterus, shoulder dystocia, vasa previa.<br>• Complications of third stage<br>  ▪ PostpartumHemorrhage<br>  ▪ Atonic uterus<br>  ▪ Injuries to the birth canal<br>  ▪ Retained placenta and membranes<br>  ▪ Inversion of uterus | 10 | • Lecture cum discussion<br>• Demonstration<br>• Bed-side clinic<br>• Videos and charts<br>• Clinical teaching<br>• IMPAC module of WHO<br>• MCPC module of Government of India | • Short answers<br>• Objective type<br>• Essay type<br>• Assessment of skill using checklist |
| X | • Describe the puerperal complications<br>• Demonstrate skill in the management of complica-tions of puer-perium | **Management of complications of puerperium**<br>• Puerperal pyrexia<br>• Puerperal sepsis<br>• Thrombophlebitis and embolism<br>• Breast engorgement, mastitis, breast abscess<br>• Puerperal psychosis | 4 | • Lecturer cum discussion<br>• Demonstration<br>• Clinical teaching MCPC module of Government of India | • Short answers<br>• Objective type<br>• Essay type |
| XI | • Describe the management of high-risk and sick newborn<br>• Demonstrate skills in caring for high-risk and sick newborns | **High-risk and sick newborn**<br>• Assessment<br>• Nursing care<br>• Management of newborn with:<br>  ▪ Hyperbilirubinemia<br>  ▪ Neonatal hypoglycemia<br>  ▪ Hypothermia<br>  ▪ Neonatal convulsions<br>  ▪ Rh incompatability<br>  ▪ Small for dates<br>  ▪ Low birth weight<br>  ▪ Preterm<br>  ▪ Asphyxia, RDS<br>  ▪ Sepsis | 10 | • Lecturer cum discussion<br>• Demonstration Clinical teaching IMNCI module SBA module<br>• NSSK module | • Short answers<br>• Objective type<br>• Essay type<br>• Assessment of skill using checklist |

*Contd...*

| Unit No. | Learning objectives | Contents | Hrs | Teaching learning activities | Assessment methods |
|---|---|---|---|---|---|
| | | ▪ Birth injuries cephalohematoma caput succedaneum facial and Erb's palsy to torticollis hemorrhage<br>▪ Congenital anomalies<br>• Newborn of HIV positive mother, diabetic mother<br>• Levels of care in NICU | | | |
| XII | Describe the obstetric operations and midwife role in assisting with each one | **Obstetric operations**<br>• Definition, indication and care of women undergoing<br>▪ Induction of labor<br>▪ Manual removal of placenta<br>▪ Version<br>▪ Forceps delivery<br>▪ Vacuum extraction<br>▪ Cesarean section<br>▪ Sterilization<br>▪ Destructive surgeries<br>▪ Amnio infusion<br>▪ Manual vaccum aspiration, dilatation and evacuation, dilatation and curettage<br>• Post abortion care | 10 | • Lecture cum discussion<br>• Clinical teaching Videos<br>• Post abortion care module of GoI | • Short answers<br>• Objective type<br>• Essay type<br>• Assessment of skill using checklist |
| XIII | Describe the midwife's role in the administration of drugs for women during pregnancy labor and post-postpartum period | **Drugs used in obstetrics**<br>• Indication, dose, action, contraindication, side effects and responsibilities in the administration of:<br>▪ Oxytocin<br>▪ Uterotonics<br>▪ Tocolytics<br>▪ Antihypertensives<br>▪ Anticonvulsants<br>▪ Anesthesia and analgesia<br>• Drugs used for newborn<br>• Teratogens—effects of drugs on mother and baby | 4 | • Lecture cum discussion<br>• Drug presentation | • Short answers<br>• Objective type<br>• Essay type |
| XIV | Describe the ethical and legal issues related to midwifery | **Ethical and legal aspects related to midwifery**<br>• Maternal and newborn death review<br>• Mother and child tracking system | 2 | • Lecture cum discussion<br>• Presentation | • Short answers<br>• Objective type |

# GYNECOLOGIAL NURSING

## Course Objective

The students shall be able to identify different gynecological disorders and diseases and gain skills in providing nursing care to women suffering from them.

**Total Hours: 20**

| Unit No. | Learning objectives | Contents | Hrs | Teaching learning activities | Assessment methods |
|---|---|---|---|---|---|
| I | • Define the terms used in gynecology<br>• Demonstrate the skills of gynecology history taking, conducting examination and investigation | **Introduction**<br>• Definition of terms<br>• History<br>• Examination<br>• Investigation | 2 | • Lecture cum discussion<br>• Demonstration Videos | • Short answers<br>• Objective type<br>• Essay type<br>• Return demonstra-tion |
| II | Describe the physiology, psychology and pathology of puberty | **Puberty**<br>• Definition<br>• Development of sex organs in females and sexuality<br>• Review of menstrual cycle<br>• Premenstrual syndrome<br>• Disorders of menstruation, dysmenorrhea, cryptomenorrhea, dysfunctional uterine bleeding | 3 | • Lecture cum discussion<br>• Clinical teaching<br>• Videos<br>• Charts | • Short answers<br>• Objective type<br>• Essay type |
| III | Describe the management of couples with fertility related problems | **Fertility and infertility**<br>• Definition<br>• Causes—both in male and female<br>• Investigation<br>• Management<br>• Artificial reproductive techniques | 2 | • Lecture cum discussion<br>• Clinical teaching<br>• Videos<br>• Role play | • Short answers<br>• Objective type<br>• Essay type |
| IV | Demonstrate skills in the management of clients with various pelvic infections | **Pelvic infections**<br>• Vulva—vulvitis, bartholinitis<br>• Vagina—vaginitis, trichomonas vaginitis, moniliasis<br>• Metritis, salpingitis, oophritis<br>• Cervical erosions<br>• Pelvic abscess<br>• Chronic infection<br>• Pelvic inflammatory disease<br>• Pelvic tuberculosis | 4 | • Lecture cum discussion<br>• Clinical teaching<br>• Videos<br>• Prevention of STI module of NACO | • Short answers<br>• Objective type<br>• Essay type |

*Contd...*

| Unit No. | Learning objectives | Contents | Hrs | Teaching learning activities | Assessment methods |
|---|---|---|---|---|---|
| | | • Sexually transmitted diseases<br> ▪ Syphilis<br> ▪ Gonorrhea<br> ▪ Warts<br> ▪ HIV<br>• Syndromic case management | | | |
| V | Describe the care of women with gynecological disorders | **Gynaecological disorders**<br>• Retroversion, retroflexion<br>• Fistulas<br>• Uterine displacement and prolapse (Procidentia)<br>• Uterine malformations<br>• Cysts and fibroids<br>• Uterine polyps<br>• Tumors of the reproductive tract—benign and malignant<br>• Palliative care and rehabilitation | 5 | • Lecture cum discussion<br>• Case presentation<br>• Demonstration | • Short answers<br>• Objective type<br>• Essay type |
| VI | Describe the care of the woman with breast disorders | **Breast disorders**<br>• Review mastitis, breast engorgement, breast abscess<br>• Tumors of the breast benign and malignant | 2 | • Lecture cum discussion<br>• Clinical teaching<br>• Videos<br>• Role play | • Short answers<br>• Objective type<br>• Essay type |
| VII | Describe the care of women with menopause | **Menopause**<br>• Definition and physiological changes<br>• Signs and symptoms<br>• Health education and counseling<br>• Hormone replacement therapy<br>• Surgical menopause | 2 | • Lecture cum discussion<br>• Case histories | • Short answers<br>• Objective type<br>• Essay type |

# Contents

## SECTION I: MIDWIFERY

# SECTION II:   GYNECOLOGICAL NURSING

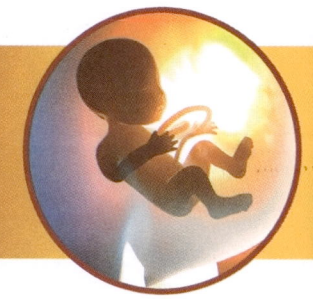

# Midwifery

## Section Outline

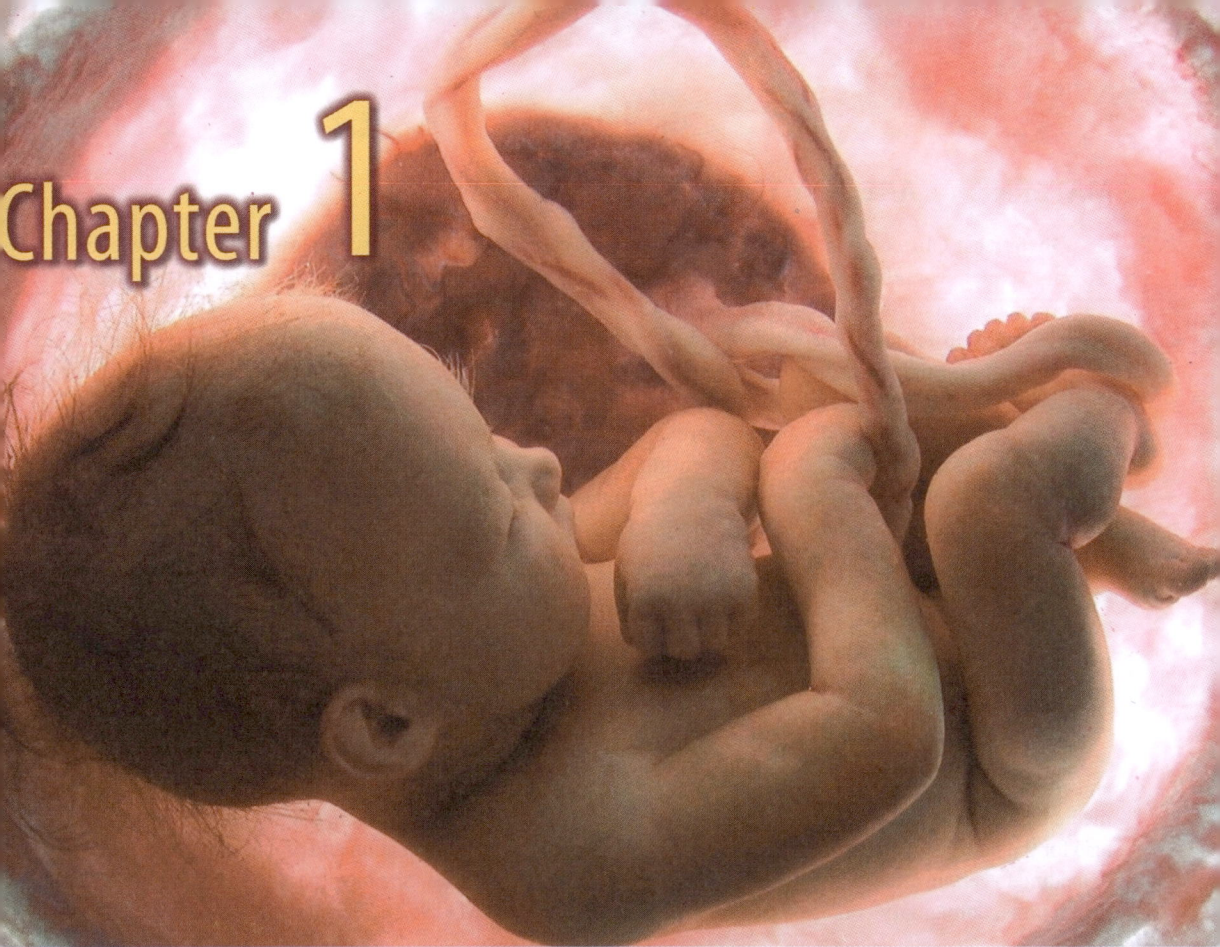

# Chapter 1

# Introduction

## MATERNITY CARE: KEY TERMS AND CONCEPTS

- **Obstetrics:** Obstetrics is defined as the branch of medicine that deals with parturition, its antecedents and sequel. Therefore, obstetrics is principally concerned with the phenomenon and management of pregnancy, labor and the puerperium under normal and abnormal circumstances.

  The word obstetrics is derived from obstetrician, meaning midwife. The Latin word 'obsto' means 'to stand by.' In England and the United States, this branch of medicine was called midwifery until the latter part of the 19th century, when the term obstetrics came to the forefront.
- **Midwifery:** Midwifery is a healthcare profession in which midwives provide care to childbearing women during pregnancy, labor and childbirth, and also during postpartum period. They also help in care of the newborn for their healthy growth and development.
- **Midwife:** The term midwife is derived from middle English word Midwife, which literally means "with the women" (Mid = with and wife = women).

Midwife is a person "who has been admitted to a regular midwifery educational program, duly recognized by the country in which it is located and has successfully completed the prescribed course of studies in midwifery, and has acquired the requisite qualifications to be registered and/or legally licensed to practice midwifery." Furthermore, "she must be able to give necessary supervision, care, and advice to the woman during pregnancy, labor and the postpartum period; conduct deliveries on her own; and provide care for the newborn and infant. This care includes preventive measures, detection of abnormal conditions in the mother and child, the procurement of medical assistance and the execution of emergency measures in the absence of medical help. A midwife has an important task in health counseling and education, not only for the women, but also for the family and community. The work should involve antenatal education and preparation of parenthood extending to certain areas of gynecology, family planning and child care. She may practice in hospitals, clinics, health units, domiciliary conditions, or in any other services." [ICM (1952), FIGO (1991), WHO (1992)]*.

## MIDWIFERY

### Scope of Midwifery

The role of a nurse in obstetrical care is diverse—the difference lies in the scope of practice and responsibilities. These are described here:

- **Teacher/educator:** Assesses educational needs of mothers and infants based on the data collected for health promotion, maternal care, infant care, postnatal care and family planning throughout the childbearing age.
- **Nurse manager:** Prioritizes client's needs, gives care with minimum input and maximum output, coordinates health care facilities and maintains midwifery care standards.
- **Nurse advocate:** Acts as a liaison/advocate between the client and the healthcare delivery system and encourages client awareness, talks about rights and responsibilities, makes informed choices and ensures utilization of available healthcare resources.
- **Nurse researcher:** Encourages evidence-based practice in midwifery, participates and conducts midwifery research and evaluates current protocols and recent research findings for their applications in practice.
- **Clinical nurse specialist:** Clinical nurse specialist is an expert in maternity nursing who serves as a role model of excellence in knowledge and clinical practice of midwifery. She provides high-quality individualized care to women and newborn and performs the role of a neonatal nurse in neonate intensive care unit (NICU), high-risk pregnancy units and gynecological units.

*__*Abbreviations:__ ICM, International Confederation of Midwives; FIGO, International Federation of Gynecology and Obstetrics; WHO, World Health Organization*

- **Political activist:** As a political activist, a midwife serves as an active member of professional organization. She implements all governmental programs for maternal and child health (MCH) care at the grass root level. She also keeps a track of the current health care policies regarding women's health.
- **Change agent:** As a change agent, she encourages women empowerment and stimulates awareness among women.

The **International Confederation of Midwives (ICM) recognizes the scope of midwifery practice to include:**

- Education and counseling on sexual health and provision of contraceptive methods
- Provision of support, care and advice during pregnancy, labor and postpartum period
- Conducting births is the responsibility of the midwife
- The provision of care for the newborn and the infant. Midwifery care may be provided in any setting including the home, community hospital, clinic or health unit, depending on how maternity care is organized within a given country. Midwifery care is linked with the care provided by health providers in referral centers (doctor, nurses and specialists). Midwifery care is provided with consideration given to the context care; i.e. the health care system in which she practices, and the special circumstances of the country of practice, its specific health concerns and epidemiological challenges [e.g., human immunodeficiency virus (HIV)/acquired immunodeficiency syndrome (AIDS)].

## History of Midwifery

Midwifery is as old as the history of human species. Archeological evidence of a woman squatting in childbirth supported by another woman from behind demonstrates the existence of midwifery in 500 BC. In the Bible, in the Old Testament, genesis 35:7. "It came to pass, where she was in hard labor; that the midwife said unto her, fear not Rachael, it is another boy." In Exodus 1:15, it is recorded that King of Egypt spoke to a Shiphrah and Puah, the two midwives, who helped Hebrew women during childbirth. These two midwives are the first midwives who are mentioned in the literature.

Hippocrates (460 BC), the father of scientific medicine, organized training and supervised midwives. Hippocrates believed that the fetus had to fight its way to come out of the womb and membranes.

Aristotle (384–382 BC), the father of embryology, described the uterus and female pelvic organs. He also discussed the essential qualities of the midwives.

Soranus, in the second century, was the first to specialize in obstetrics and gynecology. He used a vaginal speculum and advised on cord care. In 1513, the first book on midwifery was printed in Germany based on the teachings of Soranus.

From 5th to 15th centuries, which was the period of decline of Roman Empire, untrained midwives controlled the practice of midwifery.

Leonardo da Vinci (1452–1519) made anatomical drawings of pregnant uterus. Ambroise Paré (1510–1590) laid the foundation of modern obstetrics. He performed internal podalic version. He was the first to help a woman deliver a baby in bed rather than a stool. He also sutured perineal lacerations. Ambroise Paré founded a school for midwives in Paris, France. Louise Bourgeois, midwife trained by Pare, attended the ladies of the French court. She warned midwives against getting infected with syphilis and transmitting it to other women. She recommended induction of labor for pelvic contraction.

William Harvey (1578–1657), the father of British midwifery, wrote the first English textbook on midwifery. He described the fetal circulation and placenta, and was the first to deliver the placenta by massaging the uterus. He described the raw placental surface and initiated the study of uterine sepsis. Women remained largely reluctant to be delivered by men during this period. Midwives did not usually seek medical aid until the labor was hopelessly obstructed, as in the case of gross pelvic deformities. The resultant death of mother or newborn gave physician unwarranted reputation.

Julius Caesar Aranzi wrote the first book for Italian midwives, which ran up to 17th edition. He advised cesarean section for contracted pelvis. The French King Louise XIV, in 1663, employed a surgeon from Paris to attend one of his mistresses and pleased with the result, the king honored the surgeon with the title "accoucheur." William Smellie (1697–1763) is called the Father of British midwifery. Charles White, in 1773, stated puerperal fever was infectious. He used lime as disinfectant and clean linen, and isolation, adequate ventilation and sitting posture to facilitate drainage.

Laennec, in 1816, invented a stethoscope. James Young Simpson in 1847 used chloroform in obstetrics for anesthesia for the first time. Florence Nightingale, in 1862, organized a small training school in connection with King's College Hospital, where she conducted training for midwives. Louis Pasteur, in 1879, wrote a thesis on puerperal sepsis demonstrating the presence of streptococci in the lochia, blood and in fatal cases in the peritoneal cavity. Spencer and Ballantyne promoted the concept of antenatal care for pregnant women. The first antenatal clinic was started about the time of the First World War. In 1876, Porro formed subtotal hysterectomy. Max Sanger in 1882, first sutured the uterine walls.

In 1912, Kronig introduced lower segment vertical incision and it was popularized by DeLee (1922). Munro Kerr in 1926, introduced the present technique of lower segment cesarean operation and popularized it. In 1940, the first book was translated into English. For a century and half, it was the only book on midwifery in English. During this period, doctors were rigidly excluded from labor rooms and midwives assisted women in labor.

Vesalius, in 1953, opened the full-term pregnant uterus in a lower animal, extracted the fetus and demonstrated uterus as a single chamber organ. The history of cesarean section dates back to 715 BC and the operation derives its name from the notification *lex caesarea* → a Roman law, which was followed even during Caesar's reign. The law provided for an abdominal delivery either in a dying woman with a hope to get a live baby or to perform postmortem abdominal delivery for a separate burial. The operation does not derive its name from the birth of Caesar, as his mother lived long time, after his birth. The origin of the word "cesarean" is also related to a Latin verb *caedere* which means 'to cut'. Chamberlain, in 1975, designed obstetric forceps.

## Introduction to Midwifery

The provision of midwifery is witnessing long-awaited increase in global attention. Recognizing the significant contribution made by midwives worldwide, many countries are giving center stage to midwives in order to improve quality of care, reduce "over-medicalization" during childbirth and increase efficient use of resources.

### What is Midwifery?

"Skilled, knowledgeable and compassionate care for childbearing women, newborn, infants and families across the continuum throughout prepregnancy, pregnancy, birth, postpartum and the early weeks of life. Core characteristics include optimizing normal biological, psychological, social and cultural processes of reproduction and early life; timely prevention and management of complications; consultation with and referral to other services; respect for women's individual circumstances and views; and working in partnership with women to strengthen women's own capabilities to care for themselves and their families." (Lancet Series on Midwifery, 2014)

### Who is a Midwife?

"A midwife is a person who has successfully completed a midwifery education program that is duly recognized by the country where it is located and that is based on the International Confederation of Midwives (ICM), Essential Competencies for Basic Midwifery Practice and the framework of the ICM, Global Standards for Midwifery Education; who has acquired the requisite qualifications to be registered and/or legally licensed to practice midwifery and use the title 'midwife' and who demonstrates competency in the practice of midwifery." (International Confederation of Midwives, 2015)

## MIDWIFERY IN INDIA

### Why does India Need Midwifery?

Global evidence has shown that the introduction of midwifery care has been historically translated into the increased availability of quality maternal and newborn health services, and significantly aided the reduction of maternal and newborn mortality and morbidity.

The State of the World's Midwifery Report 2014, which examined the midwifery workforce data across 73 low- and middle-income countries, calls for urgent investment in high-quality midwifery care. The 73 countries represented in the report account for 96% of global maternal deaths, 91% of stillbirths and 93% of newborn deaths. However, these countries have only 42% of the world's doctors, midwives and nurses. Of the 73 countries, only four have the workforce needed to provide the care needed by women and their newborns and for reduction of maternal and newborn mortality and morbidity.

The WHO Statement on C-Section Rates (2015) describes that C-Sections are effective in saving maternal and infant lives, but only when they are required for medically indicated reasons. At population level, C-Section rates higher than 10% are not associated with reductions in maternal and newborn mortality rates. This means that approximately 85% of pregnancies and births do not require specialized obstetric intervention. The Lancet Series on Midwifery (2014) notes that 87% of services can be provided by midwives, when educated to international standards. Midwifery care includes the entire continuum of care for women as well as newborn care, breastfeeding, family planning and screening women for HIV infection, tuberculosis and malaria. As midwives are often the first point of contact for women with the health system, early signs of noncommunicable diseases can be detected through routine antenatal check-ups.

A Cochrane Review on "Midwife-led continuity models vs other models of care for childbearing women" (2016) provides evidence that midwife-led continuity of care can result in a 24% reduction in preterm birth, a significant reduction in episiotomy, instrumental birth or use of pain relief while increasing psychological support for women.

In summary, "Midwifery is associated with improved efficient use of resources, and outcomes when provided by midwives who are educated, trained, licensed and regulated, and that midwives were most effective when integrated into the health system in the context of effective teamwork, referral mechanisms and sufficient resources" (Lancet Series of Midwifery, 2014). Thus, midwifery care introduces a system level shift from fragmented maternal and newborn care focused on identification and treatment of pathology, to skilled and compassionate woman-centric care.

### Introducing Midwifery in India

Several attempts have been made to formally introduce midwives into India's health system. A post-basic course, known as the Nurse Practitioner in Midwifery (NPM) course, was instituted by the Indian Nursing Council (INC). In 2000–2003, with support from the 'India–Australia Training and Capacity Building Project', a curriculum for the NPM was prepared, with the aim to provide nurses with advance knowledge, skills and attitudes, which allow them to become safe and competent NPMs who can practice independently in rural areas. The duration of the course was 18 months (including 6 months' internship) and was developed using the essential competencies set out by the ICM. The INC also developed midwifery practice and clinical standards. This initiative was pilot-tested in the State of West Bengal. Two batches of training were conducted and 12 candidates who passed out of this course were posted as NPMs and were offered a remuneration equivalent to that of Assistant Nursing Superintendent.

The "Inter-Institutional Collaboration between Institutions in India and Sweden for Improving Midwifery and Emergency Obstetric Care (EmOC) Services in India" Project 2007–13 was carried out by collaboration between State governments, the Indian Institute of Management—Ahmedabad (IIM-A), the Society of Midwives, India (SOMI), the Trained Nurses Association, India (TNAI), the Advanced Nursing Society (ANS), the White Ribbon Alliance, India (WRAI) supported by the Swedish International Development Agency (SIDA), the Karolinska Institute, and the Swedish Midwifery Association. The objectives of the project were: capacity building to improve midwifery skill; research and advocacy; pilot testing to develop a midwifery focused model of care; policy analysis, and networking. Five Centers for Advanced Midwifery Trainings (CAMT) were established in four States with advance skills laboratories, training equipment, mannequins, audio-visual teaching aids and well-equipped libraries. Fifteen senior faculty members (9 in 1st batch and 6 in 2nd batch) teaching midwifery and maternal health-related subjects were nominated by the State governments and were given three-months training, part of which was in Sweden. In addition, the tutors were regularly mentored and given additional skill training on site. The project was successful in increasing visibility of midwifery care at policy level and was partially successful in bringing midwifery to the focus of program managers in the four States. Adequate mechanisms were not put in place for sustainability and scaling-up for systemic integration into the health system.

Recently, the INC reintroduced the Post-Basic Diploma in Nurse Practitioner in Midwifery, a one-year course in midwifery post-BSc nursing training. The course was adopted by the States of West Bengal and Gujarat. Examples of past experiences and current on-going midwifery trainings from various States are indicated in Table 1.

**TABLE 1:** Examples of midwifery training courses in India from various states

| State | Project | Current situation |
|---|---|---|
| West Bengal (2002/2011) | **India-Australia Training and Capacity Building Project**.<br>• In 2002, the first course of 18-months training in Nurse Practitioner Midwifery started under the India-Australia AID project, based on curriculum developed by INC. Twelve posts of NPM sanctioned by the State Government. Total two batches of training conducted.<br>• In 2011, West Bengal implemented the One-Year Post Basic Diploma in Nurse Practitioner in Midwifery. | Training stopped after two batches. Twelve candidates posted in PHCs and BPHCs. |
| Andhra Pradesh (AP), West Bengal (WB), Gujarat and Tamil Nadu | Beginning with the NPM course in two States (West Bengal and Gujarat), five CAMT centers were established in four States with 12-months training course. Fifteen senior faculties underwent a three-month advanced tutor course, some of which was in Sweden. In Gujarat, training of NPM for one year led to a separate cadre of NPM equal to Matron class 3. | Midwifery visibility increased, however, the initiative was not started up. |
| Telangana (2011/2014/2017) | • In 2011, the Professional Midwifery Education and Training Program were conducted by Fernandez Hospital.<br>• In 2014, Fernandez Hospital was accredited to initiate the Post-Basic Diploma in NPM with 10 seats.<br>• In 2017, the Government of Telangana initiated a tripartite partnership between State Government, UNICEF and Fernandez Hospital to train nursing students in midwifery using 18-months course based on ICM competencies. Training of first batch is going on. Training is supported by NHM. Total 126 posts of midwives created by the State Government. | Training is going on. |
| Madhya Pradesh | Eighteen-months training on Midwifery is going on for four nurses at private institute, Choithram Hospital, based on ICM competencies. No involvement of State Government. | Training is going on. |

# TRENDS OF MATERNITY SERVICES IN INDIA

Since last few decades, enormous changes have taken place in the delivery of nursing care to the mother and the newborn. In yesteryears, most babies were delivered at home by an untrained woman, neighbor, relative or friend or for the fortunate few by a physician or trained midwife. All the family members and dear ones used to provide proper care to the mother and her newborn.

In the second half of 20th century, most of the deliveries were conducted in the hospital setting. Most of the care to the mother and newborn was provided by medical professionals. At that point, childbearing became much more than merely a family affair. The mother and newborn remained isolated from the family for a week to 10 days, when family had only visiting privileges.

Nursing was separated into three specialties, with one nurse caring for the mother during labor and delivery, another handling postpartum mother and third caring for the baby.

In the 1940s, "Rooming In" concept was devised. Full-term infants were placed in a crib at their mother's bedside. This not only established the mother-child relationship but the mother also got conversant with the art of baby care so that she can take full care of the baby while at home. The advantages of the system included a reduction in neonatal infection from cross contamination, increased confidence and independence for the mother and successful breastfeeding.

In the 1960s, the focus changed from the person giving care to the person receiving the care. It led to the change of terminology and obstetrical care become maternity care. The broadened scope includes both prenatal and postnatal care and promotes the health and wellbeing of the mother, the newborn and the entire family.

World Health Organization (WHO) defined maternity care as "the objective of maternity care is to ensure that every expectant and nursing mother maintains good health, learns the art of childcare, has a normal vaginal delivery and bears healthy children."

## Current Trends

- **Technological advances:** Advances in technology have revolutionized the diagnosis and treatment of many health conditions for both the mother and the baby. Because of these advances, it became necessary for nursing personnel to become well conversant with the procedures and protocols developed for use of the advanced equipment and treatment. Although there is a concern that the technological advances discourage the "Hand-on care" of the client, the nursing process must remain the foundation of quality nursing care.
  - Fetal monitoring has progressed from the use of fetoscope to electronic fetal monitors (EFM), which allow observation of the baby's heart beat during pregnancy and throughout labor, even during uterine contractions.
  - The strength of labor contractions can now be measured by means of an internally placed catheter attached to a monitor.
  - Telemetry using radio transmission now makes it possible to monitor contractions and fetal heartbeat even when the mother is not in the same room in which the monitor is. This new development allows more comfort and mobility during labor.
- **Increased cost of high-tech care:** As the high and sophisticated technology is being introduced into today's world, the costs are also increasing. For the procedure such as ultrasound, fetal monitoring, etc. the couple has to pay good amount of money. Gradually, obstetric care is becoming a business for the care providers.
- **Changing patterns of childbirth and their effects on maternal infant mortality statistics:** Increasing numbers of working women defer motherhood until they are in their 30s. As early marriage practices

continue, teenage pregnancies continue to occur. At both ends of the spectrum, the older and younger mother face increased risk of complications during pregnancy such as preterm delivery, low-birth-weight babies, maternal and fetal morbidity, and mortality. In addition, women in increasing numbers are working outside the home during pregnancy and shortly after delivery compounding the risks to themselves and the fetus by exposure to toxic chemicals, excessive noise and workplace stress.

- **Family-centered care:** This concept was introduced in obstetrics by Wiedenbach. It is a system for the provision of quality midwifery care that is adapted to the physical and psychological needs of the mother, newborn and her family. It enhances social support, develops parental self-esteem and competence and upgrades the level of midwifery practice.

- **Rising cesarean birth rates:** The use of fetal monitoring and ultrasound for prenatal evaluation of fetal condition has increased rate of cesarean birth rates. Many physicians nowadays because of financial gains conduct cesarean section, therefore eventually increasing cesarean birth rates.

- **Increasing the number of intensive care units:** Over the past 20 years, care of infant and children has become extremely technical. Many infants nowadays are born with low-birth-weight and who are sick. Such infants are transferred to NICU. For this, opportunities for advanced practice nurses also have increased.

- **Epidural analgesia in labor:** Epidural analgesia provides better pain relief in labor. However, it is not associated with improved maternal satisfaction. It does not increase lower segment cesarean section (LSCS) rates. Risk of postpartum backache is not increased. It increases the risk for vaginal instrumental delivery and also prolongs the second stage of labor.

- **Positions during second stage of labor:** Earlier, lithotomy position was used during second stage of labor. Now various studies have proved that upright or sitting positions are good for childbirth because it enhances gravity and also allows the coccyx to move backwards as the baby passes through the birth canal. In case of lithotomy position, the coccyx is pressed against the hard bed and not able to move back and thus not allowing the pelvic outlet to widen.

- **Team midwifery practice:** Every pregnant mother is allocated a small group of three or four midwives who are responsible for the total care of the woman throughout the complete maternity cycle. Continuity of care with cost effectiveness, short-term hospitalization, freedom of choice for the place of delivery, avoidance of unnecessary obstetrical intervention, professional autonomy and better utilization of midwifery skills are some of the benefits of team midwifery practices.

- **Complementary and alternative medicine (CAM):** The following therapies are used in obstetric and gynecological care by nurses:
  - Aroma therapy
  - Music therapy
  - Acupuncture
  - Acupressure
  - Hot packs
  - Infrared lamp therapy for episiotomy wound healing
  - Yoga and meditation
  - Massage therapy

- **Natural childbirth:** It is a method of childbirth in which medical interventions are minimized. The mother uses birthing positions according to her comfort and practices breathing and relaxation techniques to decrease pain, which make the delivery easier.

- **Water births:** Water birth has several benefits. Contractions cause less discomfort as the warmth of water is maintained. This method promotes relaxation of the abdominal and uterine muscles. The first stage of labor duration is also shortened.

- **Early discharge:** During earlier days, women were hospitalized for longer duration and physical activity was increased gradually. Over the years now, however, health care personnel have realized the early return to normal activities is the best course for uncomplicated births.

- **Role of father:** With increased societal emphasis on shared parenting and the recognition of parental bonding, many fathers are active in care giving and are enjoying the closeness with the baby.
- **Midwifery (a separate profession):** Nursing and midwifery care are becoming attractive career options among women. Like nursing graduates, midwifery graduates demonstrated competencies in midwifery practice, care of the mother and their babies, and are eligible for advanced education. Midwifery leaders believe that midwifery is a specialization, it has a body of knowledge and many countries have recognized midwifery as a separate profession, like nursing profession.
- **Entry to midwifery practice: A degree in midwifery from university:** In order to meet the global standard to establish educational criteria, a task force committee decided that nursing and midwifery practice should be a degree, and therefore a degree program for midwives was devised. It is believed that this will make the midwives more competent and will help them perform high quality of maternal and child care resulting in positive maternal and birth outcome.
- **Independent nurse midwifery practice:** This program establishes independent midwifery practitioner. Here, midwives enjoy more autonomy focusing on mother and newborn in a particular population, this enables them to bring better birth outcome.

## VITAL STATISTICS

### Definition

Vital statistics refers to quantitative data relating to birth, death, marriages, health and disease.

### Purpose

The use of statistics enables the health policy makers and healthcare providers to discern trends and events in the health arena; thus, they are able to predict and plan to minimize or control health outcomes.

Government of India promulgated the Central Birth and Death Registration Act in 1969. The Act came into force in 1970. The Act provides compulsory registration of births and deaths throughout the country, and compilation of vital statistics in the state to ensure uniformity and comparability of data. The time limit for registering the event of birth is 14 days and that of death is 7 days. In case of any default, some amount of fine can be imposed.

### Comparison of Vital Statistics in World and India

| Vital statistics | In World | In India |
|---|---|---|
| Birth rate | 19.95 | 20.97 |
| Death rate | 8.12 | 7.48 |
| Maternal mortality rate (MMR) | 251.00 | 212.00 |
| Infant mortality rate (IMR) | 41.61 | 47.57 |
| Neonatal mortality rate | 16.19 | 44.00 |
| Perinatal mortality rate | 20.00 | 39.00 |
| Total fertility rate | 2.47 | 2.62 |

- **Birth rate:** Birth rate is defined as "the number of live births per 1000 in the estimated mid-year population in a given year"

$$\text{Birth rate} = \frac{\text{Number of live births during the year}}{\text{Estimated mid-year population}} \times 1000$$

- **Maternal Mortality Rate (MMR):** MMR is expressed as an annual number of female deaths per 1000 live births.

$$MMR = \frac{\begin{array}{c}\text{Total number of female deaths in an area, due to complications} \\ \text{of pregnancy, childbirth, or within 42 days of delivery} \\ \text{from puerperal causes during a given period}\end{array}}{\text{Total number of live births in the same area and year}} \times 1000$$

- **Infant Mortality Rate (IMR):** IMR is defined as the ratio of infant deaths registered in a given year to the total number of births registered in the same year. It is usually expressed as a rate per 1000 live births.

$$IMR = \frac{\text{Number of deaths of children less than 1 year of age in a year}}{\text{Number of live births in the same year}} \times 1000$$

- **Neonatal Mortality Rate (NMR):** NMR is the number of neonatal deaths in a given year per 1000 live births in that year.

$$NMR = \frac{\text{Number of deaths of children under 28 days of age in a year}}{\text{Total live births in the same year}} \times 1000$$

- **Perinatal Mortality Rate (PMR):** It is defined as death among fetuses weighing over 1000 g at birth, which die before or during delivery or within the first 7 days of delivery (late fetal and early neonatal deaths). The PMR is expressed in terms of such deaths per 1000 total births.

$$PMR = \frac{\begin{array}{c}\text{Late fetal deaths (28 weeks of gestation or more)} \\ \text{plus early neonatal deaths (1 week)}\end{array}}{\text{Live births in the same year}} \times 1000$$

## Prevention of Maternal/Infant Morbidity and Mortality (Fig. 1)

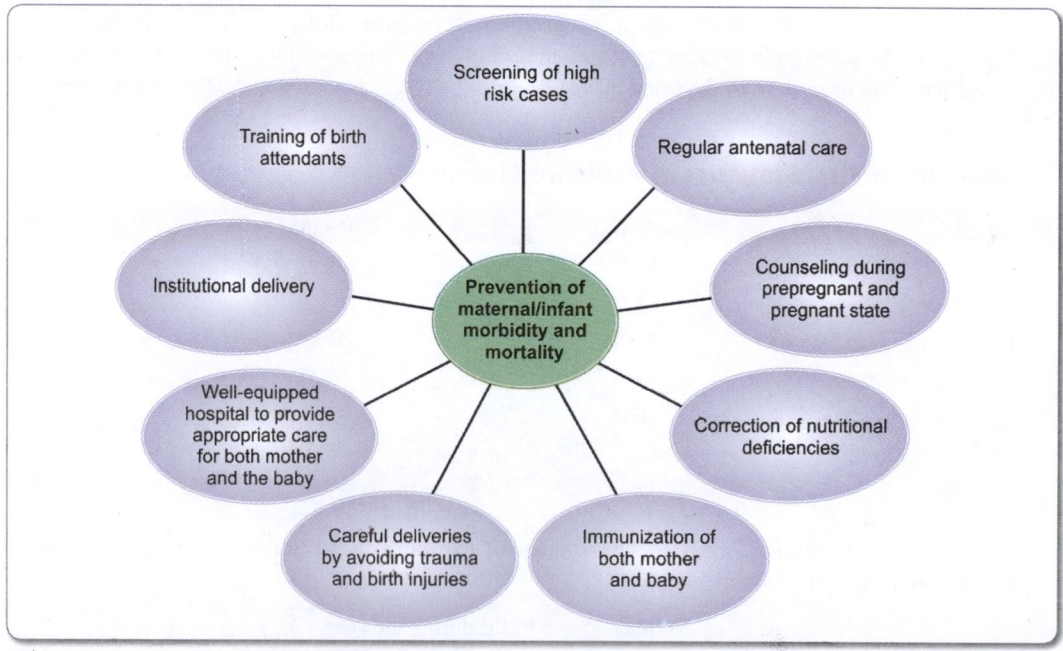

**Fig. 1:** Prevention of maternal/infant morbidity and mortality

- **General Fertility Rate (GFR):** It is the number of live births per 1000 women in the reproductive age group (15–45 years) in a given year.

$$\text{GFR} = \frac{\text{Number of live births in an area during the year}}{\text{Midyear female population age (15–44 years) in the same area in same year}} \times 1000$$

- **Total Fertility Rate (TFR):** It represents the average number of children that would be born per woman if all women lived to the end of the child bearing years and bore children according to a given fertility rate at each age group.

## BASIC COMPETENCIES OF NURSE MIDWIVES

**Competency (midwifery):** A combination of knowledge, professional behavior and specific skills that are demonstrated at a defined level of proficiency in the context of midwifery education and practice.

According to International Confederation of Midwives (2010), Essential Competencies for Basic Midwifery Practice are discussed as follows.

### Competency # 1: Competency in Social, Epidemiologic and Cultural Context of Maternal and Newborn Care

Midwives have the requisite knowledge and skills from obstetrics, neonatology, the social sciences, public health and ethics that form the basis of high quality, culturally relevant, appropriate care for women, newborns, and childbearing.

#### Knowledge

**The midwife has the knowledge and/or understanding of:**

- The community and social determinants of health (e.g., income, literacy and education, water supply and sanitation, housing, environmental hazards, food security, disease patterns, common threats to health)
- Principles of community-based primary care using health promotion and disease prevention and control strategies
- Direct and indirect causes of maternal and neonatal mortality and morbidity in the local community and strategies for reducing them
- Methodology for conducting maternal death review and near miss audits
- Principles of epidemiology, community diagnosis (including water and sanitation), and how to use these in care provision
- Methods of infection prevention and control, appropriate to the service being provided
- Principles of research, evidenced-based practice, critical interpretation of professional literature, and the interpretation of vital statistics and research findings
- Indicators of quality health care services
- Principles of health education
- National and local health services and infrastructures supporting the continuum of care (organization and referral systems), how to access needed resources for midwifery care
- Relevant national programs (provision of services or knowledge of how to assist community members to access services, such as immunization and prevention or treatment of health conditions prevalent in the country)

- The concept of alarm (preparedness), resources for referral to higher health facility levels, communication and transport (emergency care) mechanisms
- The legal and regulatory framework governing reproductive health for women of all ages, including laws, policies, protocols and professional guidelines
- Human rights and their effects on health of individuals (includes issues such as domestic partner violence and female genital mutilation [cutting])
- Advocacy and empowerment strategies for women
- Local culture and beliefs (including religious beliefs, gender roles)
- Traditional and modern health practices (beneficial and harmful)
- Benefits and risks of available birth settings (birth planning)
- Strategies for advocating women for a variety of safe birth settings.

## Professional Behaviors

**The midwife:**

- Is responsible and accountable for clinical decisions and actions
- Acts consistently in accordance with professional ethics, values and human rights
- Acts consistently in accordance with standards of practice
- Maintains/updates knowledge and skills, in order to remain current in practice
- Uses universal/standard precautions, infection, prevention and control strategies, and clean technique
- Behaves in a courteous, nonjudgmental, nondiscriminatory, and culturally appropriate manner with all clients
- Is respectful of individuals and of their culture and customs, regardless of status, ethnic origin or religious belief
- Maintains the confidentiality of all information shared by the woman; communicates essential information between/among other health providers or family members only with explicit permission from the woman and compelling need
- Works in partnership with women and their families, enables and supports them in making informed choices about their health, including the need for referral or transfer to other health care providers or facilities for continued care when health care needs exceed the abilities of the midwife provider, and their right to refuse testing or intervention
- Works collaboratively (teamwork) with other health workers to improve the delivery of services to women and families.

## Skills and/or Abilities

**The midwife has the skill and/or ability to:**

- Engage in health education discussions with and for women and their families
- Use appropriate communication and listening skills across all domains of competency
- Assemble, use and maintain equipment and supplies appropriate to setting of practice
- Record and interpret relevant findings for services provided across all domains of competency, including what was done and what needs follow-up
- Comply with all local reporting regulations for birth and death registration
- Take a leadership role in the practice arena based on professional beliefs and values.

# Competency # 2: Competency in Prepregnancy Care and Family Planning

Midwives provide high quality, culturally sensitive health education and services to all in the community in order to promote healthy family life, planned pregnancies and positive parenting.

## Knowledge

**The midwife has the knowledge and/or understanding of:**

- Growth and development related to sexuality, sexual development and sexual activity
- Female and male anatomy and physiology related to conception and reproduction
- Cultural norms and practices surrounding sexuality, sexual practices, marriage and childbearing
- Components of health history, family history and relevant genetic history
- Physical examination content and investigative laboratory studies that evaluate potential for a healthy pregnancy
- Health education content targeted to sexual and reproductive health (e.g., sexually transmitted infections, human immunodeficiency virus (HIV), newborn and child health)
- Basic principles of pharmacokinetics of family planning drugs and agents
- Culturally acceptable and locally available natural family planning methods
- Contemporary family planning methods, including barrier, steroidal, mechanical, chemical and surgical methods of contraception, mode of action, indications for use, benefits and risks; rumors and myths that affect family planning
- Medical eligibility criteria for all methods of family planning, including appropriate time frames for the use of method
- Methods and strategies for guiding women and/or couples needing to make decisions about methods of family planning
- Signs and symptoms of urinary tract infection and sexually transmitted infections commonly occurring in the community/country
- Indicators of common acute and chronic disease conditions specific to a geographic area of the world that present risks to a pregnant woman and the fetus (e.g., HIV, tuberculosis, malaria) and referral process for further testing and treatment including postexposure preventive treatment
- Indicators and methods for advising and referral of dysfunctional interpersonal relationships, including sexual problems, gender-based violence, emotional abuse and physical neglect
- Principles of screening methods for cervical cancer, (e.g., visual inspection with acetic acid [VIA], Pap test, and colposcopy).

## Skills and/or Abilities

**The midwife has the skill and/or ability to:**

- Take a comprehensive and obstetric, gynecologic and reproductive health history
- Engage the woman and her family in preconception counseling, based on the individual situation, needs and interests
- Perform a physical examination, including clinical breast examination, focused on the presenting condition of the woman
- Order and/or perform and interpret common laboratory tests (e.g., hematocrit, urinalysis dipstick for proteinuria)
- Request and/or perform and interpret selected screening tests such as screening for tuberculosis, HIV, sexually transmitted infections (STIs)

- Provide care, support and referral or treatment for the HIV positive woman and HIV counseling and testing for women who do not know their status
- Prescribe, dispense, furnish or administer (however, authorized to do so in the jurisdiction of practice) locally available and culturally acceptable methods of family planning
- Advise women about management of side effects and problems related to use of family planning methods
- Prescribe, dispense, furnish or administer (however, authorized to do so in the jurisdiction of practice) emergency contraception medications, in accord with local policies, protocols, law or regulation
- Provide commonly available methods of barrier, steroidal, mechanical, and chemical methods of family planning
- Take or order cervical cytology (Pap) test.

## Competency # 3: Competency in Provision of Care during Pregnancy

Midwives provide high quality antenatal care to maximize health during pregnancy and that includes early detection and treatment or referral of selected complications.

### Knowledge

**The midwife has the knowledge and/or understanding of:**

- Anatomy and physiology of the human body
- The biology of human reproduction, the menstrual cycle, and the process of conception
- Signs and symptoms of pregnancy
- Examinations and tests for confirmation of pregnancy
- Methods for diagnosis of an ectopic pregnancy
- Principles of dating pregnancy by menstrual history, size of uterus, fundal growth patterns and use of ultrasound (if available)
- Components of health history and focused physical examination for antenatal visits
- Manifestations of various degrees of female genital mutilation (cutting) and their potential effects on women's health, including the birth process
- Normal findings [results] of basic screening laboratory tests defined by need of area of the world, (e.g., iron levels, urine test for sugar, protein, acetone, bacteria)
- Normal progression of pregnancy: body changes, common discomforts, expected fundal growth patterns
- Implications of deviation from expected fundal growth patterns, including intrauterine growth retardation/ restriction, oligo- and polyhydramnios, multiple fetuses
- Neonatal risk factors requiring transfer of women to higher levels of care prior to labor and birth
- Normal psychological changes in pregnancy, indicators of psychosocial stress, and impact of pregnancy on the woman and the family
- Safe, locally available nonpharmacological substances for the relief of common discomforts of pregnancy
- How to determine fetal well-being during pregnancy including fetal heart rate and activity patterns
- Nutritional requirements of the pregnant woman and fetus
- Health education needs in pregnancy (e.g., information about relief for common discomforts, hygiene, sexuality, work inside and outside the home)
- Basic principles of pharmacokinetics of drugs prescribed, dispensed or furnished to women during pregnancy
- Effects of prescribed medications, street drugs, traditional medicines, and over-the-counter drugs on pregnancy and the fetus

- Effects of smoking, alcohol abuse and illicit drug use on the pregnant woman and fetus
- The essential elements of birth planning (preparation for labor and birth, emergency preparedness)
- The components of preparation of the home/family for the newborn
- Signs and symptoms of the onset of labor (including women's perceptions and symptoms)
- Techniques for increasing relaxation and pain relief measures available for labor
- Signs, symptoms and potential effects of conditions that are life-threatening to the pregnant woman and/or her fetus, (e.g., preeclampsia/eclampsia, vaginal bleeding, premature labor, severe anemia, Rh isoimmunization, syphilis)
- Means and methods of advising about care, treatment and support for the HIV positive pregnant woman including measures to prevent maternal-to-child transmission (PMTCT) (including feeding options)
- Signs, symptoms and indications for referral of selected complications and conditions of pregnancy that affect either mother or fetus (e.g., asthma, HIV infection, diabetes, cardiac conditions, malpresentations/abnormal lie, placental disorders, preterm labor, postdated pregnancy)
- Measures for prevention and control of malaria in pregnancy, according to country disease pattern, including intermittent preventive treatment (IPT) and promotion of insecticide-treated bednets (ITN)
- Pharmacologic basis of deworming in pregnancy (if relevant to the country of practice)
- The physiology of lactation and methods to prepare women for breastfeeding.

## Skills and/or Abilities

**The midwife has the skill and/or ability to:**

- Take an initial and ongoing history at each antenatal visit
- Perform a physical examination and explain findings to the woman
- Take and assess maternal vital signs including temperature, blood pressure, pulse
- Assess maternal nutrition and its relationship to fetal growth; give appropriate advice on nutritional requirements of pregnancy and how to achieve them
- Perform a complete abdominal assessment including measuring fundal height, lie, position, and presentation
- Assess fetal growth using manual measurements
- Evaluate fetal growth, placental location, and amniotic fluid volume, using ultrasound visualization and measurement (if equipment is available for use)
- Listen to the fetal heart rate; palpate uterus for fetal activity and interpret findings
- Monitor fetal heart rate with Doppler (if available)
- Perform a pelvic examination, including sizing the uterus, if indicated and when appropriate during the course of pregnancy
- Perform clinical pelvimetry (evaluation of bony pelvis) to determine the adequacy of the bony structures
- Calculate the estimated date of birth
- Provide health education to adolescents, women and families about normal pregnancy progression, danger signs and symptoms, and when and how to contact the midwife
- Teach and/or demonstrate measures to decrease common discomforts of pregnancy
- Provide guidance and basic preparation for labor, birth and parenting
- Identify variations from normal during the course of the pregnancy and institute appropriate first-line independent or collaborative management based upon evidence-based guidelines, local standards and available resources for:

- Low and/or inadequate maternal nutrition
- Inadequate or excessive uterine growth, including suspected oligo- or polyhydramnios, molar pregnancy
- Elevated blood pressure, proteinuria, presence of significant edema, severe frontal headaches, visual changes, epigastric pain associated with elevated blood pressure
- Vaginal bleeding, multiple gestation, abnormal lie/malpresentation at term
- Intrauterine fetal death
- Rupture of membranes prior to term
- HIV positive status and/or acquired immunodeficiency syndrome (AIDS)
- Hepatitis B and C positive

- Prescribe, dispense, furnish or administer (however, authorized to do so in the jurisdiction of practice) selected, life-saving drugs (e.g., antibiotics, anticonvulsants, antimalarials, antihypertensives, antiretrovirals) to women in need because of a presenting condition
- Identify deviations from normal during the course of pregnancy and initiate the referral process for conditions that require higher levels of intervention.

## Competency # 4: Competency in Provision of Care during Labor and Birth

Midwives provide high quality, culturally sensitive care during labor, conduct a clean and safe birth and handle selected emergency situations to maximize the health of women and their newborns.

### Knowledge

**The midwife has the knowledge and/or understanding of:**

- Physiology of first, second and third stages of labor
- Anatomy of fetal skull, critical diameters and landmarks
- Psychological and cultural aspects of labor and birth
- Indicators of the latent phase and the onset of active labor
- Indications for stimulation of the onset of labor, and augmentation of uterine contractility
- Normal progression of labor
- How to use the partograph
- Measures to assess fetal well-being in labor
- Measures to assess maternal well-being in labor
- Process of fetal passage (descent) through the pelvis during labor and birth; mechanisms of labor in various fetal presentations and positions
- Comfort measures in first and second stages of labor (e.g., family presence/assistance, positioning for labor and birth, hydration, emotional support, nonpharmacological methods of pain relief)
- Pharmacological measures for management and control of labor pain, including the relative risks, disadvantages, safety of specific methods of pain management, and their effect on the normal physiology of labor
- Signs and symptoms of complications in labor (e.g., bleeding, labor arrest, malpresentation, eclampsia, maternal distress, fetal distress, infection, prolapsed cord)
- Principles of prevention of pelvic floor damage and perineal tears
- Indications for performing an episiotomy
- Principles of expectant (physiologic) management of the 3rd stage of labor
- Principles of active management of 3rd stage of labor
- Principles underpinning the technique for repair of perineal tears and episiotomy

- Indicators of need for emergency management, referral or transfer for obstetric emergencies (e.g., cord prolapse, shoulder dystocia, uterine bleeding, retained placenta)
- Indicators of need for operative deliveries, vacuum extraction, use of forceps or symphysiotomy (e.g., fetal distress, cephalopelvic disproportion).

## Skills and/or Abilities

**The midwife has the skill and/or ability to:**

- Take a specific history and maternal vital signs in labor
- Perform a focused physical examination in labor
- Perform a complete abdominal assessment for fetal position and descent
- Assess the effectiveness of uterine contractions
- Perform a complete and accurate pelvic examination for dilatation, descent, presenting part, position, status of membranes, and adequacy of pelvis for birth of baby vaginally
- Monitor progress of labor using the partograph or similar tool for recording
- Provide physical and psychological support for woman and family and promote normal birth
- Facilitate the presence of a support person during labor and birth
- Provide adequate hydration, nutrition and nonpharmacological comfort measures during labor and birth
- Provide pharmacologic therapies for pain relief during labor and birth
- Provide for bladder care including performance of urinary catheterization when indicated
- Promptly identify abnormal labor patterns and initiate appropriate and timely intervention and/or referral
- Stimulate or augment uterine contractility, using nonpharmacologic agents
- Stimulate or augment uterine contractility, using pharmacologic agents
- Administer local anesthetic to the perineum when episiotomy is anticipated or perineal repair is required
- Perform an episiotomy if needed
- Perform appropriate hand maneuvers for a vertex birth
- Perform appropriate hand maneuvers for face and breech deliveries
- Clamp and cut the cord
- Institute immediate, life-saving interventions in obstetrical emergencies (e.g., prolapsed cord, malpresentation, shoulder dystocia, and fetal distress) to save the life of the fetus, while requesting medical attention and/or awaiting transfer
- Manage a cord around the baby's neck at birth
- Support expectant (physiologic) management of the 3rd stage of labor
- Conduct active management of the 3rd stage of labor
    - Administer uterotonic drug within one minute of birth of infant
    - Perform controlled cord traction
    - Perform uterine massage after delivery of placenta
- Inspect the placenta and membranes for completeness
- Perform fundal massage to stimulate postpartum uterine contraction and uterine tone
- Provide a safe environment for mother and infant to promote attachment (bonding)
- Estimate and record maternal blood loss
- Inspect the vagina and cervix for lacerations
- Repair an episiotomy if needed.
- Repair 1st and 2nd degree perineal or vaginal lacerations
- Manage postpartum bleeding and hemorrhage, using appropriate techniques and uterotonic agents as indicated

- Prescribe, dispense, furnish or administer (however, authorized to do so in the jurisdiction of practice) selected, life-saving drugs (e.g., antibiotics, anticonvulsants, antimalarials, antihypertensives, antiretrovirals) to women in need because of a presenting condition
- Perform manual removal of placenta
- Perform internal bimanual compression of the uterus to control
- Perform aortic compression
- Identify and manage shock
- Insert intravenous line, draw blood for laboratory testing
- Arrange for and undertake timely referral and transfer of women with serious complications to a higher level health facility, taking appropriate drugs and equipment and arranging for a companion care giver on the journey, in order to continue giving emergency care as required
- Perform adult cardiopulmonary resuscitation.

## Competency # 5: Competency in Provision of Care for Women during the Postpartum Period

Midwives provide comprehensive, high quality, culturally sensitive postpartum care for women.

### Knowledge

**The midwife has the knowledge and/or understanding of:**

- Physical and emotional changes that occur following childbirth, including the normal process of involution
- Physiology and process of lactation and common variations including engorgement, lack of milk supply, etc.
- The importance of immediate/early/exclusive breastfeeding for mother and child
- Maternal nutrition, rest, activity and physiological needs (e.g., bowel and bladder) in the immediate postpartum period
- Principles of parent-infant bonding and attachment (e.g., how to promote positive relationships)
- Indicators of subinvolution (e.g., persistent uterine bleeding, infection)
- Indicators of maternal breastfeeding problems or complications, including mastitis
- Signs and symptoms of life-threatening conditions that may first arise during the postpartum period (e.g., persistent vaginal bleeding, embolism, postpartum preeclampsia and eclampsia, severe mental depression)
- Signs and symptoms of selected complications in the postnatal period (e.g., persistent anemia, hematoma, depression, thrombophlebitis; incontinence of feces or urine; urinary retention, obstetric fistula)
- Principles of interpersonal communication with and support for women and/or their families who are bereaved (maternal death, stillbirth, pregnancy loss, neonatal death, congenital abnormalities)
- Approaches and strategies for providing special support for adolescents, victims of gender-based violence (including rape)
- Principles of manual vacuum aspiration of the uterine cavity to remove retained products of conception
- Principles of prevention of maternal to child transmission of HIV, tuberculosis, hepatitis B and C in the postpartum period
- Methods of family planning appropriate for use in the immediate postpartum period (e.g., lactational amenorrhea, progestin—only oral contraceptives)
- Community-based postpartum services available to the woman and her family, and how they can be accessed.

## Skills and/or Abilities

**The midwife has the skill and/or ability to:**

- Take a selective history, including details of pregnancy, labor and birth
- Perform a focused physical examination of the mother
- Provide information and support for women and/or their families who are bereaved (maternal death, stillbirth, pregnancy loss, neonatal death, congenital abnormalities)
- Assess for uterine involution and healing of lacerations and/or repairs
- Initiate and support uninterrupted (immediate and exclusive) breastfeeding
- Teach mothers how to express breast milk, and how to handle and store expressed breast milk
- Educate mother on care of self and infant after childbirth including signs and symptoms of impending complications, and community-based resources
- Educate a woman and her family on sexuality and family planning following childbirth
- Provide family planning services concurrently as an integral component of postpartum care
- Provide appropriate and timely first-line treatment for any complications detected during the postpartum examination (e.g., anemia, hematoma, maternal infection), and refer for further management as necessary
- Provide emergency treatment of late postpartum hemorrhage, and refer if necessary.

## Competency # 6: Competency in Postnatal Care of the Newborn

Midwives provide high quality, comprehensive care for the essentially healthy infant from birth to two months of age.

### Knowledge

**The midwife has the knowledge and/or understanding of:**

- Elements of assessment of the immediate condition of newborn (e.g., Apgar scoring system for breathing, heart rate, reflexes, muscle tone and color)
- Principles of newborn adaptation to extrauterine life (e.g., physiologic changes that occur in pulmonary and cardiac systems)
- Basic needs of newborn: airway, warmth, nutrition, attachment (bonding)
- Advantages of various methods of newborn warming, including skin-to-skin contact (Kangaroo mother care)
- Methods and means of assessing the gestational age of a newborn
- Characteristics of low-birth-weight infants and their special needs
- Characteristics of healthy newborn (appearance and behaviors)
- Normal growth and development of the preterm infant
- Normal newborn and infant growth and development
- Selected variations in the normal newborn (e.g., caput, molding, Mongolian spots)
- Elements of health promotion and prevention of disease in newborns and infants (e.g., malaria, tuberculosis, HIV), including essential elements of daily care (e.g., cord care, nutritional needs, patterns of elimination)
- Immunization needs, risks and benefits from infancy through young childhood
- Traditional or cultural practices related to the newborn
- Principles of infant nutrition and infant feeding options for babies (including those born to HIV positive mothers).

- Signs and symptoms of selected newborn complications (e.g., jaundice, hematoma, adverse molding of the fetal skull, cerebral irritation, nonaccidental injuries, hemangioma, hypoglycemia, hypothermia, dehydration, infection, congenital syphilis).

### *Skills and/or Abilities*

**The midwife has the skill and/or ability to:**

- Provide immediate care to the newborn, including cord clamping and cutting, drying, clearing airways, and ensuring that breathing is established
- Assess the immediate condition of the newborn (e.g., Apgar scoring or other assessment method)
- Promote and maintain normal newborn body temperature through covering (blanket, cap), environmental control, and promotion of skin-to-skin contact
- Begin emergency measures for respiratory distress (newborn resuscitation), hypothermia, hypoglycemia.
- Give appropriate care including kangaroo mother care to the low-birth-weight baby, and arrange for referral if potentially serious complications arise, or very low-birth-weight
- Perform a screening physical examination of the newborn for conditions incompatible with life
- Perform a gestational age assessment
- Provide routine care of the newborn, in accord with local guidelines and protocols (e.g., identification, eye care, screening tests, administration of vitamin K, birth registration)
- Position infant to initiate breastfeeding as soon as possible after birth and support exclusive breastfeeding
- Transfer the at-risk newborn to emergency care facility when available
- Educate parents about danger signs in the newborn and when to bring infant for care
- Educate parents about normal growth and development of the infant and young child, and how to provide for day-to-day needs of the normal child
- Assist parents to access community resources available to the family
- Support parents during grieving process for loss of pregnancy, stillbirth, congenital birth defects or neonatal deaths
- Support parents during transport/transfer of newborn or during times of separation from infant [e.g., neonatal intensive care unit (NICU) admission]
- Support and educate parents who have given birth to multiple babies (e.g., twins, triplets) about special needs and community resources
- Provide appropriate care for baby born to an HIV positive mother (e.g., administration of antiretroviral drugs and appropriate feeding)

## Competency # 7: Competency in Facilitation of Abortion-related Care

Midwives provide a range of individualized, culturally sensitive abortion-related care services for women requiring or experiencing pregnancy termination and loss that are congruent with applicable laws and regulations and in accord with national protocols.

### *Knowledge*

**The midwife has the knowledge and/or understanding of:**

- Policies, protocols, laws and regulations related to abortion-care services
- Factors involved in decisions relating to unintended or mistimed pregnancies
- Family planning methods appropriate for use during the postabortion period
- Medical eligibility criteria for all available abortion methods

- Care, information and support which are needed during and after miscarriage or abortion (physical and psychological) and services available in the community
- Normal process of involution and physical and emotional healing following miscarriage or abortion
- Signs and symptoms of sub-involution and/or incomplete abortion (e.g., persistent uterine bleeding)
- Signs and symptoms of abortion complications and life-threatening conditions (e.g., persistent vaginal bleeding, infection)
- Pharmacotherapeutic basics of drugs recommended for use in medication abortion
- Principles of uterine evacuation via manual vacuum aspiration (MVA).

## *Skills and/or Abilities*

**The midwife has the skill and/or ability to:**

- Assess gestational period through query about last menstrual period, bimanual examination and/or urine pregnancy testing
- Inform women who are considering abortion about available services for those keeping the pregnancy and for those proceeding with abortion, methods for obtaining abortion, and to support women in their choice
- Take a clinical and social history to identify contraindications to medication or aspiration abortion
- Educate and advise women (and family members, where appropriate), on sexuality and family planning post-abortion
- Provide family planning services concurrently as an integral component of abortion-related services
- Assess for uterine involution; treat or refer as appropriate
- Educate mother on care of self, including rest and nutrition and on how to identify complications such as hemorrhage
- Identify indicators of abortion-related complications (including uterine perforation); treat or refer for treatment as appropriate.

23

Chapter 1  Introduction

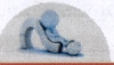

## ASSESS YOURSELF

### FREQUENTLY ASKED QUESTIONS IN EXAMS

1. Describe the current trends of midwifery practice in India.
2. Explain the scope of midwifery practice.
3. Discuss the basic competencies of a midwife.
4. Define the terms:
   a. Obstetrics
   b. Midwifery
   c. Infant mortality rate
   d. Maternal mortality rate
   e. Neonatal mortality rate

### MULTIPLE CHOICE QUESTIONS

1. The time limit for registering the event of birth is:
   a. 7 days
   b. 14 days
   c. 10 days
   d. 21 days
2. Mortality means:
   a. Death
   b. Birth
   c. Disease
   d. Fertility
3. Time limit for the registration of death is:
   a. 7 days
   b. 21 days
   c. 14 days
   d. 24 days
4. The period immediately before and after birth is called:
   a. Antenatal period
   b. Intranatal period
   c. Postnatal period
   d. Perinatal period
5. The branch of medicine that deals with the parturition, its antecedents and its sequels is called:
   a. Sociology
   b. Pharmacology
   c. Obstetrics
   d. Biology
6. Which of the following is in the scope of midwifery?
   a. Nurse researcher
   b. Nurse advocate
   c. Nurse educator
   d. All of the above
7. Number of deaths of children less than 1 year to the total number of births registered in the same year is called:
   a. Neonatal mortality rate
   b. Infant mortality rate
   c. Neonatal morbidity rate
   d. Infant morbidity rate
8. The death of the baby before, during delivery or within the first 7 days of birth is called:
   a. Neonatal mortality rate
   b. Infant mortality rate
   c. Perinatal mortality rate
   d. None of the above
9. ICM stands for:
   a. International Council of Midwives
   b. International Confederation of Midwives
   c. Integrated Child Management
   d. None of the above
10. The cause of perinatal death is:
    a. Preterm birth
    b. Elderly primigravida
    c. Closely spaced birth
    d. All of the above

### Answer Key

| 1. b | 2. a | 3. d | 4. d | 5. c | 6. d | 7. b |
|------|------|------|------|------|------|------|
| 8. c | 9. b | 10. d | | | | |

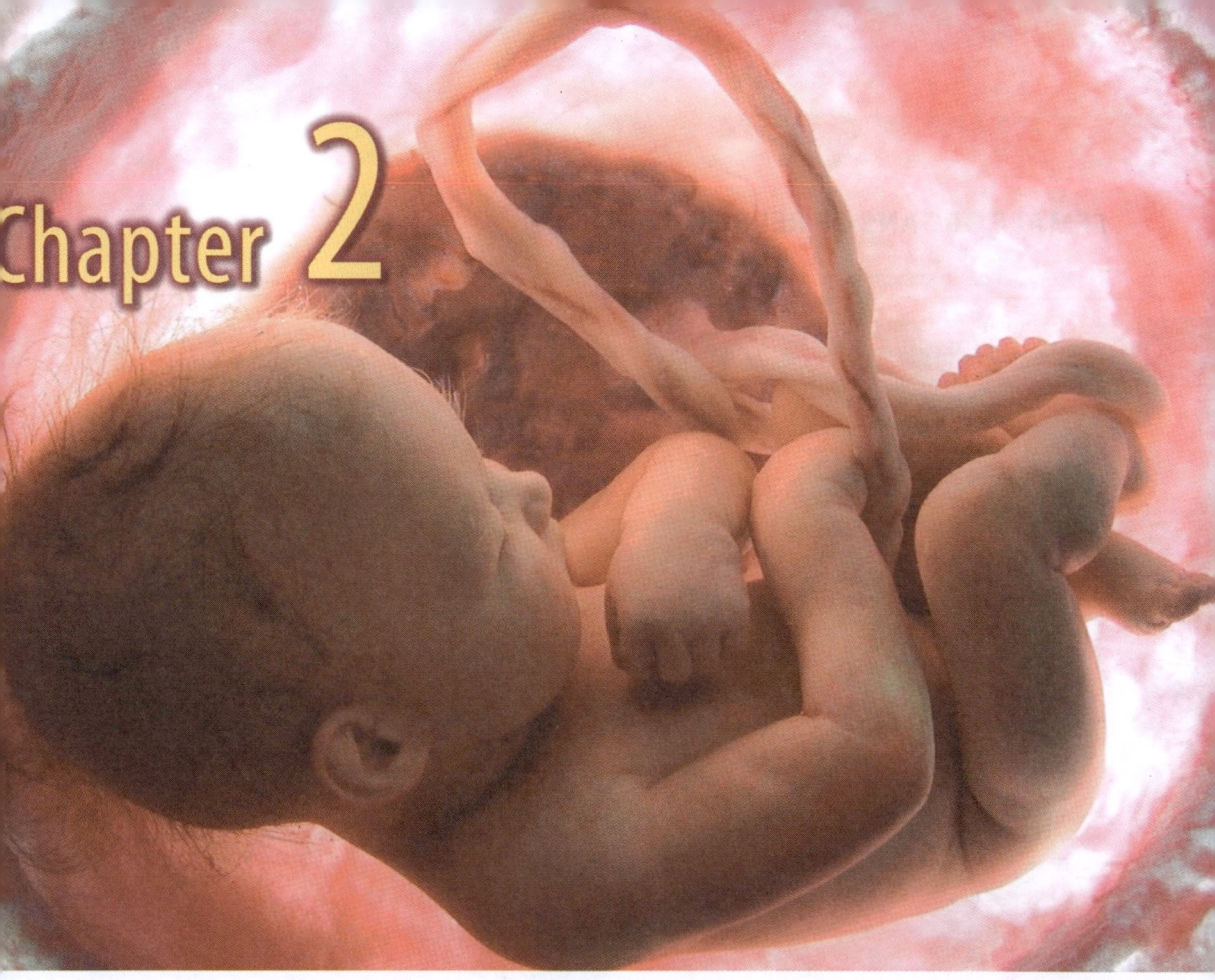

# Chapter 2

# Reproductive System

## Learning Objectives

**Upon completing this chapter, the learner will be able to:**

- ➥ Enlist the different parts of female reproductive system
- ➥ Describe the functions of female reproductive organs
- ➥ Evaluate the structure, types and diameters of pelvis

## Chapter Outline

- ▲ Female Organs of Reproduction
- ▲ Female Pelvis

# FEMALE ORGANS OF REPRODUCTION

The reproductive system consists of:

- External genitalia
- Internal genitalia
- Accessory reproductive organs

## External Genitalia

External genitalia are also referred to as vulva or pudendum. External genitalia include, mons pubis, labia majora, labia minora, clitoris and glands within the vestibule (Fig. 1).

**The external genitalia have three main functions:**

1. Enable entry of sperms into the body
2. Protect internal genital organs from infectious organisms
3. Provide sexual pleasure

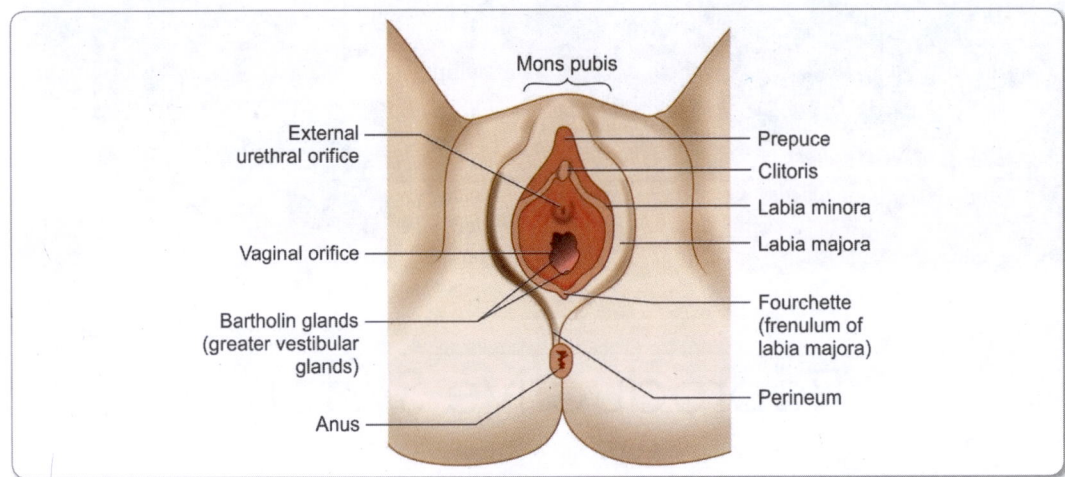

**Fig. 1:** Female external genitalia

### Mons Pubis

It is the pad of subcutaneous adipose connective tissue lying in front of the pubis and in adult female is covered by inverted triangular pattern of hair.

### Labia Majora (Greater Lips)

- The labia majora are two symmetrical folds of skin, which protect the urethral and vaginal orifices.
- The skin on the outer convex surface is pigmented and covered with hair follicles. The labia majora are homologous to the scrotum in males.

### Labia Minora (Lesser Lips)

- The labia minora are thin, delicate folds of fat free hairless skin, located between the labia majora.

- The inner surface of labia minora is pinkish in color. It contains many sensory nerve endings, sebaceous glands and erectile muscle fibers. Anteriorly, they divide to enclose the clitoris and unite with each other in front and behind the clitoris to form the prepuce and frenulum, respectively.

## Clitoris

- It is a small cylindrical erectile body, measuring about 1.5–2 cm, situated in the most anterior part of the vulva.
- It consists of glans, a body and two crura. It is homologous with the penis and is an erectile organ.
- It is highly sensitive and very important in the sexual arousal of a female.

## Vestibule

It is a triangular space bounded anteriorly by the clitoris, posteriorly by fourchette and on either side by labia minora. There are four openings into the vestibule:

### 1. Urethral Opening

The opening is situated in the midline just in front of the vaginal orifice about 1–1.5 cm below the pubic arch.

### 2. Vaginal Orifice

It lies in the posterior end of the vestibule. In virgins and nulliparae, the opening is closed by labia minora. But in parous, it may be exposed. It is incompletely closed by a septum of mucus membrane called hymen.

### 3. Opening of Bartholin Ducts

There are two Bartholin glands, one on each side. They are situated in the superficial perineal pouch, close to the posterior end of the vestibular bulb. They are pea-sized and yellowish in color. During sexual intercourse, they secrete mucus which helps in lubrication. They are homologous to the bulb of the penis in males.

### 4. Opening of Skene's Glands

These are the largest paraurethral glands and are homologous to the prostate gland in the male.

## Perineum

It is the short stretch of skin starting at the bottom of the vulva and extending to the anus. It is diamond-shaped area between the symphysis pubis and coccyx. In clinical obstetrics, it is the area between anal and vaginal orifice.

# Internal Genitalia

These include vagina, uterus, fallopian tubes and the ovaries (Fig. 2).

## Vagina

It is the fibrovascular membranous sheath communicating the uterine cavity with the exterior at the vulva. It is located between the rectum and urinary bladder.

### Functions of Vagina

- Forms the birth canal for parturition
- Receives male penis during sexual intercourse
- Provides the passage route for uterine secretions and menstrual blood.

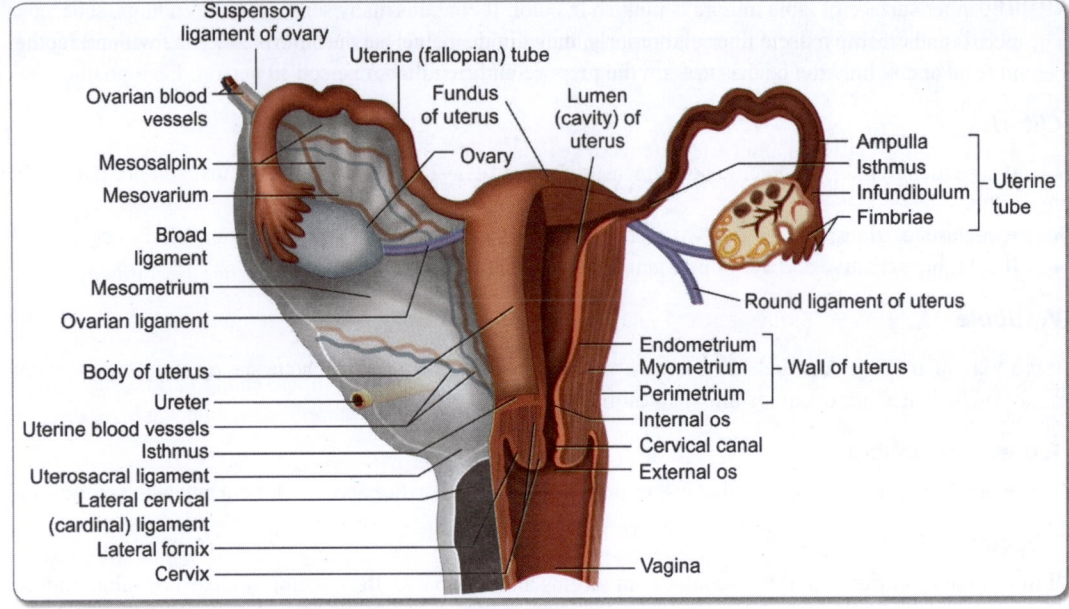

**Fig. 2:** Female internal genitalia

## Structure

- Vagina has an anterior, a posterior and two lateral walls. The length of anterior wall is about 7 cm and that of the posterior wall is about 9 cm. The vaginal wall has many small folds called rugae, which allow vaginal walls to stretch during intercourse and childbirth. The upper part of vagina is called vault. The places, where the cervix projects into it, the vault forms circular recesses, called fornices.
- There are four fornices: One anterior, one posterior and two lateral.

### Layers of Vagina

Layers from within outwards are:

- Mucus layer
- Submucus layer
- Muscular layer
- Fibrous layer

### Relations of Vagina with other Genital Structures

- **Anterior:** Bladder and urethra
- **Posterior:** Pouch of Douglas, the rectum and the perineal body
- **Lateral:** The upper two-thirds are pelvic fascia and ureters, which pass beside the cervix; the lower third are the muscles of pelvic floor
- **Superior:** The uterus
- **Inferior:** The external genitalia

## Uterus

The uterus is a thick-walled muscular organ capable of expansion to accommodate a growing fetus. It is connected distally to the vagina, and laterally to the uterine tubes.

## Position

The uterus is a hollow pyriform muscular organ situated in the pelvis between the bladder in front and rectum behind. The actual position of the uterus within the pelvis varies from person to person. Each position has its own name:

- **Anteverted uterus:** An anteverted uterus tips slightly forward.
- **Retroverted uterus:** A retroverted uterus bends slightly backward.

## Measurement and Parts

It is about 8 cm long, 5 cm wide and 1.25 cm thick. Weight varies from 50 g to 80 g. It has the following parts:

- **Fundus:** Upper part of the uterus is fundus. It is broad and curved. Fallopian tubes are attached to the uterus just below the fundus.
- **Corpus:** The main body of the uterus is corpus. It is muscular and can stretch enough to accommodate a developing fetus. The muscular walls of the corpus contract during labor to help push the baby through the cervix and vagina.

  A mucus membrane called the endometrium lines the corpus. During each menstrual cycle, this membrane responds to reproductive hormones by changing its thickness. If fertilization takes place, it attaches to the endometrium. If no fertilization occurs, the endometrium sheds its outer layer of cells, which are released during menstruation.

- **Isthmus:** It is situated between the body and cervix. It is a constricted part measuring about 0.5 cm in length.
- **Cervix:** The cervix is the lowest part of the uterus. It connects the uterus to the vagina and is lined with a smooth mucus membrane. Glands in the cervical lining usually produce a thick mucus. However, during ovulation, this becomes thinner to allow sperm to easily pass into the uterus.

  Three main parts of the cervix are:
  - **Endocervix:** It is the inner part of the cervix that leads to the uterus.
  - **Cervical canal:** The cervical canal links the uterus to the vagina.
  - **Exocervix:** The outer part of the cervix that protrudes into the vagina is exocervix. During childbirth, the cervix dilates to allow the baby to pass through the birth canal.

  During childbirth, the cervix dilates (widens) to allow the baby to pass through the birth canal.

## Layers of Uterus

Uterus has three layers:

1. **Perimetrium:** It is the outer peritoneal layer of the uterus.
2. **Myometrium:** It is the thickest layer, consisting of thick bundles of smooth muscle fibers held by connective tissues and are arranged in various directions. During pregnancy, three distinct layers can be identified–outer longitudinal, middle interlacing and the inner circular.
3. **Endometrium:** It is the inner layer, directly apposed to the muscle coat, as there is no submucosal layer. It is 1–10 mm thick, depending on hormonal situation.

## Relation of Uterus with Other Structures

- **Anterior:** The uterovesical pouch and bladder
- **Posterior:** Rectouterine pouch of Douglas and the rectum

- **Lateral:** The broad ligaments, the uterine tubes and the ovaries
- **Superior:** The intestines
- **Inferior:** The vagina

### Ligaments of the Uterus

- Transcervical ligament
- Uterosacral ligament
- Pubocervical ligament
- Ovarian ligament
- Broad ligament
- Round ligament

### Blood Supply of Uterus

It is primarily supplied by a pair of uterine arteries.

### Lymphatic Drainage

It occurs via iliac, sacral, aortic and inguinal lymph modes.

### Functions of Uterus

- Helpful for periodic menstrual bleeding till menopause
- Provides canal for transmission of sperm to fallopian tube
- Bears the growing fetus during pregnancy
- Supplies nutrients and oxygen to fetus through placenta
- Expels the fetus from uterine cavity to exterior at the time of birth
- The uterus has a rich supply of blood vessels that extend to the female genitalia, and is essential for women to achieve orgasm during sexual activity.

## Uterine (Fallopian) Tubes

- The uterine tubes (or fallopian tubes, oviducts, salpinx) are muscular 'J-shaped' tubes, found in the female reproductive tract. They lie in the upper border of the broad ligament, extending laterally from the uterus, opening into the abdominal cavity, near the ovaries.
- The uterine tubes are paired structures, measuring about 10 cm and situated at the upper corners of the uterus. Each tube has two openings, one communicating with the lateral angle of uterine cavity called uterine opening and measures 1 mm in diameter; the other is at the lateral end of tube, called pelvic opening and measures about 2 mm in diameter.

### Parts

Uterine tube is divided into four parts (Fig. 3).

### Infundibulum

- It is the funnel-shaped lateral or distal end of the uterine tube, measuring 1.25 cm.
- It is closely related to ovary.
- It is opening into peritoneal cavity and is called abdominal ostium.
- Abdominal ostium is surrounded by a number of radiating fimbriae (20–25).
- One of the fimbriae is longer than rest and is attached to the outer pole of the ovary called ovarian fimbria.

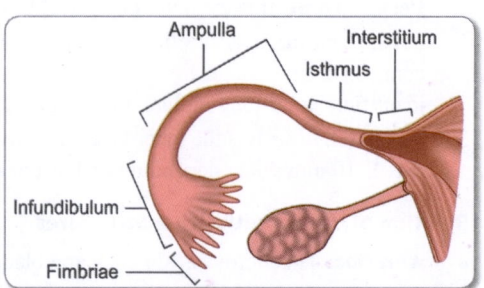

**Fig. 3:** Structure of fallopian tubes

- During ovulation, the fimbriae trap the oocyte and sweep it through the abdominal ostium into the ampulla.

### Ampulla
- It begins at the medial end of infundibulum.
- It is the tortuous part where fertilization occurs.
- Ampulla is the widest and longest part of the uterine tube, making up over half of its length.

### Isthmus
- It is short (2.5 cm), narrow, thick-walled part of the uterine tube.
- The lumen is 1–2 mm in diameter.

### Interstitium
- It is the narrowest part and measures 1.25 cm in length.

### Structure of Fallopian Tube
It consists of three layers:
1. Serous
2. Muscular
3. Mucus layer: Mucus membrane is lined by:
   - Columnar ciliated epithelial cells
   - Secretory columnar cells
   - Peg cells

### Relations to other Structures
- **Anterior, posterior and superior:** The peritoneal cavity and intestines.
- **Lateral:** The sidewalls of pelvis.
- **Inferior:** The broad ligament and ovaries.
- **Medial:** The uterus lies between two uterine tubes.

### Blood Supply of Uterine Tubes
The blood supply is via uterine and ovarian arteries, returning by the corresponding veins.

### Lymphatic Drainage of the Uterine Tubes
This is through the lumbar glands.

### Functions of Fallopian Tubes
- Transportation of gametes
- The site for fertilization
- To facilitate survival of zygote through its secretion. (Secretion of fallopian tube contains pyruvate for nourishment of ovum).

## Ovaries

Ovaries are paired sex glands or gonads in females. Each gland is oval in shape and pinkish grey in color, and surface is scarred during reproductive period. It measures about 3 cm in length, 2 cm in breadth and 1 cm in thickness. Each ovary presents two ends: Tubal and uterine; two surfaces: Medial and lateral.

## Structure

The ovaries are covered on the outside by a layer of simple-cuboidal epithelium called germinal (ovarian) epithelium. This is actually the visceral peritoneum that envelops the ovaries. Underneath this layer, there is dense connective tissue capsule, the tunica albuginea. The substance of the ovaries is distinctly divided into an outer cortex and inner medulla.

- **Cortex:** Appears dense and more granular due to presence of numerous ovarian follicles. Each follicle contains an oocyte, a female germ cell.
- **Medulla:** It is composed of the loose connective tissue with abundant blood vessels, lymphatic vessels and nerve fibers.

## Blood Supply

The blood supply is from the ovarian arteries and venous drainage is from ovarian veins.

## Lymphatic Drainage

It occurs via lumbar glands.

## Functions

- Germ cell maturation, storage and its release.
- Steroidogenesis (Production of sex hormones, namely estrogen and progesterone).

# Accessory Reproductive Organs

It includes pelvic floor muscles, pelvic fascia, pelvic cellular tissue, female urethra, urinary bladder, pelvic ureter and the breast. The description of most important accessory reproductive organ, i.e. breast is as follows:

## Breast

The breasts are modified sebaceous glands. They constitute as accessory reproductive organs as the glands are concerned with lactation following childbirth.

The shape of the breast varies in women and also during different periods of life. But the size of the base of the breast is fairly constant. It usually extends from 2nd to 6th rib in the midclavicular line.

## Structure

- **Areola** is placed about the center of breast and is pigmented. It is about 2.5 cm in diameter.
- **Montgomery glands** are accessory glands located around the periphery of the areola. They can secrete small amount of breast milk, but they mostly produce a natural, oily substance that cleans and lubricates the nipple and areola.
- **Nipple** is a muscular projection covered by pigmented skin. It is vascular and surrounded by non-striated muscles which make it erectile. It has about 15–20 lactiferous ducts and their openings. Each milk duct dilates to form lactiferous sinus at about 5–10 mm away from its opening in the nipple. During sucking by newborn, milk from the sinuses squeezes into oropharynx of infant. Structure of breasts are shown in Figure 4.

## Blood Supply

- Lateral thoracic branches of the axillary artery
- Internal mammary
- Internal costal arteries

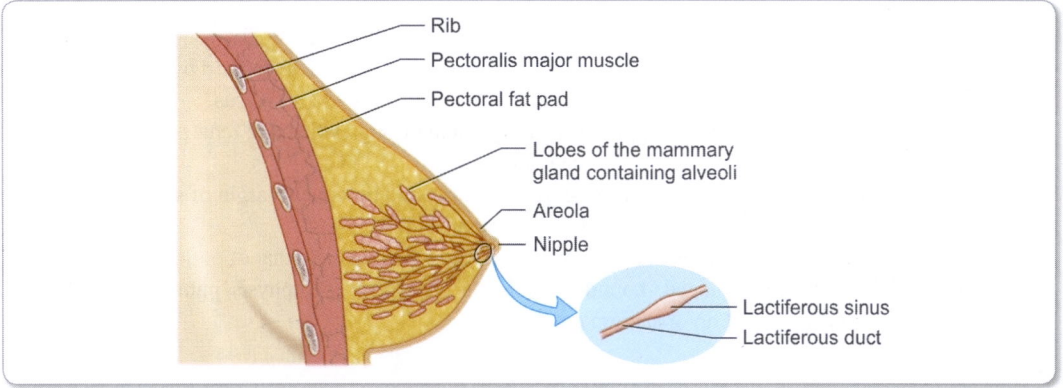

**Fig. 4:** Structure of breast

### Nerve Supply

The nerve supply is from 4th, 5th and 6th intercostal nerves.

### Development

The parenchyma of the breasts is developed from the ectoderm. The connective tissue stroma is from the mesoderm.

## FEMALE PELVIS

The pelvis is a skeletal ring often referred to as pelvic girdle formed by two innominate (hip) bones, the sacrum and the coccyx.

- **Innominate (hip) bones:** Each innominate (hip) bone is made up of three bones: Ilium, Ischium and Pubis.
  - **Ilium** is the large flared out part. The concave inner surface is iliac fossa and curved upper border is the iliac crest. At the front of iliac crest, there is bony prominence known as anterior superior iliac spine and below is anterior inferior iliac spine. On posterior side of iliac crest, similar bony prominence called posterior superior and posterior inferior iliac spine are located.
  - **Ischium** forms parts of acetabulum above and the thick lower part is the ischial tuberosity. The slight projection behind and just above the tuberosity is called ischial spine. Ischial spine helps to assess the station of the head during labor.
  - **Pubis** is a small bone that has a body and two projections called superior ramus and the inferior ramus. Two pubic bones meet at the symphysis pubis. Two inferior rami form the apex of pubic arch.
- **Sacrum:** The sacrum is a wedge-shaped bone consisting of five fused vertebrae and lies between the two iliums on each side. The prominent upper border is known as sacral promontory. The smooth concave anterior surface is referred to as hollow of the sacrum and the areas on either side are the alae or wings.
- **Coccyx:** It is a small triangular bone which articulates with the lower end of the sacrum. During labor the coccyx moves backwards to enlarge the pelvic outlet.

## Divisions of Pelvis

- **False pelvis:** It is the part of the pelvis situated above the pelvic brim. It is formed by upper flared –out portions of the iliac bones. Function of false pelvis is to support the gravid uterus.

- **True pelvis:** Lies below the pelvic brim. It is the bony canal through which the fetus passes during labor. It is divided into three planes: Brim, cavity and outlet.
  - **Brim:** It is the upper boundary of true pelvis. It is bounded by upper margin of symphysis pubis in front; linea terminalis on sides and sacral promontory at back.
  - **Cavity:** It is circular in shape and is the space between the brim and that of outlet.
  - **Outlet:** It is diamond-shaped, bounded by lower margin of symphysis pubis in front, ischial tuberosities on sides and tip of sacrum posteriorly.

## Pelvic Joints

Four pelvic joints are (Fig. 5):

- **Sacroiliac joints - two:** It is two highly movable joints formed where the ilium joins with the first two sacral vertebrae on either side.
- **Symphysis pubis - one:** It is a cartilaginous joint between the two pubic bones.
- **Sacrococcygeal joint - one:** It is a hinge joint between the sacrum and coccyx.

## Pelvic Ligaments

**The pelvic ligaments are (Fig. 6):**

- Sacroiliac ligament
- Pubic ligament
- Sacrotuberous ligament
- Sacrospinous ligament

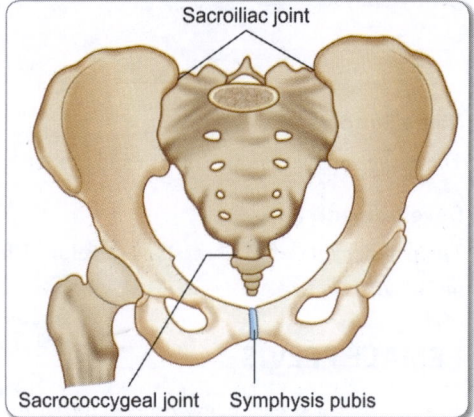

**Fig. 5:** Pelvic joints

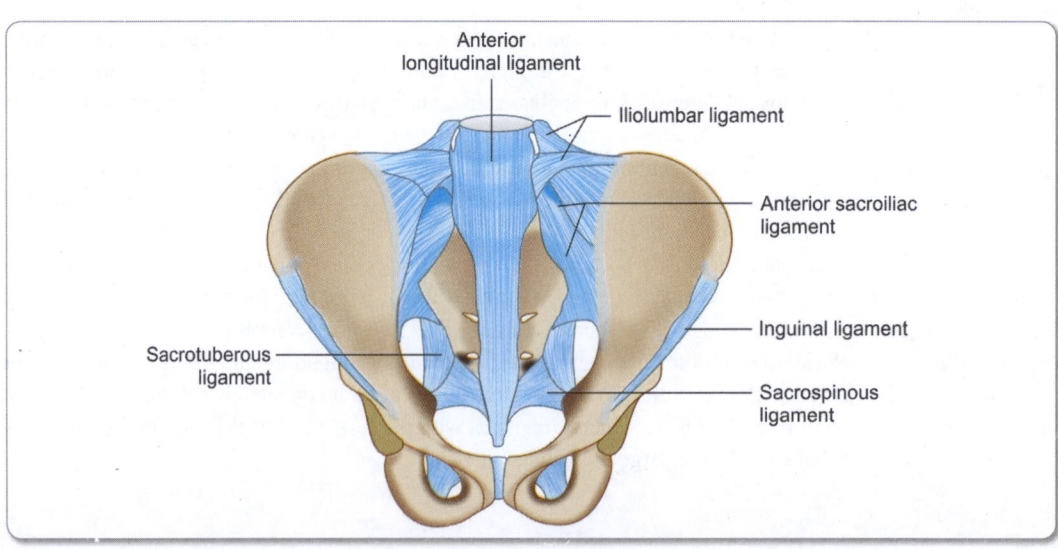

**Fig. 6:** Pelvic ligaments

## Landmarks of Pelvis

There are nine landmarks of pelvis (Fig. 7):

1. Sacral promontory
2. Ala or wings of sacrum
3. Sacroiliac joint
4. Iliopectineal line
5. Iliopubic eminence
6. Pectineal line
7. Pubic tubercle
8. Pubic crest
9. Symphysis pubis

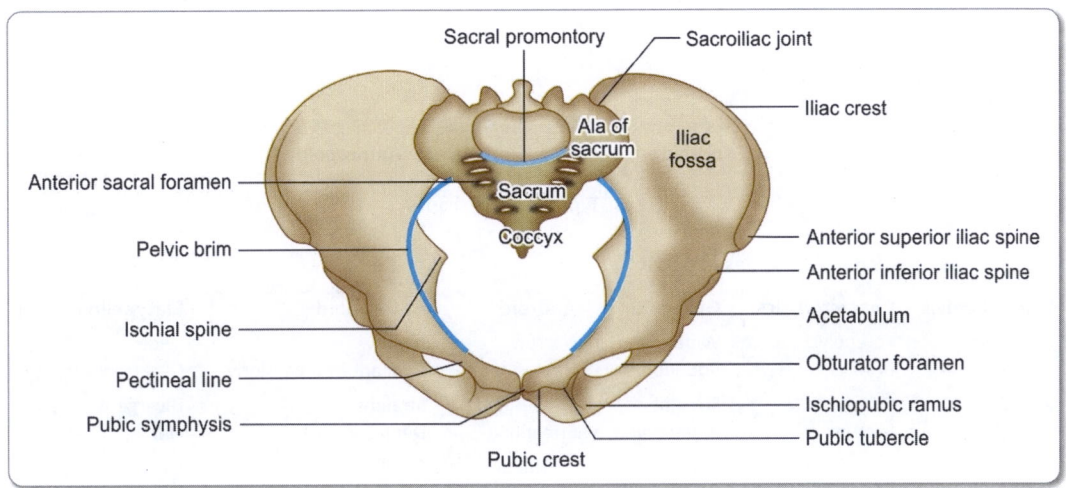

**Fig. 7:** Landmarks of pelvis

## Types of Pelvis Shapes

There are four types of pelvis shapes (Fig. 8 and Table 1):

1. **Gynecoid pelvis:** It is oval at the inlet, has a generous capacity and has wide subpubic arch. It is the typical female pelvis. Pelvic brim is a transverse ellipse and is most favorable for delivery.
2. **Android pelvis:** It is triangular in shape at the inlet with narrow subpubic arch. It is a male type pelvis. Pelvic brim is triangular.
3. **Anthropoid pelvis:** It has an oval inlet but the long axis is oriented vertically rather than side to side. It favors occiput posterior position. Pelvic brim is an anteroposterior ellipse.
4. **Platypelloid pelvis:** It is flattened at the inlet and has a prominent sacrum. It favors transverse presentations. It is very short.

Chapter 2 ◑ Reproductive System

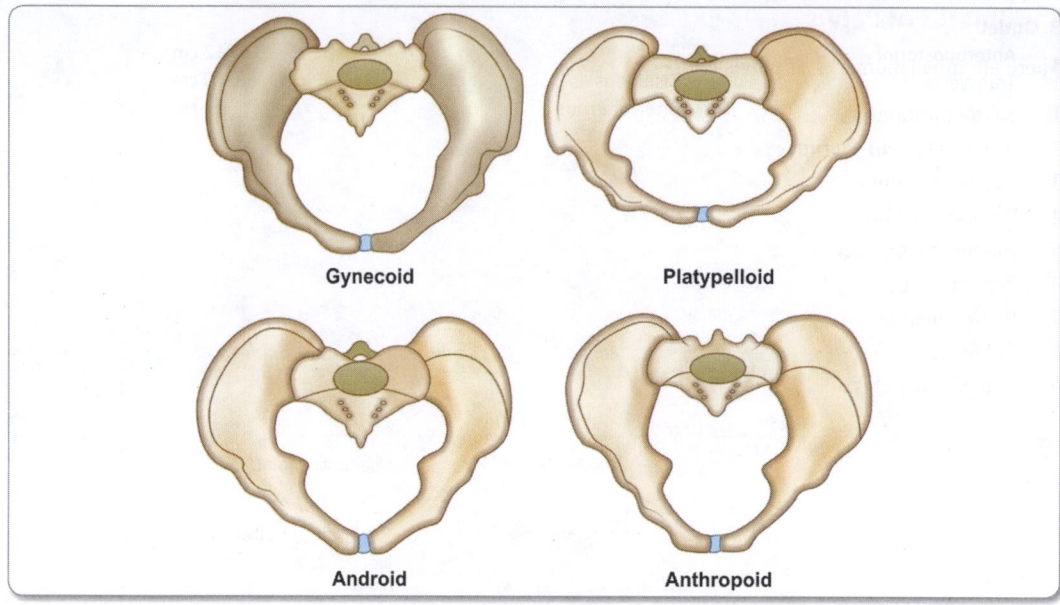

Gynecoid

Platypelloid

Android

Anthropoid

**Fig. 8:** Types of pelvis shapes

**TABLE 1:** Description of four types of pelvis

| | Place of pelvis | Characteristics | Gynecoid | Android | Anthropoid | Platypelloid |
|---|---|---|---|---|---|---|
| 1. | Brim | Forepelvis Brim | Wide Rounded | Narrow Heart-shaped | Narrow Oval anteroposteriorly | Wide Oval transversely |
| 2. | Cavity | Side walls Sacrum | Straight Well-curved | Convergent Straight | Straight Deep concave | Divergent Flat |
| 3. | Outlet | Ischial spine Subpubic arch | Blunt Wide, 90° | Prominent Narrow, <90° | Blunt Wide >90° | Blunt Wide >90° |
| 4. | Bone structure | | Medium | Heavy | Medium | Medium |
| 5. | Incidence | | 50% | 20% | 25% | 5% |

## Diameters of Pelvis (Table 2 and Fig. 9)

**TABLE 2:** Diameters of pelvis

| 1. Brim/Inlet | | |
|---|---|---|
| ▪ Anteroposterior | • True conjugate/Anatomical conjugate | 11 cm |
| | • Obstetric conjugate | 10 cm |
| | • Diagonal conjugate | 12 cm |
| ▪ Oblique diameter | • Right oblique | 12 cm |
| | • Left oblique | 12 cm |
| ▪ Transverse diameter | – | 13 cm |
| 2. Cavity | | |
| ▪ Anteroposterior | – | 12 cm |
| ▪ Transverse | – | 13 cm |

*Contd...*

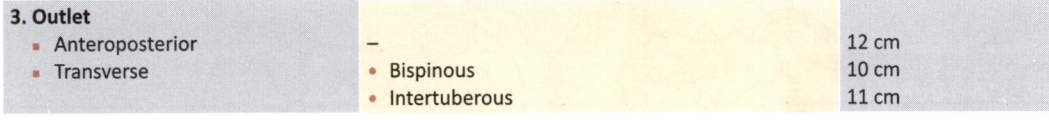

| 3. Outlet | | | |
|---|---|---|---|
| ▪ Anteroposterior | – | | 12 cm |
| ▪ Transverse | • Bispinous | | 10 cm |
| | • Intertuberous | | 11 cm |

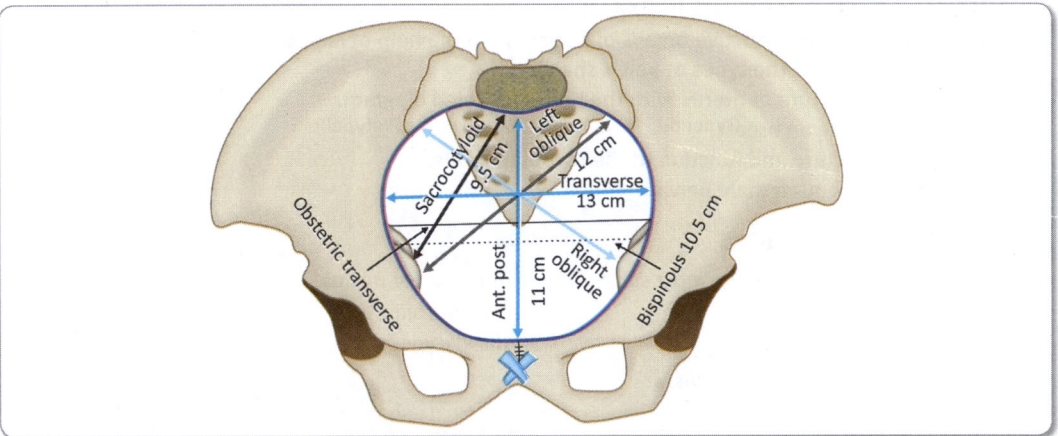

**Fig. 9:** Diameters of pelvis

## Brim or Inlet

- **Anteroposterior diameter**
    - ▪ **True conjugate/Conjugate vera/Anatomical conjugate (11 cm):** It is the distance between the midpoint of the sacral promontory to the inner margin of the upper border of symphysis pubis.
    - ▪ **Obstetric conjugate (10 cm):** Distance between midpoints of sacral promontory to the middle inner surface of symphysis pubis.
    - ▪ **Diagonal conjugate (12 cm):** Distance between the lower border of symphysis pubis to the midpoint on the sacral promontory.
- **Oblique diameter (12 cm):** Distance between one sacroiliac joint to the opposite iliopubic eminence. Right or left denotes the sacroiliac joint from which it starts.
- **Transverse diameter (13 cm):** It is the distance between the two farthest points on the pelvic brim over the iliopectineal lines.

## Cavity

- **Anteroposterior (12 cm):** It measures from the midpoint on the posterior surface of the symphysis pubis to the junction of second and third sacral vertebrae.
- **Transverse (12 cm):** Cannot be measured as the points lie over the soft tissue covering the sacrosciatic notches and obturator foramen.

## Outlet

- **Anteroposterior (12 cm):** It extends from the lower border of symphysis pubis to the tip of coccyx.
- **Transverse:** There are two transverse diameters.
    - i. **Bispinous (10 cm):** It is the distance between the tips of two ischial spines.
    - ii. **Intertuberous (11 cm):** It is the distance between the inner borders of ischial tuberosities.

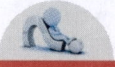

## ASSESS YOURSELF

### FREQUENTLY ASKED QUESTIONS IN EXAMS

1. Describe internal reproductive organs of female with the help of labeled diagram.
2. Briefly explain about the types of pelvis shapes.
3. Describe the structure of uterus with the help of labeled diagram.
4. Write a short note on breast.
5. Explain the structure and function of the fallopian tubes.
6. Write in detail about female pelvis.

### MULTIPLE CHOICE QUESTIONS

1. Which of the following is the most suitable type of pelvis for normal vaginal delivery?
   - a. Gynecoid
   - b. Android
   - c. Anthropoid
   - d. Platypelloid

2. Shape of brim of gynecoid pelvis is:
   - a. Rounded
   - b. Heart-shaped
   - c. Oval
   - d. Diamond

3. Joint between pubic bones is:
   - a. Sacroiliac joint
   - b. Sacrococcygeal joint
   - c. Sacrospinous joint
   - d. Symphysis pubis

4. All diameters of the cavity are to be:
   - a. 12 cm
   - b. 13 cm
   - c. 14 cm
   - d. 10 cm

5. True conjugate diameter of brim is:
   - a. 10 cm
   - b. 11 cm
   - c. 8 cm
   - d. 12 cm

6. Pelvis consists of:
   - a. 4 joint
   - b. 5 joints
   - c. 6 joints
   - d. 8 joints

7. Station of fetal head is detected from:
   - a. Iliac crest
   - b. Ischial spines
   - c. Iliopubic eminence
   - d. Symphysis pubis

8. During sitting, weight of whole body bears on:
   - a. Ischial tuberosities
   - b. Iliac crest
   - c. Ischial spines
   - d. None of the above

9. Innominate bones consist of:
   - a. Ilium
   - b. Ischium
   - c. Pubis
   - d. All of the above

10. Sacrum consists of:
    - a. 5 vertebrae
    - b. 6 vertebrae
    - c. 7 vertebrae
    - d. 4 vertebrae

11. **Which is the longest and widest part of the fallopian tube?**
    a. Isthmus
    b. Ampulla
    c. Infundibulum
    d. Interstitium

12. **Which is the thickest layer of uterus?**
    a. Perimetrium
    b. Myometrium
    c. Endometrium
    d. All of the above

13. **All of the following are parts of the uterus, except:**
    a. Body
    b. Cervix
    c. Ampulla
    d. Isthmus

14. **Weight of nonpregnant uterus is:**
    a. 50–80 g
    b. 200 g
    c. 150–180 g
    d. 500 g

15. **Which of the following is the least vascular part of uterus?**
    a. Lateral
    b. Middle
    c. Upper
    d. Lower

16. **The length of fallopian tube is:**
    a. 8–10 cm
    b. 10–12 cm
    c. 15 cm
    d. None

17. **Narrowest part of fallopian tube is the:**
    a. Infundibulum
    b. Isthmus
    c. Ampulla
    d. Interstitial portions

18. **External genitalia of female help in all of the following functions except:**
    a. Enabling sperm to enter the body
    b. Providing sexual pleasure
    c. Protecting the fetus
    d. Protecting internal genital organs

19. **Supports of uterus are:**
    a. Uterosacral ligament
    b. Round ligament of uterus
    c. Mackenrodt's ligament
    d. None of the above

20. **External genitalia include all, except:**
    a. Vagina
    b. Mons pubis
    c. Clitoris
    d. Labia majora

## 🔑 Answer Key

| | | | | | | |
|---|---|---|---|---|---|---|
| 1. a | 2. a | 3. d | 4. a | 5. b | 6. a | 7. b |
| 8. a | 9. d | 10. a | 11. b | 12. b | 13. c | 14. a |
| 15. b | 16. b | 17. d | 18. c | 19. d | 20. a | |

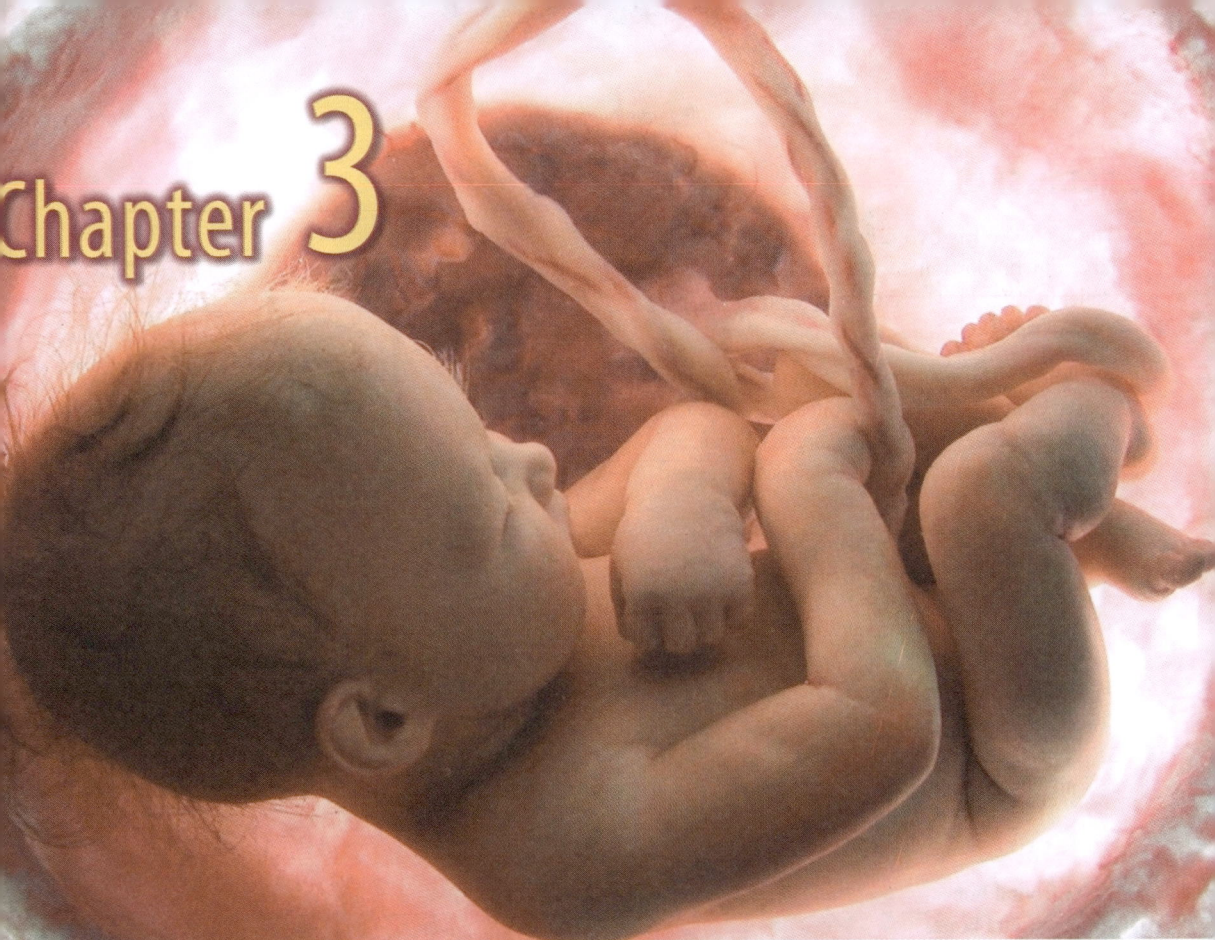

# Chapter 3

# Embryology and Fetal Development

## FETAL SKULL

The fetal skull is ovoid in shape. At term it is larger in proportion to the other parts of the skeleton (Fig. 1). The skull may be divided into three parts:

1. **Vault:** The vault which contains the brain is composed of five bones: two frontal, two parietal and one occipital. These are united by membranes known as sutures and fontanels.
2. **Base:** The base of skull is composed of five bones: two temporal, one ethmoid, one sphenoid and a part of occipital bone. These are firmly fused together. At the base of the skull is an opening known as Foramen magnum through which the spinal cord passes.
3. **The face** is composed of 14 bones and all are fused together.

### Bones of Fetal Skull (Fig. 2)

- 2 frontal bones
- 2 parietal bones
- 2 temporal bones
- 1 occipital bone

### Sutures

The area where two skull bones join together is called suture. There are four sutures of obstetrical importance:

1. **Frontal suture:** Between two frontal bones
2. **Sagittal suture:** Between two parietal bones
3. **Coronal suture:** Between the frontal bone and parietal bones
4. **Lambdoid suture:** Between the parietal and occipital bones

#### Importance of Sutures

- Permits gliding movement of one bone over the other during molding of fetal head during labor.
- Digital palpation of sagittal suture during vaginal examination in labor gives idea of engagement of head, degree of internal rotation of head and degree of molding of head.

### Fontanels

The area where two or more sutures join is called fontanel. There are six fontanels on skull but only two are of obstetrical importance:

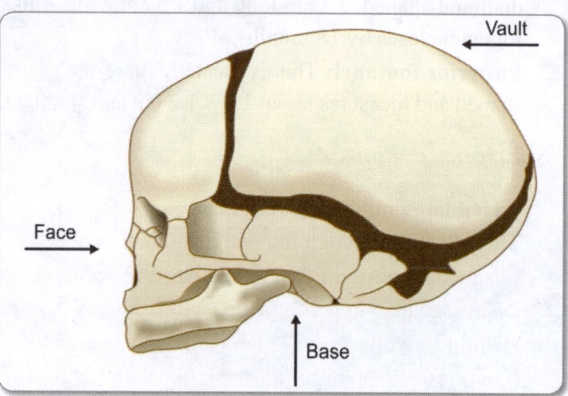

**Fig. 1:** Fetal skull

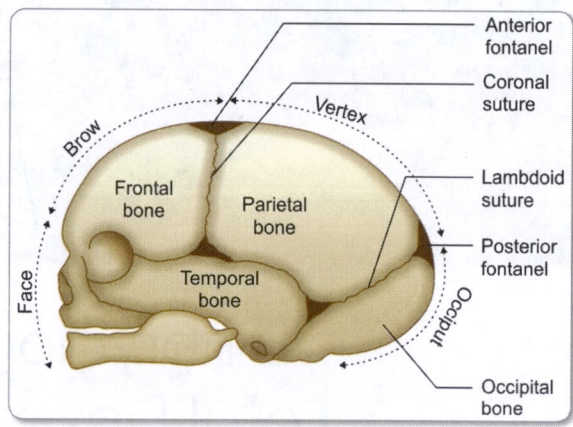

**Fig. 2:** Parts of fetal skull

1. **Anterior fontanel:** It is the largest fontanel. It is the junction of sagittal, frontal and coronal suture. It is diamond-shaped, 2.5 cm long and 1.5 cm wide. Pulsations of cerebral vessels can be felt through it. The fontanel closes by 18 months of age.
2. **Posterior fontanel:** This is located where the sagittal suture meets the lambdoid suture. It is triangle-shaped and measures about 1.2 × 1.2 cm and smaller than anterior fontanel. It closes by six weeks of age.

## Importance of Fontanels

- It facilitates molding of fetal head
- The palpation through internal examination denotes degree of flexion of head
- It is membranous after birth and helps in accommodating marked brain growth
- Depressed in dehydration, elevated in case of raised intracranial pressure (ICP)
- Helpful for collection of blood and exchange transfusion
- Cerebrospinal fluid can be drawn through fontanels

## Diameters of Fetal Skull

Fetal skull has:

- Four transverse diameters
- Six anteroposterior diameters

### Transverse Diameters

For memorizing transverse diameters, learn the mnemonic "Miss Tina So Pretty".

**Miss** = Bimastoid diameter
**Tina** = Bitemporal diameter
**So** = Super subparietal diameter
**Pretty** = Biparietal diameter

- **Bimastoid diameter (7.5 cm):** Distance between the tips of mastoid processes.
- **Bitemporal diameter (8 cm):** Distance between anteroinferior ends of coronal suture.
- **Super subparietal diameter (8.5 cm):** Extends from a point placed below one parietal eminence to a point placed above other parietal eminence of the opposite side.
- **Biparietal diameter (9.5 cm):** Distance between two parietal eminences.

### Anteroposterior Diameters

- **Suboccipitobregmatic (9.5 cm):** Extends from the nape of neck to center of bregma.
- **Suboccipitofrontal (10 cm):** Extends from nape of neck to the anterior end of anterior fontanel or center of sinciput.
- **Occipitofrontal (11.5 cm):** Extends from the occipital eminence to the root of nose (glabella)
- **Mentovertical (14 cm):** Extends from midpoint of the chin to the highest point on the sagittal suture.
- **Submentovertical (11.5 cm):** Extends from junction of floor of the mouth and neck to the highest point on the sagittal suture.
- **Submentobregmatic (9.5 cm):** Extends from junction of floor of mouth and neck to the center of the bregma.

Chapter 3 ❖ Embryology and Fetal Development

# EMBRYOLOGY

Embryology is the branch of biology that studies the prenatal development of gametes (sex cells), fertilization and development of embryo and fetus.

The embryonic stages between conception and birth are given in Figure 3:

The stage after conception is zygote and upon cell division, it becomes morula. The morula becomes blastocyst and attaches to the uterus and six to twelve days after conception, the blastocyst turns into embryo. At 10 weeks, the fetal period begins and embryo is termed as a fetus.

(**Note:** Detailed explanation of each step is given in fetal development)

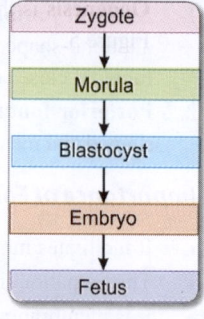

**Fig. 3:** Embryonic stages

## Fetal Development

Various processes or developmental stages occur before the development of fetus. They are as follows:

- Gametogenesis
  - Spermatogenesis
  - Oogenesis
  - Ovulation
- Fertilization

- Implantation
- Decidua
- Development of fertilized ovum/embryo
- Development of fetus

### Gametogenesis

It is the process of formation of male and female gametes in gonads.

- **Spermatogenesis** is the process of formation of spermatozoa in testis. The process is described in Figure 4.

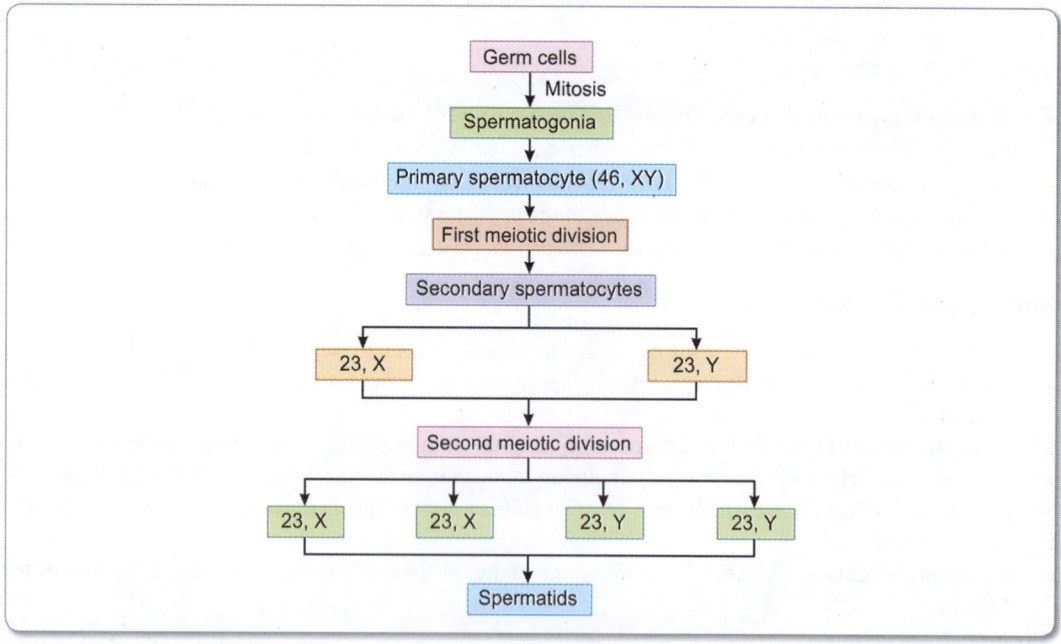

**Fig. 4:** Spermatogenesis

- **Oogenesis** is the process of formation of mature ovum (egg) in the ovary. The process is discussed in Figure 5.

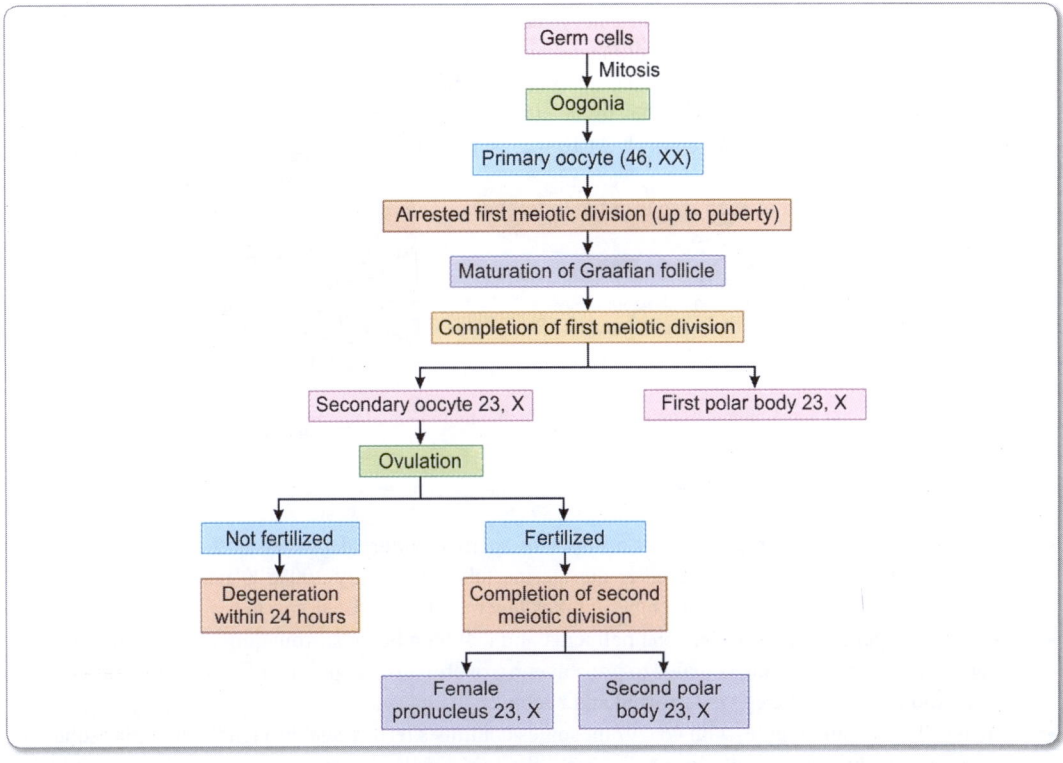

**Fig. 5:** Oogenesis

- **Ovulation:** Ovulation is a process whereby a secondary oocyte is released from the ovary following rupture of a mature Graafian follicle and becomes available for conception. Only one secondary oocyte is likely to rupture in each ovarian cycle which starts at puberty and ends in menopause.
  - **Mechanism:**
    - Ovulation, prompted by luteinizing hormone from anterior pituitary occurs when the mature follicle ruptures and release secondary oocyte into peritoneal cavity.
    - The ovulated secondary oocyte, ready for fertilization is still surrounded by zona pellucida and few layers of cells called corona radiata.
    - If not fertilized, secondary oocyte degenerates in a couple of days.
    - If a sperm passes through corona radiata and zona pellucida and enters the cytoplasm of the secondary oocyte, the second meiotic division resumes to form a polar body and a mature ovum.

## Fertilization (Fig. 6)

- It is the process of fusion of the spermatozoon with the mature ovum.
- Fertilization is most likely to occur if intercourse takes place around the time of ovulation. In most of the cases fertilization occurs in the ampullary part of the uterine tubes/fallopian tubes.

Chapter 3 ◑ Embryology and Fetal Development

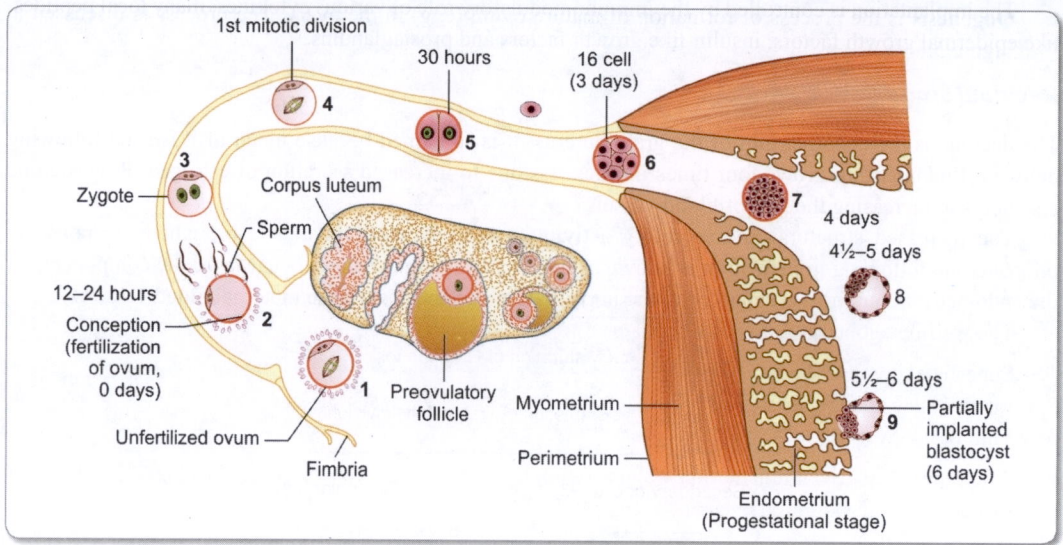

**Fig. 6:** Stages of development—early embryo

- During ejaculation, out of hundreds of millions of sperms that are deposited in the vagina, only a few thousand capacitated spermatozoa enter the uterine tube while only 300–500 reach the ovum due to muscular contractions of the uterine tube. It takes few minutes for the sperm to reach the fallopian tube.
- The mature sperm penetrates the zona pellucida and cell membrane surrounding ovum. After the entry of one sperm, the membrane is sealed to prevent entry of any further sperm. Following penetration of the sperm into the ovum, the egg is fertilized and becomes an embryo.
- The fertilized ovum (zygote) with 46 chromosomes continues its passage through the fallopian tubes and undergoes division into 2 cells → 4 cells → 8 cells → 16 cells and so on, until a mulberry-like ball of cells is formed, called morula.
- On 4th day, morula reaches the uterine cavity.
- On 4th–5th day, morula is covered by a film of mucus. The fluid passes through the canaliculi of the zona pellucida which separates the cells of the morula and is called blastocyst.
- At this point, cells of zygote differentiate into two distinct types:
  i.   **Embryoblast cells:** These cells continually divide into what will become the embryo, the fetus itself.
  ii.  **Trophoblast:** These cells form the placenta that is attached against the uterine wall to nourish the embryo.

## Implantation

Implantation is the process of the embryo attaching itself to the uterine wall.

Implantation occurs in the endometrium of the anterior or posterior wall of the body of uterus near the fundus on 6th day which corresponds to the 20th day of a regular menstrual cycle. If implantation is successful, the developing placenta will begin to produce beta hCG that is easily detectable in the urine and blood.

Implantation occurs through four stages:
1. Apposition
2. Adhesion
3. Penetration
4. Invasion

The implantation is controlled by the immunomodulatory role of various cytokines, many local peptides, like epidermal growth factors, insulin-like growth factors and prostaglandins.

## Decidual Stage

The decidua is the endometrium of the gravid uterus. It is so named because much of it is shed following delivery. Endometrium grows four times in thickness due to increased secretion of estrogen. Progesterone also helps in increasing the size of blood vessels.

The increased structural and secretory activity of the endometrium that is brought in response to progesterone following implantation is known as decidual reaction. Changes occur in all the components of the endometrium but most are marked at the implantation site and around the maternal blood vessels.

The well-developed decidua differentiates into three layers:

1. Superficial compact layer
2. Intermediate spongy layer
3. Thin basal layer

After the interstitial implantation of blastocyst into the compact layer of the decidua, the different portions of the decidua are renamed as:

- **Decidua basalis:** It lies between the blastocyst and uterine muscle. This part later forms placenta.
- **Decidua capsularis:** This is the superficial compact layer which overlies blastocyst. With fetal growth, the decidua capsularis bulges into the uterine cavity and fuses with the decidua parietalis.
- **Decidua parietalis:** This is the decidua lining the rest of the uterine cavity.

## Development of Fertilized Ovum/Embryo

After the blastocyst embeds into endometrium, outer trophoblastic cells proliferate to form three layers:

1. **Syncytiotrophoblast:** It is the outer layer, which makes nutrients in the maternal blood accessible to the developing embryo.
2. **Cytotrophoblast:** Inner layer, which produces beta hCG hormone.
3. **Mesoderm:** The third layer, which develops to chorionic vesicle with its membrane is called chorion. It forms body stalk and umbilical cord.

The trophoblast develops to form the placenta and inner cell mass develops to form fetus. The cells differentiate into three layers: Ectoderm, endoderm and mesoderm.

1. **Ectoderm:** Develops into central and peripheral nervous system and the epidermis.
2. **Endoderm:** Forms the dermis, skeleton, urinary bladder, skeletal and smooth muscles.
3. **Mesoderm:** Forms heart, blood vessels, liver, pancreas, bones and muscles.

### Embryo

The word embryo (Greek: swelling within) refers to the growing organism from the second to the eighth week of life. During this time, it develops from a tiny cell cluster into a little growth of about 1 inch in length.

As this development proceeds, the placenta, a special organ of interchange, begins to grow between the embryo and uterus. The embryo is connected to the placenta by the umbilical cord. The placenta acts as filter and barrier. It allows the embryo (and later the fetus) to absorb food and oxygen from mother's blood and to eliminate $CO_2$ and other waste from its own blood in return. At the same time, however, the two blood systems remain completely separate.

## Development of Fetus

- **First trimester:** During first 3 months of pregnancy, the product of conception grows from just visible speck to the fertilized ovum to a lively embryo. At the end of first trimester, the following changes occur:
  - All organs are formed and heart starts to beat.
  - The fetus becomes less vulnerable to the effect of most of the drugs, infections after embryonic period.
  - Facial features form and there is rapid development of brain. The fetus becomes human in appearance.
  - External sex organs are visible, but positive sex identification is difficult.
  - Well-defined neck, nail beds begin to form, nose, mouth and eyelids become visible; tooth buds form.
  - Rudimentary kidneys excrete small amounts of urine into the amniotic sac.
  - Fetus is about 2.9 inches long and weighs about 45 g.
- **Second trimester:** During these months, the fetus grows fast. At the end of 2nd trimester
  - FHR can be heard with stethoscope.
  - Eyes remain closed and body growth accelerates.
  - Vernix caseosa is present; the skin of the fetus is wrinkled, translucent and appears pink.
  - Sex is visible.
  - Skeleton is calcified.
  - After birth survival is possible, but the fetus is at serious risk.
  - Production of lung surfactant occurs.
  - Average crown-rump length is around 20 cm and weight is 560 g.
- **Third trimester:** During these months, fetus gains maturity.
  - Skin is whitish pink.
  - Sucking reflex is stronger and eyes begin to open and shut.
  - Skull is formed.
  - Testes are in the scrotum, if a male child.
  - Lightening occurs.
  - Fetal Hb begins to convert to adult Hb.
  - Kicks rapidly.
  - Fetus is about 31 cm long and weighs about 3000 grams.

The postfertilization events have been summarized in Table 1.

**TABLE 1: Postfertilization events**

| 0 hour | Fertilization | 0 hour | Fertilization |
|---|---|---|---|
| 24 hours | 2 cell stage of zygote | 12th day | Primary villi |
| 42 hours | 4 cell stage | 16th day | Secondary villi |
| 72 hours | 12 cell stage | 21st day | Tertiary villi |
| 96 hours | Morula enters uterine cavity | 21–22 day | Fetal heart, fetoplacental circulation |
| 5th day | Blastocyst | 21–40 day | Chorion frondosum |
| 7th day | Implantation | 40–50 day | Cotyledons |
| 11th day | Implantation completed | 71–267 day | Fetal stage |

## FETAL MEMBRANES

It consists of two layers outer chorion and inner amnion (Fig. 7).

### Chorion

It is formed out of chorion leave and ends at placental margin. Chorion is thick, opaque, friable membrane. It consists of two layers:
1. Outer layer is formed by primitive ectoderm or trophoblast.
2. Inner layer is formed by somatic mesoderm with which amnion is attached.

### Amnion

It is the inner layer of fetal membranes. This is the smooth, slippery, glistening innermost

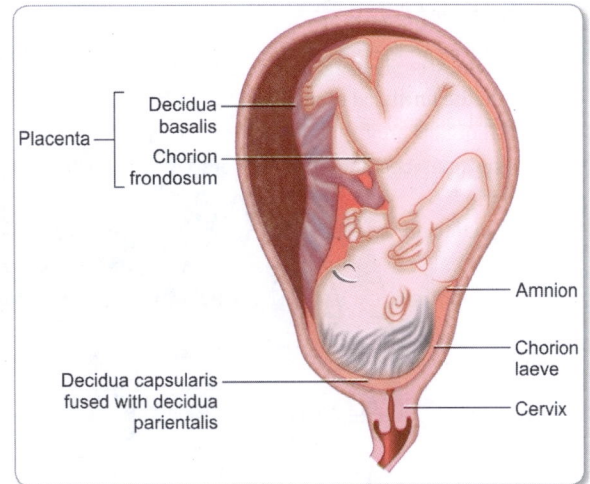

**Fig. 7:** Fetal membranes

membrane that lines the amniotic space. It is filled with fluid and is called "Bag of waters". The fetus floats and moves in the amniotic cavity. When first formed, the amnion is in contact with the body of the embryo, but about the 4th or 5th week, fluid (liquor amnii) begins to accumulate within it.

This fluid increases in quantity and causes the amnion to expand and ultimately to adhere to the inner surface of the chorion.

### Functions

- Contribute to the formation of liquor amnii.
- Intact membranes prevent ascending uterine infections.
- Facilitate dilatation of the cervix during the labor.
- Plays important role in the enzymatic activities for steroid hormone's metabolism.
- Rich source of glycerophospholipids containing arachidonic acids, which is a precursor of prostaglandin.

## PLACENTA

The human placenta is:
- **Discoid:** Because of the shape.
- **Hemochorial:** Because of direct contact of the chorion with the maternal blood.
- **Deciduate:** Because of connection between the mother and fetus through the umbilical cord.

### Structure

Placenta is a disc-like spongy fleshy structure, thick at center and thin at edges. Fully developed placenta (at term) is reddish in color. It is formed from the layers of blastocyst (Figs 8A and B).
- **Average weight of placenta:** 500 g (approximately 1/6th of fetal weight)
- **Diameter:** 15–20 cm
- **Thickness:** 2–2.5 cm at center thinning towards periphery
- The umbilical cord is attached to the center of fetal surface of the placenta.
- **Diameter of cord:** 1–2.5 cm

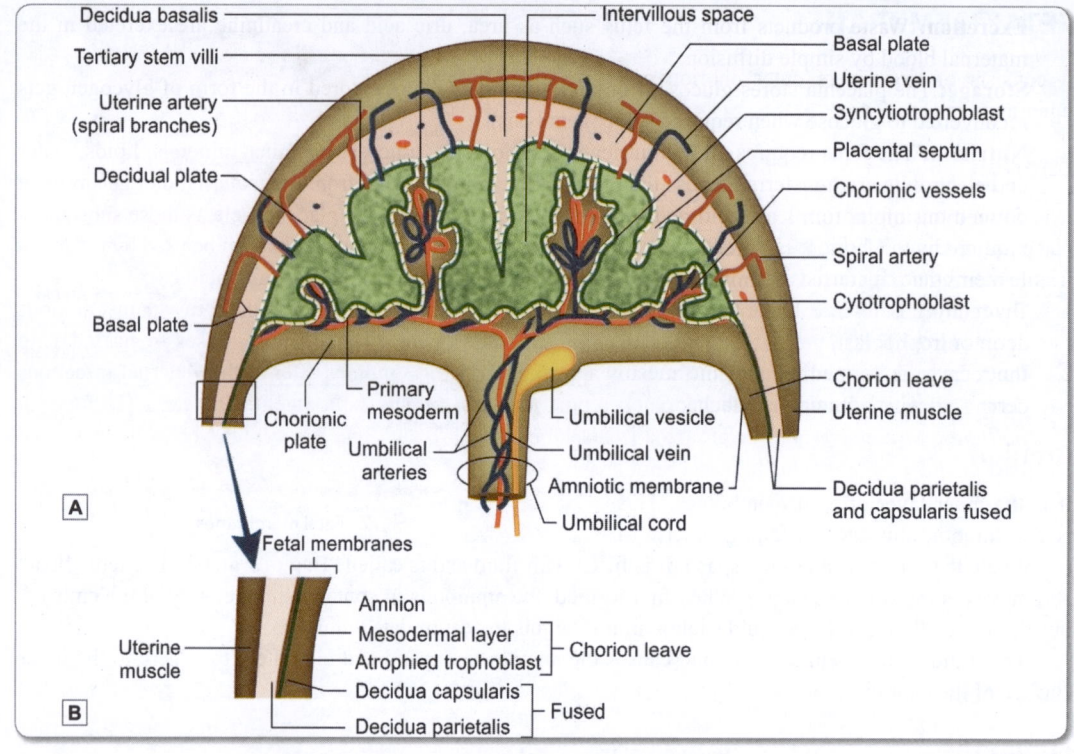

Decidua basalis — Intervillous space
Tertiary stem villi — Basal plate
Uterine artery — Uterine vein
(spiral branches) — Syncytiotrophoblast
Decidual plate — Placental septum
— Chorionic vessels
— Spiral artery
Basal plate — — Cytotrophoblast
Primary — Chorion leave
Chorionic mesoderm — Umbilical vesicle Uterine muscle
plate Umbilical — Umbilical vein
arteries Amniotic membrane — Decidua parietalis
and capsularis fused
A — Umbilical cord
Fetal membranes
— Amnion
Uterine — Mesodermal layer ⎤ Chorion leave
muscle — Atrophied trophoblast ⎦
— Decidua capsularis ⎤ Fused
B — Decidua parietalis ⎦

**Figs 8A and B:** Structure of placenta

- **Length:** 30–100 cm (average)
- Covering of cord from outside to inside are amnion, mucoid embryonic connective tissue and Wharton's jelly
- **Blood vessels:** 2 arteries +1 vein

## Placental Surfaces

- **Fetal surface:** It is smooth, shiny, transparent, and umbilical cord is attached at or near the center. Branches of umbilical vessels can be seen on this surface, radiating from umbilical cord. The underlying chorion can be seen through glistening amniotic membrane. Amniotic membrane can be peeled off from underlying chorionic plate except at umbilical cord.
- **Maternal surface:** It looks dull red in color and surface is divided into 15–30 cotyledons, separated by sulci. Small calcified white infarcts can be seen on the maternal surface.

## Functions of Placenta

The placenta truly is an organ of life with a number of functions to protect the fetus. Its functions include:

- **Respiration:** Fetus obtains oxygen and excretes $CO_2$ through the placenta. Oxygen from the mother's body passes into the fetal blood by simple diffusion and similarly fetus gives off $CO_2$ into maternal blood.

- **Excretion:** Waste products from the fetus such as urea, uric acid and creatinine are excreted in the maternal blood by simple diffusion.
- **Storage:** The placenta stores glucose, iron and vitamins. Glucose stored in the form of glycogen gets reconverted to glucose when required (glycogenolysis)
- **Nutrition:** The fetus requires all the nutrients. Amino acids, glucose, vitamins, minerals, lipids, water and electrolyte are transferred across the placental membrane. Food from the maternal diet gets broken down into simpler forms by the time it reaches the placental site. The placenta selects those substances required by the fetus. It can breakdown complex nutrients into compounds that can be used by the fetus. Proteins get transferred as amino acids; carbohydrates as glucose and fats as fatty acids.
- **Protection:** Fetal membrane has long been considered as protective barrier to the fetus against noxious agents circulating in the maternal blood. Certain antibodies, which the mother possesses are passed on to the fetus to provide immunity for the baby approximately for 3 months after birth. Maternal infections during pregnancy by virus (rubella, chicken pox, measles, mumps, poliomyelitis), bacteria (*Treponema pallidum*, *Mycobacterium*) or protozoa (malarial parasite, *Toxoplasma gondii*) may cross the placental barrier and affect the fetus in utero. Similarly, certain drugs can also cross the placental barrier and may have deleterious effects on the fetus.
- **Enzymatic functions:**
  - Diamine oxidase which inactivates the circulatory precursor amines
  - Oxytocinase which neutralizes the oxytocin
  - Phospholipase A$_2$ which synthesizes arachidonic acid
- **Endocrine functions:** Placenta secretes the following four hormones:
  i. **Beta hCG:** Cytotrophoblastic layer of chorionic villi produces hCG.
  ii. **Estrogens:** These are produced by placenta in large amount throughout the pregnancy. The estrogen production is an index of fetoplacental well-being also.
  iii. **Progesterone:** It is produced in the syncytial layer of placenta in increasing quantities until immediately before the onset of labor, then its level falls gradually.
  iv. **Human placental lactogen:** It is another hormone produced by placenta and is involved in lactogenic and metabolic processes in pregnancy.
- **Immunological functions:** The fetus and the placenta contain paternally determined antigens, which are foreign to the mother. In spite of this, there is no evidence of graft rejection. Placenta probably offers immunological protection against rejection.

## Abnormalities of Placenta

There is a marked variation in the morphology including size, shape and weight of the placenta, on the basis of which, abnormalities of placenta are described as follows (Figs 9A to E):
- **Succenturiate placenta/succenturiata placentae:** One or more separate accessory lobes in the membranes are present at a variable distance away from the main placental mass. These accessory lobes are usually connected to the main placental mass. This condition is managed by exploration of uterus and removal of lobe under general anesthesia.
- **Extrachorial placenta:** A placental anomaly is observed on the fetal surface as a thick white ring, which gives the impression that central portion is somewhat depressed.
  There are two varieties of extrachorial placenta:
  i. **Circumvallate placenta:** The ring is situated at a variable distance between the margin and center of the placenta. A double fold of both chorion and amnion with fibrin and degenerated decidua forms the ring giving it a raised appearance.

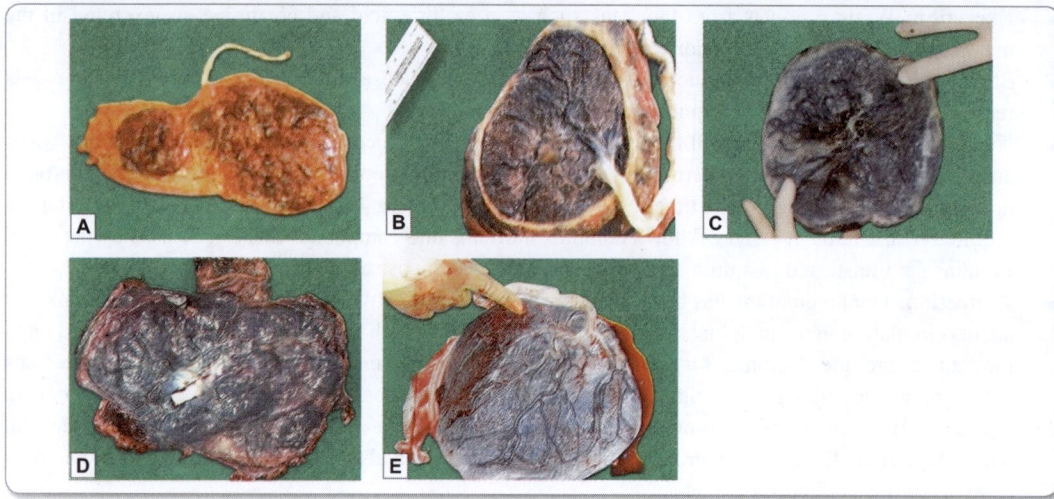

**Figs 9A to E:** Abnormalities of placenta; **A.** Succenturiate placenta; **B.** Circumvallate placenta; **C.** Placenta marginata; **D.** Placenta membranacea; **E.** Membranous placenta

    ii. **Placenta marginata/circummarginate placenta:** The ring is located at the edge or margin of the placenta and is raised by the presence of degenerated decidua and fibrin.

- **Lobulated placenta:** It appears to be multiple placenta for a single baby. In fact, it is one placenta divided into two or more parts either completely separated or joined in part. The lobes are held together by one set of membranes and blood vessels. The number of lobes determines the name as bipartite (placenta duplex) and tripartite placenta (placenta triplex).
- **Placenta membranacea:** The placenta is unduly large and thin. Placenta does not develop from chorion frondosum but from chorion leave so that whole of the ovum is practically covered by the placenta.
- **Larger and heavier placenta:** It is as seen in large-sized fetuses, fetal syphilis and erythroblastosis.
- **Smaller and lighter placenta:** It may occur with general systemic diseases or local uterine conditions that cause undernourishment of placenta and lead to intrauterine growth retardation (IUGR).
- **Light-colored placenta:** May be due to fetal anemia in case of erythroblastosis.
- **Tumor formation:** Associated with prematurity and polyhydramnios.
- **Infarct of cotyledons:** Due to diseases such as maternal hypertension and eclampsia that reduce placental circulation leading to IUGR and eventually fetal death.
- **Edematous placenta:** It is characterized by mushy, thick and pale, and fluid can be squeezed from this type of placenta. It is due to maternal diabetes, heart disease, nephritis or severe erythroblastosis that cause fetal death.

## LIQUOR AMNII (AMNIOTIC FLUID)

**Definition:** Amniotic fluid (liquor amnii) is faintly alkaline watery content of the amniotic sac, which allows growth and free movement of the fetus. It is the nourishing and protecting liquid contained by the amnion of pregnant woman (Fig. 10).

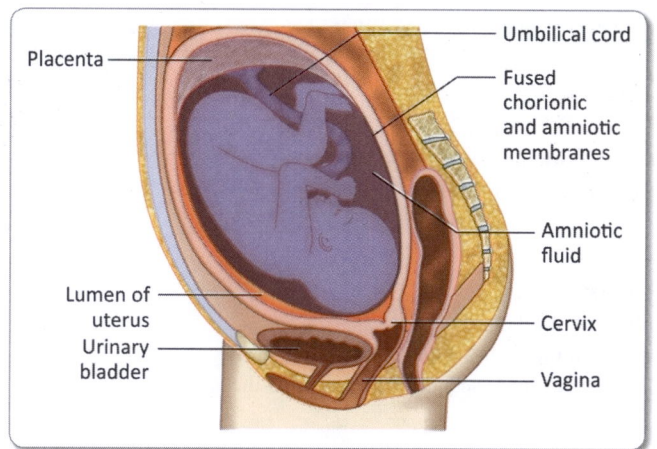

**Fig. 10:** Amniotic fluid

## Volume

Amniotic fluid volume is related to gestational age. It is about 50 mL at 12 weeks; 400 mL at 20 weeks and 1 L at 36–38 weeks.

Thereafter it diminishes, till at term it measures about 600–800 mL. At post term, reduction occurs to the extent of 200 mL at 43 weeks.

## Physical Features

- Faintly alkaline with low specific gravity of 1.010.
- In early pregnancy, it is colorless, but near term it becomes pale straw.
- Abnormal color of liquor is seen in the following cases:
  - **Green:** Meconium stained.
  - **Golden:** Rh incompatibility, due to hemolysis of fetal RBC.
  - **Green yellow (saffron):** Post maturity.
  - **Dark colored:** Concealed hemorrhage.
  - **Dark brown:** Intrauterine death.

## Composition

In first half of pregnancy, the composition is identical to plasma. But in late pregnancy, the composition is altered. It includes:

- Water 98–99%
- Solid (1–2%): The following are solid constituents:
  - **Organic:** Proteins, glucose, urea, uric acid, creatinine, lipids and hormones
  - **Inorganic:** Sodium, chloride, potassium
  - **Suspended particles:** Lanugo, epithelial cells, vernix caseosa, cast off amniotic cells

## Functions

### During Pregnancy

- Acts as shock absorber and protects fetus from injuries.
- Maintains even temperature (hemostasis).
- Allows free movement of fetus within the uterus.

### During Labor

- Helps in cervical dilatation.
- Guards against umbilical cord compression.
- Flushes the birth canal at the end of 1st stage of labor.
- Protects the fetus and prevents ascending infection to the uterine cavity due to aseptic and bacterial action.

## Clinical Importance

- Gives information regarding maturity of fetus.
- Intra-amniotic instillation of chemicals is used as a method for induction of abortion.
- Excess or less volume of liquor amnii is assessed by amniotic fluid index (AFI).
- Rupture of membranes with drainage of liquor is a helpful method in induction of labor.

## UMBILICAL CORD

The umbilical cord or funis forms the connecting link between the fetus and the placenta through which the fetal blood flows to and from the placenta. It extends from the fetal umbilicus to the fetal surface of the placenta (Fig. 11).

- It contains blood vessels—two arteries and one vein.
- Umbilical cord is protected by gelatinous substance called Wharton's jelly, which is formed from mesoderm.
- It is developed from body stalk of the mesodermal tissue stretching between embryonic disc and chorion.

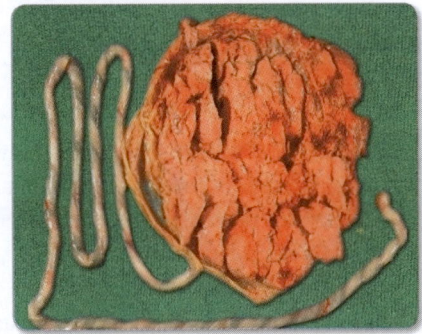

**Fig. 11:** Umbilical cord

## Structure

The cord is bluish white in color and is about 40 cm in length with usual variation of 30–100 cm. Average diameter is 1.5 cm. The cord is twisted spirally and, in some cases, may be wrapped around neck or body of the fetus. There can be swelling at some places due to collection of Wharton's jelly called false knots.

## Functions

Umbilical cord acts as a lifeline between placenta and fetus by providing oxygen and nutrients to fetus and disposing the fetal waste products.

## Cord Abnormalities

- **Battledore placenta:** The cord is attached to the margin of the placenta. It is associated with low implantation of placenta; there is a chance of cord compression in vaginal delivery leading to fetal anoxia or death (Figs 12A to G).

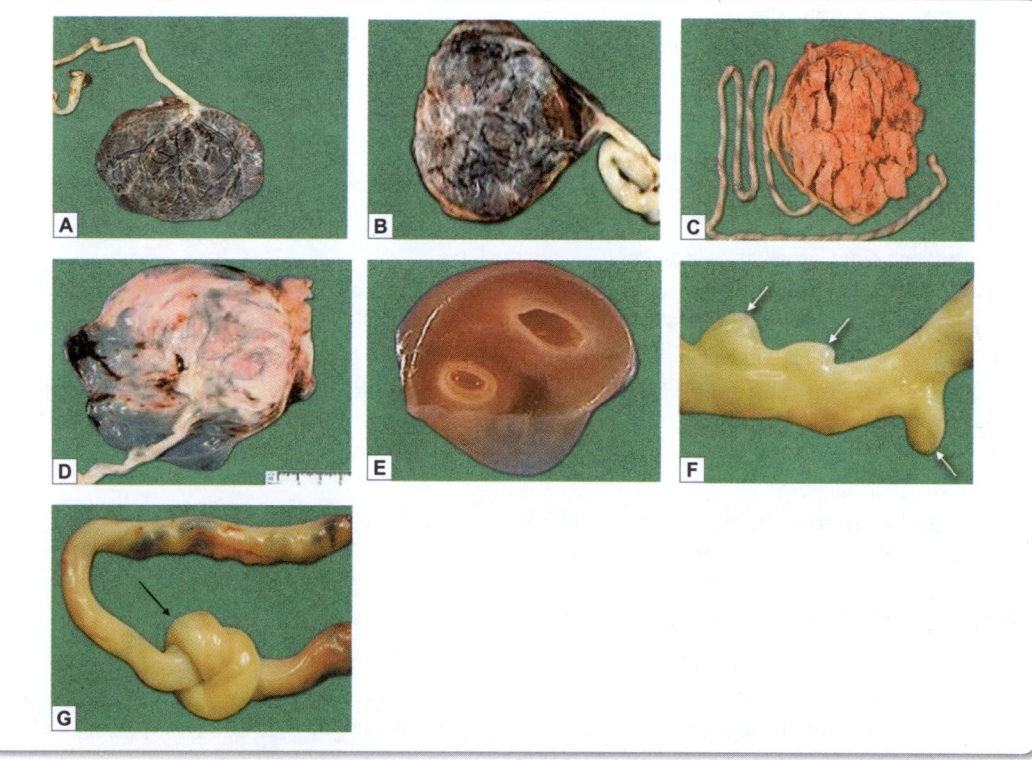

**Figs 12A to G:** Abnormalities of umbilical cord; **A.** Battledore insertion; **B.** Velamentous insertion; **C.** Abnormal cord length; **D.** Short cord; **E.** Single umbilical artery; **F.** Multiple false knots; **G.** True knot

- **Velamentous placenta:** The cord is attached to the membranes. The unsupported umbilical vessels in velamentous placenta, lies below the presenting part and runs across the cervical Os called vasa previa. These vessels are torn spontaneously or during rupture of membrane leading to profuse vaginal bleeding and finally fetal death.
- **Short cord:** When the length of cord is <30 cm. A short cord may be causative factor in failure of the fetus to descend. It may cause abruptio placenta, umbilical hernia, fetal distress and rupture of cord.
- **Long cord:** Where the length of cord is >100 cm (average cord length 30–100 cm). In some cases, long cord becomes looped around fetal body or neck.

## Cord Knotting

- **False knot:** When cord appears to be knotted, but instead has kinking of blood vessels within the cord or accumulation of Wharton's jelly on the cord.
- **True knot:** When real knot has been created and interferes with circulation.
- **Single umbilical artery:** Normally in umbilical cord, there are two arteries and one vein. About one-third of babies are born with only one umbilical artery because of which they will have multiple and severe congenital malformations.
- **Other rare conditions:** Other conditions that may occur in the umbilical cord are hematoma, tumor, cysts and edema.

# FETAL CIRCULATION

Fetal circulation differs from adult circulation in several ways and is designed to ensure a high oxygen blood supply to the brain and myocardium.

## Structures

Fetal circulation contains some unique structures:

- **Umbilical vein:** Carries oxygen and nutrients to the fetus.
- **Two umbilical arteries:** Carry deoxygenated blood and waste products from the fetus to the mother.
- **Ductus venosus (from a vein to a vein):** Shunts blood from the umbilical vein to the inferior vena cava, bypassing the liver and organs of digestion.
- **Foramen ovale (oval opening):** Shunts blood from the right atrium to the left atrium, bypassing the lungs.
- **Ductus arteriosus (from an artery to an artery):** Shunts blood from the pulmonary artery to the aorta, bypassing the lungs.
- **Hypogastric arteries:** Blood from descending aorta returns to the placenta through the two hypogastric arteries, which become umbilical arteries, when they enter the umbilical cord.

## Pattern of Blood Flow (Fig. 13)

- Umbilical vein carries oxygenated blood from the placenta then blood enters the inferior vena cava through the ductus venosus.
- In this way, most of the highly oxygenated blood goes directly into the right atrium, bypassing the liver
- From the right atrium blood flows directly into the left atrium through the foramen ovale.
- From left atrium, blood flows into the left ventricle and then to aorta and through the subclavian arteries, to the cerebral and coronary arteries.
- As a result, brain and heart receive most highly oxygenated blood.
- Through the superior vena cava deoxygenated blood returns from head and arms, enters the right atrium and passes into the right ventricle.
- From right ventricle blood flows into pulmonary artery. Because fetal lungs are collapsed, most of the blood passes into the distal aorta through the ductus arteriosus. From the aorta, blood flows to the rest of the body.

## Changes in Circulation after Birth

After the umbilical cord is clamped, the blood supply from maternal side is cut off and oxygenation takes place in the newborn's lungs. When the lungs expand with air, the pulmonary artery pressure decreases and circulation to lungs increases. Because of this, the following structural changes occur in the newborn vascular system.

- Closure of umbilical arteries
- Closure of ductus arteriosus
- Closure of the umbilical vein
- Closure of ductus venosus
- Closure of foramen ovale

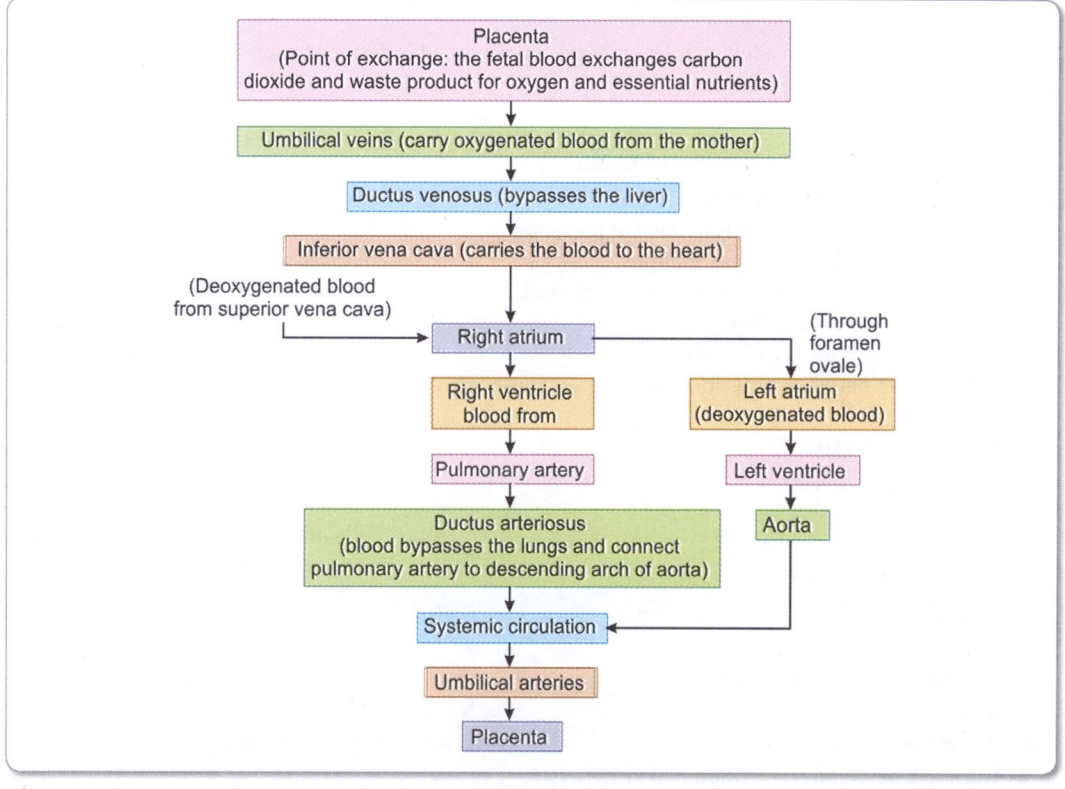

**Fig. 13:** Fetal circulation

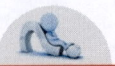

## ASSESS YOURSELF

### FREQUENTLY ASKED QUESTIONS IN EXAMS

1. Discuss in detail about fetal circulation.
2. Describe the structure and functions of placenta.
3. Explain about placental abnormalities.
4. Describe the sutures and fontanels of fetal skull.
5. Enlist the cord abnormalities.
6. Explain the diameters of fetal skull.
7. Differentiate between anterior and posterior fontanels.

### MULTIPLE CHOICE QUESTIONS

1. Fertilization occurs in:
   a. Uterus
   b. Ovaries
   c. Fallopian tubes
   d. Vagina
2. In regular 28-days cycle, ovulation is on:
   a. 14th day
   b. 18th day
   c. 10th day
   d. 12th day
3. Transition of blastocyst into:
   a. Embryo
   b. Morula
   c. Zygote
   d. Fetus
4. The stage between conception and growth is:
   a. Zygote
   b. Morula
   c. Blastocyst
   d. Fetus
5. Implantation stages are:
   a. Apposition
   b. Adhesion
   c. Penetration
   d. All of the above
6. Which decidual layer forms placenta in later stages?
   a. Decidua basalis
   b. Decidua capsularis
   c. Decidua parietalis
   d. None of the above
7. Fetal heart starts to beat at:
   a. First trimester
   b. Second trimester
   c. Third trimester
   d. After the birth of baby
8. Umbilical cord contains:
   a. 2 arteries and one vein
   b. 2 veins and 1 artery
   c. 2 arteries only
   d. One vein and one artery
9. The other name of umbilical cord is:
   a. Funis
   b. Amnion
   c. Chorion
   d. Decidua
10. Fertilization occurs in which part of the fallopian tubes?
    a. Isthmus
    b. Fundus
    c. Ampulla
    d. Infundibulum

11. **Average length of umbilical cord is:**
   a. 30–100 cm
   b. 50–60 cm
   c. <30 cm
   d. >100 cm

12. **Shape of human placenta is:**
   a. Discoid
   b. Globular
   c. Oval
   d. Irregular

13. **Functions of placenta are:**
   a. Respiratory
   b. Excretory
   c. Storage
   d. All of the above

14. **Sagittal suture is in between:**
   a. Frontal bones
   b. Parietal bones
   c. Temporal bones
   d. Occipital bones

15. **Fetal skull consists of how many bones?**
   a. 7 bones
   b. 6 bones
   c. 5 bones
   d. 8 bones

16. **Anterior fontanel ossifies at:**
   a. 18 months
   b. 8 months
   c. 24 months
   d. 6 months

17. **Shape of anterior fontanel is:**
   a. Diamond
   b. Triangular
   c. Oval
   d. Globular

18. **Lambdoid suture is in between:**
   a. Parietal and occipital bones
   b. Between two parietal bones
   c. Between two frontal bones
   d. Between parietal and temporal bones

19. **Suboccipitobregmatic diameter is:**
   a. 9.5 cm
   b. 10 cm
   c. 12 cm
   d. 14 cm

20. **Largest diameter of fetal skull is:**
   a. Mentovertical diameter
   b. Occipito bregmatic diameter
   c. Submentobregmatic diameter
   d. Occipitofrontal diameter

## Answer Key

| 1. c | 2. a | 3. a | 4. a | 5. d | 6. a. | 7. a |
| 8. a | 9. a | 10. c | 11. a | 12. a | 13. d | 14. b |
| 15. a | 16. a | 17. a | 18. a | 19. a | 20. a | |

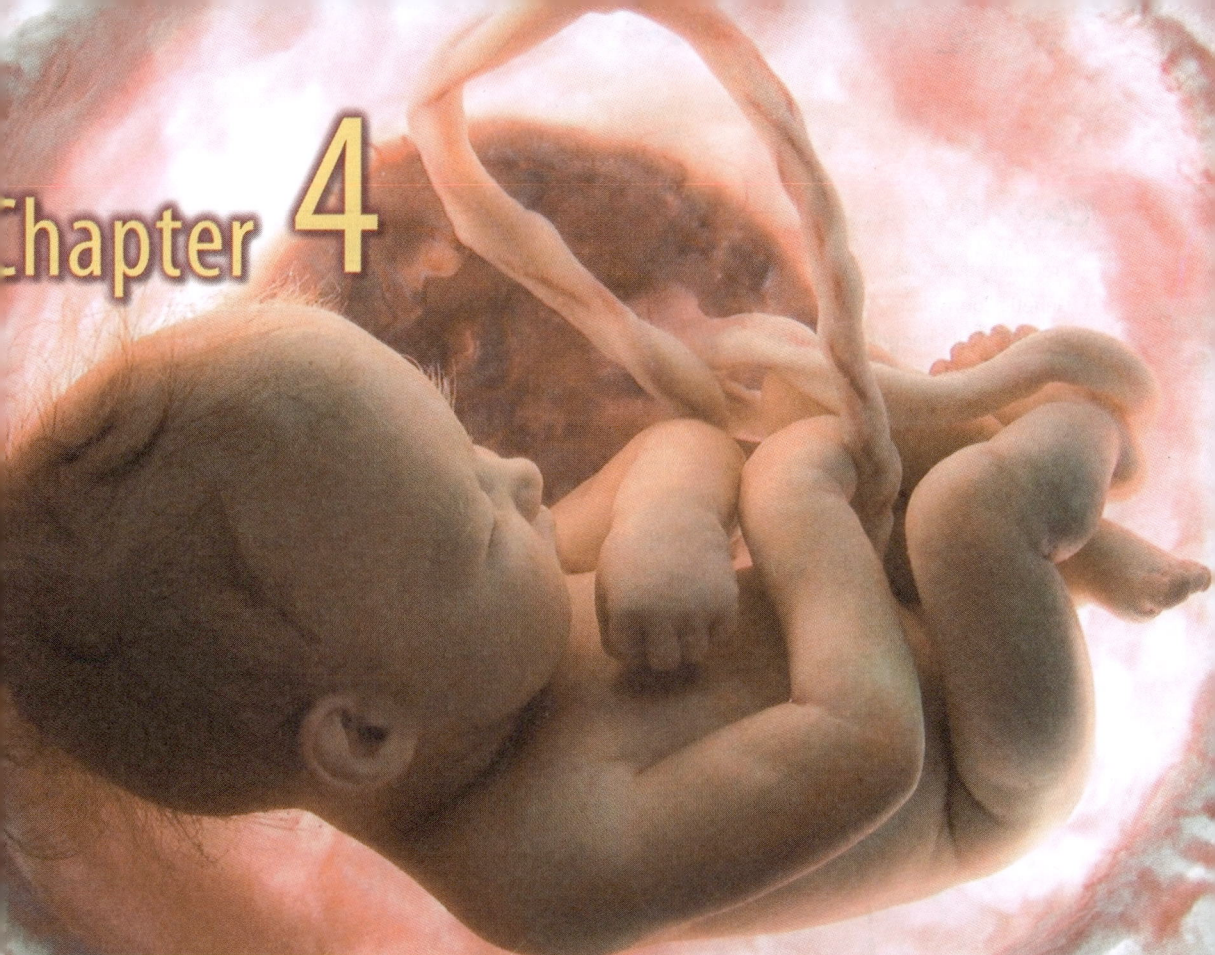

# Normal Pregnancy and its Management

**Upon completing this chapter, the learner will be able to:**

- Explain the importance of genetic counseling during antenatal period
- Describe the physiological changes during pregnancy
- Discuss the diagnostic tests of pregnancy
- Calculate the expected date of delivery
- Describe the minor disorders of pregnancy and their management

## PRECONCEPTION CARE

Preconception care is the provision of biomedical, behavioral and social health interventions to women and couples before conception or pregnancy (Fig. 1).

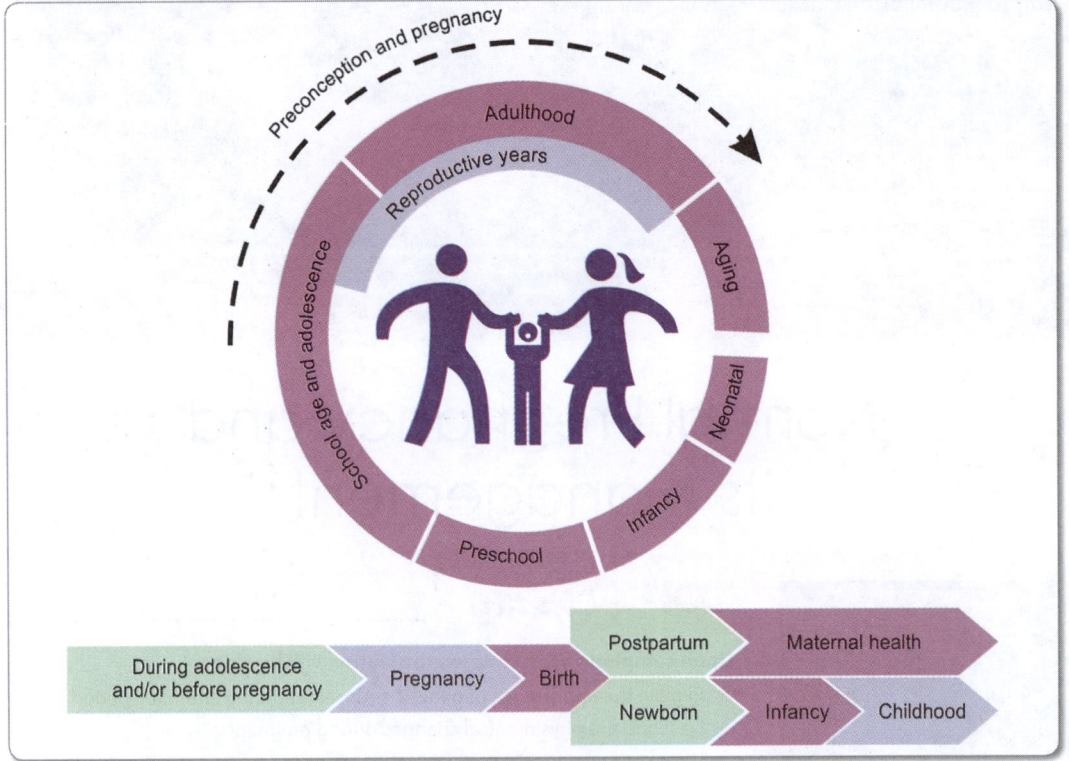

**Fig. 1:** Preconception care

### Aims of Preconception Care

- Improving health status of mother and reducing behaviors of individual and environmental factors that contribute to poor maternal and child health outcome.
- Its ultimate aim is to improve maternal and child health in both the short- and long-term.

- Even if preconception care aims primarily at improving maternal and child health, it brings health benefits to the adolescents, women and men, irrespective of their plans to become parents.

## Objectives

- To reduce maternal and infant mortality rates
- To prevent unintended pregnancies
- To prevent complications during pregnancy and after delivery
- To prevent stillbirths, preterm birth and low-birth-weight
- To reduce birth defects
- To decrease the risk of neonatal infections
- To prevent vertical transmission of HIV/STIs
- To prevent underweight and stunting
- To prevent the risk of some forms of childhood cancers

## Preconception Care Package

Domains of the preconception care package is given in Figure 2.

The package of preconception care interventions has been given in tabular form (Table 1).

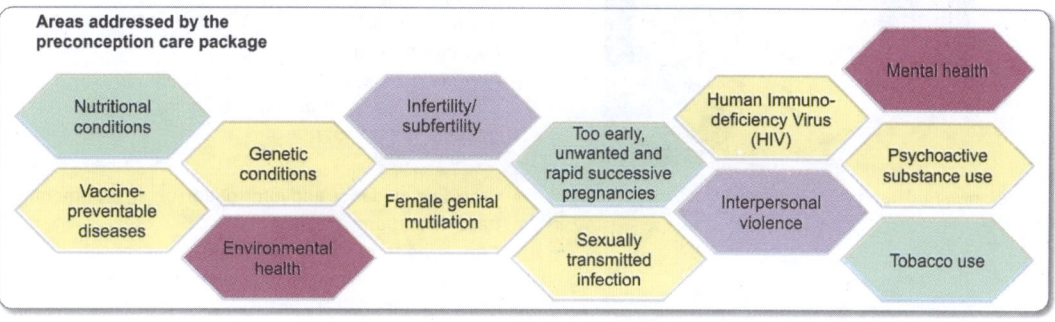

**Fig. 2:** Domains of preconception care package

**TABLE 1:** Package of preconception care interventions

| Areas addressed by the preconception care package | Examples of evidence-based interventions |
|---|---|
| Nutritional conditions 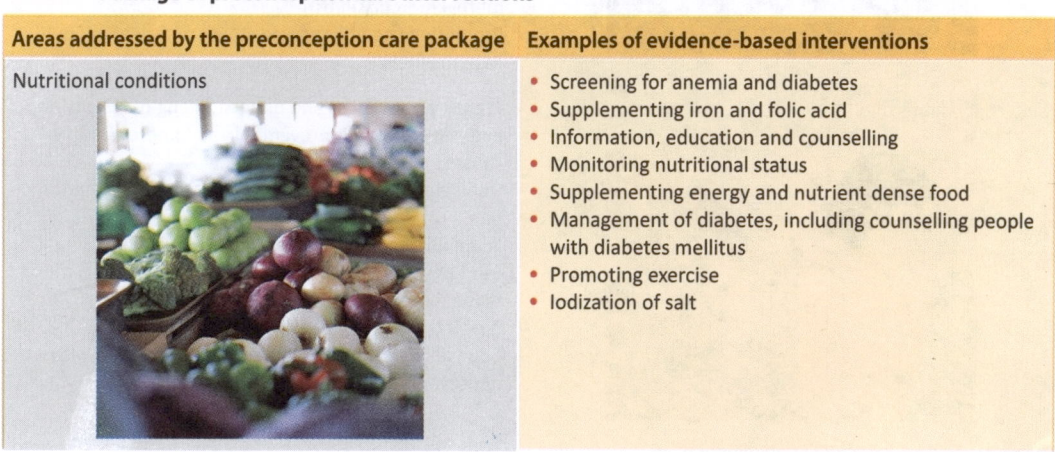 | • Screening for anemia and diabetes<br>• Supplementing iron and folic acid<br>• Information, education and counselling<br>• Monitoring nutritional status<br>• Supplementing energy and nutrient dense food<br>• Management of diabetes, including counselling people with diabetes mellitus<br>• Promoting exercise<br>• Iodization of salt |

*Contd...*

| Areas addressed by the preconception care package | Examples of evidence-based interventions |
|---|---|
| Tobacco use<br>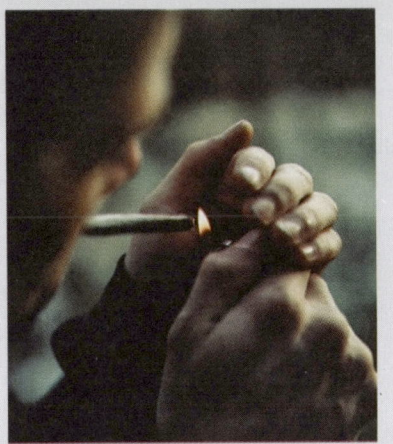 | • Screening of women and girls for tobacco use (smoking and smokeless tobacco) at all clinical visits using "5 As" (ask, advise, assess, assist, arranges)<br>• Providing brief tobacco cessation advice, pharmacotherapy (including nicotine replacement therapy, if available) and intensive behavioral counselling services<br>• Screening of all nonsmokers (men and women) and advising about harm of second-hand smoke and harmful effects on pregnant women and unborn children |
| Genetic conditions<br>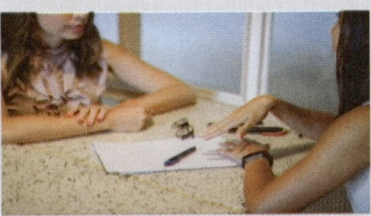 | • Taking a thorough family history to identify risk factors for genetic conditions<br>• Family planning<br>• Genetic counselling<br>• Carrier screening and testing<br>• Appropriate treatment of genetic conditions<br>• Community-wide or national screening among populations at high risk |
| Environmental health<br>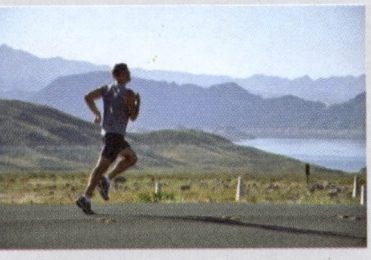 | • Providing guidance and information on environmental hazards and prevention<br>• Protecting from unnecessary radiation exposure in occupational, environmental and medical settings<br>• Avoiding unnecessary pesticide use/providing alternatives to pesticides<br>• Protecting from lead exposure<br>• Informing women of childbearing age about levels of methyl mercury in fish<br>• Promoting use of improved stoves and cleaner liquid gaseous fuels |
| Infertility/subfertility<br>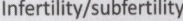<br>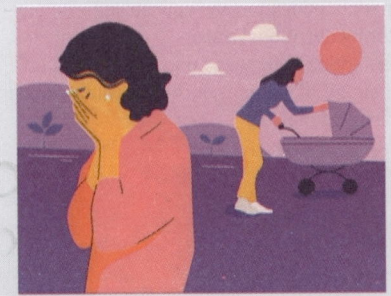 | • Creating awareness and understanding of fertility and infertility and their preventable and unpreventable causes<br>• Defusing stigmatization of infertility and assumption of fate<br>• Screening and diagnosis of couples following 6–12 months of attempting pregnancy, and management of underlying causes of infertility/sub-fertility, including past STIs<br>• Counselling for individuals/couples diagnosed with unpreventable causes of infertility/subfertility |

*Contd...*

Textbook of Midwifery and Gynecological Nursing

| Areas addressed by the preconception care package | Examples of evidence-based interventions |
|---|---|
| Interpersonal violence 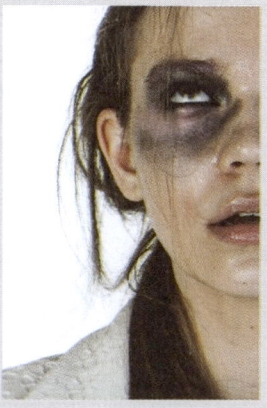 | • Health promotion to prevent dating violence<br>• Providing age-appropriate comprehensive sexual education that addresses gender equality, human rights and sexual relations<br>• Combining and linking economic empowerment, gender equality and community mobilization activities<br>• Recognizing signs of violence against women<br>• Providing health care services (including postrape care), referral and psychosocial support to victims of violence<br>• Changing individual and social norms regarding drinking, screening and counselling of people who are problem drinkers, and treating people who have alcohol use disorders |
| Too-early, unwanted and rapid successive pregnancies 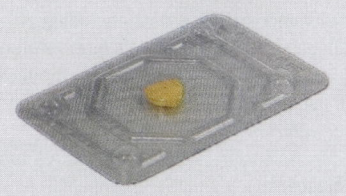 | • Keeping girls in school<br>• Influencing cultural norms that support early marriage and coerced sex<br>• Providing age-appropriate comprehensive sexual education<br>• Providing contraceptives and building community support for preventing early pregnancy and contraceptive provision to adolescents<br>• Empowering girls to resist coerced sex<br>• Engaging men and boys to critically assess norms and practices regarding gender-based violence and coerced sex<br>• Educating women and couples about the dangers to the baby and mother of short birth intervals |
| Sexually transmitted infections (STIs) 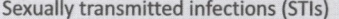 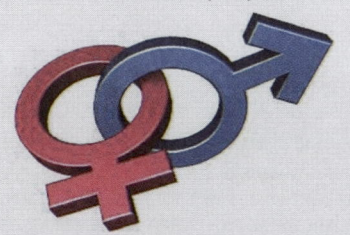 | • Providing age-appropriate comprehensive sexual education and services<br>• Promoting safe sex practices through individual, group and community-level behavioral interventions<br>• Promoting use of condoms for dual protection against STIs and unwanted pregnancies<br>• Ensuring increased access to condoms<br>• Screening for STIs<br>• Increasing access to treatment and other relevant health services |
| HIV 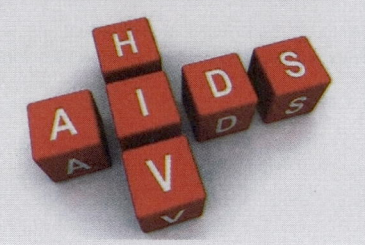 | • Family planning<br>• Promoting safe sex practices and dual method for birth control (with condoms) and STIs control<br>• Provider-initiated HIV counselling and testing, including male partner testing<br>• Providing antiretroviral prophylaxis for women not eligible for, or not on, antiretroviral therapy to prevent mother-to-child transmission<br>• Determining eligibility for lifelong antiretroviral therapy |

*Contd...*

| Areas addressed by the preconception care package | Examples of evidence-based interventions |
|---|---|
| Mental health assessment 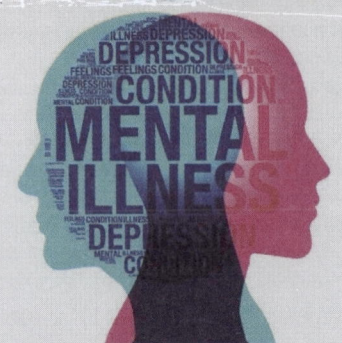 | • Assessing psychosocial problems<br>• Providing educational and psychosocial counselling before and during pregnancy<br>• Counselling, treatment and managing depression in women planning pregnancy and other women of childbearing age<br>• Strengthening community network and promoting women's empowerment<br>• Improving access to education for women of childbearing age<br>• Reducing economic insecurity of women of childbearing age |
| Psychoactive substance use 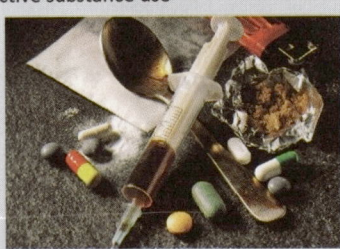 | • Screening for substance use<br>• Providing brief interventions and treatment when needed<br>• Treating substance use disorders, including pharmacological and psychological interventions<br>• Providing family planning assistance for families with substance use disorders (including postpartum and between pregnancies)<br>• Establishing prevention programs to reduce substance use in adolescents |
| Vaccine-preventable diseases 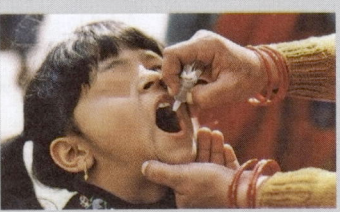 | • Vaccination against rubella<br>• Vaccination against tetanus and diphtheria<br>• Vaccination against hepatitis B |
| Female genital mutilation (FGM) 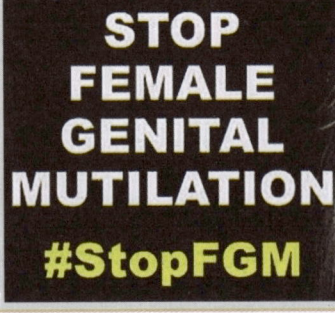 | • Discussing and discouraging the practice with the girl and her parents and/or partner<br>• Screening women and girls for female genital mutilation to detect complication<br>• Informing women and couples about complications of FGM and about access to treatment<br>• Carrying out defibulation of infibulated or sealed girls and women before or early in pregnancy<br>• Removing cysts and treating other complications |

## An Agenda for Action: Learning from Experience, Supporting Change

In February 2012, World Health Organization (WHO) meeting brought together researchers, practitioners and program managers with experience in preconception care, as well as United Nations Agencies and partner organizations to achieve a global consensus on the place of preconception care as part of an overall strategy to prevent maternal and childhood mortality and morbidity.

An agenda for action was agreed upon at the meeting, including actions to:

- Build regional and national capacity to plan, implement and monitor preconception care programs and services.
- Stimulate and support country action.
- Carry out demonstration projects in selected countries.
- Document and disseminate good preconception care practices.

The "Draft action plan for the prevention and control of noncommunicable diseases 2013–2020," which were discussed at 66th World Health Assembly in May 2013, calls governments to reduce modifiable risk factors for noncommunicable diseases and underlying social determinants. Preconception care, as part of the National Policy framework, is recognized as an important contributor to noncommunicable disease prevention and control (Fig. 3).

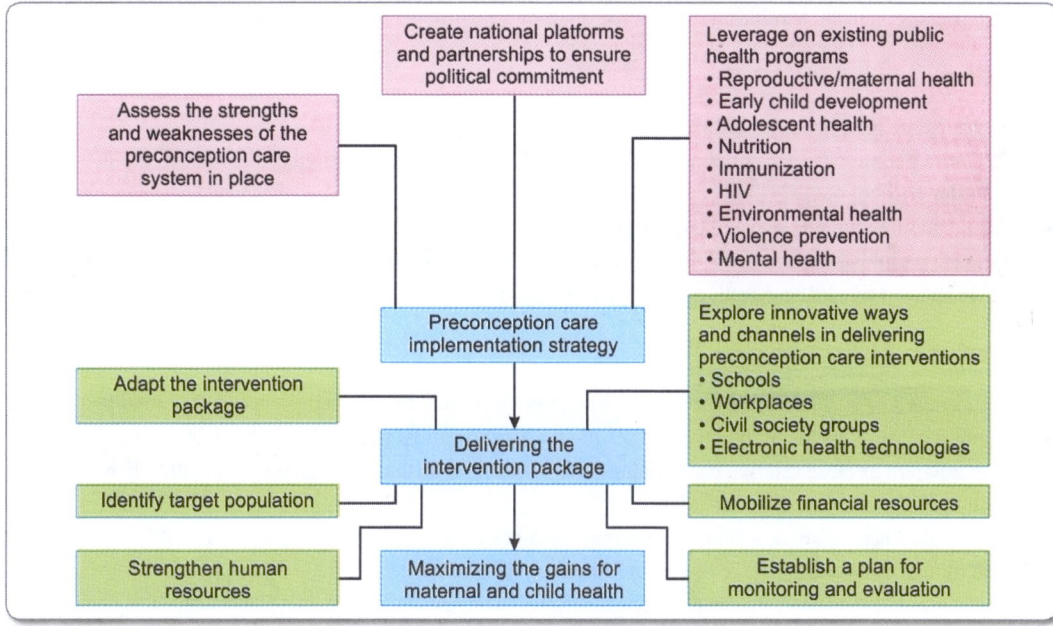

**Fig. 3:** A strategy for country action

## WHO Support to Countries

WHO supports regions and countries in implementing a step-by-step process to improve availability of and access to preconception care interventions:

- Create regional/national platforms and partnerships to advance preconception care interventions.
- Introduce professionals in countries to international experience, research, evidence and good practices.

- Provide a methodology to analyze and understand the strengths and weaknesses of the preconception care system in place, and opportunities for improvement.
- Explore various delivery strategies for preconception care interventions, and their comparative advantages in terms of coverage, feasibility, acceptability and cost.
- Adapt the package of preconception care interventions to regional and country priorities, and health systems contexts.
- Explore and document innovative ways to deliver preconception care outside the traditional maternal and child health programs, while recognizing the importance of integrated delivery mechanisms.
- Develop a roadmap to make changes over time.
- Monitor, evaluate and document progress.

## GENETIC COUNSELING

### Definition

- According to American Society of Human Genetics, "Genetic counseling is a communication process, which deals with human problems associated with the occurrence or the risk of occurrence of a genetic disorder in a family."
- Smith (1955) defined counseling as, "a process in which the counselor assists the counselee to make interpretations of facts relating to a choice, plan or adjustments which he needs to make."

### Purposes

- Provide concrete, accurate information about inherited disorders.
- Reassure people who are concerned that their child may inherit a particular disorder, to the fact that the disorder will not occur.
- Allow people who are affected by inherited disease to make informed choice about future reproduction.
- Educate people about inherited disorder and the process of inheritance.
- Offer support by skilled health professionals to people who are affected by genetic disorders.

### Indications

- If a standard prenatal screening test (such as alpha-fetoprotein [AFP] test) yields an abnormal result.
- It amniocentesis yields an unexpected result (such as chromosomal defect in the unborn baby)
- Either parent or close relative has an inheritance disease or birth defect, either parent already has children with birth defect or genetic disorders.
- The mother has had two or more miscarriage or a baby dies in infancy.
- The mother is 35 years of age or above (elderly primigravida).
- The partner is in blood relation (consanguineous marriage).

### Prenatal Tests during Genetic Counseling Include

- Level II ultrasound
- Maternal serum AFP/triple test
- Chorionic villus sampling (CVS)
- Amniocentesis

## Steps of Genetic Counseling

An accurate diagnosis of disorder is made. To complete an accurate diagnosis, the following procedures should be followed:

- **History:**
  - This includes both present and relevant past history.
  - Family history includes siblings and other relatives also.
  - Obstetric history includes exposure to drugs, X-ray in pregnancy. History of abortion or stillbirth if any, should be recorded and reported.
  - Enquiry should be made about consanguinity as it increases the risk, especially in autosomal recessive disorders.
- **Pedigree charting:**
  At a glance this offers, in a concise manner, the state of disorder in a family. Constructing a pedigree with proper interrogation (though time consuming), is ultimately rewarding. It forms an indispensable step towards counseling.
- **Estimation of risk:** To estimate it, one requires to take into account the following points:
  - Mode of inheritance
  - Analysis of pedigree or family tree
  - Results of various tests
- **Transmitting information:** The next important step is communicating this information to the consultant/ expert.
- **Psychology of the patient:**
  - Emotional stress under prevailing circumstances
  - Attitude of family members towards the patient
  - Educational, social and financial background of the family
  - Gain confidence of consultant in subsequence meetings during follow-up
  - Ethical, moral and legal implications involved in process
  - Above all, communication skills to transmit facts in an effective manner, i.e. making them more acceptable and palatable.
- **Management:** In genetics, "Treatment" implies a very restricted scope. It naturally aims for prevention rather than cure. In fact, for most of the genetic disorders cure is unknown. Treatment is therefore directed towards minimizing the damage by early diagnosis and preventing further irreversible damage.

## Role of Nurse in Genetic Counseling

- Guiding a woman or couple through prenatal diagnosis.
- Helping parents to make decision regarding to abnormal prenatal diagnostic results.
- Assisting parents who have had a child with a birth defect to locate needed services and support system.
- Providing support to help the family deal with the emotional impact of birth defect.
- Coordinative services of other professionals, such as social workers, physical and occupational therapists, psychologists and dieticians are essential.

# PHYSIOLOGICAL CHANGES IN PREGNANCY

During pregnancy, physiological and anatomical changes occur in many organs. This is due to metabolic demands of the fetus, placenta and uterus due to increased level of hormones or because of enlarged uterus.

## Reproductive System

### Uterus

Refer to Figure 4 in this regard:

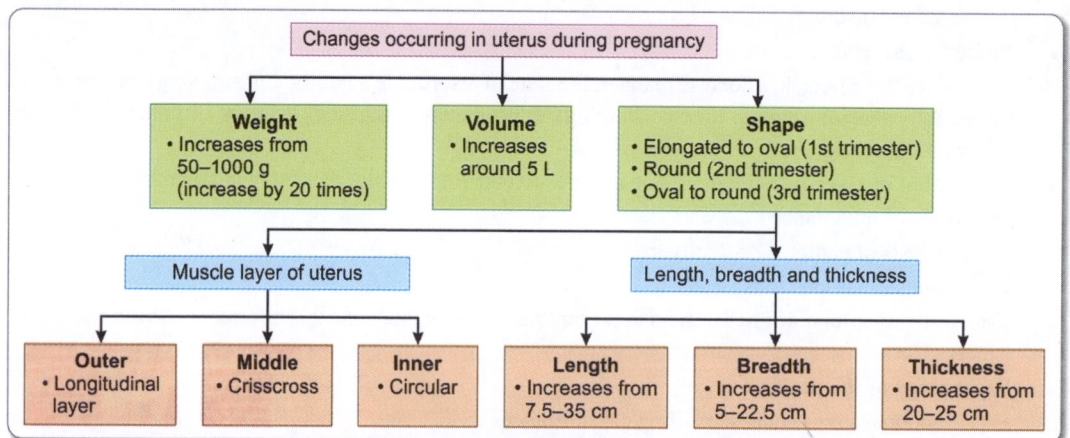

**Fig. 4:** Changes in uterus during pregnancy

### Cervix

- Length constant, about 2.5 cm.
- Width increases due to hygroscopic effect of estrogen.
- Increased vascularity and looks purple in color.
- Softens in late pregnancy due to Braxton-Hicks contractions.
- Local release of prostaglandins helps in ripening of cervix.

### Vagina

- Increased vascularity
- Feels soft
- Vaginal secretions become acidic, which were alkaline earlier.

### Ovaries and Fallopian Tubes

- Hypertrophy of fallopian tubes and increased vascularity is common
- Corpus luteum produces progesterone that forms endometrial lining.
- Ovaries produce certain hormones that maintain and regulate pregnancy. For example, estrogen, follicle stimulating hormone (FSH) and progesterone.

## Breast

- Breast becomes more vascular
- Weight increase (0.4 kg)
- Secretion of colostrum
- Pigmentation of areola
- Development of Montgomery's tubercles
- Development of secondary areola (In 2nd trimester) (Fig. 5)

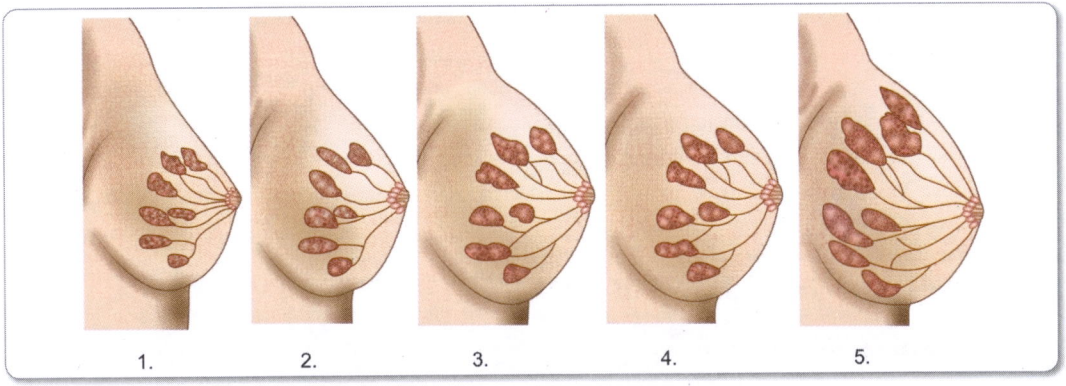

**Fig. 5:** Breast changes during pregnancy

## Weight Gain

A pregnant woman gains around 12 kg of weight. Refer to Figure 6 in this regard.

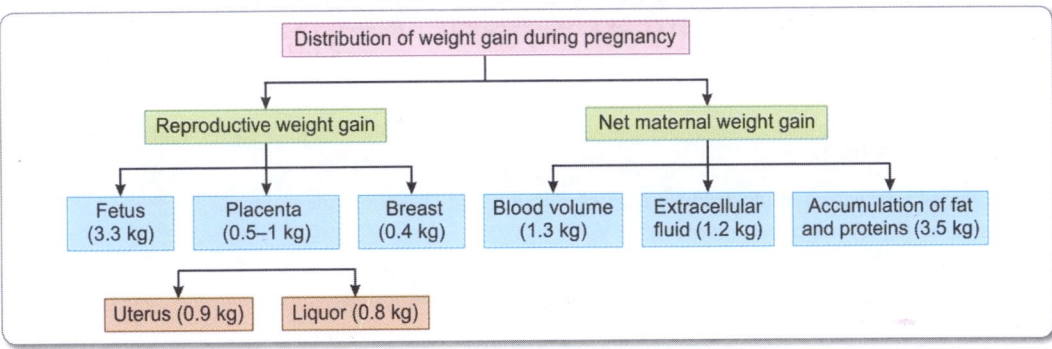

**Fig. 6:** Distribution of weight gain during pregnancy

## Cardiovascular System

- **Size of heart:** Increases about 12%
- **Cardiac capacity:** Increases 70–80 mL
- **Cardiac output:** Increases by 30–40% till 30 weeks; thereafter continues to increase up to 15% till term.
- **Clotting time:** From 12 minutes to 8 minutes

- Blood pressure
  - **Systolic:** Slight change or same
  - **Diastolic:** Reduced 5–10 mm Hg at about 12–26 weeks and by 36 weeks comes to prepregnancy level.

## Respiratory System

- Increased tidal volume, minute ventilation, minute $O_2$ uptake and airway conductance.
- Respiratory rate, vital capacity and maximum breathing capacity: Remains unchanged.
- Residual volume, total lung capacity and functional residual capacity decrease in pregnancy.

## Urinary System

- **Kidney:** Increase in length by 1–1.5 cm.
- **Ureters:** Elongate, widen and are curved that result in increased urinary stasis.
- **Bladder:** Vascularity increases; muscle tone decreases; bladder mucosa becomes edematous and increased frequency of urination.
- **Glomerular Filtration Rate (GFR):** Increases by 50%.
- **Renal plasma flow rate:** Increases by 25–50%.

## Gastrointestinal System

- **Oral cavity:** Increase salivation.
- **Saliva becomes acidic:** Causes tooth decay.
- Gums may swell and bleed easily, due to increased vascularity.
- Change in sense of taste.
- Increased craving for bizarre substances, for example, mud, pencil, etc.
- **Stomach and esophagus:** Due to increased hormonal levels (progesterone and relaxin) causing muscles of digestive tract become relax and causing frequent gastric reflux.
- **Gastrointestinal motility:** Increase in progesterone decreases gastrointestinal motility and causes constipation.

## Metabolic Changes

- Increased total serum lipids, triglycerides, cholesterol and phospholipids.
- Increased (15%) calorie requirements.
- Increased (50%) protein requirements.
- Increased requirements for folate, calcium, phosphorus, magnesium, iron, vitamin A and C, zinc and iodine.

## Musculoskeletal System

- Gravid uterus leads to alteration in body posture and hence, lordosis occurs (Fig. 7).
- Increase in estrogen and progesterone relaxes/softens pelvic joints and ligaments.

## Skin Changes

- **Linea nigra:** Dark hairy line that runs from umbilicus to symphysis pubis becomes dark (Fig. 8A).
- **Chloasma:** Brownish hyperpigmentation of skin over face and forehead also; called mask of pregnancy.

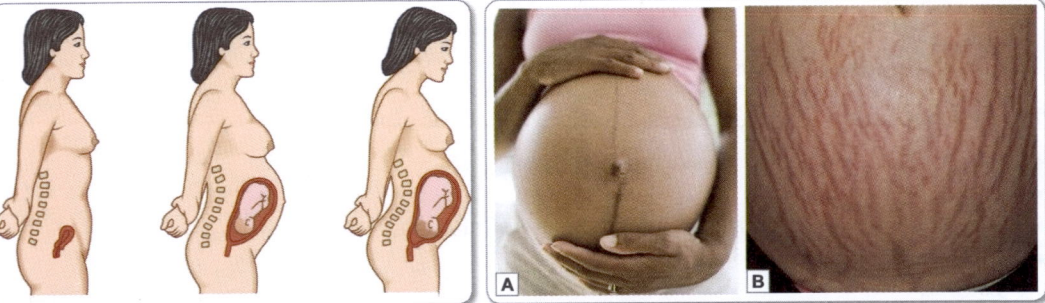

**Fig. 7:** Lordosis due to gravid uterus      **Figs 8A and B: A.** Linea nigra; **B.** Striae gravidarum

- Striae gravidarum → stretch marks on abdomen, thighs and breasts (Fig. 8B).
- Vascular spiders → minute red elevations on face, neck, arms and chest.

## Hematological Changes

- Increased blood volume (30–40%), red blood cells (20–30%) and plasma volume (40–50%) and viscosity of blood is decreased.
- Hb increases but Hb concentration/hematocrit is decreased.
- Increased blood fibrinogen.
- Fibrinolytic activity depressed.
- Increased level of all coagulation factors except factor XI and factor XII.
- Increased erythrocyte sedimentation rate (ESR) (about four times)
- Decreased hematocrit
- Neutrophilic leukocytosis occurs.

## Endocrine System

- Syncytiotrophoblast secretes beta human chorionic gonadotropin (hCG).
- Placenta secretes human placental lactogen.
- Pituitary gland enlarges and compresses optic nerve that causes headache.
- Follicle Stimulating Hormone (FSH) and Luteinizing Hormone (LH) are inhibited during pregnancy.
- Thyroid gland enlarges leading to increase in basal metabolic rate.
- Increased adrenocorticotropic hormone (ACTH) and cortisol level.
- Hyperinsulinism occurs if mother is diabetic.

## DIAGNOSIS OF PREGNANCY

Pregnancy may be diagnosed by the woman herself even before she has missed a period because she feels certain changes, such as changes in breasts can occur as early as 5–6 weeks after conception.

Diagnosis of pregnancy in the first trimester and early second trimester is based on a combination of presumptive and probable signs of pregnancy. Pregnancy is self-evident in later gestation when the positive signs are readily observed.

## Signs of Pregnancy

### *Presumptive Signs of Pregnancy*

These are the maternal physiological changes which the woman experiences.

- Amenorrhea (cessation of menstruation): 4 weeks.
- Nausea and vomiting from 4th to 14th week.
- Tingling, tenseness and enlargement of breast from 3rd to 4th week.
- Frequency of micturition (6–12 weeks) increases.
- Fatigue
- Breast changes include darkening of nipples, primary and secondary areolar changes and appearance of Montgomery tubercles.
- Presence of colostrum in the nipples.
- Excessive salivation.
- Quickening is the first movement of fetus felt by the mother around 18–20th week.
- Skin pigmentation and condition such as chloasma, breast and abdominal striae, linea nigra and palmar erythema.

### *Probable Signs*

These are maternal physiological changes other than presumptive signs which are detected upon examination and documented by the examiner.

- Enlargement of the uterus.
- Presence of hCG in blood from 6 to 12 weeks.
- Vaginal discharge: Copious nonirritating mucoid discharge which appears at 6th week.
- Hegar's sign: Softening and compressibility of the isthmus from 6th to 10th week.
- Jacquemier's sign/Chadwick's sign: Violet blue discoloration of the vaginal membrane due to increased vascularity by 8th week.
- Osiander's sign: Increased pulsation felt in the lateral fornices from 8th week onwards.
- Palmer's sign: Regular and rhythmic uterine contractions resembling systole and diastole of heart that can be elicited during bimanual examination as early as 48 weeks.
- Goodell's sign: Softening of the cervix from a nonpregnant state of firmness similar to the tip of nose to the softness of lips of mouth in the pregnant state by 6th week.
- Globular enlargement of uterus with soft consistency.
- Palpation of Braxton Hick's contraction.
- Ballottement of fetus from 16th to 28th weeks.

### *Positive Signs*

Positive signs are those signs which are directly attributable to the fetus as detected and documented by the examiner.

- Visualization of fetus by ultrasound from 6th week onwards.
- Visualization of fetal skeleton by 16th week.
- Fetal heart rate (FHR) assessed by ultrasound from 6th week onwards.
- Palpable fetal movements from 22nd week onwards.

- Visible fetal movements in later pregnancy.
- Palpation of fetal parts from 24th week onwards.

**Pregnancy Tests**

- **Immunologic test:** This test is based on the production of hCG by the syncytiotrophoblastic cells during early pregnancy. hCG is secreted into the maternal bloodstream and then excreted in mother's urine. Specific antisera are mixed with urine from the woman suspected of being pregnant. If the urine contains hCG, it will neutralize the antibodies in the antiserum and inhibit agglutination indicating a positive pregnancy test.
  If the urine does not contain hCG, agglutination will occur indicating negative pregnancy test.
- **Radioimmunoassay test:** Blood is tested to detect the beta hCG subunit. These are extremely sensitive tests, able to detect hCG at far lower levels than other tests. The test known as betapreg can be used as early as one week after conception, if laboratory facilities are available.
- **Biological tests of pregnancy:** Biological tests were done in the past using mice and frogs. The tests included Aschheim-Zondek test, Friedman test, Frank test and Hogben test.
- **Ultrasonography:** Ultrasonography of abdomen can diagnose the pregnancy as follows:
  - **At 5th week:** Spherical gestation sac is visible
  - **At 6th week:** Fetal pole can be seen
  - **At 7th week:** One can see crown-rump length
  - **At 10th week:** Fetal heart sound heard by ultrasound Doppler
  - **At 12th week:** Biparietal diameter (2.1 cm) is seen
  **Transvaginal ultrasonography** can diagnose earlier than abdominal sonography.
  - **At 4th week:** Visualization of gestational sac.
  - **At 5th week:** Yolk sac and fetal cardiac motion.

# ANTENATAL CARE

Antenatal care refers to the care given to an expectant mother from the time of the conception until the beginning of labor.

## Objectives

The objectives of prenatal care are to:

- Promote, protect and maintain the health of the mother during pregnancy.
- Detect high risk pregnancies and give special attention.
- Foresee complications and take preventive measures.
- Remove anxiety and fear associated with pregnancy and outcome
- Reduce maternal and infant morbidity and mortality.
- Teach the mother elements of nutrition, personal hygiene and newborn care.
- Sensitize the mother to the need of family planning.
- Prepare the mother for motherhood.

The importance of regular visits to the prenatal clinic must be emphasized to help the mother, have an optimum outcome of pregnancy that is "healthy mother with healthy baby".

## Assessment

**History taking:** Ideally the mother should visit the antenatal clinic once a month during the first seven months (28 weeks) twice a month during the eight month (up to 32 weeks) and thereafter once a week if everything is normal. The first visit irrespective of when it occurs should include the client's health history, obstetric history, physical and pelvic examinations and laboratory examinations.

### Antenatal History Format

I. **Patient profile:**

| | |
|---|---|
| Full name | : |
| Age (in years) | : |
| Hospital No. | : |
| I.P. No. | : |
| Marital status | :       Married/unmarried/divorced/separated |
| Education status | : |
| Occupation | : |
| Husband's name | : |
| Age (in years) | : |
| Education status | : |
| Occupation | : |
| Type of family | : |
| Per capita income | : |
| Date of booking | : |
| Date of last antenatal visit | : |
| Date of admission | : |
| Obstetric score | : |
| Gravida | |
| Para | |
| Abortion | |
| MTP | |
| Living | |

II. **Reasons for hospitalization/chief complaints:**
- Onset
- Duration
- Severity
- Relieving factors
- Aggravating factors

III. **Menstrual history:**
- Age at menarche
- Duration of cycles
- Regularity

- Flow—heavy/moderate scanty
  - Clots
  - Number of days
- Any dysmenorrhea
- Relief measures
- Last menstrual period
- Period menstrual period

IV. **Obstetric history:**

**Present obstetric history**
- Is pregnancy confirmed: Yes/No
- When, where and how it was confirmed
- What test was done for confirmation
- Quickening
- Immunization

Other complaints like: Vomiting, hemorrhoids, heart burn, backache, bleeding, varicose vein, constipation, leg cramps, fever, leucorrhea, anorexia, insomnia.

**Past obstetric history**

| Sl. no. | Date of delivery | Place of birth | Duration of pregnancy | Method of delivery | Course of pregnancy | Labor | Puerperium | Baby | |
|---------|------------------|----------------|-----------------------|--------------------|--------------------|-------|------------|------|---|
| | | | | | | | | Sex | Wt. |
| | | | | | | | | | |

V. **Family history:**
- Congenital diseases
- Any hereditary diseases
- Multiple pregnancy
- Diabetes
- Heart disease
- Any mental retardation
- Hypertension or PIH (in mother/sisters)
- Twin pregnancy
- If yes, in whom? Mother/Father?

VI. **Medical-surgical history:**
- Childhood disease
- Chronic disease, like asthma, diabetes, epilepsy
- Previous surgery
- Injuries, especially of back and pelvis
- Hepatitis, STD, HIV
- History of anemia
- Any medication taken at present or past
- Reason for use, date stopped
- Blood transfusion, allergic reaction

VII. **Nutrition:**
- General nutrition—veg/nonveg
- Appetite—decreased/increased
- Any eating disorders 24 hours recall

VIII. **Partner's health history:**
- Genetic abnormalities
- Chronic diseases
- Infections
- Use of drugs such as cocaine, alcohol
- Smoking habits: tobacco, cigarette
- Sexually transmitted diseases—HIV/AIDS
- Blood type

IX. **Psychosocial history:**
- Emotional changes experienced
- Women's and family's reactions to present pregnancy
- Family support system—Family members and friends
- Coping strategies
- Lifestyle change
- Social relationships with the neighbors
- Financial support

# Examination and Investigation

## Physical Examination

Refer to Figure 9 in this regard.

### General Appearance

A complete screening physical examination is done during the initial antenatal examination in order to ascertain if the woman has any medical disease or abnormalities. General observation includes appearance, emotional state, posture and apparent state of health. The components of physical examination are:

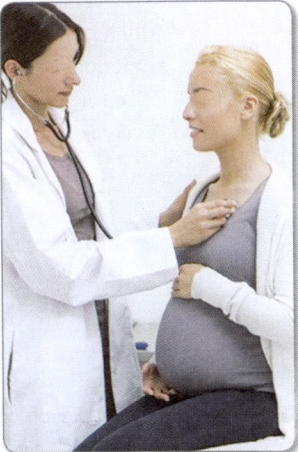

- **Built:** Obese/average/thin
- **Nutrition:** Good/average/poor
- **Height:** Short or long stature (below 5 feet); short stature is likely to be associated with a small pelvis.
- **Weight:** Repeated weight checking at each visit by same weighing machine.
- **Pallor:** Sites noted are conjunctiva, dorsum of tongue and nail beds.
- **Jaundice:** Sites noted are conjunctiva, under surface of tongue, hard palate and skin.
- **Teeth, tongue, gums** and **tonsils:** Evidence of malnutrition is evident from glossitis and stomatitis.

**Fig. 9:** Physical examination

- **Neck:** Neck veins, thyroid gland or lymph nodes are checked for any abnormality.
- **Edema of legs:** Sites noted are medial malleolus and anterior surface of the lower one-third of the tibia.
- Check the pulse and blood pressure, respiration and temperature of the woman.
- **Review of systems:** Heart, lungs, liver and spleen:- assess both anatomically and physiologically.
- **Breast:** Note the skin condition of areola.
- **Nipples:** Cracked/depressed (inverted)

### Abdominal Examination

It is the process of examination of a pregnant woman to determine the normalcy of fetal growth in relation to the gestational age, position of the fetus in uterus and its relationship to the maternal pelvis (Fig. 10).

### Purposes

- To measure the abdominal girth and fundal height
- To determine the abdominal muscle tone
- To determine the fetal lie, presentation, position, variety (anterior or posterior), engagement and attitude
- To determine the possible location of the fetal heart sound (FHS)
- To observe the signs of pregnancy
- To detect any deviation from normal

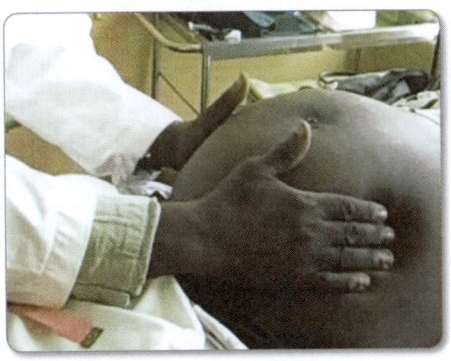

**Fig. 10:** Abdominal examination

### Articles

- Fetoscope/stethoscope
- Measuring tape/pelvimeter

### Procedure

| Nursing action | Rationale |
|---|---|
| • Explain to the woman what will be done and how she may cooperate during the procedure | To reduce anxiety and promote relaxation during the procedure |
| • Instruct the woman to empty her bladder | To avoid discomfort during palpation |
| • Draw curtains around the bed | To provide privacy |

| Inspection | |
|---|---|
| • Position the woman for examination (knees flexed)<br> ▪ Place a pillow under her head and shoulders<br> ▪ Have her arms by her sides | Promote relaxation of abdominal muscles |
| ▪ Expose her abdomen from below the breasts to the symphysis pubis | Enable visualization of the whole abdomen |
| • Inspect abdomen for the following: Scars, diastasis recti, hernia, linea nigra, striae gravidarum, contour of the abdomen, state of umbilicus and skin condition | |
| • Determine the fundal height using the ulnar side of the palm<br>**12 weeks:** Level of symphysis pubis<br>**16 weeks:** Midway between symphysis pubis and umbilicus<br>**20 weeks:** 1–2 finger breadth below umbilicus<br>**24 weeks:** Level of umbilicus<br>**32 weeks:** Halfway between umbilicus and xiphoid process<br>**36 weeks:** At level of xiphoid process<br>**40 weeks:** 2–3 finger breadth below the xiphoid process if lightening occurs | In order to estimate whether fetal growth corresponds to the gestational period |

Fundal height at various weeks of gestation

*Contd...*

| Nursing action | Rationale |
|---|---|
| • Measure fundal height using any one of the following methods:<br>  ▪ Using measuring tape:<br>  Place zero line of the tape measure on the upper border of the symphysis pubis and stretch the tape across the contour of the abdomen to the top of the fundus along the midline<br>  ▪ Caliper method (Pelvimeter):<br>  ○ Place one tip of the caliper on the upper border of the symphysis pubis and the other tip at the top of the fundus. Both placements are in the midline<br>  ○ Read the measurement on the centimeter scale located on the arc, close to the joint. The number of centimeters should be equal approximately to the weeks of gestation after about 22–24 weeks. | 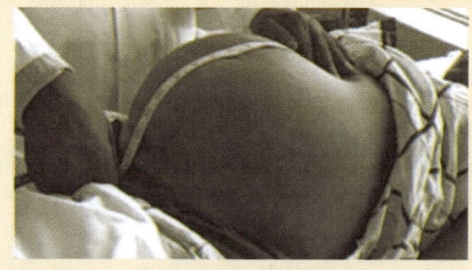<br>Measuring fundal height<br><br>The number of centimeters measured should be approximately equal to the weeks of gestation after about 22–24 weeks<br>This method is more accurate. |
| • Measure the abdominal girth by encircling the woman's abdomen with a tape measure at the level of the umbilicus. (It is measured in inches.) | Normally the measurement is 2 inches (5 cm) less than the weeks of gestation.<br>E.g., 32 inches at 34 weeks gestation. Measurements more than 100 cm (39.5 inches) are abnormal at any week of gestation. |

### Abdominal - Palpation or Leopold's Maneuvers (Figs 11A to D)

| | |
|---|---|
| • Instruct the woman to relax her abdominal muscles by bending her knees slightly and doing deep breathing<br>• Be sure your hands are warm before beginning to palpate, rest your hand on the mother's abdomen lightly while giving explanation about the procedure<br><br>• For the technique of palpation<br>  ▪ Use the flat palmar surface of fingers and not finger tips. Keep fingers of hands together and apply smooth, deep pressure as firm as necessary to obtain accurate findings<br>• Perform the first maneuver (fundal palpation)<br>  ▪ Face the woman's head<br>  ▪ Place your hands on the sides of the fundus and curve the fingers around the top of the uterus<br>  ▪ Palpate for size, shape, consistency and mobility of the fetal part in the uterus<br>• Do the second maneuver (lateral palpation)<br>  ▪ Continue to face the woman's head<br>  ▪ Place your hands on both sides of the uterus about midway between the symphysis pubis and the fundus<br>  ▪ Apply pressure with one hand against the side of the uterus pushing the fetus to the other side and stabilizing it there. | These steps reduce the stretching and tension of abdominal muscles<br>Cold hands may cause muscle contraction and discomfort. Resting hands on mother's abdomen would help her to become accustomed to your touch and dissipate muscle tightening<br>These measures would aid in gathering greatest amount of information with least discomfort to the woman<br><br><br>Round, hard, readily, movable part, ballotable between the fingers of both hands is indicative of head nonengagement.<br><br>Irregular, bulkier, less firm and not well- defined or movable part is indicative of breech<br>Neither of the above indicates transverse lie<br><br><br>A firm convex, continuously smooth and resistant mass extending from breech to neck is indicative of fetal back. Small knobby, irregular mass, which moves when, pressed or may kick or hit your examining hand is limbs of the fetus |

*Contd...*

| Nursing action | Rationale |
|---|---|
| ▪ Palpate the other side of the abdomen with the examining finger from the midline to the lateral side and from the fundus using smooth pressure and rotatory movements.<br>▪ Repeat the procedure for examination of opposite side of the abdomen | Indicative of the fetal small parts. Small parts all over the abdomen are indicative of a posterior position. |
| • Third maneuver (Pawlik's grip)<br>  ▪ Continue to face the woman's head and make sure the woman has her knees flexed/bent.<br>  ▪ Grasp the portion of the lower abdomen immediately above the symphysis pubis, if movable, it is indicative of an engaged head. It is done with one hand only | Avoids discomfort<br><br>If the fetal head is above the brim, it will be readily movable and ballotable. If not readily movable, it is indicative of an engaged head |
| • Fourth maneuver (pelvic palpation)<br>  ▪ Turn and face the woman's feet (make sure the woman's knees are bent)<br>  ▪ Place your hands on the sides of the uterus, with the palm of your hands just below the level of umbilicus and your fingers directed towards the symphysis pubis<br>  ▪ Press deeply with your fingertips into the lower abdomen and move them toward the pelvic inlet<br>  ▪ Converge the hand around the presenting part when head is not engaged<br>  ▪ The hands will diverge away from the presenting part and there will be no mobility if the presenting part is engaged or dipping. | Avoids pain with the maneuver<br><br><br><br>Cephalic prominence on the same side as the fetal small parts indicates vertex presentation with well-flexed head cephalic prominence on the same side as the fetal back may be occiput in a face presentation with extended head prominences are felt on both sides (brow presentation) |

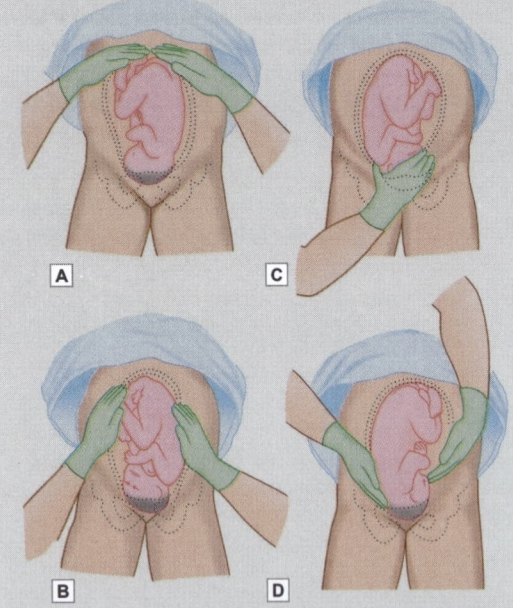

**Figs 11A to D:** Leopold's maneuvers. **A.** Fundal palpation; **B.** Lateral palpation; **C.** Pawlik's grip; **D.** Pelvic palpation

*Contd...*

| Nursing action | Rationale |
|---|---|
| **Auscultation** | |
| • Place fetoscope or stethoscope over the convex portion of the fetus closest to the anterior uterine wall (Table 2 and Fig. 12). Count fetal heart rate for 1 complete min.<br>• Inform the mother of your finding. Make her comfortable.<br>• Replace articles and wash hands<br>• Record in the patient's chart the time, finding and remarks if any | Fetal heart sounds are heard over fetal back (scapula region) in vertex and breech presentation. Over chest in face presentation. |

**TABLE 2:** Location of the maximum intensity of the fetal heart rate

| Presentation | Location of FHR |
|---|---|
| Cephalic/vertex | Midway between umbilicus and level of anterior superior iliac spine |
| Breech | Level with or above umbilicus |
| Anterior | Close to the abdominal midline |
| Occiput transverse | In lateral abdominal area |
| Occiput posterior | In flank area |

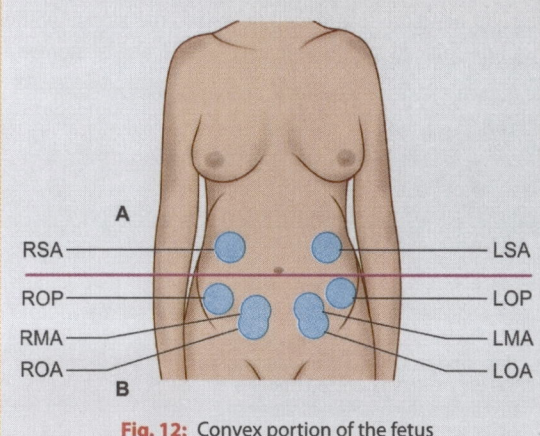

**Fig. 12:** Convex portion of the fetus

## Vaginal Examination

The vaginal examination (Fig. 13) is an intimate procedure that should be performed in the antenatal clinic when the patient attends the clinic for the first time before 12 weeks.

### Purposes

- To diagnose the pregnancy
- To corroborate the size of the uterus with the period of amenorrhea
- To exclude any pelvic pathology

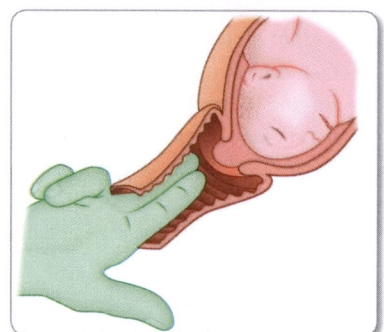

**Fig. 13:** Vaginal examination

*Contraindications*

- Previous history of miscarriage.
- Vaginal bleeding in present pregnancy (ultrasound examination preferred in this case).

*Preliminaries*

- Empty the bladder of the patient
- Draw curtains around the bed
- Provide dorsal position with thigh flexed along the buttock placed on the foot end of the table
- Wash hand with soap and water
- Dry hands
- Wear sterile gloves (usually right hand)

*Steps of Vaginal Examination*

1. **Inspection:** By separating the labia—using the left two fingers (thumb and index), the character of the vaginal discharge, if any, is noted. Presence of cystocele or uterine prolapse or rectocele is to be elicited.
2. **Speculum examination:** This should be done prior to bimanual examination, especially when the smear for exfoliative cytology or vaginal swab is to be taken. A bivalve speculum is used. The cervix and the vault of the vagina are inspected with the help of good light source placed behind. Cervical smear for exfoliative cytology or a vaginal swab from the upper vagina, in presence of discharge, may be taken.
3. **Bimanual:** Two fingers (index and middle) of the right hand are introduced deep into the vagina while separating the labia by left hand. The left hand is now placed suprapubically. Gentle and systematic examinations are to be done to note:
   - **Cervix:** Consistency, direction and any pathology.
   - **Uterus:** Size, shape, position and consistency.
   - **Adnexa:** Any mass felt through the fornix.

If the introitus is narrow, one finger may be introduced for examination. *No attempt should be made to assess pelvis at this stage.*

## Investigations

- **Blood:** Hb, hematocrit, ABO, Rh grouping, blood glucose and venereal disease research laboratory (VDRL) are done. Serology, (antibody) screening is done in selected cases only.
- **Urine:** Protein, sugar and pus cells and ketones.
- **Cervical cytology:** (Pap smear) has become a routine in many clinics. Cells are scraped from cervix and examined under a microscope to check for diseases or other problem (Fig. 14).
- Repetition of investigation:
  - Hb estimation is repeated at 28th and 36th week.
  - Urine is tested for protein and sugar at every antenatal visit.

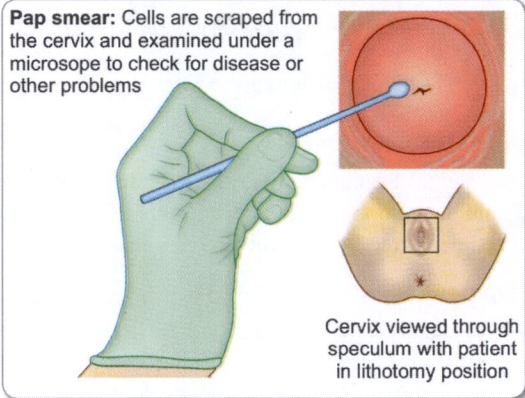

**Pap smear:** Cells are scraped from the cervix and examined under a microscope to check for disease or other problems

Cervix viewed through speculum with patient in lithotomy position

**Fig. 14:** Pap smear

## Special Investigations

### Ultrasonography

- **1st trimester scan:** Ultrasound examination helps to detect:
  - Early pregnancy
  - Accurate dating
  - Number of fetuses
  - Gross fetal anomalies
  - Any uterine or adnexal pathology
- **2nd trimester scan:** Helps to detect:
  - Detailed fetal anatomy and detect any structural abnormality including cardiac activity of the fetus
  - Placental localization

### Amniocentesis

**Amniocentesis** (Fig. 15), also referred to as **amniotic fluid test (AFT)**, is a medical procedure used in prenatal diagnosis of chromosomal abnormalities, fetal infections and also for sex determination, in which a small amount of amniotic fluid, which contains fetal tissues, is sampled from the amniotic sac surrounding a developing fetus, and then the fetal deoxyribonucleic acid (DNA) is examined for genetic abnormalities. The most common reason to have an amniocentesis is to determine whether a baby has certain genetic disorders or a chromosomal abnormality, such as Down's syndrome.

Amniocentesis is usually done when a woman is between 14 and 16 weeks of gestation.

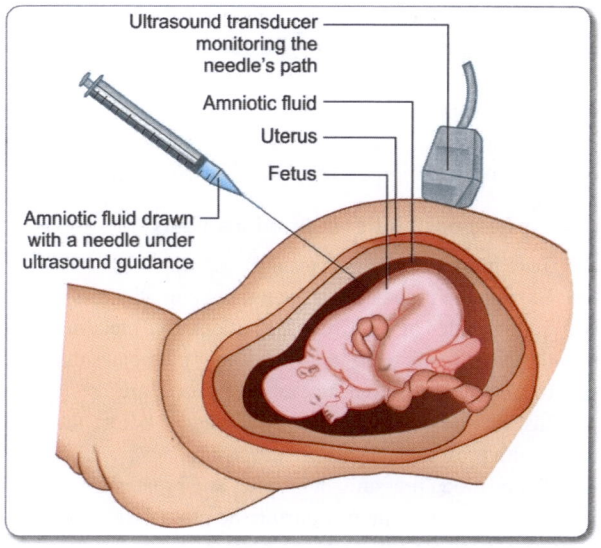

**Fig. 15:** Amniocentesis

### Procedure

- Before starting the procedure, a local anesthetic can be given to the mother in order to relieve the pain felt during the insertion of the needle which is used to withdraw the fluid.
- After the local anesthetic is in effect, a needle is usually inserted through the mother's abdominal wall, then through the wall of the uterus, and finally into the amniotic sac.
- With the aid of ultrasound-guidance, a physician punctures the sac in an area away from the fetus and extracts approximately 15–20 mL of amniotic fluid.

### Genetic Diagnosis

Early in pregnancy, amniocentesis is used for diagnosis of chromosomal and other fetal problems such as:

- Down's syndrome (trisomy 21)
- Trisomy 13
- Trisomy 18
- Fragile X
- Rare, inherited metabolic disorders
- Neural tube defects (anencephaly and spina bifida) by AFP levels in amniotic fluid.

## Other Uses

Amniocentesis can also be used to detect:

- Infection, in which amniocentesis can detect a decreased glucose level, a Gram stain showing bacteria or an abnormal differential count of white blood cells
- Rh incompatibility
- Decompression of polyhydramnios (it should be gradual otherwise there is an increased risk of abruptio placenta)
- Amniocentesis can predict fetal lung maturity, which is inversely correlated to the risk of infant respiratory distress syndrome.

## Risks/Drawback

- Preterm labor and delivery
- Fetal respiratory distress syndrome
- Postural deformities of fetus
- Chorioamnionitis
- Fetal trauma
- Alloimmunization of the mother (rhesus disease).

## Nurse's Responsibilities in Amniocentesis

- Take informed consent from the patient.
- Explain the procedure to the patient and why this test is needed.
- Take detailed history from the patient, like bleeding disorders or patient taking any anticoagulant (blood-thinning) medicines, aspirin, or other medicines that affect blood clotting. In this case, inform the patient to stop these medicines before the procedure.
- Instruct the patient to empty the bladder before the procedure and also follow the instructions given by health professionals during procedure.
- Check blood pressure, heart rate, and breathing rate before and after the procedure.
- Use aseptic precautions during the procedure.
- Inform the patient about the risks associated with amniocentesis, like: cramping, bleeding or leaking of amniotic fluid from the needle puncture site or the vagina, infection, miscarriage and preterm labor.
- In case of Rh incompatibility, administer anti D gamma globulin to patient.
- Patient may feel some cramping during or after the procedure. If patient feels lightheaded, dizzy, or nauseated, tell the nurse. Instruct the patient to rest on left side.
- After the test, rest at home and avoid strenuous activities for at least 24 hours, or as directed by healthcare provider.
- Tell the patient to inform the healthcare provider if she feels any of the following:
  - Any bleeding or leaking of amniotic fluid from the needle puncture site or the vagina
  - Fever or chills
  - Severe belly pain and/or cramping
  - Changes in the activity level of your fetus (if you are past 20–24 weeks of pregnancy).

## Chorionic Villus Sampling (CVS)

It is a form of prenatal diagnosis to determine chromosomal or genetic disorders in the fetus. It entails sampling of the chorionic villus (placental tissue) and testing it for chromosomal abnormalities. CVS usually takes place at 10–12 weeks of gestation.

## Indications

- Abnormal first trimester screen results
- Increased nuchal translucency or other abnormal ultrasound findings
- Family history of any chromosomal abnormality or other genetic disorders
- Parents are known carriers for genetic disorders
- Advanced maternal age (maternal age above 35).

## Risks/Drawbacks

- Miscarriage
- Risk of infection/chorioamnionitis
- Amniotic fluid leakage resulting in oligohydramnios
- Mild risk of limb reduction defects

### *Cordocentesis*

**Percutaneous umbilical cord blood sampling (PUBS)**, also called **cordocentesis, fetal blood sampling**, or **umbilical vein sampling** is a diagnostic genetic test that examines blood from the fetal umbilical cord to detect fetal abnormalities (Fig. 16). PUBS provides a means of rapid chromosomal analysis and is useful when information cannot be obtained through amniocentesis, CVS or ultrasonography.

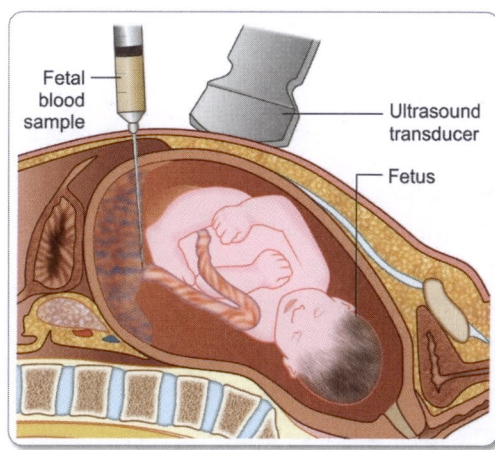

**Fig. 16:** Cordocentesis

## Indications

- Cordocentesis is performed when amniocentesis, or CVS, is unsuccessful or inconclusive in tracking fetal abnormalities. It is usually performed in later pregnancy, between 18 and 24 weeks, when the umbilical cord is sufficiently developed.
- If it is performed after 26 weeks and the baby is in distress, an emergency C-section will be performed, however this is very rare.
- Cordocentesis looks for fetal malformations; chromosomal irregularities, such as, Down's syndrome; blood disorders, fetal anemia, isoimmunization, and infections, such as toxoplasmosis.

## Advantages

Cordocentesis testing can help parents in many ways. For example, it can be used in the diagnosis of heart defects in utero. It can also help expectant mothers prepare for special needs of child, explore medical interventions that might be needed, and in some cases, it helps parents to decide whether to carry the child to term.

## Risks/Drawbacks

- Hemorrhage or bleeding
- Cord hematoma that results in sudden bradycardia
- Fetomaternal hemorrhage that may cause fetal anemia or eventually fetal death
- Infection
- Fetal loss
- Amniotic fluid leakage

### Maternal Serum Alpha-Fetoprotein (MSAFP)

The MSAFP is a screening test that examines the level of AFP in the mother's blood during pregnancy. AFP is a protein that is normally produced by the fetus liver. It is present in the fluid around the fetus (amniotic fluid) and a small amount crosses the placenta and moves into the mother's blood stream. AFP is measured in nanograms per milliliter (ng/mL). An AFP level of less than 10 ng/mL is normal for adults. An extremely high level of AFP in blood (greater than 500 ng/mL) could be a sign of liver tumors. The amount of AFP in the blood of a pregnant woman can help see whether the baby has congenital problems such as spina bifida and anencephaly.

### Contraction Stress Test (CST)

The CST is performed near the end of pregnancy to determine how well the fetus will cope with the contractions during the labor. The aim is to induce contractions and monitor the fetus to check for heart rate abnormalities using a cardiotocograph. A CST is one type of antenatal fetal surveillance technique. It has high risk for fetus and may also result in fetal distress or preterm labor.

#### Objective

To detect the degree of fetal compromise so that a suitable time can be selected to terminate the pregnancy.

#### Indications

- IUGR
- Post maturity
- Hypertensive disorders of pregnancy
- Diabetes

#### Methods

This test may be done in hospital or clinic setting. External fetal monitors are put in place and then either the nipple stimulation or intravenous pitocin (oxytocin) is used to stimulate the uterine contractions.

- **Nipple stimulation:** This test is conducted by the patient. The nurse instructs the patient on the procedure, as follows. One nipple is massaged gently through clothing until a contraction begins, or for a maximum of 2 minutes. If at least 3 contractions in 10 minutes are not achieved, then the patient rests for 5 minutes and the other nipple is stimulated in the same way. This test relies on endogenous release of oxytocin following nipple stimulation.

- **Oxytocin challenge test:** If at least 3 in 10 minutes cannot be achieved with nipple stimulation, an oxytocin challenge test may be performed. In this, intravenous oxytocin is administered to the pregnant woman. The purpose is to achieve at least three contractions in every 10 minutes.

  *Procedure:* Start intravenous infusion of oxytocin at the rate of 1 MIU/minute which is stepped up at the interval of 20 minutes until the effective uterine contractions are established. The alteration of the FHR contractions is recorded by electronic monitoring or by manual palpation. This test takes at least 1–2 hours to perform.

## Interpretation of CST (Table 3)

**TABLE 3:** Interpretation of results

| Result | Interpretation |
|---|---|
| Positive | Presence of late decelerations with at least 50% of the uterine contractions |
| Negative | No late or significant variable decelerations, with at least 3 uterine contractions (lasting 40 seconds) in 10-minute period |
| Equivocal—Suspicious | Presence of late decelerations with fewer than 50% of contractions or significant variable decelerations. Requires repeat testing on following day |
| Equivocal—Tachysystole | Presence of contractions that occur more frequently than every 2 minutes or last longer than 90 seconds in the presence of late decelerations. Requires repeat testing on following day |
| Equivocal—Unsatisfactory | Fewer than three contractions occur within 10 minutes, or a tracing quality that cannot be interpreted. Requires repeat testing on following day |

### Results

- A negative result is highly predictive of fetal wellbeing and tolerance of labor.
- A positive CST indicates high risk of fetal death due to hypoxia and is a contraindication to labor.

### Contraindications

- Any signs of premature birth
- Placenta previa
- Vasa previa
- Multiple gestations
- Previous classic cesarian section
- Previous uterine incision with scarring
- Previous myomectomy
- Premature rupture of membranes (PROM)
- Cervical incompetence

## Nonstress Test

The nonstress test is a simple, noninvasive way of checking fetal well-being. The test records baby's movement, heartbeat and contractions. It notes changes in heart rate, rhythm when fetus goes from resting to moving, or during contractions if mother is in labor. It is performed at any time after 24–26 weeks but commonly performed in third trimester, often combined with biophysical profile.

### Indications

- Gestational diabetes mellitus
- Gestational hypertension
- Baby appears to be small or not growing properly
- Baby is less active than normal
- Too much or too little amniotic fluid
- After external cephalic version
- After amniocentesis

### Interpretation

- **Reactive** (normal) is defined as the presence of two or more fetal heart rate accelerations within a 20-minute period, with or without fetal movement discernible by the pregnant woman.
- **Nonreactive** is defined as the presence of less than two fetal heart rate accelerations within a 20-minute period over a 40-minute testing period.

# HEALTH EDUCATION AND COUNSELING

Every mother needs advice regarding the importance of regular prenatal check-ups and measures to be taken to maintain or improve her health status during pregnancy in order to have a normal delivery and healthy baby.

In order to remove the fear of childbirth and to help them approach the event of labor without undue anxiety, 'child birth preparation' through explanation of physiological changes and methods of coping during labor, delivery and puerperium must be explained to the mother.

## Rest and Sleep

Pregnant woman may continue her usual activities throughout the pregnancy. Hard and strenuous activities should be avoided in the first trimester and last six weeks. The woman should have an average of 10 hours of sleep (8 hours at night and 2 hours at noon) especially in the last trimester.

In late pregnancy, lateral position in bed would be more comfortable.

## Diet

The diet during pregnancy should be adequate to maintain maternal health, meet the needs of growing fetus and provide strength during labor. During pregnancy, the calorie requirement is increased by 300 kcal. The diet should be light, nutritious, easily digestible and rich in protein, minerals and vitamins. In addition to the principal food, the mother needs additional quantity of milk, egg, green vegetables and fruits. A total of 2400 kcal are recommended generally for a pregnant woman.

## Exercise

Day-to-day domestic and social activities to be continued during pregnancy. Brisk walking in the morning and evening and specific antenatal exercises to prepare the mother's body for labor and delivery are recommended.

## Bathing and Clothing

Daily bath and wearing loose comfortable clothes are advised for the comfort of pregnant woman. Wearing high heeled shoes should be avoided in late pregnancy when the center of gravity alters and mother has lordosis.

## Breast Care

If the nipples are anatomically normal, nothing beyond ordinary cleaning is needed. If the nipples are flat or retracted, rolling of the nipples and drawing them out between thumb and forefinger, twice daily for 5 minutes must be explained. Drawing the nipples and rolling them between fingers is recommended after cleansing.

## Oral Care

Tendency to dental caries is high in pregnancy and consulting a dentist and taking required treatment must be emphasized. Mother should perform brushing two times a day.

**Alcohol and smoking** should be avoided in pregnancy since nicotine is harmful for the growing fetus and mother. Growth retardation and poor development of fetus are the possible complications of smoking and drinking.

## Care of Bowels

Regulation of diet including food containing roughage, fluids and vegetables as well as extra quantity of water are to be explained to mother.

## Coitus

It should be avoided in the first three months to prevent abortion and in the 3rd trimester to prevent premature labor and puerperal infection.

## Travel

The vehicles having jerks are to be avoided in first trimester and in last six weeks. Rail journey is preferable to bus travel and travel by aircraft offers no risk.

## Immunization

Immunization is essential against tetanus for mothers in developing countries to protect them as well as their neonates. Two doses of tetanus toxoid between 16 and 24 weeks are generally recommended.

## General Advices

The mother should be instructed to go to the hospital in the following circumstances:

- Active vaginal bleeding even if small amount
- Severe and continuous headache
- Swelling of face, fingers and toes
- Persistent vomiting
- Dimness or blurred vision
- Painful uterine contractions at interval of about 10 minutes or less for at least one hour
- Sudden gush of watery fluid per vagina
- Pain in abdomen
- Fever with chills

# DRUGS AND IMMUNIZATION

## Immunization

Fortunately, most of life-threatening epidemics are rare. In the developing countries, immunization in pregnancy is a routine for tetanus; others are given when epidemic occurs or travelling to an endemic zone or for travelling overseas.

- **Live virus vaccines** (rubella, measles, mumps, varicella and yellow fever) are contraindicated in pregnancy. Rabies, hepatitis A and B vaccines and toxoids can be given as in nonpregnant state. However, in certain circumstances, risk or benefit assessment should be made before making decisions.
- **Tetanus:** In unprotected woman, 0.5 mL tetanus toxoid is given intramuscularly at 6 weeks interval for 2 such, the first one to be given between 16 and 24 weeks. Woman who are immunized in the past, a booster dose of 0.5 mL IM is given in the last trimester.
- **Anti D Gamma globulin:** In case of Rh incompatibility, woman with pregnancy beyond 12 weeks, a full dose of 300 μg IM of anti D gamma globulin is provided to pregnant woman.

## Drugs during Antenatal Period

In routine commonly used drugs during antenatal period are:

- Iron tablets
- Folic acid tablets
- Multivitamins

Certain drugs that are contraindicated in pregnancy are:

- Lithium
- Methotrexate
- Valproic acid
- Mifepristone
- Angiotensin-converting enzyme (ACE) inhibitors
- Danazol
- Radioactive substances and others

Table 4 enlists the FDA risk categories for drugs and medications to be followed during pregnancy.

**TABLE 4:** Food and drug administration (FDA) risk categories for drugs and medication: FDA drug bulletin 1994

| Category | Definitions |
|---|---|
| A | Well-controlled studies in pregnant women; have failed to demonstrate a fetal risk. |
| B | **No evidence of risk in humans:** Well-controlled studies in pregnant women have not shown any increased risk of fetal malformation despite adverse findings in animals. The chances of fetal harm are remote but still remain a possibility. |
| C | **Risk cannot be ruled out:** Adequate, well-controlled human studies are lacking. Animal studies have shown a risk to the fetus or are lacking as well. Potential benefit may outweigh the risk. |
| D | **Positive evidence of risk:** Studies in humans have demonstrated fetal risk. Potential benefits from the use of the drug may outweigh the potential risk. |
| X | **Contraindicated in pregnancy:** Proven fetal risks clearly overweigh any possible benefit. Drugs are alcohol, lithium, methotrexate, valproic acid, mifepristone, ACE inhibitors, danazol, radioactive substances and others. |

Teratogens cause permanent alteration in the structure and function of an organ during embryonic or fetal life. The teratogens may be chemical agents (drugs) or physical agents (radiations, heat). The dose (amount) and duration of teratogen exposure may cause variable response from no effect level to lethal level. Final results of abnormal development are:

- Death
- Malformation
- Growth restriction
- Functional disorder.

# MINOR DISORDERS OF PREGNANCY AND THEIR MANAGEMENT

## Digestive System

### Nausea and Vomiting

Nausea and vomiting upon getting up in the morning are experienced by some woman, especially primigravidae in the first trimester. Normally these subside automatically after first trimester (Fig. 17).

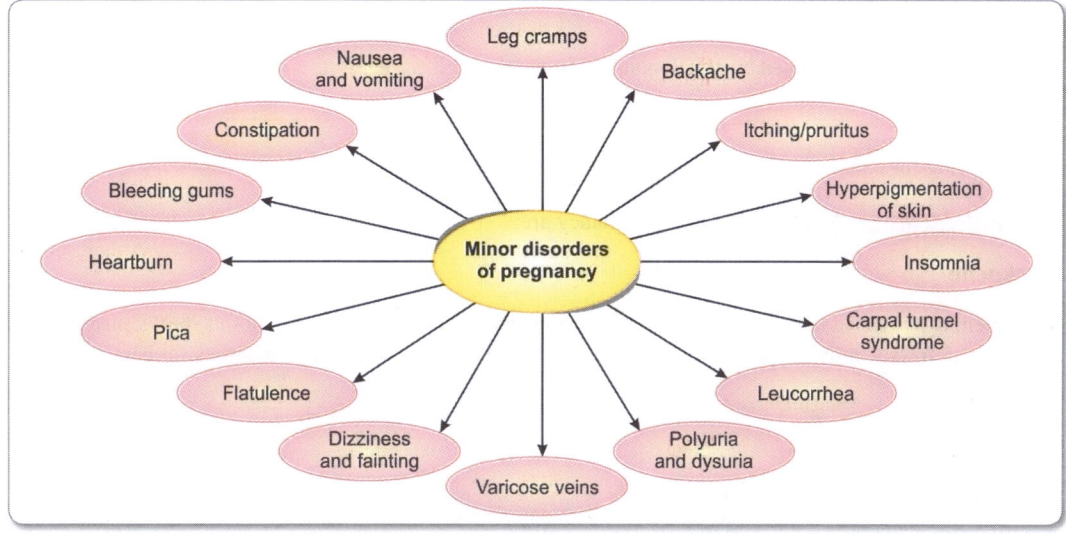

**Fig. 17:** Minor disorders of pregnancy

## Treatment

- Avoid fatty food and fluid in empty stomach.
- Take dry toast or biscuit before rising out of bed.
- Antiemetic drugs can be taken with plenty of glucose drink.

## Constipation

This is common problem in pregnancy due to the effect of progesterone on the intestines and diminished physical activity, gravid uterus reduces the gastrointestinal motility.

### Treatment

- Regular bowel habits
- Take plenty of fluids/vegetables/milk and milk products
- Mild laxative if required

## Heartburn

It is due to the effect of progesterone, which relaxes the cardiac sphincter during pregnancy. The stomach is compressed and pushed up by the gravid uterus. As a result, digestion is impaired in the stomach and takes longer to empty the food.

### Treatment

- Avoid taking heavy meals
- Eat small, frequent meals
- Avoid spicy/fatty foods
- Avoid eating before sleeping
- Take pillow during sleep
- Avoid drinking lot of liquids with meals.

## Bleeding from Gums

It is due to increased blood supply to the gums and higher blood level of progesterone. Soft brushes should be used to prevent bleeding from gums.

### Flatulence

Increase gas in bowels, caused by swallowing air in order to relieve nausea.

### Pica

It is a craving for certain foods or unnatural substances, such as mud, or pencil, etc.

## Musculoskeletal System

### Backache

A problem experienced in the last trimester by some woman. Relaxation of pelvic joints, faulty posture, shift of center of gravity, muscle spasm and urinary infection are some of the common causes for backache.

**Treatment**

- Advice rest in hard bed
- Massaging back
- Analgesics
- Wearing well-fitted pelvic girdle belt during walking

### Leg Cramps

Leg cramps often occur due to deficiency of serum calcium, elevation of serum phosphorus and pressure of gravid uterus on pelvic nerves.

**Treatment**

- Instruct the patient to elevate her legs periodically
- Avoid lying with toes pointed
- Take calcium and vitamin B complex substances
- Take warm baths at bed time
- Wear elastic stockings
- Regular exercise

## Circulatory System

### Dizziness and Fainting

Dizziness and fainting occur mainly because of fall in blood pressure as progesterone relaxes the muscles of blood vessels or gravid uterus puts pressure on the inferior vena cava and diminishes blood return to the heart.

**Treatment**

- Advice mother to lie in left lateral position
- Avoid long periods of standing

### Varicose Veins

Varicose veins in the legs, vulva or rectum appears in the later month of pregnancy due to the effect of progesterone that relaxes the smooth muscles of veins which results in diminished circulation. Gravid uterus also compresses the pelvic nerves.

**Treatment**

- Elevation of legs while resting
- Wear elastic crepe bandage during walking
- Perform circulatory exercise for toes and ankles
- For hemorrhoids mild laxative, regular bowel habits and hydrocortisone ointment can be used

## *Ankle Edema*

Ankle edema occurs due to retention of fluid during pregnancy, hot weather and because of long standing period.

**Treatment**

- Not to sit with feet hanging down
- Elevation of legs while resting
- Not sit near the edge of chair

# Genitourinary System

## *Polyuria and Dysuria*

Two main causes:
1. Gravid uterus puts pressure on the bladder
2. Kidneys function efficiently and the urine production increases

**Treatment**

- Take more fluids during day time
- Avoid holding the urine
- Early treatment of urinary tract infection

## *Leucorrhea*

During pregnancy, there is increased white, nonirritant vaginal discharge, due to change in vaginal pH and flora.

**Treatment**

- Instruct woman for local cleanliness of genitals
- Presence of any vaginal infection treated with medication such as metronidazole or miconazole
- Avoid tight/synthetic underwear

# Integumentary System

## *Itching/Pruritus*

The skin of abdomen stretches during 3rd trimester and becomes dry and itchy. There are stretch marks on breasts, abdomen and thighs.

**Treatment**

- Drink plenty of fluids
- Apply any moisturizing lotion

### Depigmentation of Skin

The three main areas of the darkening of the skin are: around the nipples, around navel and between external genitalia and anus. It is believed to be due to higher level of estrogen in pregnancy.

## Nervous System

### Carpal Tunnel Syndrome

Due to retention of fluids during pregnancy, edema causes pressure on the median nerve. Woman feels numbness, 'pins and needles' in the fingers and hands (Fig. 18).

**Treatment**

Restrict salt intake in the diet. Rest the hands on pillow while sleeping wear splint at night. Perform circulatory exercise such as flexing and extending of fingers and wrist.

### Insomnia

It is due to uncomfortable posture during pregnancy, frequency of micturition, fetal movements, etc.

**Treatment**

- Lie in left lateral position.
- Provide comfortable environment.
- Wear loose/cotton clothes at night.
- Pass urine before going to bed. Do not drink fluids before sleeping.

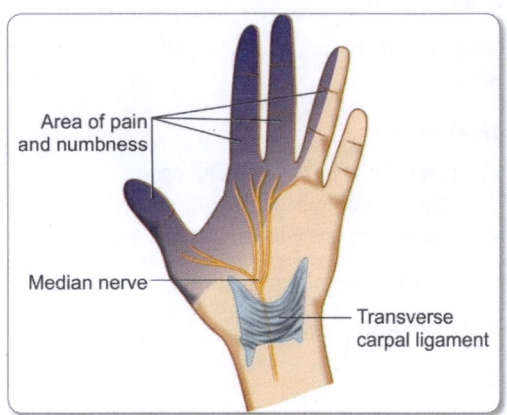

**Fig. 18:** Carpal tunnel syndrome

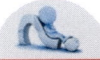

## ASSESS YOURSELF

### FREQUENTLY ASKED QUESTIONS IN EXAMS

1. Describe the physiological changes in pregnancy.
2. Explain various methods for the diagnosis of pregnancy.
3. Enlist the minor disorders of pregnancy and its management.
4. Write short notes on:
    i. Genetic counseling
    ii. Preconception care

### MULTIPLE CHOICE QUESTIONS

1. According to Naegele's rule, if a woman had regular 28-days menstrual cycle and LMP is 2–2–18 then EDD is on:
    a. 8–12–18
    b. 9–11–18
    c. 7–10–18
    d. 10–11–18
2. The most commonly performed test in case of genetic disorders is:
    a. Maternal serum fetoprotein
    b. Amniocentesis
    c. X-ray
    d. Both A and B
3. Which injection is given as a routine to pregnant woman during antenatal period?
    a. Hepatitis B
    b. Tetanus toxoid
    c. Iron injection
    d. PPD injection
4. What is the average weight gain during pregnancy?
    a. 11–12 kg
    b. 15–16 kg
    c. 8–10 kg
    d. 4–5 kg
5. How much dose of woman tetanus toxoid is given to pregnant woman?
    a. 0.5 mL
    b. 1 mL
    c. 2 mL
    d. 0.1 mL
6. What is the purpose of genetic counseling?
    a. To reduce morbidity and mortality
    b. To improve maternal and fetal well being
    c. To reduce the occurrence of fetal malformations
    d. All of the above
7. In case of abdominal examination during antenatal period, the 2nd grip or Leopold's maneuver is called:
    a. Fundal grip
    b. Lateral grip
    c. Pelvic grip
    d. Pawlik's grip
8. The presence of which hormone in the urine indicates pregnancy:
    a. FSH
    b. hCG
    c. LH
    d. Estrogen
9. The total duration of pregnancy is:
    a. 270 days
    b. 280 days
    c. 290 days
    d. 276 days

10. **Quickening can be felt at:**
    a. 14 weeks
    b. 16 weeks
    c. 20 weeks
    d. 15 weeks

11. **Commonest type of vertex presentation is:**
    a. Left occipito transverse
    b. Left occipito anterior
    c. Right occipito anterior
    d. Right occipito posterior

12. **What do you mean by Chadwick sign?**
    a. Bluish discoloration of vagina
    b. Pulsations felt in the vagina
    c. Softening of cervix
    d. Intermittent uterine contractions

13. **Osiander's sign means:**
    a. Pulsations felt in lateral vaginal fornices
    b. Bluish discoloration of vagina
    c. Softening of cervix
    d. Fetal parts felt on abdominal examination

14. **Quickening means:**
    a. Fetal movement in the womb
    b. Softening of cervix
    c. Fetal parts felt on examination
    d. Changes in vagina mucosa

15. **Amniocentesis gives best result if performed at:**
    a. 14–16 weeks
    b. 8–10 weeks
    c. 20–22 weeks
    d. 18–20 weeks

16. **Cardiac activity of the fetus is seen by ultrasound at:**
    a. 4 weeks
    b. 6 weeks
    c. 5 weeks
    d. 7 weeks

17. **High level of maternal serum fetoprotein (MSAFP) indicates:**
    a. Neural tube defects
    b. Fetal cardiac defects
    c. Cleft lip/palate
    d. Nervous system defect

18. **According to JSY, how many iron tablets are to be consumed by a pregnant woman:**
    a. 100 tablets
    b. 50 tablets
    c. 80 tablets
    d. 30 tablets

19. **What are the warning signs of pregnancy?**
    a. Leakage of fluid per vaginum
    b. Disappearance of FHR
    c. Blurred vision
    d. All of the above

20. **Best investigation to diagnose fetal age is:**
    a. Serial ultrasound
    b. Amniocentesis
    c. X-ray
    d. MSAFP

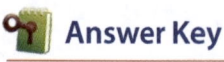

## Answer Key

| 1. | b | 2. | d | 3. | b | 4. | a | 5. | a | 6. | d | 7. | b |
|----|---|----|---|----|---|----|---|----|---|----|---|----|---|
| 8. | b | 9. | b | 10. | b | 11. | b | 12. | a | 13. | a | 14. | a |
| 15. | a | 16. | b | 17. | a | 18. | a | 19. | d | 20. | a | | |

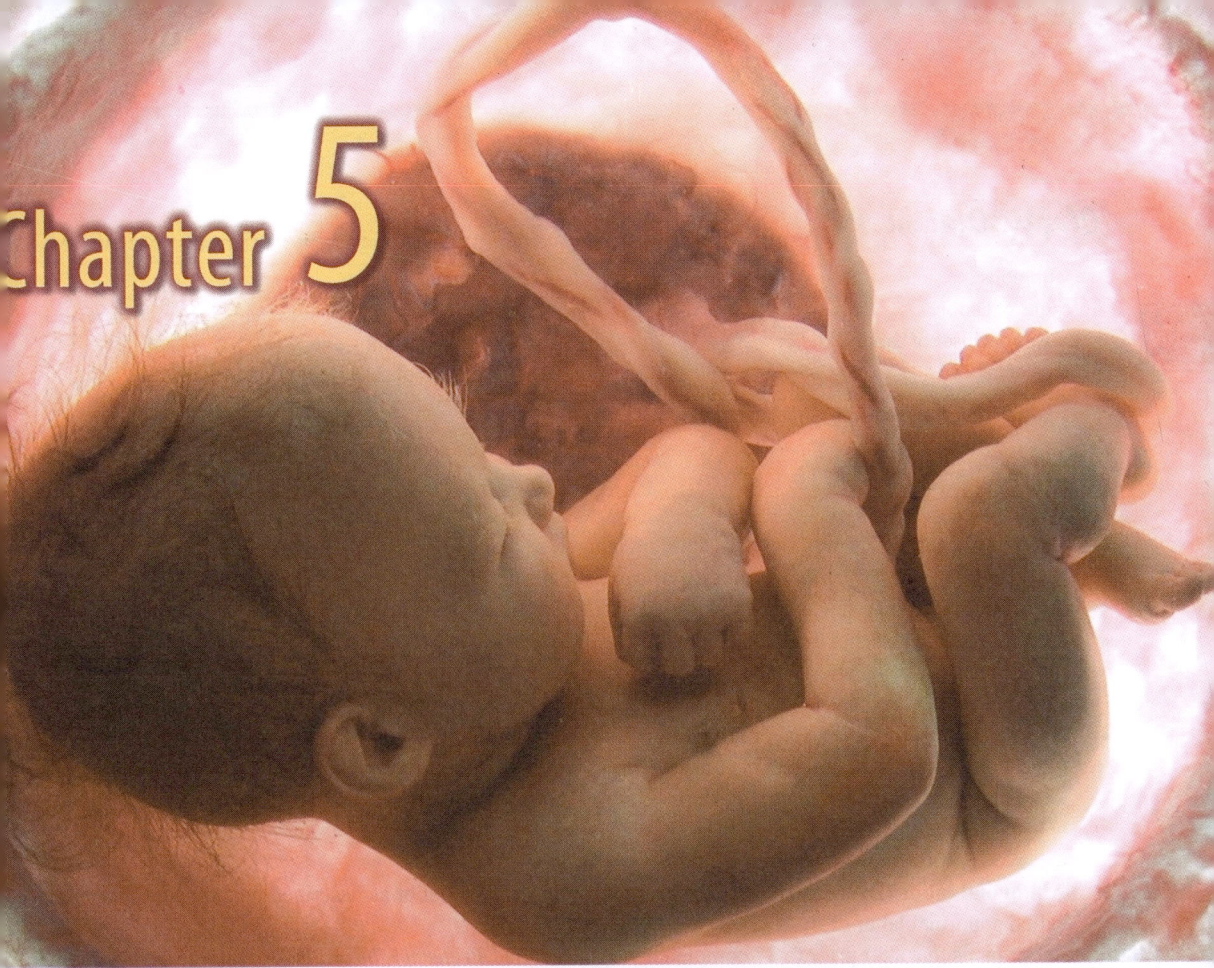

# Chapter 5

# Normal Labor and its Management

## Learning Objectives

**Upon completing this chapter, the learner will be able to:**

➡ Explain various stages of labor and the physiological events in different stages of labor
➡ Describe the mechanism of normal labor
➡ Demonstrate placental examination
➡ Discuss in detail for episiotomy, its risks and benefits
➡ Enumerate the nursing care steps during each stage of labor

## DEFINITIONS

- **Prelabor:** Means the premonitory signs of labor (*i.e. lightening, cervical ripening, taking up of the cervix and false labor pains*) that occur prior to the onset of true labor pains, is called Prelabor. It may last from few days to few weeks and is associated with increased oxytocin receptors in myometrium.
- **Labor:** The process that involves a series of events that take place in the genital organs in order to propel the products of conception (fetus, placenta and membranes) out of the uterus through the birth canal is called labor.
- **Normal labor (Eutocia):** Labor is said to be normal if:
  - Spontaneous in nature and occurs at term.
  - Fetus is in vertex presentation. Completed in normal time period. Natural termination (minimal use of instrumental aids).
  - No complications to mother and fetus.
- **Abnormal labor (Dystocia):** Any change in criteria of normal labor as described in above definition is called abnormal labor or dystocia.

  Labor pains that start prior to 37 completed weeks is called ***Preterm labor***. If labor pains occur between 38 and 42 weeks, it is ***termed labor***. ***Post-term labor*** occurs after completing 42 weeks.

## STAGES OF LABOR

- **First stage:** It starts with onset of true labor pains and ends with full dilatation of cervix (10 cm) approximately. ***Duration is approximately 12 hours in primipara and 6 hours for multipara.***
- **Second stage:** It starts from full dilatation of cervix till expulsion of fetus from birth canal. It has two phases:
  i. **Propulsive phase:** Starts from full dilatation of cervix up to the descent of the presenting part to the pelvic floor.
  ii. **Expulsive phase:** It is characterized by maternal bearing down efforts and ends with expulsion of fetus from birth canal.

  *Duration of second stage is approximately 2 hours in primipara and 30 minutes for multipara.*
- **Third stage:** It starts after the expulsion of fetus from birth canal and ends with expulsion of placenta and membranes.

  *Duration is approximately 15 minutes in both primipara and multipara, however its duration is reduced to 5 minutes with active management. Nowadays active management is encouraged.*
- **Fourth stage:** It is the observational stage in which both mother and baby are observed for at least 1 hour to ensure the wellbeing of both.

## CAUSES OF ONSET OF LABOR

The exact cause is unknown. Some of the hypotheses are as listed below:

- **Uterine distension:** The stretching effect on the myometrium by growing fetus and liquor amnii can initiate the labor pains.
- **Pressure of the presenting part** on the nerve ending in the cervix may stimulate a nerve plexus known as cervical ganglion that can initiate the onset of labor.
- **Myometrial involvement:** Estrogen increases oxytocin receptors in myometrium and decidua.
- **Oxytocin stimulation theory:** The uterus becomes increasingly sensitive to oxytocin as pregnancy progresses and its maximum at term (37 weeks)
- **Estrogen stimulation theory:** Estrogen increases the release of oxytocin from maternal posterior pituitary. It stimulates irritability of uterine muscles and enhances uterine contractions.
- **Progesterone withdrawal theory:** In pregnancy, progesterone inhibits contractions, but at term progesterone synthesis falls and estrogen increases. There is a change in estrogen: progesterone ratio, which stimulates prostaglandin synthesis.
- **Prostaglandin stimulation theory:** Prostaglandin stimulates smooth muscles to contract, therefore initiate the labor.
- **Fetal cortisol theory:** Estrogen level increases due to the effects of fetal cortisol in late pregnancy.
- **Fetoplacental contribution:** Due to unknown factors, fetal pituitary is stimulated that increases the release of adrenocorticotropic hormone (ACTH) and stimulates the fetal adrenal to secrete cortisol that further accelerates the production of estrogen and prostaglandins from the placenta.

## SIGNS OF LABOR

### Prelabor or Premonitory Signs of Labor

- It may begin 2–3 weeks prior to the onset of true labor in primipara and a few days before in multipara. These signs are lightening, cervical changes, taking up of cervix, increased frequency of micturition, appearance of false labor pains, gastrointestinal upset, premature rupture of membranes (PROM) and energy spurt.
  - **Lightening:** A few days/weeks prior to the onset of labor, presenting part sinks into the true pelvis. It is a welcome sign as it rules out cephalopelvic disproportion and other conditions preventing the head from entering the pelvic inlet (Fig. 1).

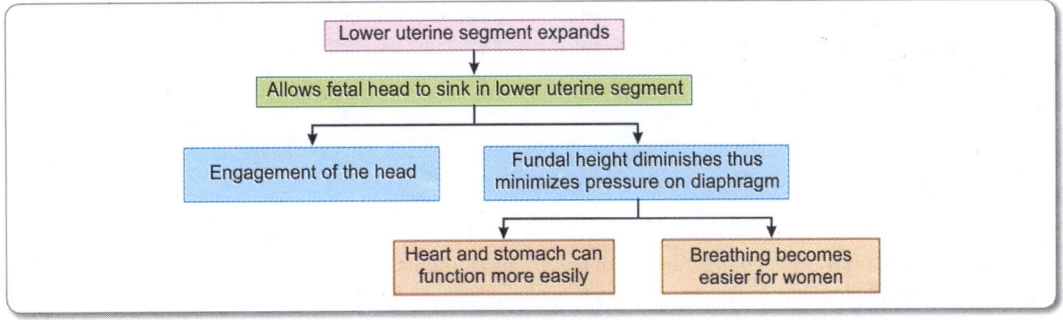

**Fig. 1:** Lightening

- **Cervical changes:** The cervix becomes ripe. A ripe cervix is soft, less than 1.3 cm in length, allows to admit one finger and is dilatable.
- **Cervical effacement:** It is a process by which muscular fibers of the cervix are pulled upward and merge with the fibers of the lower uterine segment. In primigravidae, effacement precedes dilatation of the cervix, whereas in multipara, both occur simultaneously.
- **Frequency of micturition:** It means frequent urination. It is due to pressure by engaged presenting part (Fig. 2).

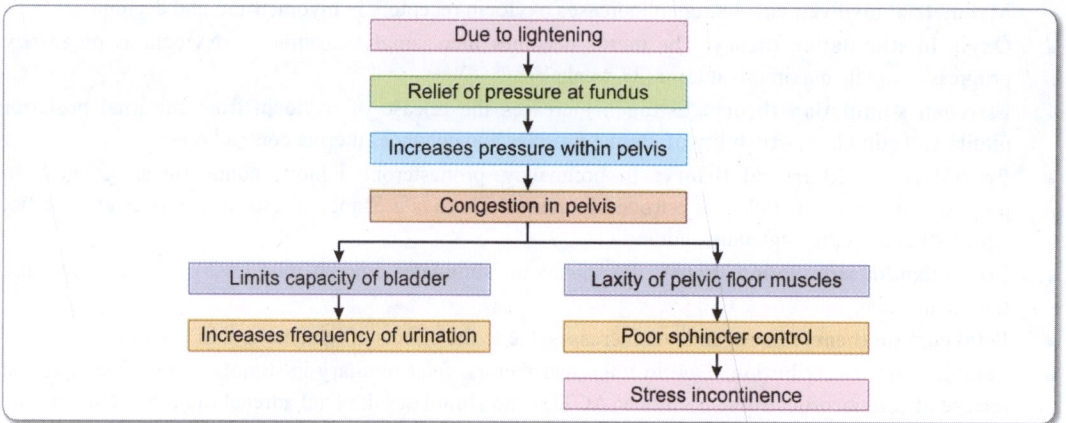

**Fig. 2:** Process leading to increased frequency of micturition

- **Appearance of false labor pains:** False labor pains consist of painful uterine contractions that have no measurable progressive effect on the cervix. It may be due to the stretching of cervix and lower uterine segment with consequent irritation of the neighboring ganglia. It may occur by 1–2 weeks prior to onset of true labor pains in primipara and by a few days in multipara.
- **Gastrointestinal upset:** In the absence of any causative factors for occurrence of diarrhea, indigestion, nausea and vomiting, it might be indicative of impending labor. No explanation for this is known, but some women do experience one to all of these signs.
- **PROM:** Normally membranes rupture at the end of 1st stage of labor but in about 12% of woman it may rupture before the onset of labor. Approximately, 80% of woman with PROM have spontaneous onset of labor within 24 hours.
- **Energy spurt:** Many women experience an energy spurt approximately 24–48 hours before the onset of labor. There is no known explanation for this, other than it is a nature's way of giving energy needed for labor. A woman should be informed about this and advised to conserve it for labor.
- **Late pregnancy feeling:** Mood swings-both elation and depression in later weeks occur just prior to onset of labor.

## True Labor

The features of true labor pains are:

- Painful, rhythmic uterine contractions with hardening of uterus.
- Progressive dilatation and effacement of cervix.
- Descent of the presenting part.

- Appearance of "show" blood stained mucoid discharge.
- Formation of bag of waters.
- True labor pain is not relieved by enema and sedatives.

Table 1 enlists the differences between true and false labor pains.

**TABLE 1:** Differences between true and false labor pains

| Features | True labor pains | False labor pains |
| --- | --- | --- |
| Location of pain | Lower abdomen and back, radiating to thighs | Lower abdomen only |
| Characteristics of pain | Intermittent in nature with increased intensity, frequency and duration | Pain is continuous without any rhythmicity |
| Uterine changes | Hardening of uterus due to retraction of muscle fibers | No hardening of uterus |
| Cervical changes (dilatation and effacement) | Present | Absent |
| Bag of waters | Formed | Not formed |
| Show | Present | Absent |
| Relief with enema/sedation | No | Yes |
| Cause of pain | Due to uterine contraction | Due to loaded rectum |

# FIRST STAGE OF LABOR

It starts from the onset of true labor pains and ends till full dilatation of the cervix (10 cm). Duration is approximately 12 hours for primi- and 6 hours for multipara.

The first stage is divided into three phases:

1. **Latent phase:** It is defined as the period between the onset of true labor pains and ends with cervical dilatation of 3–4 cm. Rate of cervical dilatation is about 0.35 cm/hr.
   - **Duration:** In primigravida average duration is 8 hours and in multipara it is 5 hours.
   - **Frequency and interval:** During this phase, initially contraction comes at interval of 15–30 minutes with duration of about 30 seconds. But gradually the interval becomes shortened with increasing intensity and duration, and contraction comes at interval of 5–7 minutes and lasts for about 40 seconds.
2. **Active phase:** The active phase of labor begins when the cervix is 3–4 cm dilated and ends when cervical dilatation is of 8 cm. During this phase, contraction occurs every 3–5 minutes and lasts up to 60 seconds.
   - **Duration:** In primigravida 6 hours and multigravida 4 hours.
   - **Dilatation rate:** 1.2–1.5 cm/hr
3. **Transition phase:** The last and shortest part of 1st phase of labor is transition; it is more intense phase of a laboring woman. Contractions occur every 2–3 minutes lasting 60–90 seconds.
   - *Duration*: In primigravida it lasts for 2 hours and in multigravida the duration is 1 hour.

## Signs and Symptoms

- Contraction and retraction of uterine muscles.
- Formation of upper and lower uterine segments.
- Development of retraction ring (Bandl's ring)
- Cervical dilatation and effacement

- Bloody show
- Formation of bag of waters
- Rupture of membranes.

**Note:** *All these points are discussed in detail in physiology of 1st stage of labor.*

# Physiology

Physiology of labor has three components and the brief summary is as follows:

1. **Uterine changes**
   - Fundal dominance
   - Polarity
   - Contraction and retraction
   - Formation of upper and lower uterine segment
   - Development of retraction ring (Bandl's ring)

2. **Cervical changes**
   - Cervical ripening
   - Cervical effacement
   - Cervical dilatation
   - Bloody show

3. **Mechanical factors**
   - Formation of bag of waters
   - General fluid pressure
   - Rupture of membranes
   - Fetal axis pressure
   - Descent of the presenting part

## Uterine Changes

- **Fundal dominance:** Each uterine contraction starts in the fundus near one of the cornua and spreads across downwards. The contraction lasts longest in the fundus where it is also most intense, but the peak is reached simultaneously over the whole uterus and the contraction fades from all parts together (Fig. 3).

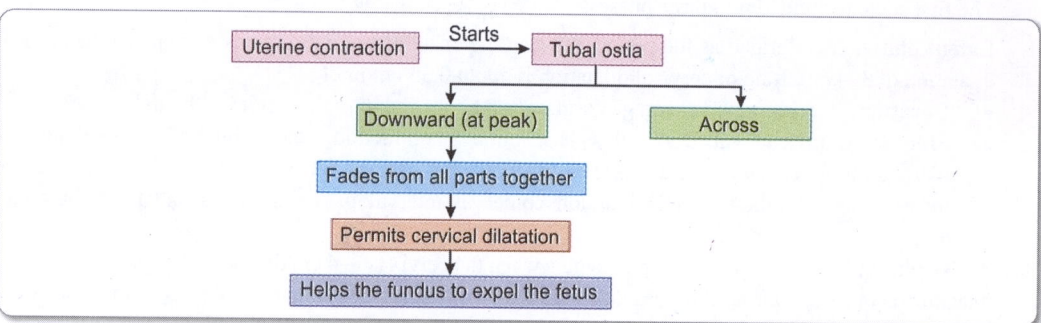

**Fig. 3:** Fundal dominance during labor

- **Polarity:** It is the neuromuscular harmony between upper and lower pole of uterus throughout the labor (Fig. 4).

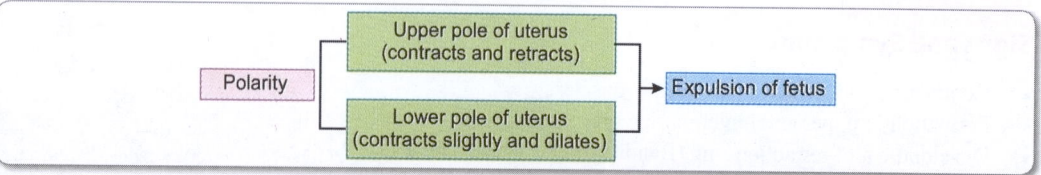

**Fig. 4:** Phenomenon of polarity

- **Contraction and retraction:** Contraction is temporary shortening of muscle fibers followed by relaxation. Relaxation is regaining of original length of muscle fibers. Retraction is a phenomenon of the uterus in labor in which muscle fibers are permanently shortened once and for all (Fig. 5).

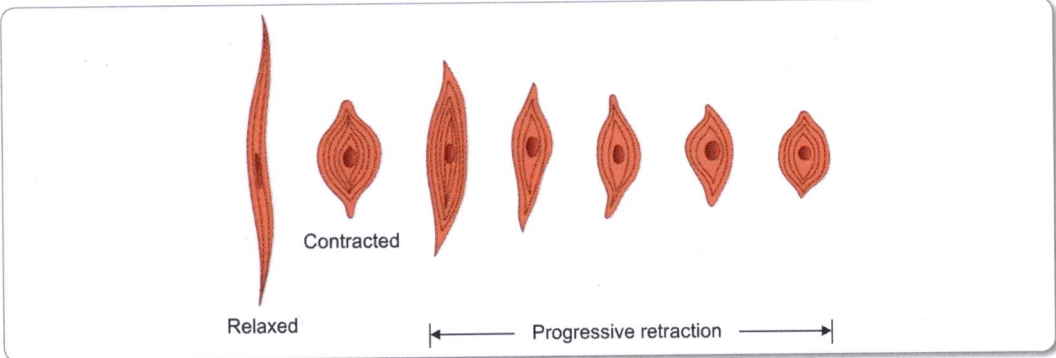

**Fig. 5:** Muscle fibers showing contraction and retraction

- **Formation of upper and lower uterine segments:** Before the onset of labor, there is no complete anatomical or functional division of the uterus. During labor, the demarcation of an active upper segment and a relative passive lower segment is more pronounced. The wall of the upper segment becomes progressively thickened with progressive thinning of the lower segment. This is pronounced in late first stage, especially after rupture of the membranes and attains its maximum in second stage (Fig. 6).

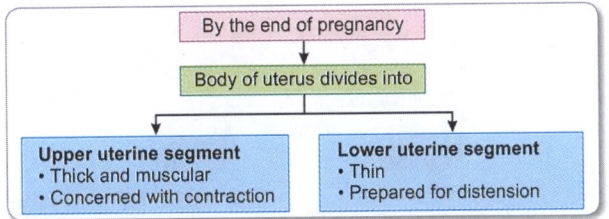

**Fig. 6:** Formation of upper and lower uterine segments

- **Development of retraction ring (Bandl's ring):** When upper uterine segment contracts and retracts, the lower segment thins out to accommodate the presenting part and the ridge is formed between upper and lower uterine segment called Bandl's ring (Fig. 7).

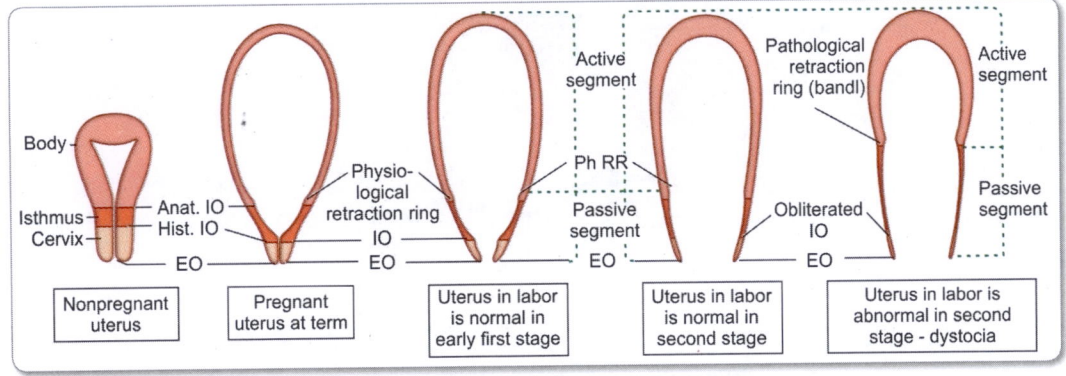

**Fig. 7:** Formation of retraction ring or Bandl's ring

*Abbreviations:* EO, external OS; Hist, histological internal OS; IO, internal OS; Ph RR, physiological retraction ring

### Cervical Changes

- **Cervical ripening:** It refers to the softening of the cervix that typically begins prior to the onset of labor and is necessary for cervical dilatation and the passage of the fetus (Fig. 8).

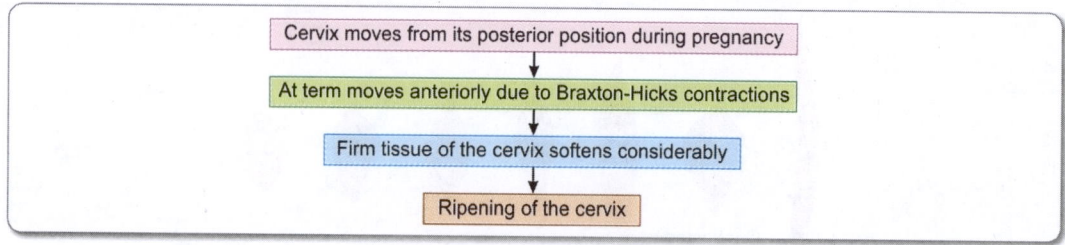

**Fig. 8:** Process of ripening of cervix

- **Cervical effacement:** It is defined as the thinning of the cervix and shortening of the cervical canal (normal length of 2–3 cm) (Fig. 9).

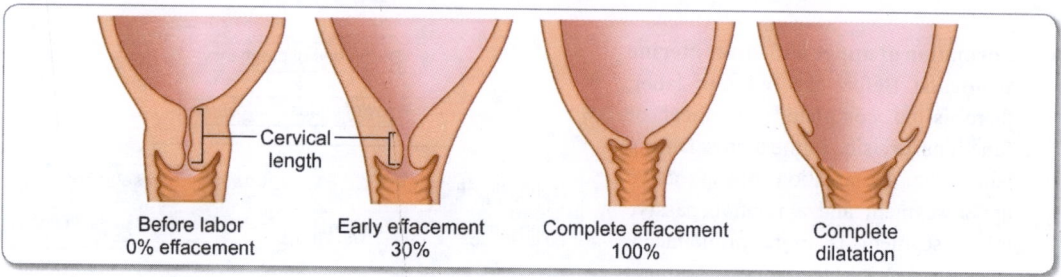

**Fig. 9:** Cervical effacement and dilatation

- **Cervical dilatation:** It is the process of enlargement of external os from closed external os to permit passage of fetal head. Full dilatation of cervix is 10 cm.
- **Bloody show:** It is defined as expulsion of mucus plug stained with blood (Fig. 10). It is caused by separation of the membranes due to over stretching of the lower uterine segment.

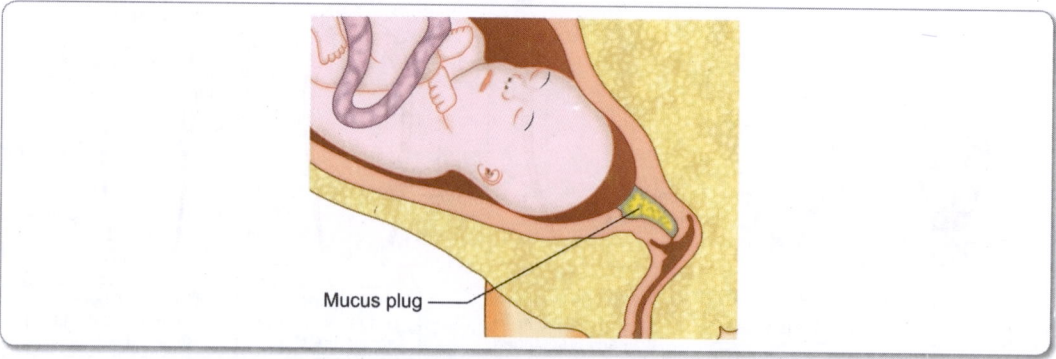

**Fig. 10:** Mucus plug (removal of this plug leads to bloody show)

## Mechanical Factors

- **Formation of bag of waters**

  Process of formation of bag of water have been discussed in Figures 11 and 12.

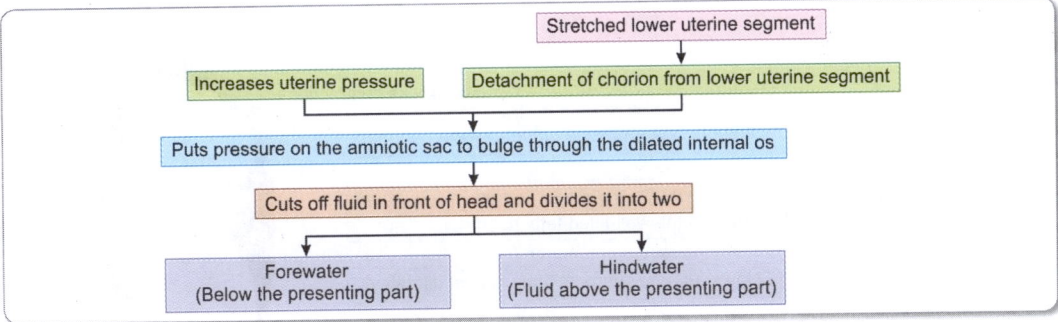

**Fig. 11:** Process of formation of bag of waters

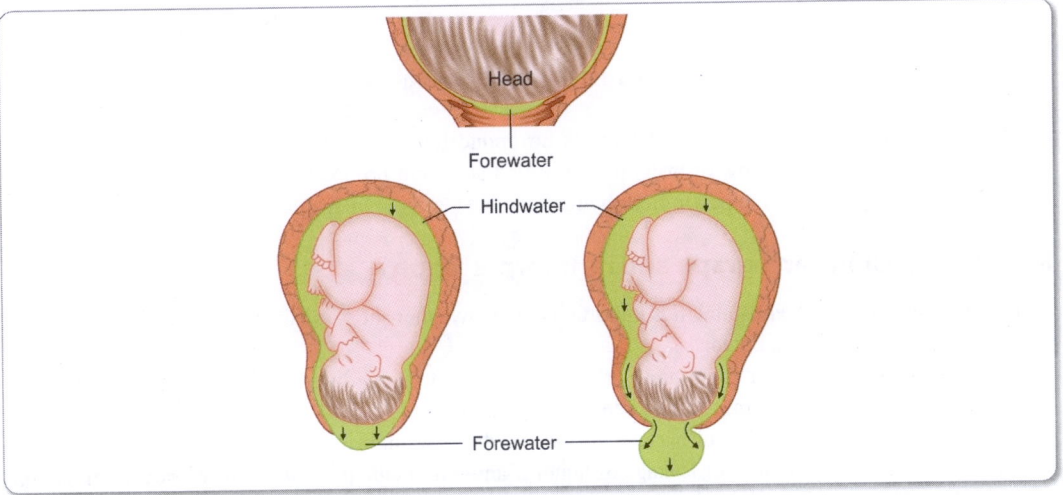

**Fig. 12:** Bag of waters

- **General fluid pressure:** While the membranes remain intact, the pressure of the uterine contractions is exerted on the fluid and as fluid is not compressible, the pressure is equalized throughout the uterus and the fetal body; it is known as general fluid pressure or fetal axis pressure (Fig. 13).

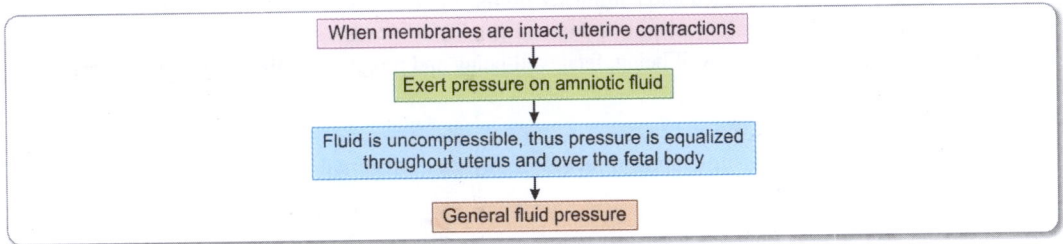

**Fig. 13:** Formation of general fluid pressure

- **Rupture of membranes:** It is a term used during pregnancy to describe rupture of the amniotic sac. Normally, it occurs spontaneously at full term either during or at the beginning of labor. Rupture of membranes is also known as "breaking the water" or as one's "water is breaking".
- **Fetal axis pressure** (Figs 14A and B):

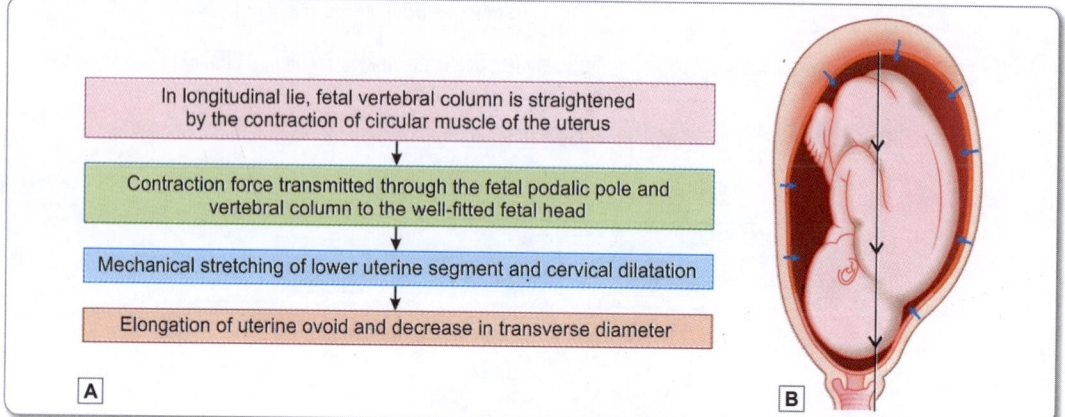

**Figs 14A and B:** Formation of fetal axis pressure

- **Descent of the presenting part:** If there is no undue bony or soft tissue obstruction, descent is a continuous process. It is slow or insignificant in first stage but pronounced in second stage. Presenting part is expected to reach the pelvic floor by the time the cervix is fully dilated.

## Monitoring using Partograph and its Interpretation

When a woman comes to the hospital, it is important to note whether she is in labor or not. During assessment the following points are to be noted:

- Admit the mother in labor room and perform the complete procedures, such as changing to hospital gown, applying identification band and completing charts.
- **History taking:** This consists of basic evaluation of the past clinical conditions. Enquiry is to be made about the onset of labor pains or leakage of liquor if any. Thorough, general and obstetrical examinations including vaginal examination are to be carried out and recorded. Records or antenatal visits, investigation reports and any specific treatment given, if available, are to be reviewed.
- Orient patient to labor and delivery rooms.
- Explain admission protocol, labor process and management plans.
- Carry out perineal shave and administer enema if not contraindicated.
- Start intravenous line if indicated and administer fluids.
- Provide physical and psychological care and attend to comfort needs.
- Monitor and evaluate maternal well-being, fetal well-being and progress of labor by using partograph.

### Partograph

Partograph (Fig. 15) is a composite graphical record of key data (maternal and fetal) during labor, entered against time on a single sheet of paper.

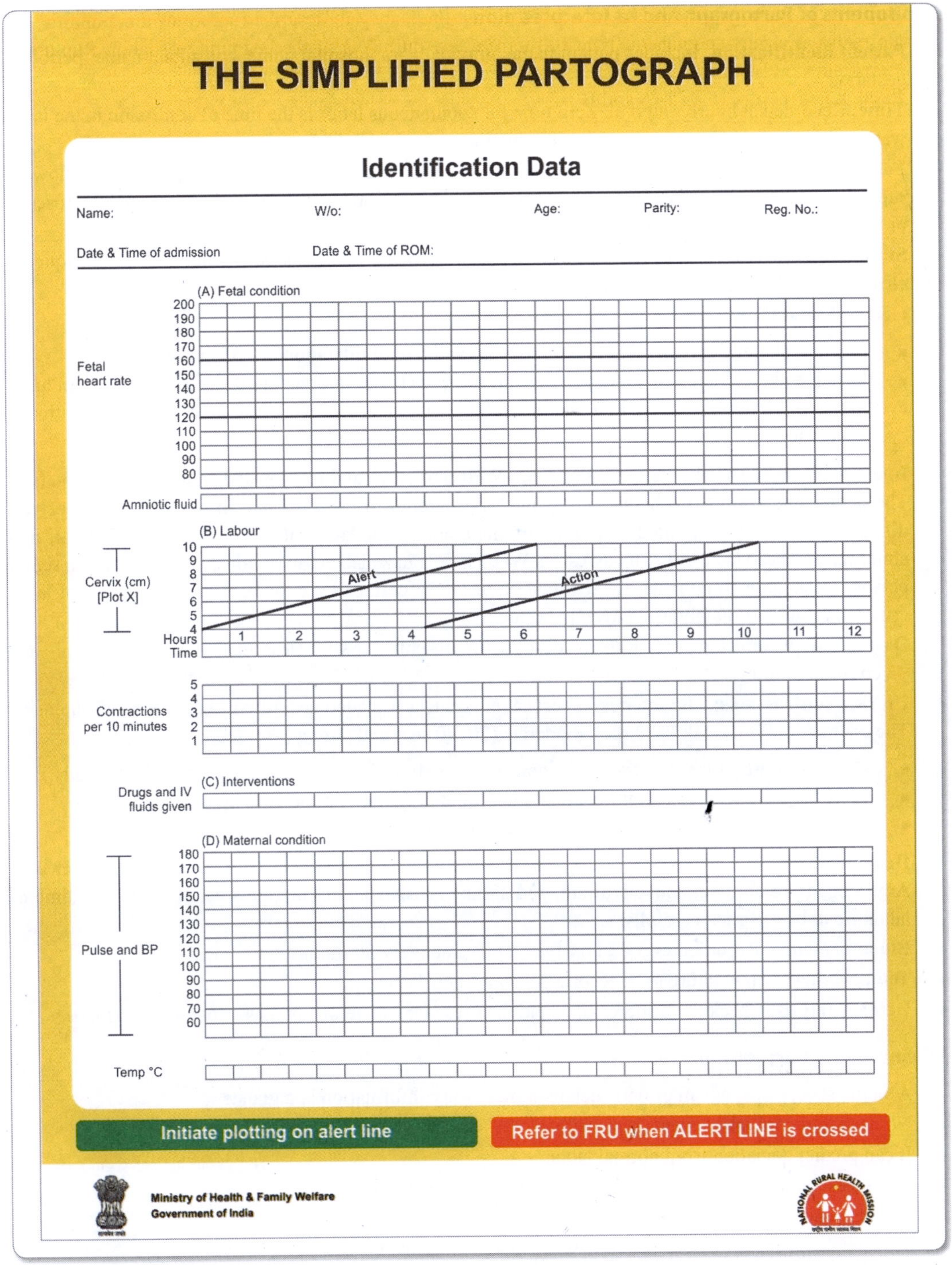

# THE SIMPLIFIED PARTOGRAPH

## Identification Data

Name:                W/o:                Age:        Parity:        Reg. No.:

Date & Time of admission        Date & Time of ROM:

**(A) Fetal condition**

Fetal heart rate
200
190
180
170
160
150
140
130
120
110
100
90
80

Amniotic fluid

**(B) Labour**

Cervix (cm)
[Plot X]
10
9
8
7
6
5
4

Alert        Action

Hours
Time        1    2    3    4    5    6    7    8    9    10    11    12

Contractions per 10 minutes
5
4
3
2
1

**(C) Interventions**

Drugs and IV fluids given

**(D) Maternal condition**

Pulse and BP
180
170
160
150
140
130
120
110
100
90
80
70
60

Temp °C

**Initiate plotting on alert line**        **Refer to FRU when ALERT LINE is crossed**

Ministry of Health & Family Welfare
Government of India

Chapter 5 ● Normal Labor and its Management

**Fig. 15:** Partograph

## Components of Partograph and its Interpretation

- **Patient identification**: Includes patient name, gravida, para, hospital name, consultant name, period of gestation.
- **Time:** Recorded at hourly interval. Zero time for spontaneous labor is the time of admission in the labor ward and for induced labor is the time of induction.
- **Fetal heart rate:** Recorded every half hourly in 1st stage and every 15 minutes in 2nd stage or following rupture of membranes. Normal fetal heart rate (FHR) is 110–150 beats per minute measured by fetoscope or Doppler ultrasonic cardiography.
- **State of membranes and color of liquor:** If membranes are intact, mark 'I', ruptured 'R'. If liquor is clear, mark 'C', if meconium stained, mark 'M'.
- **Cervical dilatation:**
  - In latent phase: Cervical dilatation up to 4 cm and rate of dilatation is 0.35 cm/hr.
  - In active phase: Start with dilatation of 4 cm and ends till 8 cm. Rate of dilatation is 1.2–1.5 cm/hr.
  - In transition phase: Start with dilatation of 8 cm and ends with 10 cm. Rate of critical dilatation is 1.5 cm/hr.

  **In cervicograph:** The alert line starts at 4 cm (WHO) of cervical dilatation and ends at 10 cm dilatation. The action line is drawn 4 hours to the right and parallel to the alert line. In normal labor, cervical dilatation (cervicograph) should be either on the alert line or left to it. When it falls on Zone 2, it is abnormal and need to be critically assessed. When it falls in zone 3, case should be reassessed by a senior person. Decision is to be made for termination of labor [cesarean section/or for augmentation of labor artificial rupture of membranes (ARM)/Oxytocin]

  **Descent of presenting part:** Rate of descent of presenting part is less than 1 cm/hr in primi- and <2 cm/hr in multipara.
- **Uterine contractions:** The squares in vertical columns are shaded according to duration and intensity. The contractions are weak (<20 sec), moderate (20–40 sec) and strong (>40 sec).
  - **During latent phase:** Contractions come at interval of 15–30 minutes and last for 30 seconds.
  - **In active phase:** Contractions come at interval of 3–5 minutes and lasts up to 60 seconds.
  - **In transition phase:** Contractions occur every 2–3 minutes lasting 60–90 seconds
- **Drugs and fluids:** Concentration of oxytocin in the upper box and dose (mIU/min) in the lower box. Any drugs (like diuretic, anticonvulsant, and antihypertensive, etc.) or fluids given during the time of labor are to be recorded carefully.
- **Blood pressure:** Recorded every 2 hourly and pulse at every 30 minutes.
- **Temperature:** Temperature to be recorded every 4 hourly.
- **Urine Analysis:** Check the urine volume and the presence of acetone bodies, proteins and glucose.

## Advantages of Partograph

- A single sheet of paper can provide details of necessary information at a glance.
- No need to record labor events repeatedly.
- It can predict deviation from normal labor.
- It reduces the incidence of prolonged labor and cesarean section rate.
- It saves time.
- Transfer of information becomes easy when labor status changes.
- Helpful to reduce maternal morbidity and mortality, perinatal morbidity and mortality rates.

## Care of Mother: Physical and Psychological

- **General:**
  - Aseptic precautions should be taken throughout the labor process.
  - Continuous emotional support, encouragement and assurance are to be given to keep up the morale of the mother
  - Constant supervision is required.
- **Careful examination:** A complete and careful examination of the woman is important. Physical and pelvic examination is carried out and laboratory tests are also performed.
- **Prevention of infection:** To prevent infection, aseptic technique should be followed during vaginal examination and hygiene of the woman should be maintained throughout the labor.
- **Perineal preparation:** Shave the perineal area for easy viewing. Vulval toileting is also to be done.
- **Rest:** Generally, a woman in early normal labor may not to be confined to bed. While in bed she may take any comfortable position, advise the mother not to lie down in dorsal supine position so as to prevent aortocaval compression.
- **Ambulation:** If the membranes are intact, the patient is allowed to walk. This prevents venacaval compression and encourages descent of the head.
- **Bowel:** During vaginal examination if rectum feels loaded, soap and water enema is given in early stage to prevent soiling of the perineum during the time of delivery. Loaded bowel also inhibits uterine contractions.
- **Bladder care:** Mother is encouraged to pass urine by herself as full bladder often inhibits uterine contractions and may lead to infection or injury to the urinary bladder itself. If the woman cannot go to toilet, provide bedpan or catheterization should be done with strict aseptic precautions.
- **Diet:** There is delayed emptying of the stomach in labor so advise the woman not to take solid food during active labor. Fluid in the form of plain water, ice chips or fruit juice may be given in early labor. In case of prolonged labor, 5% dextrose may be started.
- **Relief of pain:** Pethidine is an effective analgesic. Dose given during labor: 50–100 mg IM. Metoclopramide 10 mg IM is commonly given to combat vomiting due to pethidine.
- **Vital signs:**
  - **Maternal:** Pulse is recorded every 30 minutes and is marked with dot (.) in the partograph. Blood pressure is recorded at every 1 hour and marked with (↑) Temperature is recorded at every 2 hours.
  - **Fetal:** Fetal vital signs should be noted every half hour in the first stage and every 15 minutes in second stage or following rupture of membranes. Fetal heart rate should be recorded immediately after uterine contractions. The count should be made for 60 seconds. Normal FHR ranges from 110 to 150 beats/minutes.
- **Abdominal palpation:**
  - Note the frequency, intensity and duration of contractions. The number of contractions in 10 minutes and duration of each contraction in seconds are recorded in the partograph.
  - Note the position and presentation of the fetus.
  - Note the descent of the presenting part.
- **Vaginal examination:** Vaginal examination should be kept as minimum (at least 4 hourly) to avoid risk of infection and the following points are to be noted:
  - Dilatation of the cervix
  - Position of head and degree of flexion
  - Station of head
  - Color of liquor
  - Degree of molding of head.

- **Intake and output:** Careful recording of intake/output chart is to be done. Maintain intake/output chart every 4 hourly.
- **Emotional support:**
  - Mother is supported emotionally.
  - She should be guided and informed about the observations and actions.
  - Maintain good interpersonal relations with the mother so that she can verbalize her feelings during the time of labor.
  - Allow any family member/husband to stay with the mother, with which mother feels comfortable.

## Pain Management

It is by nature that delivery takes place with labor pains and the pains are so intense that sometimes a woman becomes anxious. Labor pain is experienced by most of the women with satisfaction at the end of a successful labor. Pain during labor results from a combination of uterine contractions and cervical dilatation. The most distressing time during the whole labor is just prior to full dilatation of the cervix. Antenatal classes, sympathetic care and encouraging environment during labor can reduce the need of analgesia. The factors which affect the intensity and amount of pain experienced by a woman in labor are:

- Duration and intensity of uterine contractions
- Degree of dilatation of cervix
- Distention of perineal tissues
- Parity (primipara needs pain management more frequently than multipara)
- Pain threshold of the woman
- Coping mechanisms
- Communication pattern
- Cultural characteristics
- Surrounding environment

### Methods of Pain Relief

#### Pharmacological Methods

- **Sedatives and analgesics:** Commonly used sedatives and analgesics in labor are shown in Table 2:

**TABLE 2:** Commonly used sedatives and analgesics

| Drug | Usual dose | Route | Frequency | Neonatal half-life (approx) |
|------|-----------|-------|-----------|-----------------------------|
| Pethidine | 50–100 mg | IM | 4 hours | 13–20 hours |
| Fentanyl | 50–100 µg | IV | 1 hour | 5 hours |
| Morphine | 10 mg | IM | 4 hours | 7 hours |
| Meperidine | 5–25 mg | IV/IM | 4 hours | – |

- **Inhalational agents:** Commonly used inhalational agents used during labor are entonox, halothane and methoxyflurane. Ethnox is made up of 50% nitrous oxide and 50% oxygen, and is administered by face mask or inhaler. Halothane is helpful for uterine relaxation but causes respiratory depression and postpartum hemorrhage.

#### Anesthesia

- **Regional anesthesia:** In regional anesthesia, injection is given to block the transmission of painful stimuli from the uterus, cervix, vagina and perineum to the thalamic pain center in the brain. Injection of the local anesthetic can be given once or continuously. The methods used are as follows:

- **Paracervical block:** In this, local anesthetic injection is given transvaginally, near the outer rim of the cervix. It is helpful to relieve pain caused by cervical dilatation.
  - **Side effects:** In mother, it causes systemic toxic reaction and hematoma reaction.
  - **In fetus:** Bradycardia, acidosis and even death. It is the responsibility of the nurse to check the vital signs of the mother and FHR periodically.
- **Pudendal nerve block:** In this, injection is given around the pudendal nerve. It is given prior to episiotomy suturing or forceps delivery (Fig. 16).
  - **Side effect:** Vulval hematoma.

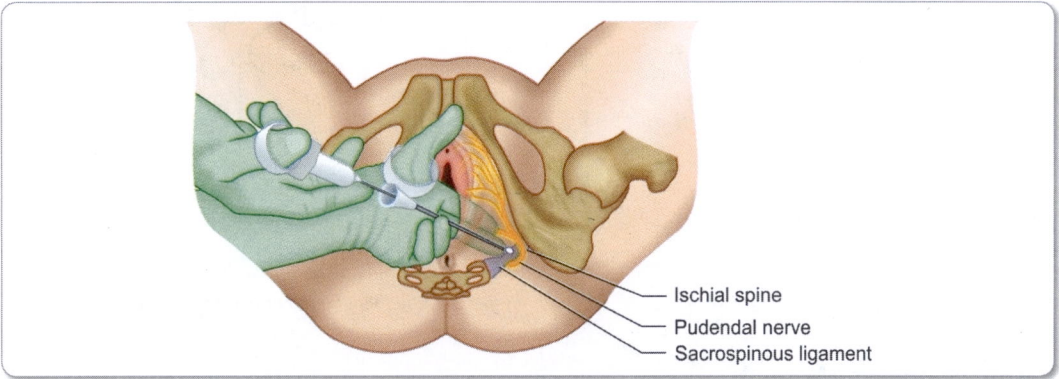

Ischial spine
Pudendal nerve
Sacrospinous ligament

**Fig. 16:** Pudendal nerve block

- **Epidural analgesia:** When complete relief of pain is needed throughout labor, epidural analgesia (Fig. 17) is the safest and simplest method for procuring it. A lumbar puncture is made between $L_2$ and $L_3$ with the epidural needle. Bupivacaine 0.5% is injected in epidural space. For complete analgesia a block from $T_{10}$ to $S_5$ is needed.
  - **Nursing responsibility:** Check blood pressure, pulse and FHR every 15 minutes.
  - **Side effects:** Hypotension, pain at the site of insertion, back pain, post spinal headache, injury to nerves, convulsions, pyrexia.

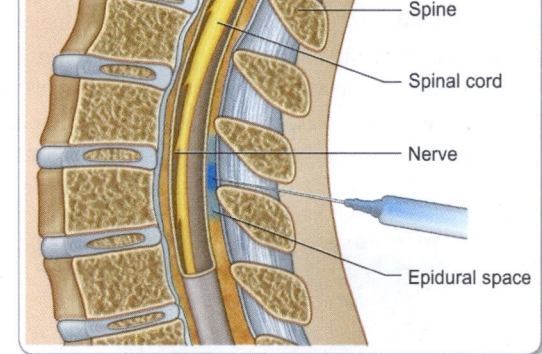

Spine
Spinal cord
Nerve
Epidural space

**Fig. 17:** Epidural analgesia

- **Spinal anesthesia:** Spinal anesthesia (Fig. 18) is obtained by injecting the drug into the subarachnoid space of third or fourth lumbar interspace with the patient lying on her side with a slight head up tilt. Bupivacaine 5–10 mg or lignocaine 25–50 mg is used.

  **Nursing responsibility:** Blood pressure and respiratory rate should be recorded every 3 minutes for the first 10 minutes and every 5 minutes thereafter. $O_2$ should be given for respiratory depression and hypotension.

- **Perineal infiltration:** This procedure is done 2–5 minutes before performing episiotomy. In this, 10 mL of 1% lignocaine is infiltrated in a fanwise manner on the proposed episiotomy site. Each time prior to infiltration, aspiration to exclude blood is mandatory (Fig. 19).

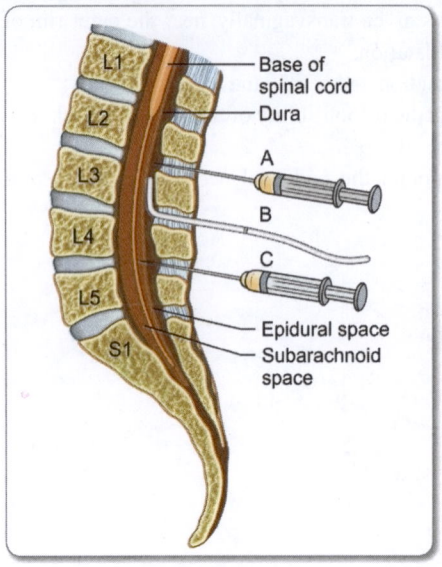

**Fig. 18:** Spinal anesthesia

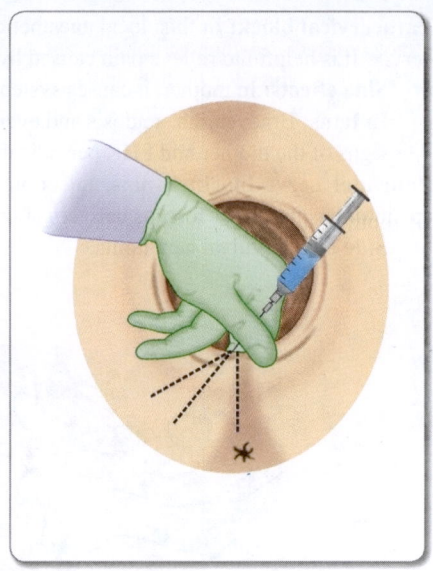

**Fig. 19:** Perineal infiltration

## Nonpharmacological Methods

- **Transcutaneous electric nerve stimulation (TENS):** In this, pain is relieved during labor by electrical nerve stimulation. Electrodes are placed over the level of $T_{10}$–$L_1$ and $S_2$–$S_4$. Current strength can be adjusted according to pain. It works by inhibiting transmitter release through interneuron level (Fig. 20).
- **Disadvantages:** Allergy caused by the use of electrodes and risk of interference with fetal monitoring.
- **Acupuncture:** In this pressure is put on the various points on the body by insertion of needles which can produce sedation and analgesia through the release of beta-endorphins.
- **Acupressure:** In this, massage is given on the specific points and it also releases endorphins in the body. During labor, it provides relaxation, helps in concentration and rhythmic breathing (Fig. 21).
- **Meditation:** Meditation and yoga also relaxe the mother and cause distraction from the pain.

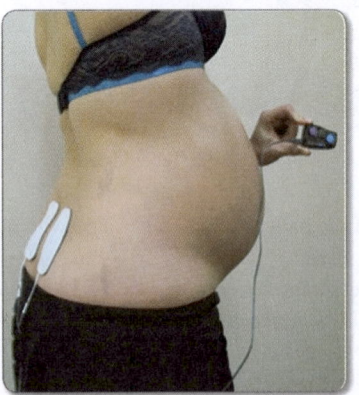

**Fig. 20:** Transcutaneous electric nerve stimulation

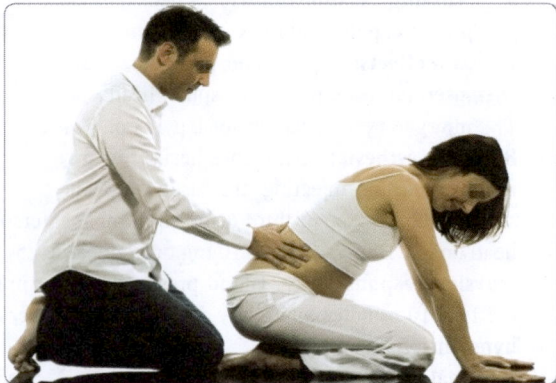

**Fig. 21:** Acupressure

## Psychoprophylaxis

It is a psychological method of antenatal preparation designed to prevent or at least to minimize pain and difficulty during labor. Relaxation and motivation can reduce the fear and apprehension to some extent. Every case of labor does not require analgesia and only sympathetic explanation is required.

## Setting up of the Labor Room including Newborn Corner

A labor room is an area in a hospital that is equipped for delivering babies.

- The obstetrical unit should be located in a manner so as to prevent unrelated traffic through the unit and to provide reasonable protection of mother from infection and from cross infection.
- An emergency communication system connected to the operations and control station should be provided by the facility.
- Resuscitation facilities for neonate should be provided within the obstetrics unit and convenient to the delivery room.
- A labor room should meet the following requirements:
    - A minimum of 80 sq.ft. of area should be provided per labor bed.
    - The labor room should be located so as to permit visual observation of each room from the nurses' working station.
    - Labor room should afford privacy and should be conveniently located with reference to the delivery room.
    - If labor room also serves as birthing room, it should be equipped to handle obstetrics and neonatal emergencies.
    - A labor room should contain facilities for medication, hand washing, charting and storage for supplies and equipment.
    - At least one shower with direct access within the delivery unit should be provided.
    - At least two labor beds with adjacent toilet should be provided for each delivery room.
    - No more than two beds may be located in one labor room.
- A toilet with hand washing facilities should be provided for the staff.
- A separate recovery room may be omitted with less than 1500 births per year.
  When provided, the recovery room should meet the following requirement:
    - A recovery room should contain not less than 2 beds and should have charting facilities located so as to permit visual observation of all beds.
    - Provisions for medicine dispensing, hand washing, clinical sink with bedpan washer and storage for supplies and equipment should be provided.
- Delivery room should be properly cleaned to reduce the spread of infection and for keeping it ready to use.
- Delivery table, mattress and mackintosh on the delivery table should be thoroughly cleaned after each use.
- Visitors and unnecessary people should not be allowed to enter in the labor room.
- There should be good source of light in the labor room. (Use special lights with each labor table).
- Prearrangement of all the articles, drugs and healthcare team members including: anesthetist, pediatrician, obstetrician and nursing officer.

## Articles for Normal Vaginal Delivery (NVD)

### For Mother

**A sterile delivery tray containing:**

- Articles for cutting and suturing an episiotomy.
    - A pair of straight, blunt-ended scissor–to cut down suture thread.

- ■ Episiotomy scissor–1
- ■ Artery clamp–3
- ■ Tissue forceps–1
- ■ Needle holder–1
- ■ Syringe and needle for infiltration—10 cc.
- Scissors for cutting the cord–1
- Bowl containing antiseptic solution
- Basin to receive placenta
- Cotton balls for cleaning the perineum
- Gauze pieces (sizes 4 × 4 pieces)
- Sterile gown, apron, gloves and mask (delivery kit).
- Sterile perineal pads

### Newborn Corner

- Flannel clothes: one to receive and dry the baby of excess secretion and another to wrap the baby
- Suction machine
- Mucous sucker
- Radiant warmer
- Cord clamp/thread
- Measuring tape
- Rectal thermometer
- Oxygen source with tubing
- Identification band (blue for male baby, pink for female baby)
- Baby clothes
- Baby blanket
- Injection Vitamin K (10 mg)
- Needle and syringe
- Neonatal resuscitation equipment should be checked and kept ready for use in case of emergency.

### Clean Tray Containing

- Antiseptic lotion–Savlon or Dettol
- Suture material
- Oxytocic drugs
- Sterile gloves
- Methergine
- Lignocaine
- Syringes and needles for injection

## SECOND STAGE OF LABOR

**Definition:** It starts with full dilatation of cervix and ends with expulsion of fetus from birth canal. *Duration is 2 hours in primipara and 30 minutes in multipara.*

It has two phases.

1. **Propulsive phase:** It starts from full dilatation up to the descent of presenting part to the pelvic floor.
2. **Expulsive phase:** It is characterized by maternal bearing down effort and ends with delivery of the fetus.

## Signs and Symptoms

- **Uterine contraction:** Contraction comes at interval of 2–3 minutes and lasts for about 1–1½ minutes.
- **Descent:** Descent of presenting part can be assessed either vaginally or by abdominal palpation. On vaginal examination, descent of head is assessed in relation to ischial spines. On abdominal examination, descent of presenting part can be estimated by number of "fifths" of the head above the brim. If it is one fifth above, only sinciput can be felt abdominally and fifth means head has almost entered in the pelvic cavity and cannot be felt abdominally.
- **Bearing down effort:** It is the additional voluntary expulsive efforts that appear during 2nd stage of labor. During the height of uterine contractions, a woman is instructed to exert downward pressure as done during defecation for the expulsion of fetus from the birth canal.
- **Rupture of membranes:** Usually the membranes rupture during this stage spontaneously and gush of amniotic fluid escapes out. This allows the hard, round fetal head to be directly applied to the vaginal tissue and helps in distention. Presenting part also stimulates nerve receptors in the pelvic floor and the woman experiences need to push.
- **Soft tissue displacement:** As the hard fetal head descends, the soft tissues of the pelvis get displaced. Bladder is pushed upward into abdomen and rectum becomes flattened into sacral curve. Levator ani muscles dilate and are displaced laterally; perineal body is flattened, stretched and thinned.
- **Dilatation, gaping of anus and perineal bulging:** Due to deep engagement of presenting part and premature bearing down effort, this may occur during later part of first stage.
- **Visibility of fetal head at introitus:** Due to uterine contraction and bearing down effort by mother, the fetal head becomes visible at the vulva, advancing with each contraction and receding during resting phase until crowning takes place and the head is born.
- **Congestion of the vulva:** Enthusiastic premature pushing may cause congestion of vulva.
- **Maternal vital signs:**
  - **Blood pressure:** Rises 15–20 mm Hg during contractions. A rise of 10 mm Hg between contractions, when a woman has been pushing normally.
  - **Pulse rate:** Increases during each pushing effort. Tachycardia may develop at the time of delivery.
  - **Temperature:** Increase of 0.5°–1°C is normal.
- **Fetal effects:** Slowing FHR during contraction but comes to normal after contraction is over.
- **Metabolism:** Metabolic rate also increases during 2nd stage. The maternal pushing efforts add further skeletal muscle activity that contributes to increase in metabolism.
- **Gastrointestinal changes:** Gastric motility and absorption decreases. Nausea and vomiting usually subside in 2nd stage but in some women it may persist.

## Physiology of Second Stage of Labor

The physiology of second stage of labor is summarized in Figure 22.

## Mechanism of Labor

### Definition

It is the series of movements that occur on the head and trunk of the fetus in the process of adaptation, when it passes through the birth canal.

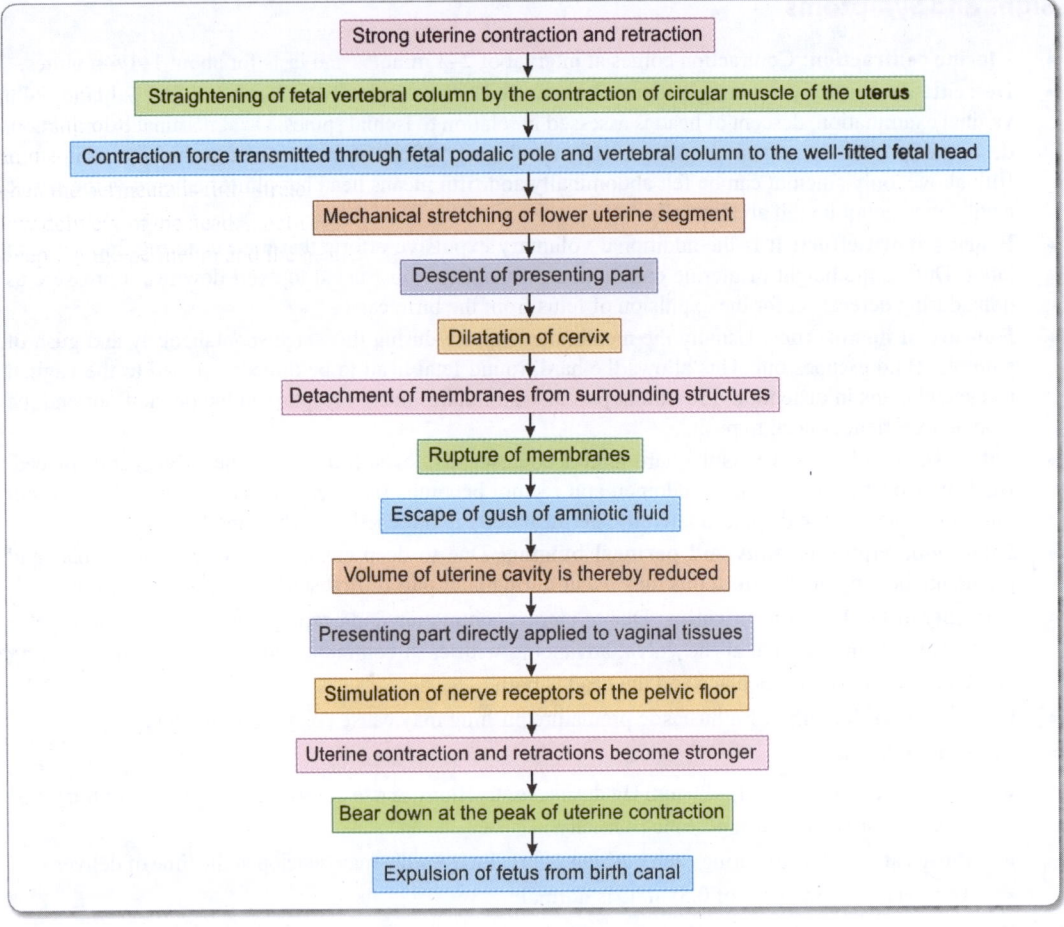

**Fig. 22:** Physiology of second stage of labor

## Common Terms used in Mechanism

- **Lie:** It is the relationship of the long axis of the fetus with long axis of the mother's uterus, for example, longitudinal, transverse and oblique.
- **Attitude:** It is the relationship of fetal limbs and head to its trunk. Normal attitude is well flexed.
- **Position:** The relationship of the denominator to the six parts of the pelvic brim is known as position or areas of the brim, for example, left anterior, right anterior, right lateral, right posterior, left posterior and left lateral. In vertex presentation, occiput is the denominator. If occiput points to the left side on the anterior side of the brim, it is known as left occipitoanterior (LOA) position.
- **Presentation:** It is the part of the fetus which lies in the lower pole of the uterus, or at the pelvic brim. For example, vertex, brow, face, shoulder cord presentation.
- **Presenting part:** It is the part of the fetus, which lies over the os during labor. For example, in LOA position of the vertex, the presenting part is posterior part of the right parietal bone.

- **Denominator:** It is the part of the presentation that determines or indicates the position. For example, in vertex presentation, the occiput; in breech presentation the sacrum, in face presentation, the mentum, in shoulder presentation, the acromion process of the scapula.

In normal labor, the most common presentation is vertex and position is either left or right occipitoanterior. The fetus is normally situated in the position as follows:

- The lie is longitudinal
- The presentation is vertex
- The position is right or left occipitoanterior
- Attitude is well flexed
- Denominator is occiput
- Presenting part is posterior part of the anterior parietal bone

Series of cardinal movements which occur in sequence as described in Figures 23 and 24.

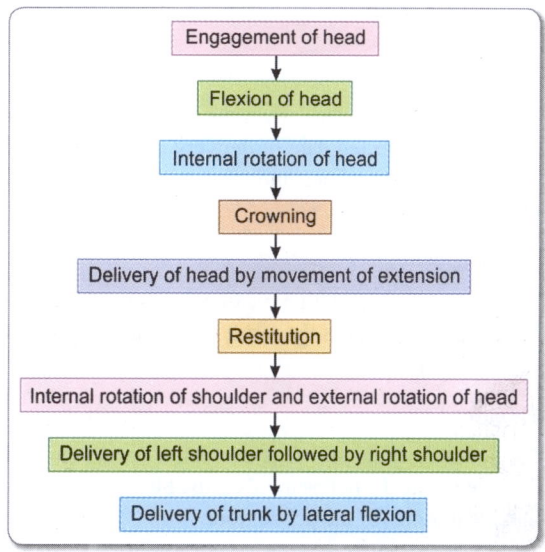

**Fig. 23:** Cardinal movement occurring in left occipitoanterior position

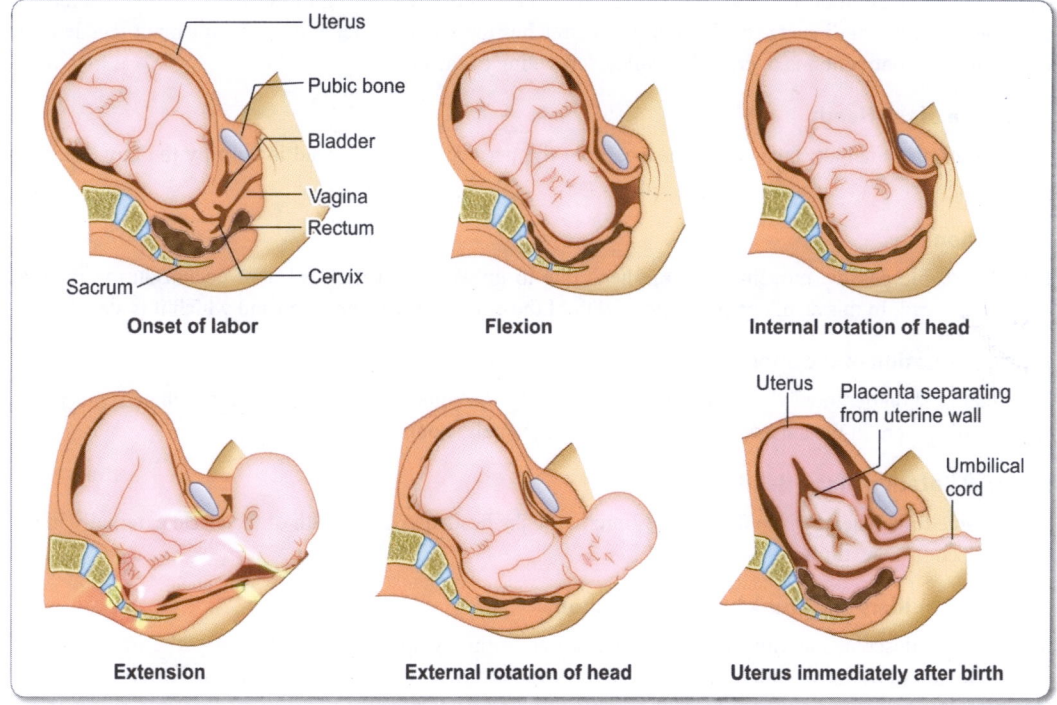

**Fig. 24:** Mechanism of labor

## Mechanism

### Engagement

Engagement takes place when the fetal head enters the pelvic brim. In primigravida, it occurs few weeks prior to the expected date of delivery but in multipara, it may take place until labor actually begins. Most commonly (70%) suboccipitobregmatic diameter (9.5 cm) of the fetal head engages in the transverse diameter of the maternal pelvis.

### Descent

Descent takes place with increased flexion and it is a continuous process until fetus is expelled out from the birth canal. Descent is the result of a number of forces including uterine contractions and maternal bearing down efforts.

### Flexion

Flexion is essential to further descent. It occurs throughout labor, resulting in smaller presenting diameter 50 as to negotiate the pelvis more easily. Flexion is achieved either due to resistance offered by undilated cervix and the muscles of the pelvic floor.

### Internal Rotation of the Head

The occiput touches the iliopubic eminence and sinciput points towards opposite sacroiliac joint. The occiput moves 1/8th of the circle anteriorly and comes under the symphysis pubis.

### Crowning

After internal rotation of the head, further descent occurs until the subocciput lies under the pubic arch. At this point, maximum diameter of the fetal head stretches the vulval outlet and the head cannot recede back even after the contraction is over, and is called "crowning of the head."

### Extension of the Head

In this step, the sinciput, face and chin sweep out the perineum and the head is born by the movement of extension.

### Restitution

It is the visible passive movement of the head due to untwisting of the neck that occurs during internal rotation of head. In this step, occiput moves 1/8th of the circle towards the side from which it is started.

### Internal Rotation of the Shoulder

The anterior shoulder moves 1/8th of the circle anteriorly and comes under the symphysis pubis. At this point, fetal shoulders are in the anteroposterior diameter of the pelvic outlet.

### External Rotation of the Head

At the same time when the shoulder moves internally, the head also turns 1/8th of the circle externally in the same direction as restitution.

### Birth of Shoulders and Trunk by Lateral Flexion

With further descent, anterior shoulder escapes below the symphysis pubis first. By the movement of lateral flexion of the spine, the posterior shoulder sweeps out the perineum. The trunk is born by the lateral flexion.

# Conduction of Normal Delivery

## Principles

- To assist in natural expulsion of fetus slowly and steadily
- To provide immediate care to the newborn
- To prevent perineal injuries
- To prevent intrapartum complications

## Preparation for Delivery

- Assess the progress of labor in terms of uterine contraction and station of fetal head.
- Note FHR after every 5 minutes.
- Assess the maternal vital signs.
- Vaginal examination is carried out to note the position, presentation, station of fetal head and to detect any abnormality.
- When the delivery is to be imminent, transfer the mother to the delivery table.
- Assist the mother in assuming comfortable position (example semi-sitting, squatting, side-lying, birthballing, etc.) Dorsal position with 15° left lateral tilt is most suitable for delivery as it prevents aortocaval compression.
- The accoucheur scrubs up and wears sterile gown, gloves and mask.
- Clean the external genitalia and inner surface of the thighs with Savlon or Dettol solution.
- Spread sterile sheet under the buttocks and one over the abdomen. Provide sterilized leggings or sterile perineal sheets.
- If bladder is full, catheterization should be done.
- Keep the trolley near the delivery table, in which articles are to be neatly placed for delivery.

## Instruments

Figure 25 shows various instruments of a normal vaginal delivery. In all, there are other articles too as given here:

- Small artery forceps
- Straight scissors
- Episiotomy scissors
- Kocher's forceps
- Sponge holding forceps
- Needle holder
- Suture material
- Sterile catheter
- Sterile gauze pieces, pads and cotton swabs
- Savlon solution
- Sterile linen
- Cord clamp
- Vital sign tray
- Drug tray (syringes, injections—oxytocin, methergine, anticonvulsant, antihypertension, xylocaine, etc.)
- Resuscitation equipment
- Instrument aids (example: forceps, ventouse)
- Radiant heat warmer
- Weighing machine
- Infantometer
- Identification band (blue and pink).

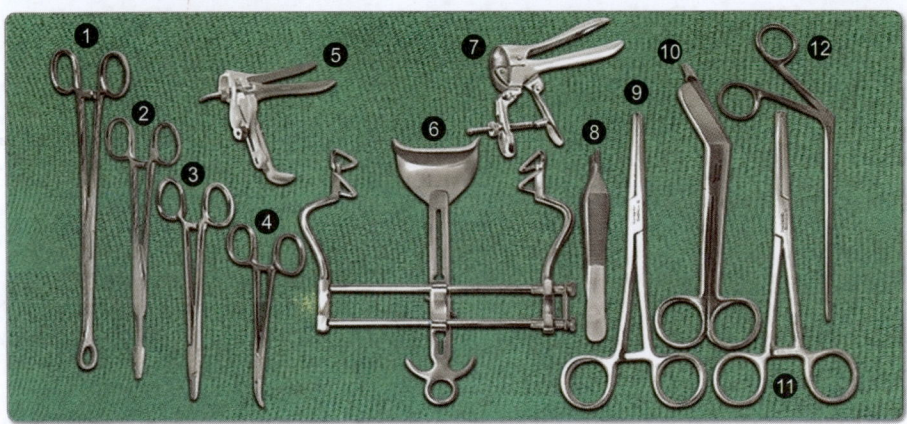

**Fig. 25:** Instruments of normal vaginal delivery. **(1)** Sponge holding forceps; **(2 to 4)** Small curved artery; **(5)** Speculum; **(6)** Retractors; **(7)** Cusco forceps; **(8)** Tooth forceps; **(9)** Vulsellum; **(10)** Episiotomy scissor; **(11)** Straight scissor; **(12)** Sponge holding curved forceps

## Team Requirement

1 obstetrician, 1 scrub nurse, 1 circulating nurse, and 1 neonatologist.

## Conduction of Delivery

The normal vaginal delivery is divided into three phases:

1. Delivery of the head
2. Delivery of shoulders
3. Delivery of trunk

### Delivery of the Head

*Principles*

- To maintain flexion of head
- To prevent early extension
- To regulate slow escape of head out of the vulval outlet

*Steps of Delivering the Head*

- To facilitate descent of the head, encourage the woman to bear down during uterine contractions.
- Due to contraction and descent of presenting part, sometimes a woman passes stool, it should be cleaned and the anal region is washed with antiseptic lotion.
- When the scalp is visible clearly from the vulval outlet, the occiput is pushed downward to maintain the flexion of the head, so that desired diameter of the head (suboccipito frontal diameter) emerges out.
- Crowning of the head occurs, when the maximum diameter of the fetal head stretches the vulval outlet and the head cannot move backward even after the contractions pass off.
- When the perineum is fully stretched, episiotomy is given prior infiltration with 10 mL of 1% lignocaine.
- Slow delivery of the head in between contractions is to be regulated. The forehead, nose, mouth and chin sweep out the perineum and the head is born by the movement of extension.

## Points to be Kept in Mind after Delivery of the Head

- After the delivery of head, the mucus and blood in mouth and pharynx are to be suctioned by mucus sucker.
- Clean the eyelids with sterile cotton swabs from inner canthus to outer canthus to prevent infection.
- Management of Nuchal Cord: If the cord is loose, slip it over the baby's head. If the cord is tight, immediately clamp (about 3 cm apart) and cut the cord at the neck before the baby is born. Tell the mother to avoid bearing down effort, while one is clamping, cutting and unwinding the cord.
- To prevent perineal lacerations/injuries:
  - Maintain flexion of head
  - Deliver the head in between contractions
  - Perform timely episiotomy
  - Provide good perineal support

## Delivery of Shoulders

- In the next contraction (after delivery of head) restitution, internal rotation of shoulders and external rotation of head usually occur.
- At this time, the bisacromial diameter is in the anteroposterior diameter of the pelvic outlet which minimizes the risk of perineal lacerations.
- A hand is place on each side of baby's head, over the ears and downward traction is applied. This allows the anterior shoulder to slip beneath the symphysis pubis, while the posterior remains in the vagina.
- When the axillary crease is seen, head and trunk is guided in upward direction to allow the delivery of the posterior shoulder.

## Delivery of the Trunk

After shoulders are delivered, the forefingers of each hand are inserted under the axillae and trunk is gently delivered by movement of lateral flexion.

## Immediate Care of the Newborn

- Receive the baby in prewarmed sterile cloth.
- Immediately after delivery of baby, mucus is drained out either by mucus sucker or by placing the infant in a tray with the head slightly downward.
- Check the Apgar score at 1 minute and at 5 minutes.
- Clamp and cut the cord by placing 2 clamps on the cord, the near one is placed 5 cm away from the umbilicus and is cut in between.
- Ligate the cord: 2 ligatures are applied on the cord, at 1 cm and 2.5 cm away from the naval.
- After cutting the cord aseptically, the baby should be dried, wrapped with dry warm clothes.
- Quick check is made to detect gross abnormality or any signs of infection.
- Apply identification band to both mother and baby.
- Show the sex of the baby to the mother.
- Check the weight, length and vital signs of the newborn.
- Put the baby on the mother's breast for feeding.
- Record the events of birth neatly and accurately, especially birth date, time, sex, examination findings, weight of newborn, etc. in the file.
- After one hour of observation, if both mother and baby are healthy, shift them in the ward.
- Sick or at risk neonate and mother need special care in special setting.

## Essential Newborn Care

Nursing care of healthy newborn baby should be provided after birth as immediate care of the neonates and daily routine care.

### Daily Routine Care

It includes the following points:

- **Warmth:**
  - Keep the baby dry and covered in adequate clothing. Ensure head and extremities are well covered.
  - Kangaroo mother care is also helpful to maintain baby's temperature.
  - Bathing is avoided for first 24 hours to prevent hypothermia.
  - Atmospheric temperature to be kept adequate (28°–32°C).
  - Temperature should be recorded frequently during initial postnatal period.
  - Warm chain should be maintained during transfer of baby.

- **Breastfeeding:**
  - Encourage the mother to initiate breastfeeding within half an hour or as soon as possible when she feels comfortable.
  - Advise the mother to breastfeed the baby on demand or every 2 hourly.
  - Educate the mother regarding importance of colostrum and exclusive breastfeeding.

- **Skin care:**
  - Baby must be cleaned of blood, mucus and meconium by gentle wiping before presenting to mother.
  - Dip bath should be avoided until the cord shed off.
  - Each baby should have own separate clothing and articles for care to prevent cross-infection.

- **Baby bath:**
  - It should be given using lukewarm water in a warm room gently and quickly.
  - Dry the baby thoroughly and wrap in warm towel. Bathing should be avoided in open spaces.
  - Perform oil massage before bath as it improves circulation and muscle tone.
  - During bathing, observe the baby for behavior and presence for any abnormalities or infections.

- **Care of umbilical cord** (Fig. 26):
  - Inspect the cord daily for any discharge, infection or bleeding.
  - No dressing should be applied and cord should be kept open and dry.
  - Educate mother that cord normally falls off after 5–10 days but may take longer in case of infection.

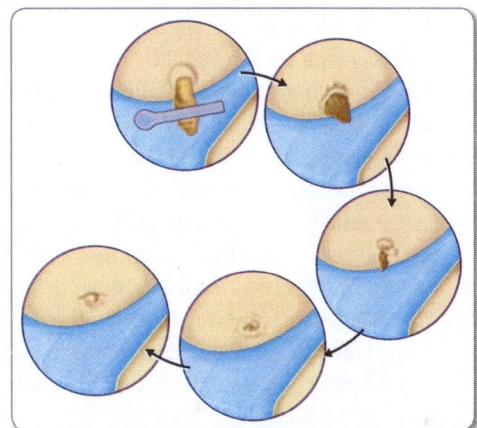

**Fig. 26:** Umbilical cord care

- **Care of eyes:**
  - Clean the eye from inner canthus to outer using single stroke.
  - Avoid applying 'Kajal' in the eyes.
  - Observe the eyes for redness, sticky discharge or excessive tearing.
- **Clothing of the baby:**
  - Baby should be dressed with loose, soft and cotton clothes.
  - Cloth should be open in the front and back for easy wearing.
  - Avoid wearing synthetic, plastic or nylon napkins.
  - Woolen clothes should not be stored with moth balls, because of chances of severe jaundice in the baby with G-6 PD deficiency.
  - Light detergent should be used for washing and baby's cloth should be washed properly and sun-dried to prevent skin-irritation.
- **General care:**
  - Promote bonding or rooming-in.
  - Gently handle the baby after proper hand washing.
  - Don't allow the infected person to touch the baby.
  - Nappies should be changed periodically.
  - Surrounding should be kept clean.
  - Allow the baby to sleep in supine position to prevent sudden infant death syndrome (SIDS).
  - Educate the mother about art of mothering.
- **Observation:**
  - Daily routine observation is essential to detect danger signs for early interventions.
  - Temperature, pulse, heart rate, feeding pattern, stool, urine and sleeping pattern should be assessed.
  - Mouth, eye, cord and skin should be checked for any infections.
- **Weight recording** (Fig. 27):
  - In the first week, there is physiological loss of baby weight.
  - After 7 days, average daily weight gain in healthy term babies is about 30 g/day in 1st month, 20 g/day in 2nd month and 10 g/day afterwards during 1st year of life.
  - Adequate breastfeeding is essential to weight gain.
- **Immunization**
  - Educate the mother regarding National Immunization Schedule.
  - Educate her regarding the importance of complete immunization and possible reaction following vaccinations.

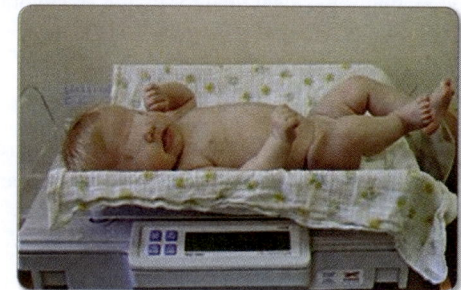

**Fig. 27:** Weighing the newborn

- **Follow-up care:**
  - Educate the mother for the follow-up of the infant, at least once every month for first 3 months and subsequently at 3-months interval till one year of age.
  - Follow-up is necessary for assessment of growth and development, early detection and management of health problems and prevention of childhood illnesses.
  - Health advice should be given to the mother regarding warmth, skin care, rooming-in, immunization and follow-up.
  - Danger signs related to childhood illnesses should be explained to mother and family members.

- Preventive measures against various child health problems should be taken.
- Harmful cultural practices should be discouraged. For example, Janam ghutti instead of colostrum.

## Episiotomy

**Definition:** It is surgically planned incision given on the perineum during second stage of labor to enlarge the vaginal introitus. It facilitates safe and easy delivery of the fetus.

### Objectives

- To enlarge the size of vaginal orifice
- To prevent perineal tear (if given on time)
- To reduce stress and strain on fetal head
- To cut-short second stage of labor
- To maintain the integrity of pelvic floor

### Indications

- Large fetus >4 kg
- Preterm or small for gestational age baby in order to minimize the risk of intracranial hemorrhage
- Presence of rigid perineum
- Face to pubis delivery, breech delivery or shoulder dystocia
- Fetal distress, to make the delivery fast
- When large lacerations seem inevitable
- In case of operative delivery, like forceps/ventouse
- Previous history of pelvic floor repair, perineal reconstructive surgery.

### Timing of Episiotomy

Bulging thinned perineum during contraction along with bearing down efforts by the mother just prior to crowning is the ideal time for giving episiotomy.

### Types

Four types of episiotomy are shown in Figure 28.

- **Mediolateral:** Incision is given downward and outwards from the midpoint of fourchette. The cut may be given either towards right or left side and about 2.5 cm.

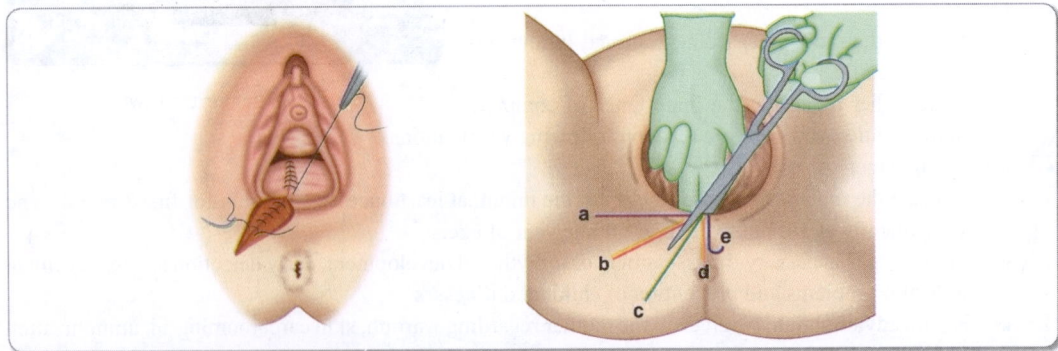

**Fig. 28:** Types of episiotomy. **a.** Lateral episiotomy; **b.** 8 o'clock episiotomy; **c.** Mediolateral episiotomy; **d.** Median episiotomy; **e.** 'J'-shaped episiotomy

- **Median/midline:** The incision is given from the center of fourchette and extends posteriorly. The cut is 2.5 cm in length.
- **Lateral:** Incision starts from about 1 cm away from the center of fourchette and extends laterally.
- **J-shaped:** The incision starts from center of fourchette and directed posteriorly about 1.5 cm and then pointed towards downward and outwards along 5 or 7 o'clock.

## Advantages

- **Maternal benefits:**
    - Clear incision is easy to repair.
    - Healing is better than lacerated wound.
    - Cut-short 2nd stage of labor.
    - Minimizes the chances of trauma to the pelvic floor-muscles.
    - Tear may be avoided.
    - There is less stretching of and less damage to the bladder, anterior vaginal wall and urethra.
- **Fetal benefits:**
    - It makes the birth safer and easier.
    - It prevents intracranial birth injuries.

## Complications

- **Immediate:**
    - Extension of episiotomy wound
    - Vulval hematoma
    - Infection
    - Rectovaginal fistula/vesicovaginal fistula
    - Wound impairment
- **Remote:**
    - Dyspareunia
    - Chances of perineal lacerations in subsequent labor
    - Scar endometriosis

### Repair of Episiotomy

**Preliminaries**

- Provide lithotomy position to the patient
- A good source of light is needed
- Instruct the mother to wide spread the thighs so that the area should be clearly visualized
- Clean the perineal area with antiseptic solution
- Patient is draped properly under aseptic precautions
- Evacuate the uterine cavity for retained clots or placenta
- Vaginal pack may be inserted and placed high up, if the wound site is obscured by oozing of blood from above, but it must be documented and removed, else may lead to sepsis

**Suture Material/Episiotomy Suturing**

Dexon or number "0" chromic catgut is usually used to repair episiotomy. It is absorbable suture. It is spontaneously shed off after 7–8 days of repair. Silk or nylon (nonabsorbable) sutures may be used and removed on 6th day (Fig. 29).

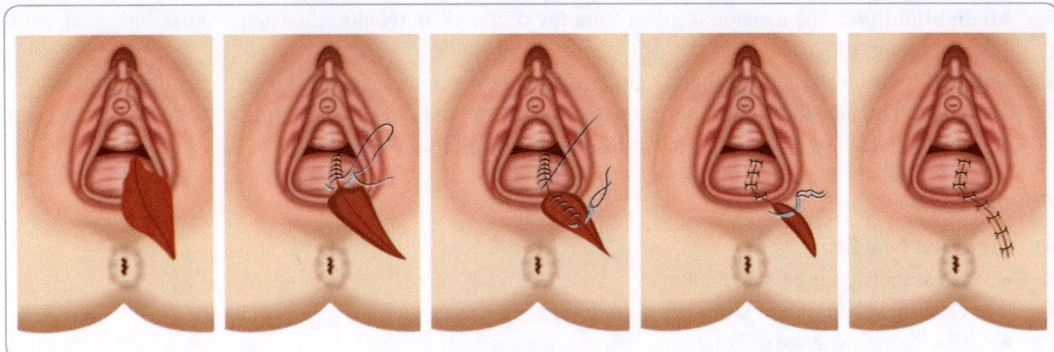

**Fig. 29:** Repair of episiotomy wound

The steps of episiotomy suturing are shown in Figure 30:

- **Vaginal mucosa** is sutured first. Firstly, inspect the apex of tear and first suture is applied just above the apex. Continuous suture is used to repair vaginal mucosa from above downwards till the fourchette is reached.
- **Perineal muscles:** Interrupted sutures are used to repair perineal muscle same from above downwards till the fourchette is reached.
- **Skin:** Mattress suture or figure of eight is used to repair skin.

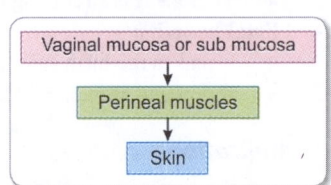

**Fig. 30:** Episiotomy suturing steps

### Episiotomy Care

- Maintenance of perineal hygiene: Instruct the patient to clean the episiotomy wound after every urination and defecation.
- Provide perineal care twice daily to the patient and clean the episiotomy wound also with antiseptic solution.
- Assess the wound healing status every time by using REEDA scale (R-Redness, E-edema, E-ecchymosis, D-discharge, A-approximation).
- If there is impaired wound healing, provide sitz bath using magnesium sulfate moist and dry heat therapy or use analgesic drugs/antibiotic therapy (local or systematic antibiotics).
- Instruct the mother, that she should not sit with crossing legs.
- Instruct the mother to ambulate to avoid stretch on the perineal wound.
- If nonabsorbable sutures are used, stitches are removed on 6th day.
- Advise the mother for abstinence of sexual activity for 6 weeks after delivery.

🧠 **Mnemonics**

**REEDA** scale
**R:** Redness
**E:** Edema
**E:** Ecchymosis
**D:** Discharge
**A:** Approximation

## THIRD STAGE OF LABOR

**Definition:** It starts after the birth of baby and ends with expulsion of placenta and membranes.

**Duration:** It is about 15 minutes in both primi and multipara, however duration is reduced to 5 minutes with active management.

## Signs of 3rd Stage of Labor

- **Pain:** Due to uterine contraction, intermittent discomfort may be felt in the lower abdomen.
- **Separation of placenta:**
  - **Before separation:**
    - Uterus is discoid in shape
    - Feels firm
    - Nonballotable
    - Fundus is below the umbilicus
    - Slight oozing of blood per vagina
    - Length of umbilical cord as visible outside remains static
  - **After separation:**
    - Uterus become globular in shape
    - Feel firm
    - Ballotable
    - Fundus is found in between symphysis pubis and umbilicus
    - Permanent lengthening of cord
    - Sudden gush of vaginal bleeding (30–60 mL)
- **Expulsion of placenta and membranes:**
  - By bearing down efforts
  - Uterine contractions
  - If required, gentle traction may be given on tags of membranes using hemostat or Kocher's clamp.
- **Maternal signs:**
  - Sudden chills
  - Shivering
  - Raise pulse rate
  - Increase blood pressure

## Physiology

The 3rd stage of labor consists of two phases:

1. Placental separation
2. Placental expulsion

### Placental Separation

**There are two ways of placental separation (Figs 31 and 32):**

1. **Schulze method (central separation):** Due to detachment of placenta resulting in opening of few uterine sinuses and accumulation of blood behind the placenta which put weight on the placenta, cause the central portion of the placenta to descend first.
2. **Matthews-Duncan (marginal separation):** Separation of placenta starts from the margin and is mostly unsupported. With subsequent uterine contraction, more and more areas get detached from the uterine wall.

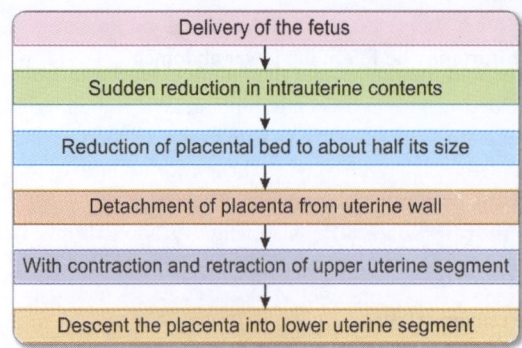

**Fig. 31:** Steps of placental separation

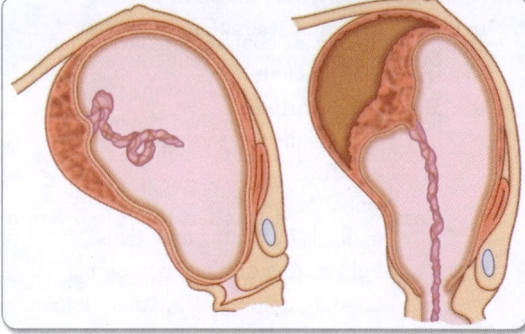

**Fig. 32:** Placental separation

## Placental Expulsion

Mechanism of placental expulsion in shown in Figure 33.

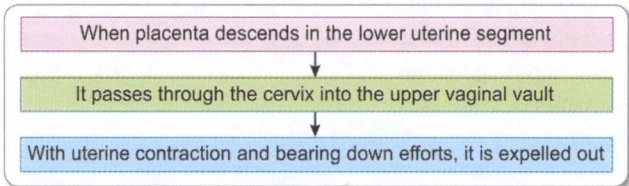

**Fig. 33:** Mechanism of placental expulsion

# Management of 3rd Stage of Labor

Management of third stage can make considerable difference due to the blood loss by the mother. Mismanaged 3rd stage is the largest single cause of postpartum hemorrhage and also causes uterine inversion and shock. Prompt nursing actions can reduce the risk of hemorrhage, infection, retained placenta and shock.

## Expectant Management

In this, placental separation and descend into vagina are allowed to occur spontaneously. Mother's efforts are used to help in expulsion. This method is practiced only if mother has not received any analgesics or oxytocic drugs.

### Steps

- A hand is placed over the fundus to feel the signs of placental separation and the state of uterine activity.
- Generally, within 15–20 minutes, placental separation takes place.
- Avoid massaging the uterus during this time.
- When signs of placental separation and descend into lower segment are confirmed, ask the client to bear down along with uterine contractions.
- As soon as the placenta passes through the introitus, it is grasped by both hands and twisted round and round so that membranes are stripped off intact.
- If there is danger of the tear of membranes, gentle traction may be given on tags of membranes using hemostat or Kocher's clamp.

## Assisted Expulsion

- In this the placental separation is not completely spontaneous but assisted.
    - **Fundal pressure:** The four fingers are placed behind the fundus and the thumb is placed in front of the uterus to use as a piston. The uterus is made to contract by gentle rubbing. When the uterus becomes hard, it is pushed downward and backward. The pressure is withdrawn as soon as the placenta expelled out through the introitus. This method is preferred when the tensile strength of the cord is less (in case of premature or macerated baby or chronic placental insufficiency).
    - **Controlled cord traction (modified Brandt Andrews method):** This method is applied only if uterus is hard and contracted and placenta is separated. In this method, left hand is placed above the symphysis pubis with the palmar surface facing towards the umbilicus to exert pressure in upward direction. The body of the uterus is displaced upwards and toward the umbilicus, while with the right hand, steady tension is given in a downward and backward direction, by holding the clamp placed on the cord until the placenta comes out of the introitus.
        - After the placenta is expelled out, examination of the placenta, membranes and cord should be done carefully.
        - Vulva, vagina and perineum should be carefully inspected for any injuries. Suture the episiotomy wound.
        - Clean the vulva and adjoining structures with antiseptic solution and sterile pad is placed over the vulva.

## Active Management

Recent guidelines recommend the active management of the third stage, so as to reduce the blood loss in 3rd stage and the management is given in Figure 34.

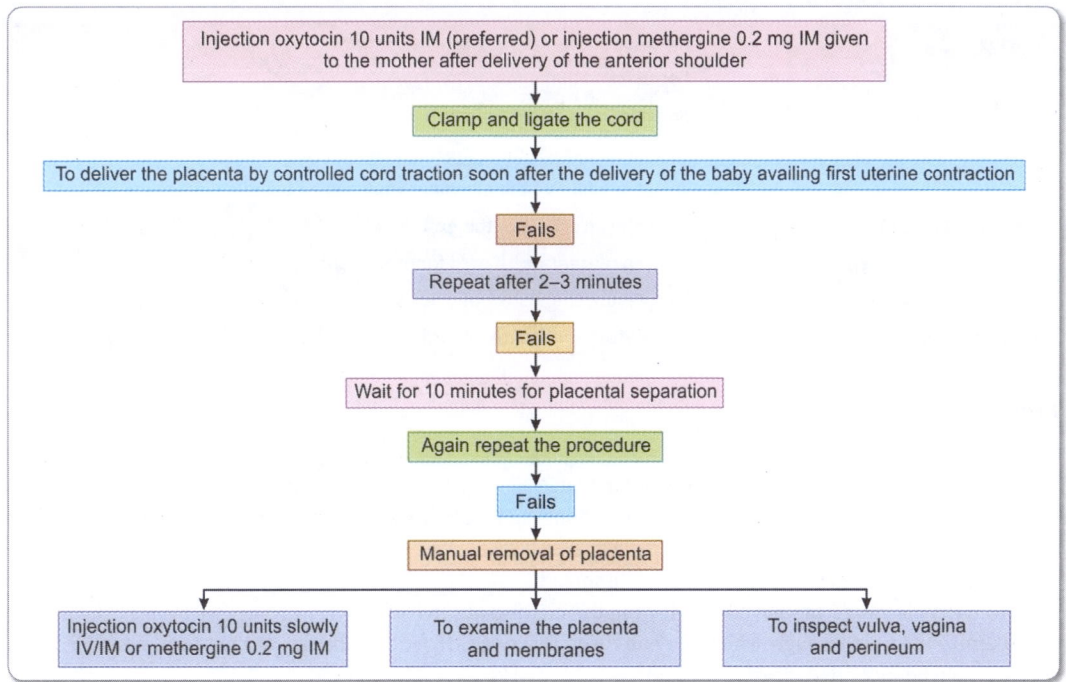

**Fig. 34:** Active management of third stage of labor

## Examination of Placenta

**Definition:** A thorough inspection and examination of the placenta and membranes, soon after expulsion, for its completeness and normalcy is advised to be done (Fig. 35).

Normally, the human placenta is:

- **Discoid**, because of its shape.
- **Hemochorial,** because of the direct contact of the chorion with the maternal blood.
- **Deciduate**, because of the connection between the mother and fetus through umbilical cord.

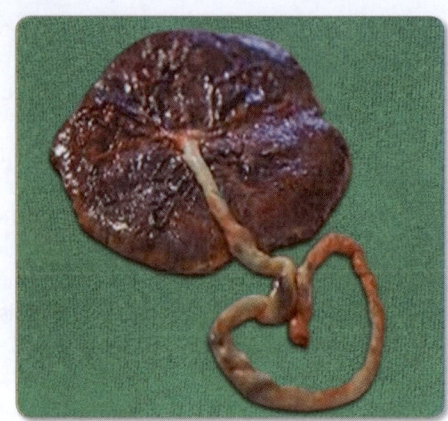

**Fig. 35:** Placental examination

### Purposes

- To assess whether the placenta is in normal size (15–20 cm in diameter), shape (discoid) and weight (1/6 of fetal weight; 500–700 g).
- To detect any abnormalities such as additional lobes, missing cotyledons (normally 15–20), infraction, etc.
- To make sure that entire membrane and placenta have been expelled out.
- To assess the length of cord (30–100 cm, 50 cm average), site of insertion of cord (at center of placenta).
- To prevent postpartum hemorrhage and infection.

### Equipment (Table 3)

**TABLE 3:** Articles and their purposes

| Article | Purpose |
|---|---|
| Placenta with cord | For examination |
| Sink with tap water | For cleaning placenta of fresh blood and blood clots |
| Gloves—1 pair | To protect the hands of the examiner |
| Mask—1 | To protect face of the examiner from spilled blood |
| Plastic Apron—1 | To protect clothing of the examiner |
| Basin with clean water—1 | To keep placenta with cord for examination |
| Mackintosh with plastic sheet | To measure the weight of placenta on weighing machine |
| Thread and tape measure | To measure the length of cord |

### Procedure

- Wear apron, gloves and mask.
- Keep placenta in basin and wash under tap water.
- Place placenta on mackintosh with paper lining and shift it on the weighing machine to measure the weight.
- Measure the length of umbilical cord with thread.
- Hold the placenta from the cord, allowing the membranes to hang.
- Identify the hole through which the baby was delivered. If the membranes are not torn, a single round hole can be identified clearly.

- Insert hand through the hole and spread out the fingers to view the membranes and blood vessels. The position of cord insertion and the course of blood vessels can be noted in this position.
- Remove the hand from inside the membranes and lay the placenta on a flat surface with the fetal surface up.
- Identify the site of cord insertion. Normally cord is inserted at the center of placenta.
- Examine the membrane, i.e. amnion and chorion for its completeness and presence of abnormal vessels and lobe. Amnion is smooth and shining but chorion is dull, rough and shaggy.
- Invert the placenta, expose the maternal surface and remove any clots present.
- Examine the maternal surface by spreading it in the palms of your two hands and placing the cotyledons in close approximation (any broken fragments must be replaced before accurate assessment is made). Ensure that no parts of placenta or membranes are left inside the uterus.
- Assess for presence of abnormalities such as infarctions, calcification or succenturiate lobes.
- Assess the umbilical cord for blood vessels (2 arteries and 1 umbilical vein)
- Place the placenta in bin for proper disposal, discard in yellow bag as it is anatomical waste.
- Clean the area used for examination of placenta and membranes, weighing scale and the bowl.
- Remove gloves, apron and mask.
- Wash hands.
- Record the findings of the placenta on mother's chart.

## FOURTH STAGE OF LABOR

**Definition:** It is the stage of observation for at least 1 hour after the expulsion of placenta and the membranes. During this period, both mother and baby are observed carefully to ensure that both are well.

### Physiology

- Uterus becomes firm and retracted (Stony hard to touch).
- When contracted, the entwining muscle fibers of the myometrium serve as ligatures to the open blood vessels at the placental site and bleeding is controlled naturally, which is also known as living ligatures.
- Thrombi form in the distal blood vessels in the decidua from where it does not get released into systemic circulation.

### Lochia

It is the vaginal discharge for 15 days to 21 days maximum. It has peculiar offensive, fishy smell and is alkaline in nature.

- It has three types: (Based on the color of the vaginal discharge)
  1. **Lochia rubra (red color):** 3–4 days, constituents are blood, decidual and trophoblastic debris.
  2. **Lochia serosa (brown ):** 5 days, consists of blood, serum, leukocytes and tissue debris
  3. **Lochia alba (white):** 10–15 days, contents are leukocytes, decidua, epithelial cells, mucus, serum and bacteria
- **Amount:** The average amount for first 5–6 days is estimated to be 250 mL.
  - Excessive lochia discharge occurs following cesarean, twin delivery and hydramnios.
  - Scanty lochia occurs following premature labor.
  - Persistent red bleeding beyond normal limit indicates subinvolution or retained products of conception.

## Care of Mother and Baby

### *Mother*

- Provide clean gown, perineal pad and comfortable position to mother.
- Check the vital signs:
  - **Temperature:** There is slight rise in temperature following delivery by 0.5°F but comes down to normal within 12 hours.
  - **Pulse:** For a few hours after normal vaginal delivery, the pulse rate is likely to be raised, which settles down to normal during 2nd day. Rise in pulse rate may be due to after-pains or excitement.
  - **Blood pressure:** It rises during delivery process which settles down gradually within 12 hours.
- **Uterus:** Immediately following delivery, the uterus becomes firm and retracted. If the uterus is soft and baggy, it means retained bits are there. Firm uterus, indicate effective uterine homeostasis. If retained bits of placenta and membranes are there, massage the uterus to remove the retained product and make them hard.
- **Vagina:** Inspect the vagina to rule out postpartum hemorrhage. If the uterus is hard, the bleeding may be due to genital tract lesions. Effective hemostasis should be maintained.
- **Hygiene:** Inspect and change pads regularly to assess the amount of blood loss during early postpartum period and maintain hygiene.
- **Fluids:** Immediately following delivery, there is increased thirst due to loss of fluids during labor, in lochia, diuresis and perspiration. Offer fluid, normally a cup of tea to the mother if not contraindicated.
- **Warmth:** Immediately following delivery, some women start shivering. Provide warm clothes and blanket and also maintain the room temperature.

### *Baby*

- **Warmth:** Keep the baby dry and wrap with adequate clothing. Ensure head and extremities are well covered. Maintain room temperature also.
- **Breastfeeding:** The baby should be put to mother's breast within half an hour or as soon as possible the mother feels comfortable. Feed the baby every 1–2 hourly or on demand of baby.
- **Umbilical cord:** Inspect cord for any bleeding.
- **Vital signs:** Check temperature, heart rate and respiration of the baby.

When fully satisfied that general condition of both mother and baby is good, shift them in the postnatal ward.

## Postpartum Family Planning

In the early postpartum period, advise the mother to adopt family planning methods for the following reasons:

- To maintain birth spacing.
- To avoid unwanted birth.
- To bring about wanted birth.
- To control the time at which birth occurs in relation to the ages of the parent.

There are several methods of contraception displayed in Figure 36:

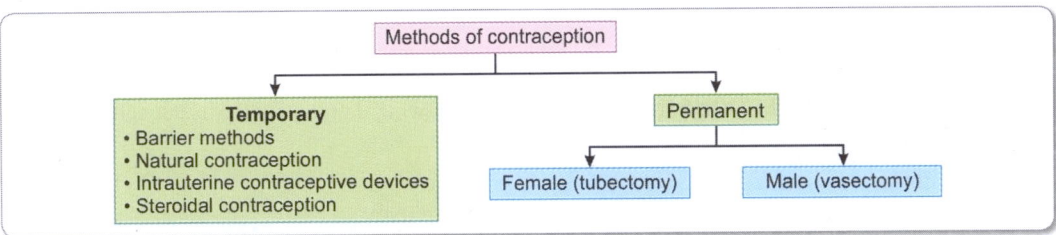

**Fig. 36:** Methods of contraception

*Note: Methods of contraception discussed in detail under Chapter 7.*

**The methods of contraception will depend upon:**

- **Breastfeeding:** Prolonged and sustained breastfeeding offers a natural protection from pregnancy. This is more effective in women who are amenorrheic than those who are menstruating. A woman who is fully breastfeeding, a contraceptive method should be used in the 3rd postpartum month and with partial or no breastfeeding, she should use it in the 3rd postpartum week. Exclusive breastfeeding provides 98% contraception. Otherwise, failure rate is 1–10%. So, additional contraceptive methods should be used such as condom, intrauterine contraceptive device (IUCD), injectables and steroids, etc.
  - Natural methods cannot be used until menstrual cycles are regular.
  - Barrier methods, like condom, diaphragm may be used.
  - **Steroidal contraception:** For nonlactating women, combined preparations are suitable from 3rd postpartum week. But in lactating women, it is avoided due to suppressive effect. Progestin is the only pill that may be a better choice for them.
  - Injectables, like DMPA/NET-EN and implants may be used.
  - Insertion of intrauterine contraceptive devices immediately following delivery is currently done. Perforation rates are less but expulsion rate is 10–20%.
- **Health status of the mother:** If mother suffers from postpartum hemorrhage, pelvic infections, etc. Intrauterine contraceptive devices should not be used. Barrier method is safe. If there is previous history of fibroids or polycystic ovarian disease, then oral contraceptives are best.
- **Number of the children:** Sterilization is suitable for those who have completed their families. Couple must be counseled adequately before adopting any permanent procedure, i.e. tubectomy or vasectomy. Individual procedure must be discussed in terms of benefits, risks, side effects, failure rate and reversibility.

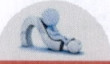

## FREQUENTLY ASKED QUESTIONS IN EXAMS

1. **Define the following:**
   a. Dystocia
   b. Show
   c. Restitution
   d. Episiotomy
   e. Labor
   f. Placenta
   g. Lightening
   h. Preterm labor
   i. Bag of membranes
   j. Primigravida
   k. Eutocia

2. **Differentiate between:**
   a. True and false labor pains
   b. Normal and abnormal labor

3. **Describe nursing management:**
   a. During 1st stage of labor
   b. During 2nd stage of labor
   c. During 3rd stage of labor

4. **Write short notes on:**
   a. Episiotomy
   b. Mechanism of normal labor
   c. Immediate care of the newborn
   d. Preparation of labor room

## MULTIPLE CHOICE QUESTIONS

1. **Delivery of baby takes place in:**
   a. 1st stage
   b. 2nd stage
   c. 3rd stage
   d. 4th stage

2. **Duration of 4th stage of labor is:**
   a. 1 hour
   b. 2 hours
   c. 8 hours
   d. 24 hours

3. **Components of partograph include all except:**
   a. Cervical dilatation
   b. Descent of head
   c. FHR
   d. Effacement

4. **Propulsive and expulsive phases occur in:**
   a. 1st stage of labor
   b. 2nd stage of labor
   c. 4th stage of labor
   d. None of the above

5. **Encourage the woman to bear down along with uterine contractions during:**
   a. 1st stage of labor
   b. 2nd stage of labor
   c. 4th stage of labor
   d. All of the above

6. **Normal duration of 2nd stage of labor in primipara is:**
   a. 2 hours
   b. 4 hours
   c. 1 hour
   d. 30 minutes

7. **Fully dilated cervix is:**
   a. 10 cm
   b. 12 cm
   c. 6 cm
   d. 8 cm

8. **Rate of cervical dilatation during active phase of labor in primigravidae is:**
   a. 0.35 cm/hr
   b. 0.5 cm/hr
   c. 1 cm/hr
   d. 1.5 cm/hr

9. **During early 1st stage of labor, duration of uterine contraction is:**
   a. 30 seconds
   b. 15 seconds
   c. 45 seconds
   d. 60 seconds

10. **When the head of the fetus is on ischial spine, the station is:**
    a. Zero station
    b. +1
    c. −1
    d. +5

11. **Episiotomy is given during:**
    a. 1st stage of labor
    b. 2nd stage of labor
    c. 3rd stage of labor
    d. None of the above

12. **Most commonly used episiotomy is:**
    a. Mediolateral
    b. Median
    c. Lateral
    d. J-shaped

13. **Blood vessels in umbilical cord:**
    a. 2 arteries and 1 vein
    b. 1 artery and 1 vein
    c. 2 arteries only
    d. 1 artery and 2 veins

14. **Weight of placenta at term is:**
    a. 1/4 of baby weight
    b. 1/6 of baby weight
    c. 1/5 of baby weight
    d. 1/10 of baby weight

15. **First stage of labor is up to:**
    a. Full dilatation of cervix
    b. Onset of true labor pains
    c. Delivery of fetus
    d. Rupture of membranes

16. **Puerperium is the period:**
    a. 1 week following delivery
    b. 4 weeks following delivery
    c. 6 weeks following delivery
    d. 2 weeks following delivery

17. **Following delivery, lochia remains for:**
    a. 10–14 days
    b. 8–9 days
    c. 4 days
    d. 21 days

18. **Lochia rubra is:**
    a. Red in color
    b. Yellow in color
    c. Pink in color
    d. Whitish discharge

19. **During the delivery of anterior shoulder, which injection is given?**
    a. Methergine
    b. Oxytocin
    c. Heparin
    d. Any from a and b

20. **Immediately after delivery, which injection is commonly given to the infant?**
    a. Vitamin A
    b. Vitamin K
    c. Heparin
    d. None of the above

21. **According to WHO, the weight of healthy newborn is:**
    a. 3 kg
    b. 2 kg
    c. 4 kg
    d. 2.5 kg

22. **Average length of umbilical cord is:**
    a. 100 cm
    b. 30 cm
    c. 50 cm
    d. 15 cm

## 🔑 Answer Key

| | | | | | | |
|---|---|---|---|---|---|---|
| 1. b | 2. a | 3. d | 4. b | 5. b | 6. a | 7. a |
| 8. c | 9. a | 10. a | 11. b | 12. a | 13. a | 14. b |
| 15. a | 16. c | 17. a | 18. a | 19. d | 20. b | 21. a |
| 22. c | | | | | | |

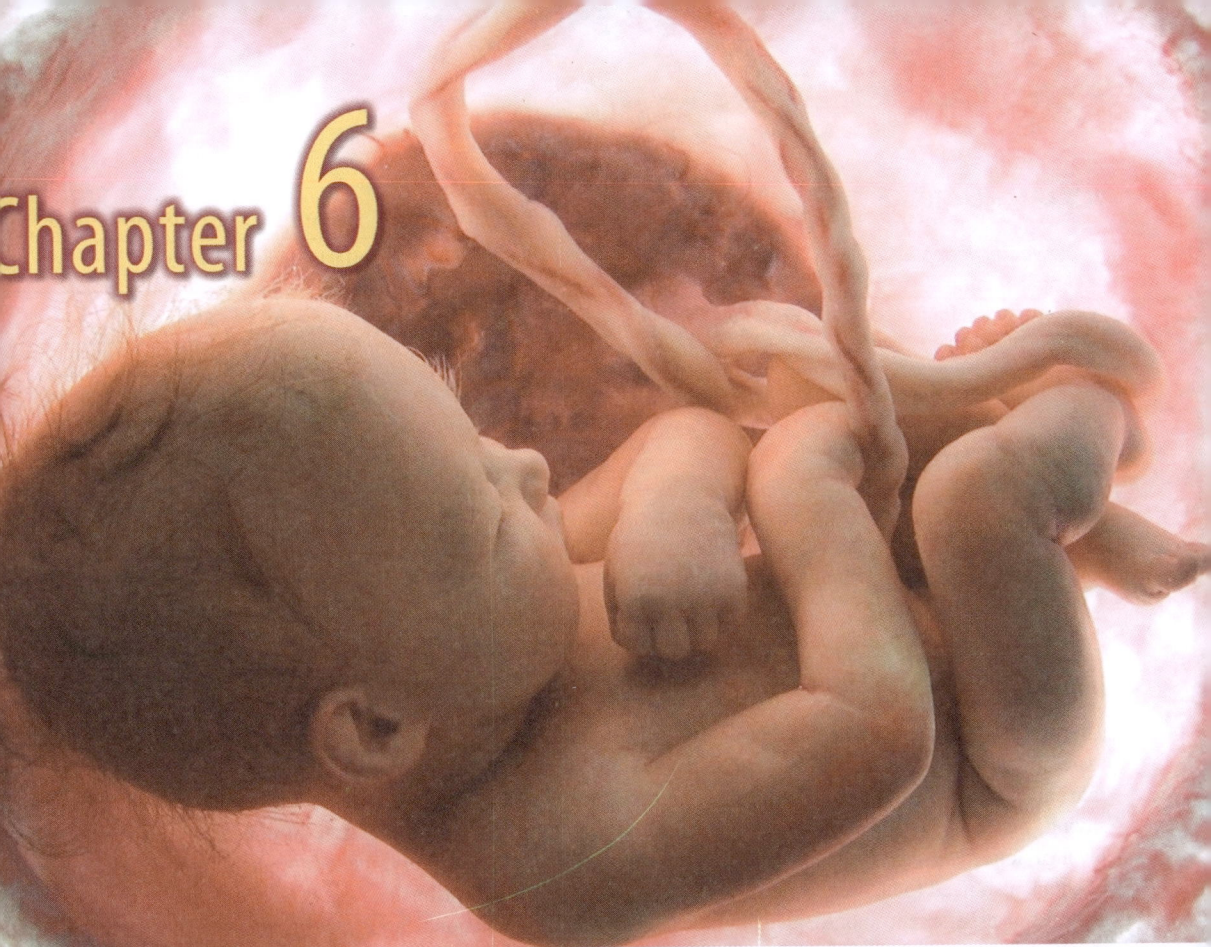

# Chapter 6

# Management of a Newborn

**Upon completing this chapter, the learner will be able to:**

➥ Describe the physiological adaptation of the newborn

➥ Explain Apgar scoring

➥ Describe the care of newborn

➥ Discuss breastfeeding and baby-friendly hospital initiative in detail

➥ Describe the minor disorders of newborn

# NEWBORN/NEONATE

The term neonate is used for a baby from birth till the first 28 days of life.

A baby born at term (between 38 and 42 weeks), has an average birth weight of 3 kg. It breathes and cries immediately after birth, establishes rhythmic respiration and adapts quickly to the extrauterine environment.

## Assessment of the Newborn

### Initial Assessment

The initial assessment of neonate is a very important activity immediately after birth. The most essential assessment is the 'First Cry'. Good cry helps in establishment of satisfactory breathing. The respiration, heart rate and skin color are the basic criteria which should be evaluated immediately to determine the need for life saving, i.e. resuscitation. The physiological status including temperature, degree of consciousness, general level of activity, gross congenital anomalies, and presence of birth injury, meconium staining and evidence of shock also need to be ascertained immediately and promptly after birth.

Initial assessment should also include assessment of gestational age, measurement of birth weight, length, head circumstance, chest circumference and detailed head to foot examination to detect the presence of congenital anomalies, like anorectal malformations, cleft lips and palate. These assessments are usually done when the baby's condition is stable.

### Goals of Initial Assessment

The goals of initial assessment of newborn are:

- To detect congenital malformations
- To protect from nosocomial infections
- To promote good health

### General Appearance

- Body symmetrical and cylindrical in shape
- Head large in proportion to the rest of the body
- Small hips
- Narrow chest
- Protruding abdomen

### Measurements

- **Head circumference:** 33–35 cm
- **Chest circumference:** 31–33 cm

- **Crown—rump length:** 35–38 cm
- **Crown—heel length:** 42–52 cm
- **Weight:** 2.5–3.0 kg (Indian baby)

## Activity

General body movements are symmetric. It includes: sneezing, yawning, sucking, rooting, swallowing, grasping, responding to sounds, blinking and crying.

## Color

- Pink body with bluish colored nail beds, palms, soles and extremities. (Acrocyanosis is normal in first few minutes after birth)
- **Temperature:** 35.5°–37.5°C

## Skin

- Covered with lanugo and vernix caseosa
- Velvet softness
- Elastic texture
- It involves other observations such as birthmark (Figs 1A and B)
    - Stork's beak mark ⎤
    - Strawberry mark    ⎟ Vascular nevi
    - Port-wine stain    ⎦
    - Pigmented skin or nonmoles (brown to black)
    - Mongolian spots

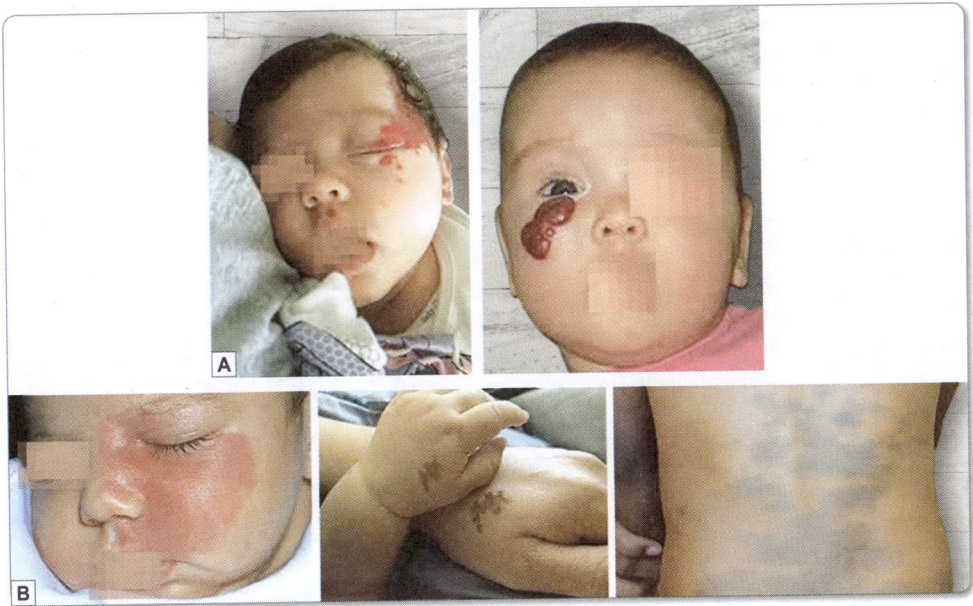

**Figs 1A and B: A.** Stork bite mark Strawberry mark; **B.** Port-wine stain brown to black mole Mongolian spots

## Head

- Slightly asymmetrical due to molding
- Caput succedaneum (swelling on the scalp)
- Cephalohematoma
- Fontanels
  - Anterior fontanel (diamond-shaped)
  - Posterior fontanel (triangular-shaped)

If fontanels are depressed conclude dehydration, bulged fontanels mean increased intracranial pressure indicating meningitis, encephalitis and hydrocephalus.

## Eyes

- Do not force to open for examination
- Puffy: Common after forceps delivery or prolonged labor
- Discharge indicates infection

## Ears

General pattern of development of both ears and position in relation to eyes (low set ears are indicative of Down's syndrome).

## Nose

- Newborn breathes through the nose
- Any flaring of nostrils may indicate respiratory distress

## Mouth

- Facial nerve paralysis
- Cleft lip/cleft palate
- Drooling of saliva (tracheoesophageal fistula)

## Neck

- Short but freely movable
- Abnormal movement to be noted

## Chest

- Assess for any discharge from nipples
- Symmetrical movements/bilateral chest expansion
- Respiratory rate of 30–60/min
- Heart rate: 120–160/min

## Abdomen

- Any distention
- Umbilical cord
  - 2 arteries and 1 vein
  - Bleeding from stump

### Liver

Normally palpable in the epigastrium

### Spleen

May be slightly palpable on occasion

### Bowel Sounds

- Sounds are audible
- Meconium may be passed soon after birth (maximum by 48 hours)

### Genitalia

- **Male baby:** Testes are palpable and descended into the scrotum (if baby is full term and in case of preterm testes may descend later also).
- **Female baby:** Edematous genitalia; labia minora and clitoris are covered by labia majora.
- **Anus:** Perforated.

### Limbs and Digits

- Length of both upper and lower extremities
- Digits: Assess for polydactylism/syndactylism
- Palms and soles creases

### Joints

Assess for range of movements for hip joints and other joints

### Back

Assess for vertebral bodies by pressing of fingers down the spines

## Newborn Reflexes

The following are newborn reflexes and some of them are shown in Figure 2.

- **Blink reflex:** When a bright light is focused on the infant's eyes, suddenly there is quick closure of the eyes. In case of impaired light perception, this reflex is absent.
- **Corneal reflex:** With a piece of cotton, cornea is touched slightly. The infant closes the eyes in response. In case of lesions of the 5th cranial nerve, this response is absent.
- **Rooting reflex:** The corner of the baby's mouth is touched with the finger. The head turns towards the stimulated side; the infant opens the mouth and tries to suck on the stimulating object.
  If baby is not hungry, the head will turn away from stimulation.
- **Palmar grasp reflex:** When any object, like finger or pencil is grasped by the flexed palm of the infant, it is called palmar reflex in case of brain damage, there is absence of the reflex.
- **Traction reflex/head lag reflex:** When pulled to an upright position by the wrists to a sitting position, the head will lag initially and then places itself right momentarily before falling forward on to the chest.
- **Tonic neck reflex:** The baby is placed on his/her back and the head is turned to one side. The arm and leg on the same side extend and the opposite arm and leg flex and the baby assumes a fencing position. If the head is turned to the opposite side, same reaction occurs. This reflex is present for 2–3 months. If persists longer than this time, it indicates neurological dysfunction.

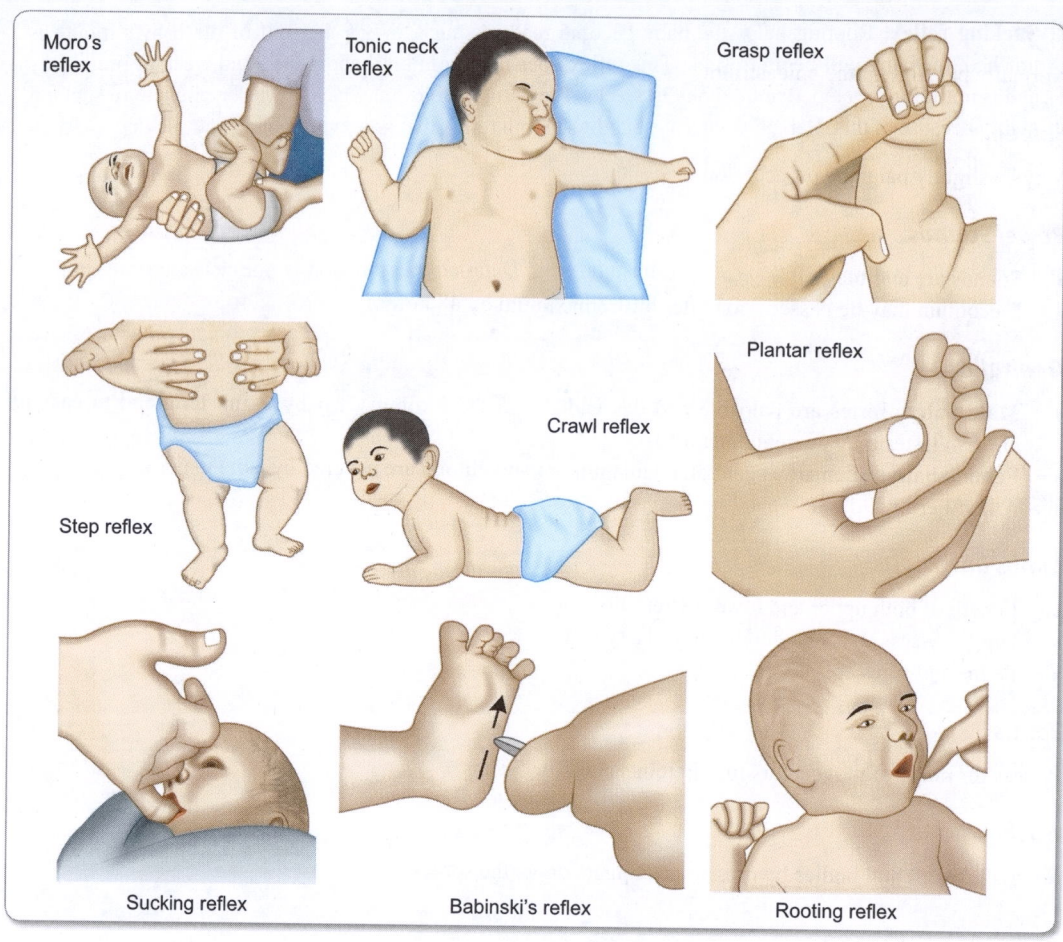

**Fig. 2:** Newborn's reflexes

- **Moro's reflex:** This reflex is elicited by sudden jerking of the cot or even a loud noise. The newborn suddenly throws his arms upwards and outwards with the hands and fingers extended with a vigorous extensor tremor of the forelimbs which rapidly subsides.
- **Walking/stepping reflex:** The baby is held so that the soles of the feet touch a flat surface. This stimulates the baby to a stepping or dancing movement with both legs. This reflex is present at birth and disappears after 3–4 weeks.
- **Plantar reflex:** When the examiner presses the balls of the infant's feet with his thumb, there is flexion of the toes. In case of defect of the lower spinal cord, this response is absent.
- **Babinski's reflex:** In this, the examiner scratches the lateral aspect of the sole of the infant's foot from heels to toes. In response, there is dorsiflexion of the toe. In case of defect of lower spinal cord, the response is absent.
- **Doll's eye reflex:** A normal response in newborns to keep the eyes stationary as the head is moved to the right or left. The reflex disappears as ocular fixation develops. It is also evaluated in comatose children for assessment of cranial nerve (III, IV, VI) function.

- **Sucking reflex:** Rooting helps the baby become ready to suck. When the roof of the baby's mouth is touched, the baby will begin to suck. This reflex does not begin until about the 32nd week of pregnancy and is not fully developed until about 36 weeks. Premature babies may have a weak or immature sucking ability because of this. Babies also have a hand-to-mouth reflex that goes with rooting and sucking and may suck on fingers or hands.

## Daily Assessment

Neonates should be observed daily during hospital stay. Detailed examination is not necessary but mother and baby should be approached two times daily and information should be collected from the mother about the feeding behavior, vomiting, passage of stool and urine, sleep and presence of any problems. The neonates should also be assessed for hypothermia, respiratory distress, jaundice and superficial infections, like conjunctivitis, umbilical sepsis, oral thrush and skin infection.

The neonates should be monitored for the danger signs. Presence of these features indicates special attention, reevaluation and early interventions. The danger signs are:

- Poor feeding, sucking and swallowing reflex
- Cold to touch or having risen in body temperature
- Poor activity and poor response to stimulation
- Excessive crying and irritability
- Rapid respiration, >60/min and presence of chest retractions
- Blue discoloration of lips or tongue
- Drooling of saliva or choking during feeding or frothiness
- Labored respiration or absence of respiration
- Jaundice appears within 24 hours and extending to palms or soles
- No urine within 48 hours and no meconium within 24 hours
- Convulsions or abnormal movements
- Bleeding from any site
- Umbilical discharge
- Superficial infections
- Diarrhea, vomiting and abdominal distention

## Physiological Adaptation

A metabolic/physiologic adjustment within the cell or tissues of an organism in response to an environmental stimulus resulting in the improved ability of that organism to cope with the changing environment is very important. In a similar way, newborn also has physiological adaptation.

### Respiratory Changes

The organ responsible for fetal respiration prior to delivery is the placenta. Upon delivery, the lungs change from a fluid-filled state to a system well-prepared for and capable of respiration. There is combination of biochemical changes and physiological changes due to other stimuli such as cold, gravity, pain, light, noise, etc. which stimulate the neonate to take the first breath.

#### Physiology of First Breath

Respiratory center is stimulated by mild hypoxia and carbon dioxide retention. During delivery baby takes the first gasp due to elastic recoil of the chest, one-third of the lung's liquid gets squeezed out through the nose during vaginal birth. Most babies cry at this time due to negative pressure of water created by elastic recoil of the chest. Lung alveoli gets filled with air and lung liquid is pushed to periphery of alveoli and gets absorbed to pulmonary circulation. With crying, lungs expand and infant breathes twice the rate of an adult.

## Circulatory Changes

- Circulatory changes begin with the clamping of the umbilical cord and the first breath is taken by the newborn. Fetal circulation alters to mature circulation due to:
  - Closure of the ductus arteriosus
  - Closure of the foramen ovale
  - Closure of the ductus venosus
  - Decreased pulmonary vascular resistance
  - Increased aortic blood pressure

  This change eliminates the placental supply of oxygen and forces the neonate to obtain oxygen from the lungs. This alters the path of blood flow and causes changes in blood volume, pressure and chemical composition. The onset of respiration increases the arterial oxygen pressure. This increase in oxygen causes vasodilatation of pulmonary arterioles and an abrupt decrease in pulmonary resistance.

## Gastrointestinal System

After around one hour of the birth, bowel sounds are present. The meconium containing bile, mucus, fatty acids and epithelial cells, are passed for 2–3 days. During the first few days, cardiac sphincter is weak which may lead to regurgitation. Physiological jaundice generally appears in the newborns due to production of glucuronyl transferase enzyme along with the red cell breakdown.

## Thermoregulatory System

As there is immaturity of hypothalamus at birth, the neonate is inefficient to maintain the optimum temperature and is at risk of hypothermia. The baby will try to maintain thermoregulation by adopting flexed posture and by peripheral vasoconstriction. The neonate is capable of producing heat through general and brown fat metabolism.

The neonate can lose heat from the body through four specific ways:

1. **Evaporation:** Whenever the skin becomes wet in a relatively dry room or incubator.
2. **Radiation:** When heat is transferred from the body to cooler objects in the environment.
3. **Convection:** With the movement of cool air passing over the surface of the body (skin).
4. **Conduction:** When heat is lost from the surface of the body to other objects in direct contact with the skin.

## Musculoskeletal System

The bones are not completely ossified, however the muscles are complete at birth. The skull bones are also not ossified completely which is mainly for the growth of brain and for helping in the molding during labor. Two fontanels which can be palpated at birth; namely, anterior fontanel (closes at around 18 months of age) and posterior fontanel (closes at around 6–8 weeks).

## Renal System

Kidney of the neonate is not adequately mature. Glomerular filtration rate (GFR) is low along with restricted tubular reabsorption. The urine of the baby is straw colored, dilute and odorless, and is passed for the first time at birth, or within 24 hours of birth.

## Reproductive System

In both the ovaries of female, primordial follicles are present. In males, there is no spermatogenesis till puberty. After the birth, there is withdrawal of the maternal hormones which can result in breast engorgement and secretion of milk in both males and females. Pseudomenstruation may occur in girls.

## Neurological System

Like other systems, nervous system is also not fully mature at birth. The brain grows rapidly after birth. Sometimes brain is not developed properly and remains immature because of which there is temperature instability and uncoordinated muscle movement. Certain reflexes are also found in baby.

(**Note:** Reflexes are already discussed in detail in the assessment of newborn at birth)

## APGAR SCORING

Dr Virginia Apgar in 1952, provided a scoring procedure that has been designed for better understanding of the clinical state of the newborn, esspecially for the circulatory, respiratory and neurological status. Five objective criteria are evaluated at one minute and 5 minutes after the birth of the baby. The criteria are: respiration, heart rate/minute, muscle tone, reflex irritability and skin color. Each of these criteria is an index of neonate's depression or lack of it at birth and is given a score of 0, 1 or 2. The score from each of the criteria is added to determine the total score. The neonate is in the best possible condition if the score is 10. Scores of 7–10 indicate no difficulty in adjustment in extrauterine life. Scores of 4–6 signify moderate difficulty and if the score is 3 or below, the neonate is in severe distress which must be treated immediately (Table 1).

**TABLE 1: Apgar score**

| Indicator | 0 | 1 | 2 |
| --- | --- | --- | --- |
| Respiration | Absent | Slow, irregular | Good, crying |
| Heart rate | Absent | Slow (below 100) | More than 100 |
| Muscle tone | Flaccid | Some flexion of extremities | Active body movements |
| Reflex response | No response | Grimace | Cry |
| Skin color | Blue, pale | Body pink, extremities blue | Completely pink |

**Total score = 10**
- No depression = 8–10
- Mild depression = 5–7
- Moderate depression = 3–4
- Severe depression = 0–3

Usually, neonates have lower score at one minute than the score at 5 minutes due to presence of depression immediately after birth. The 5-minute score has greater predictive value, since it correlates with neonatal morbidity and mortality. It also correlates more closely with the infant's neurologic status at 1 year of age.

**Note:** *If Apgar Score is less (severe depression), management of Asphyxia/respiratory distress syndrome is discussed in Chapter 11—High-risk and Sick Newborn.*

Chapter 6 ● Management of a Newborn

## EXAMINATION FOR DEFECTS

- **Head:** Head should be examined for presence of caput–succedaneum, cephalhematoma, encephalocele, widely separated or closed sutures and abnormalities of fontanels (enlarged, bulging, or sunken).
- **Face:** It should be observed for symmetry, paralysis, shape, swelling and abnormal movements
- **Eyes:** Eyes should be checked for edema, conjunctivitis, subconjunctival hemorrhages, color of sclera, Brushfield spots (Trisomy 21), strabismus, congenital cataract, pupillary size and reflex, abnormal placement of eyes (chromosomal anomalies) or abnormal distance between two eyes.
- **Nose:** Nose is examined for patency, low nasal bridge, nasal discharge, nasal flaring, etc.
- **Ears:** Ears should be examined for formation or size and shape, sufficient cartilage and position (low set ears indicate chromosomal anomalies), skin tags, preauricular sinus, etc.
- **Mouth:** Mouth should be checked for cleft palate in hard palate or soft palate, size of mouth cavity and oral opening, size of tongue, presence of natal teeth, Epstein's pearls, tongue tie, etc.
- **Neck:** Neck should be checked for mobility, fracture of clavicle, stiffness or rigidity, hyperextension, torticollis, any cyst or mass, excessive skin fold (trisomy 21) and webbing of the week.
- **Chest:** Abnormal shape and size of chest should be observed. Breast engorgement may be present due to withdrawal of maternal hormones usually at day three. Rate and rhythm of respiration, chest retractions and abnormal respiratory sound should be examined.
- **Abdomen:** Abdomen should be observed for its shape, distension (may be due to bowel obstruction, abdominal mass, enlargement of organ or infection) and synchronous movement with chest in respiration. Umbilical cord should be observed for the signs of infection, discharge, redness, and presence of hernia or any congenital anomalies (single artery). Abdomen should be palpated for any masses (Liver edge is usually felt 2 cm below costal margin and spleen tip).
- **Genitalia:** Female baby should be examined to assess whether labia majora covers labia minora and clitoris. Hymenal tag or imperforate hymen may be present. Vaginal white mucoid discharge or pink-red mucous discharge may be found due to withdrawal of maternal hormones. Full term male baby usually has both testes in scrotal sac and scrotum appears pigmented and markedly wrinkled with rugae. Penis should be examined to detect hypospadias, epispadias, phimosis or abnormal length. Ambiguous genitalia, hydrocele and inguinal hernia should be looked for.
- **Back:** Back should be checked for abnormal spinal curvature, tufts of hair or skin disruptions indicating spina bifida occults. Meningocele, meningoencephalocele and anencephaly are usually detected at initial assessment.
- **Buttocks:** It should be observed for any mass (sacrococcygeal teratoma). Perianal areas should be examined for anal opening, anal fissures or any other abnormalities
- **Hips:** Examination of hips to be done to detect congenital dysplasia. Positive Ortolani's sign and asymmetrical gluteal folds are indicative of the condition.
- **Extremities:** Extremities are examined for fractures, paralysis, range of motion and irregular position. Fingers and toes to be checked for missing digits, extra digits (polydactyly) or fused digits (syndactyly). Feet to be looked for structural or positional abnormalities mainly club foot (talipes equinovarus).
- **Neurological status:** In the neonates, neurological mechanism is immature both anatomically and physiologically which results in disturbance of temperature regulation, uncoordinated movements and lack of control over musculature. Examination of muscle tone, head control and reflexes is an essential aspect.

## BREASTFEEDING

Breastfeeding is the "Gold standard" for infant feeding. All the babies, regardless of the type of delivery, should be given early and exclusive breastfeeding up to 6 months of age. Exclusive breastfeeding means giving nothing orally other than colostrum and breast milk. Medicines and vitamins are allowed. There are several areas of biological superiority of breastfeeding and breast milk over artificial (formula) milk. Obstetricians and midwives should educate the mother during prenatal and postnatal period for the usefulness of breastfeeding.

## Colostrum

For the first 2 days following delivery, no further anatomic changes in the breast occurs. The secretion from the breast is called colostrum, which starts during pregnancy and becomes more abundant during this period.

### Composition of the Colostrum

It is deep yellow serous fluid, alkaline in reaction. It has got a higher specific gravity; a high protein, vitamin A, sodium and chloride content but has got lower carbohydrate, fat and potassium than the breast milk. It contains immunoglobulin (IgA), complements, macrophages, lymphocytes, lactoferrin and other enzymes (Lactoperoxidase).

### Advantages

- The antibodies (IgA, IgG, IgM) and humoral factors (lactoferrin) provide immunological defense to the newborn.
- It has laxative action on the baby because of large fat globules.

## Types of Breast Milk

While the content of breast milk changes over the course of baby's development, there are essentially three types of breast milk: colostrum, transitional milk, and mature milk.

1. **Colostrum:** Colostrum is the first stage of breast milk. It is the yellowish milk produced during the pregnancy and can last for several days after the baby's birth. Colostrum is very rich in nutrients and antibodies, making it the perfect food for a newborn child. Colostrum is high in protein, fat-soluble vitamins, minerals, and immunoglobulins. Immunoglobulins are antibodies that pass from the mother and provide passive immunity to the babies. Passive immunity protects babies from a wide range of bacterial and viral diseases. Two to four days after birth, colostrum will be replaced by transitional milk.
2. **Transitional milk:** Transitional milk replaces colostrum within four days after the pregnancy and lasts for about two weeks. It contains lactose, water-soluble vitamins, and high levels of fat. Transitional milk also contains more calories than colostrum does.
3. **Mature milk:** Mature milk begins to appear near the end of the second week after pregnancy. Mature milk is thinner and contains more water than transitional milk does. Water makes up to 90% of mature milk, which helps to keep the babies hydrated. The other 10% consists of carbohydrates, proteins, and fats needed for the growth of the babies. There are two types of mature milk: foremilk and hindmilk. Foremilk occurs at the beginning of the feeding and contains vitamins, water, and proteins. Hindmilk forms at the end of the feeding and contains higher levels of fat, which is necessary for the child's weight gain. Both are necessary to ensure that the baby is receiving adequate nutrition to grow up healthily.

## Benefits of Breastfeeding

### For Baby

- **Proper nutrition:** Breast milk has right amount of fat, sugar, water and proteins which are helpful for the proper growth and development of the baby.

- **Ideal composition:** Breast milk contains all required nutrients for easy digestion.
- **Higher intelligence:** Researches show that breastfed babies have higher intelligence. Breast milk affects the metabolism of fatty acids, such as docosahexaenoic acid (DHA) and arachidonic acid (AA) which are known to be linked with early brain development.

- **Long-term health effect:** Breast-fed babies have:
  - Less chances of developing diabetes
  - Less risk of obesity
  - Less risk of asthma
  - Protection against allergies
  - Protection against respiratory and intestinal infections
- **Other advantages:**
  - No need to prepare the feed
  - It has laxative action
  - Lessens the incidence of sore buttocks and atopic eczema
  - Lessens the chances of scurvy and rickets
  - Provides immunity to the baby

### For Mother

- **Acts as contraceptive:** Lactation suppresses the ovulation and delays the return of fertility through lactational amenorrhea.
- **Mother-baby bonding:** Breastfeeding promotes bonding between mother and baby.
- **Uterine involution:** During breastfeeding, there is a release of oxytocin that makes the uterus contract more quickly and reduces postpartum bleeding.
- **Weight loss:** With breastfeeding, some calories are lost that in turn reduces weight of the mother.
- **Long-term health effects:** With breastfeeding, there is less risk of breast cancer, ovarian cancer and endometrial cancer. Breastfed diabetic mother requires less insulin and there is less risk of postpartum hemorrhage.

## Different Positions used for Breastfeeding

- Cradle position:
  - Hold the baby in your arms with its back lying along your inner arm.
  - Baby's head should be on your forearm.
  - It should be facing your breast, with its mouth aligned with your nipple.
  - Pillows can be used to raise the baby's mouth to the appropriate nipple height.
  - Baby's head and bottom should be aligned with each other.
- Reverse cradle hold:
  - While sitting upright, place one or more pillows on mother's lap in order to raise the baby up to nipple's height.
  - Use the cradle hold with the opposite arm. Use your hand to support baby's head and place a pillow under your hand for support. Your free hand will support breast.
  - Baby turned on its side facing you, touch baby's lips with your nipple. When the baby opens its mouth to begin sucking, pull the baby close to you. Breast will open the baby's mouth further for bigger mouthfuls of milk.

- Clutch hold:
  - Sit upright with back and shoulders well supported.
  - Place a pillow on mother's lap, towards the side of hip.
  - Place the baby on the pillow, facing the mother.
  - Baby's mouth should be aligned with mother's nipple.
  - Tuck baby's legs and feet under mother's arm and bend the baby slightly at the waist so that its legs stretch out along mothers back.
  - The soles of baby feet should be facing the ceiling with its legs pointing upwards and its bottom resting on the pillow.
  - Do not cup baby's head; instead, place the hand under its neck.
  - Once baby begins sucking, place a pillow under the hand that is supporting the baby.
- Side-lying position:
  - Mother should lie on side. For back support; place a pillow behind the back. Use two pillows to support the head. Place a pillow under the top leg for comfort and place one pillow behind the baby.
  - Lay the baby on its side, facing mother with its mouth aligned to mother's nipple. Guide the baby's head onto mother's nipple until it latches on. Keep in mind that this is a position that is best used with babies who have already developed good latching skills.
- Laid back position:
  - Good posture and support are crucial to this position. Lie flat on the bed and elevate head and shoulders slightly with pillows.
  - Place baby face down onto your stomach with its cheeks towards breast. Baby's lips must be close enough to mother's nipple to allow the baby to suck. Adjust mother's elevation by adding or removing pillows as necessary.

## Management of Breastfeeding

- **Time of first feeding:** The baby can be put to mother's breast within half an hour after birth. The sucking reflex is the strongest in the first half hour after birth
- **Feeding schedule:** The baby should be permitted to suck freely the breast frequently and without any fixed time table (demand feeding)
- **Duration of feeding:** On first day, 2–3 minutes on each breast may be sufficient and the duration may be increased by a minute per breast per day.
  After the initial week, the baby should be fed for 7–10 minutes at each breast when baby indicates it is hungry.
- **Beginning breastfeeding:**
  - Instruct mother to clean baby's nipple and areola with wet swab or soft cloth before and after each feed.
  - Advice mother to keep clean hands, short nails and wear clean clothes.
- **Teach the technique of breastfeeding:**
  - Assume comfortable position–Sitting or lying in bed.
  - Place the nipple and areola into baby's mouth.
  - Relax and give full attention to baby while feeding and keep the baby awake while feeding.
  - Rotate breasts at the starting and ending of breastfeed for complete emptying of both breasts.
- **Burping (breaking the wind):**
  At the end of feeding from each breast, burping is done for five minutes to prevent regurgitation and vomiting. Burping helps the baby to bring out swallowed air from stomach. For burping, hold the baby

in upright position either on the shoulder or lap and gently pat the back upwards until the swallowed air is expelled.

## Difficulties Related to Breastfeeding

### *Related to Mother*

- Breast engorgement
- Inadequate supply of milk
- Poor attachment to breast
- Stress and anxiety
- Short or very large nipples

### *Related to Baby*

- Low-birth-weight baby
- Illness of the baby
- Over distention of stomach

## Contraindications to Breastfeeding

- Mothers who are taking drugs that can be harmful to baby such as cytotoxics, certain hormones and radioactive isotopes
- Infectious diseases such as typhoid fever, human immunodeficiency virus (HIV) infection and active pulmonary tuberculosis
- Chronic medical illnesses such as heart diseases, severe anemia and poorly controlled epilepsy
- Puerperal psychosis
- Mother taking high doses of antiepileptics, anticoagulants and antithyroid drugs
- Babies with cleft lip and cleft palate
- Preterm and very ill babies.

## BABY-FRIENDLY HOSPITAL INITIATIVE

### Introduction

- BFHI is a global movement, spearheaded by WHO and UNICEF that aims to give every baby the best start in life by creating a health care environment where breastfeeding is the norm.
- Maternity wards and hospitals applying the principles in the joint statement are being designated baby friendly to call public attention to their support for sound environment.
- The joint WHO/UNICEF statement on breastfeeding and maternity services has become the centerpiece of the BFHI.

### Goals of BFHI

1. To transform hospitals and maternity facilities through implementation of the "ten steps".
2. To end the practice of distribution of free and low-cost supplies of breast milk substitutes to maternity wards and hospitals.
   - BFHI has incorporated the International Code of Marketing of Breast-milk Substitutes (1981) and is aimed to protect and promote breastfeeding.

- Since the launch of initiative, more than 20,000 hospitals in 156 countries in the world have adopted it over the last 15 years.

## Steps of BFHI

The criteria for a hospital's baby friendly accreditation are as follows:

- Have a written breastfeeding policy that is routinely communicated to all health care staff.
- Train all healthcare staff in skills necessary to implement this policy.
- Inform all pregnant women about the benefits and management of breastfeeding.
- Help mothers initiate breastfeeding within half an hour of birth.
- Show mothers how to breastfeed and maintain lactation, even if they should be separated from their infants.
- Give newborn infants no food or drink other than breast milk, not even sips of water, unless medically indicated.
- Practice rooming in, i.e. allow mothers and infants to remain together 24 hours a day.
- Encourage breastfeeding on demand.
- Give no artificial teats or pacifiers (also called dummies or soothers) to breastfeeding infants.
- Foster the establishment of breastfeeding support groups and refer mothers to them on discharge from the hospital or clinic.

The program also restricts use by the hospital of free formula or other infant care aids provided by formula companies and recommends that when formula is medically needed, it should be given in a small cup or spoon, rather than a bottle and should only be used to supplement breastfeeding.

## Summary and Role of Baby-Friendly Hospitals

**Aim:** To contribute to the provision of safe and adequate nutrition for infants by:
- The protection and promotion of breastfeeding, and
- Ensuring the proper use of breast-milk substitutes, when these are necessary, on basis of adequate information and through appropriate marketing and distribution.

**Scope:** Marketing, practices-related quality and availability, and information concerning the use of:
- Breast-milk substitutes, including infant formula
- Other milk products, foods and beverages, including bottle-fed complementary foods, when intended for use as a partial or total replacement of breast milk
- Feeding bottles and teats

## Summary of the Main Points of the International Code

- No advertising of breast-milk substitutes and other products to the public
- No donations of breast-milk substitutes and supplies to maternity hospitals
- No free samples to mothers
- No promotion in the health services
- No company personnel to advise mothers
- No gifts or personal samples to health workers
- No use of space, equipment or education materials sponsored or produced by companies when teaching mothers about infant feeding.
- No pictures of infants, or other pictures idealizing artificial feeding on the labels of the products.

- Information to health workers should be scientific and factual.
- Information on artificial feeding, including that on labels, should explain the benefits of breastfeeding and the costs and dangers associated with artificial feeding.
- Unsuitable products, such as sweetened condensed milk, should not be promoted for babies.

## Global Strategy on Infant and Young Child Feeding (IYCF)

**Aim:** To improve—through optimal feeding—the nutritional status, growth and development, health, and thus the survival of infants and young children.

## Further Strengthening of BFHI

The global strategy urges that hospital routines and procedures remain fully supportive of the successful initiation and establishment of breastfeeding through the:
- Implementation of the baby-friendly Hospital Initiative
- Monitoring and reassessing already designated facilities
- Expanding the initiative to include clinics, health centers and pediatric hospitals

# CARE OF NEWBORN

(***Note:*** *Already discussed in Chapter 5 "Normal Labor and its Management" i.e. In Immediate and Essential Newborn Care*)

## Rooming-in

Rooming-in is the practice followed in hospitals and nursing homes where the baby's crib is kept by the side of the mother's bed. This arrangement gives an opportunity for the mother and father to know their baby. The bond between the parent and the child is well established in roomed-in babies. There is a better chance of success with breastfeeding in roomed-in babies. Parents do not have the fear of baby-switching while roomed-in.

Rooming-in is one of the components of baby-friendly hospitals, devised by WHO Step 7: Practice rooming-in—allow mothers and infants to remain together—24 hours a day.

### Benefits for Mother

- Cost effective
- Requires minimal equipment
- Requires no additional personnel
- Better quality sleep
- Increased confidence in handling and caring for baby
- Ability to learn what baby's cues are (sleepy, stressed, in need of quiet time, or hungry)
- Earlier identification of early feeding cues (rooting, opening mouth, and sucking on tongue, fingers, or hand)
- Improved breastfeeding experience
- Less infant crying and distress
- Less "baby blues" and postpartum depression
- Parents are better-rested and more relaxed

### Benefits for Baby

- It reduces infection
- It helps in establishing and maintaining breastfeeding
- It facilitates the bonding process which can positively affect breastfeeding duration rates
- It provides baby with better quality sleep. The baby develops a more regular sleep-wake cycle earlier, which eases the transition to day/night routines
- It helps in keeping stable body temperature
- Generally, baby feels more content, less crying because it interact with only one caregiver—mother.
- It helps in keeping more stable blood sugar
- It helps in producing lower levels of stress hormones

### Disadvantages

Handling the baby is not easy. If mother had undergone cesarean section, then she will need somebody to handle the baby and place the baby in the position for breastfeeding. After normal delivery, mother may have episiotomy. In such a case, it is very painful to sit and feed the baby with episiotomy.

## Bonding-in

**Definition:** Bonding is the formation of a mutual emotional and psychological closeness between parents (or primary caregivers) and the newborn. Babies usually bond with their parents within the minutes, hours, or days following birth.

*Bonding*, the intense attachment that develops between parents and baby, is completely natural. It is probably one of the most pleasurable aspects of *infancy*.

### Importance

When the umbilical cord is cut at birth, physical attachment to the mother ceases, and emotional and psychological bonding begins. A firm bond between mother and child affects all later development, and it influences how well children will react to new experiences, situations, and stresses. Some studies have shown that the babies were better socialized when they had their mothers to interact with. Hence, bonding is essential for survival.

> **Know it**
>
> **Kangaroo Mother Care (KMC)**
> - KMC refers to care of preterm or low-birth-weight infants by placing the infants in skin-to-skin contact with the mother or any other caregiver.
> - KMC results in keeping neonates warm and cozy. Babies get protected against cold stress and hypothermia. The heart and respiratory rates, oxygenation, sleep patterns get stabilized.
> - It significantly increases milk production in mothers and exclusive breastfeeding rates. Improves weight gain, reduces incidence of respiratory tract and nosocomial infection, it improves emotional bonding between the infant and mother.
> - KMC is indicated to all stable low-birth-weight (LBW) babies. For sick babies, short KMC sessions can be initiated during recovery with ongoing medical treatment. It can be provided while baby is being fed via Orogastric tube or on oxygen therapy.
> - All mothers can provide KMC irrespective of age, parity, education, culture and religion. Mother should be free from serious illness. A mother should receive adequate diet and supplements recommended by her physician.

Chapter 6 ❂ Management of a Newborn

### Common Problems Related to Bonding

When the interactive, reciprocal "dance" between the parent and newborn is disrupted or becomes difficult, bonding experiences are difficult to maintain. Disruptions can occur because of medical problems with the infant or the parent, the environment, or the fit between the infant and the parent.

- Problems with the newborn or the parents:
    - The parents or caregiver's behavior can also hinder bonding.
    - Maternal problems, like postpartum depression, substance abuse, or overwhelming personal problems that interfere with his/her ability to be consistent and nurturing the child.
- Environment:
    - A major impediment to healthy bonding is fear.
    - If an infant is distressed because of pain, pervasive threat, or a chaotic environment, the baby may have a difficult time engaging in a sympathetic care-giving relationship.
- Fit between the infant and the parent:
    - The fit between the infant's temperament and capabilities and those of the mother and father is important. Some parents can bond with a calm infant but are overwhelmed by an irritable infant. Understanding each other's nonverbal cues and responding appropriately is essential to preserving the bonding experiences that build healthy attachments.
    - The first phase of bonding takes place in the womb; researchers believe difficult and unwanted pregnancies and planned adoptions interfere with mother and infant bonding.
    - Teenagers and immature mothers often conceal and reject their pregnancies. This behavior and feeling may result in abandonment, neglect, and the absence of bonding at birth.
    - Mothers may have difficulty in bonding with an infant if prenatal testing suggests the child will have a birth defect or are likely to be mentally retarded and malformed.

### Ways to Develop Bonding

- Have plenty of skin-to-skin cuddle time. Touch is soothing for both mother and baby, so hold the baby often and stroke him gently.
- Give breastfeeding as it releases hormones in mother's body that promote relaxation as well as feelings of attachment and love.
- Communicate throughout the day. Look into baby's eyes, talk and sing to him.
- Play with baby every day.
- Carry the baby in a sling or front carrier. Feeling baby's warmth and looking down often to make eye contact with him can help in bonding.
- Spend plenty of close-up face time with baby. Smile at baby, and return the smile when it smiles first.
- Observe the baby every day.

## MINOR DISORDERS OF NEWBORN

### Skin

#### Baby Acne

It occurs due to pregnancy hormones which stimulate the oil glands.

**Treatment**

Wash baby's face with mild soap once a day.

## Skin Rashes

Small patches occur usually to napkin areas and may involve groins, axilla, face, legs and back.

### Treatment

Frequent care

## Birthmarks

Birthmarks are areas of discolored and/or raised skin that are present at birth or within a few weeks of birth. Birthmarks are made up of abnormal pigment cells or blood vessels (Table 2).

### Causes

The exact cause of most birthmarks is unknown, but they are thought to occur as a result of a localized imbalance in factors controlling the development and migration of skin cells. In addition, it is known that vascular birthmarks are not hereditary. Vascular birthmarks are caused by abnormal blood vessels in or under the skin, and pigmented birthmarks are caused by clusters of pigment cells. Port wine stains are thought to occur because the nerves that control the widening or narrowing of the capillaries (tiny blood vessels) do not function properly, or there are not enough of them. This means that blood is constantly supplied to the skin in that area, which makes it permanently red or purple in color.

**TABLE 2: Common birthmarks**

| Birthmark | Characteristics |
| --- | --- |
| Stork bites, angel kisses, or salmon patches | These are small pink or red patches often found on a baby's eyelids, between the eyes, upper lip, and back of the neck. The "stork bite" name comes from the marks on the back of the neck where, as the myth goes, a stork may have picked up the baby. They are caused by a concentration of immature blood vessels and may be most visible when the baby is crying. Most of these fade and disappear completely. |
| Congenital dermal melanocytosis (also known as Mongolian spots) | Congenital dermal melanocytosis refers to areas of blue or purple-colored, typically on the baby's lower back and buttocks. These can occur in darker-skinned babies of all races. The spots are caused by a concentration of pigmented cells. They usually disappear in the first 4 years of life. |
| Strawberry hemangioma | This is a bright or dark red, raised or swollen, bumpy area that looks like a strawberry. Hemangiomas are formed by a concentration of tiny, immature blood vessels. Most of these occur on the head. They may not appear at birth, but often develop in the first 2 months. Strawberry hemangiomas are more common in premature babies and in girls. These birthmarks often grow in size for several months, and then gradually begin to fade. They may bleed or get infected in rare cases. Nearly all strawberry hemangiomas completely disappear by 9 years of age. |
| Port-wine stain | A port-wine stain is a flat, pink, red, or purple colored birthmark. These are caused by a concentration of dilated tiny blood vessels called capillaries. They usually occur on the head or neck. They may be small, or they may cover large areas of the body. Port-wine stains do not change color when gently pressed and do not disappear over time. They may become darker and thicker when the child is older or as an adult. Port-wine stains on the face may be associated with more serious problems. Skin-colored cosmetics may be used to cover small port-wine stains. The most effective way of treating port-wine stains is with a special type of laser. This is done when the baby is older by a plastic surgery specialist. |
| Congenital moles | These common moles (less than 3 inches in diameter) occur in about 1 out of every 100 newborns. They increase in size as the child grows, but usually don't cause any problems. Your child's health care provider will watch them closely as rarely they can develop into a cancerous mole. |

## Complications

**Most birthmarks are harmless. But in rare cases, complications can occur that need to be treated.**

- **Hemangiomas**
- Capillary malformation (port wine stains) can lead to the following complications:
  - Glaucoma
  - **Sturge-Weber syndrome:** A rare disorder affecting the eyes and brain that is usually associated with a large port wine stain
  - Soft tissue hypertrophy
- **Klippel-Trenaunay syndrome:** A rare disorder that's present at birth where the blood vessels fail to form properly; if child has an enlarged port wine stain on their limb, they may have Klippel-Trenaunay syndrome.
- Congenital melanocytic nevi can develop into skin cancer.

## Treatment

Most birthmarks are harmless and do not require treatment. Pigmented marks can resolve on their own over time in some cases. Vascular birthmarks may require reduction or removal for cosmetic reasons. Treatments include administering oral or injected steroids, dermatological laser to reduce size and/or color, or dermatological surgery.

## *Diaper Rash Sore Buttocks*

A diaper rash is an area of inflamed skin found in the diaper area in newborn and infants. It is usually caused by skin irritation from prolonged contact with urine and feces.

A diaper rash can sometimes lead to a bacterial or fungal infection. Diapers, whether reusable or disposable, create a hot moist environment that traps diaper contents (e.g., urine and feces) against the skin, which causes irritation and infection.

## Causes

Diaper rash may be caused by a number of factors, including:

- **Contact with urine and feces:** Prolonged exposure to urine and feces can irritate the skin. Both urine and feces can cause moisture to come into contact with the skin, which makes it more prone to damage and irritation. Contact with digestive enzymes found in feces can also increase the risk of diaper rash. Although ammonia (the chemical that gives urine its smell) is irritating to the skin, the levels found in infant urine are not sufficient to cause a diaper rash. However, it can worsen skin that is already irritated and inflamed.
- **Method of feeding:** Breast-fed babies may experience fewer diaper rashes than bottle-fed babies because breast-fed babies tend to have stools of a smaller volume, which in turn are less irritating to the skin. However, the frequency of the feces increases in bottle-fed babies.
- **Friction and rubbing:** Tight-fitting diapers that chafe against the skin can lead to a diaper rash. This damage to the skin can be made worse if the skin is wet. Also, skin-to-skin contact within skin folds in the diaper area can promote a diaper rash.
- **Preexisting skin conditions:** Infants and children with preexisting skin conditions such as eczema and atopic dermatitis are more prone to develop a diaper rash.
- **Contact with irritating chemicals:** Baby's buttock's skin is very delicate. Some common chemicals that are found in fabric softeners, detergents, baby lotions, fragrances, soaps, and baby wipes can be very irritating to the skin and should be avoided. Consult pediatrician about which products to avoid.

- **Antibiotic use:** Using antibiotics can disrupt the normal balance of "good bacteria," which normally keep certain organisms such as yeast under control. Antibiotics taken by a breastfeeding mother can also affect the baby.
- **Infections:** The dark, damp, and moist environment created by a diaper is a perfect breeding ground for bacterial or yeast infections (e.g., *Candida*) on the skin. These types of infections are more common in babies who have a diaper rash. Blisters, pus, red bumps in the creases of the skin, "satellite" red areas outside the main redness, or severely swollen red areas may be signs of infection.
- **Allergy to diaper elastic chemicals:** A linear, red rash across the belly and in the skin creases can indicate an allergic reaction to chemicals in disposable diaper elastic. This is a common occurrence when there is change to a different brand of diapers. If it persists or recurs, the pediatrician should be consulted.
- **Other conditions:** Diaper rashes are not exclusive to newborn and infants. They can also affect other people with conditions such as incontinence and paralysis.

## Signs and Symptoms

- Diaper rashes often appear as redness on the skin, with shiny patches and some pimply spots.
- Skin may also be warm to the touch.
- An infant may be more irritable.
- Baby starts crying during diaper changes, especially when the skin in the diaper area is being cleaned or touched.
- An infection is usually indicated by red bumps that are present in the skin folds or creases.
- Blisters, pus, or red and severely swollen areas can also be signs of infection. "Satellite" red areas beyond the main rash are common with *Candida* yeast infection rashes.

## Treatment and Prevention

- Currently, the main treatment for diaper rash is to use a barrier cream or ointment containing ingredients such as zinc oxide and petroleum jelly.
- Avoid using products with ingredients that may irritate the skin, such as certain fragrances or lanolin.
- Use diapers that draw moisture away from the skin.
- Avoid using products that expose your child's skin to irritating chemicals (e.g., diaper wipes with alcohol, fragrances, fabric softeners and detergents).
- Change the diaper often, including throughout the night.
- Avoid using powders such as talcum powder and cornstarch. Talcum powder may cause respiratory problems in the child, and cornstarch may promote a yeast infection.
- Rinse the baby's bottom with warm water and a mild, unscented soap after each diaper change, and air- or pat-dry the area thoroughly. (Allow the area to air-dry for as long as possible.)
- Avoid using tight-fitting diapers and rubber or plastic pants, since they retain more moisture.
- Wash reusable diapers carefully to remove all the germs. Be sure to completely rinse out any soap or detergent.
- Wash the hands thoroughly after each diaper change.

## Other Skin Problems

- **Cyanosis of hands and feet:** It does not signify any abnormality. It is often visible in the first few days because of sluggish peripheral circulation in the skin.
- **Ecchymosis** or multiple minute petechial spots in the skin of the face may result from congestion of the head during labor.

- **Milia:** The multiple tiny raised white spots commonly seen on the face (especially the nose) are really hyperplastic sebaceous glands, sometimes called milia, and disappear within the month.
- **Erythema toxicum/urticarial neonatorum:** It appears about the 2nd–4th day as an eruption of blotchy red patches mainly over the trunk, face and buttock superimposed on which there are small white raised spots looking like pustules (Fig. 3). It resolves within few days without treatment.
- **Cellulitis:** It usually occurs at a traumatic skin site. Treatment includes local antibiotic ointment (Bacitracin) and systemic antibiotic (oxacillin or nafcillin and gentamicin) IV.

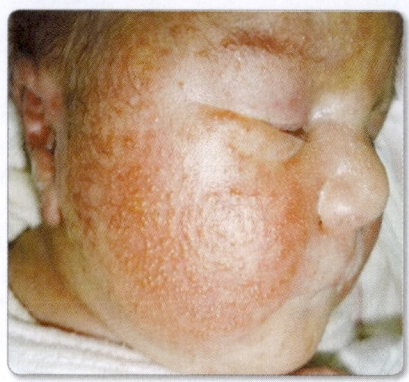

**Fig. 3:** Erythema toxicum

## Eyes

### *Subconjunctival Hemorrhage*

- Found on the sclera
- Caused by the changes in vascular tension or ocular pressure during birth

### *Pink Eyes*

Conjunctivitis or pink eyes have yellow discharge along with red irritated eyes.

#### Treatment

Cold compresses to reduce swelling. Apply antibiotic eyedrops or ointment.

### *Ophthalmia Neonatorum*

It is defined as inflammation of conjunctiva during first month of life. The clinical picture varies and the discharge may be watery, mucopurulent to frank purulent in one or both eyes. The eyelids may be sticky or markedly swollen. Cornea may be involved in some cases (Fig. 4). Treatment includes: 1% silver nitrate solution (1–2 drops to each eye), 0.5% erythromycin ophthalmic ointment, 2.5% povidone iodine solution (1 drop) each eye is administered within 1 hour of birth and continued for few days.

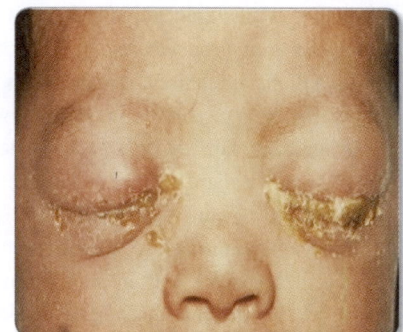

**Fig. 4:** Ophthalmia neonatorum

### *Sticky Eye*

Without purulent discharge is common during first two–three days after birth. The eyelids are swollen and stick together with redness of eyes.

## Head

### *Molding*

- The head may appear asymmetric in the newborn of a vertex birth.
- Caused by the overriding of the cranial bones during labor and birth.
- Diminishes within few days after birth.
- Head molding.

### Cephalhematoma

- Collection of blood between the cranial bone and the periosteal membrane
- Unilateral or bilateral and do not cross suture lines
- Disappears within 2–3 weeks

### Caput Succedaneum

- Collection of fluid between the periosteum and the scalp
- Overrides suture line
- Present at birth

### Forceps and Vacuum Marks

- Reddened areas over the cheeks and jaws. Disappear within 1 or 2 days
- Vacuum extractor suction marks on the scalp
- No treatment is necessary

### Plagiocephaly/Parallelogram Skull

It is of postural origin in which the baby has a preference for turning the head mainly towards one or other side when laid down. There is localized rounded swelling over one side of the head, becoming maximal in size by third or fourth day of life.

## Mouth

### Oral Thrush

Infection of the buccal mucous membranes and the tongue by the fungus *Candida albicans* is common especially in bottle fed babies (Fig. 5). Contamination by the organism occurs from the feeding bottles, teats, nurse's hands, mothers' nipple and infected vagina of the mother at the time of delivery. The fungus grows on the mucous membrane and produces milky white elevated patches resembling milk curd, which cannot be easily wiped off with gauze. Rarely, infection spread down to involve the gastrointestinal or respiratory tract.

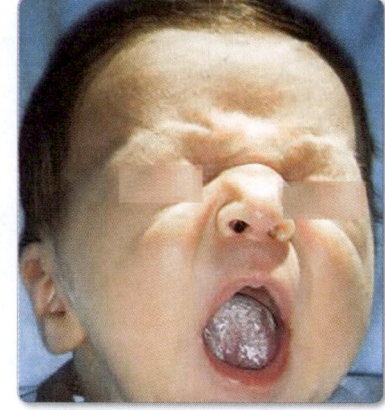

**Fig. 5:** Oral thrush

#### Management

- Local application of 1% aqueous solution of gentian violet on the oral mucous membrane twice daily after feeds for 2–3 days is quite effective.
- Nystatin oral suspension (100,000 u/mL), 1 mL is applied to each side of the mouth 4 times a day for about 2–3 weeks.
- Systemic fluconazole is highly effective in chronic mucocutaneous candidiasis.

### Precocious Teeth

The teeth are found in the mouth of the baby before birth. These are usually loose and find its way out eventually (Fig. 6).

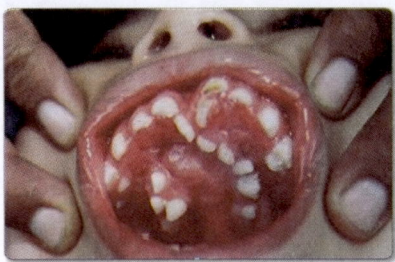

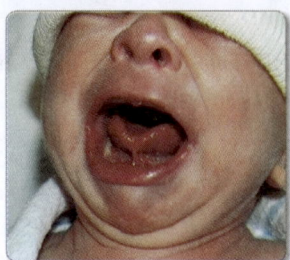

**Fig. 6:** Precocious teeth                    **Fig. 7:** Tongue tie

### Tongue-tie

Short and sometimes thickened frenulum attached more than usually anteriorly to the base of the tongue, is a common source of anxiety to mothers, who fear future speech difficulties or feeding problems (Fig. 7). Exceptionally when there is restriction of tongue protrusion beyond the alveolar margins or heavy grooving of tip of tongue, it is reasonable to advise surgical division of the frenulum in the second or third month of life, in the majority of cases.

## Chest

### Neonatal Breast Enlargement

As a result of the sudden withdrawal of maternal estrogen, it is common in both baby boys and girls (Fig. 8).

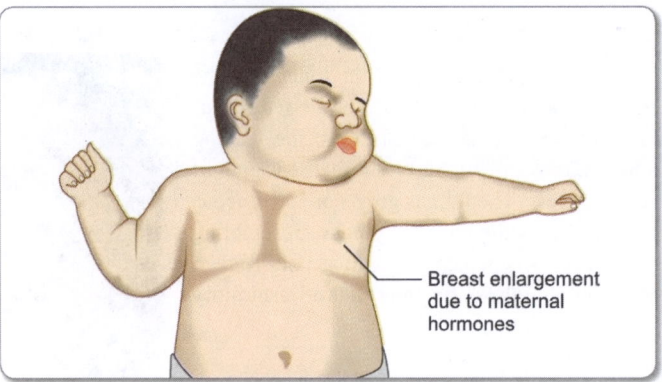

Breast enlargement
due to maternal
hormones

**Fig. 8:** Neonatal breast enlargement

## Gastrointestinal Tract

### Vomiting

It is frequently a source of worry in the first week or two. Posseting of mouthful milk soon after feeding is a normal course. The vomiting of bile always a sign of danger. Commonly vomiting is due to improper feeding technique.

### Neonatal Constipation

It occurs due to insufficient fluid or milk intake and is more common in mild fed infants.

## Management

Milk of magnesia one tea spoon twice daily. Apply lubricant over anal region.

### *Necrotizing Enterocolitis*

It is a life-threatening condition associated with ischemic and inflammatory necrosis of the relatively immature intestine (Fig. 9).

### Signs and Symptoms

- **Systemic signs:** Respiratory distress, lethargy, feeding intolerance, hypertension, acidosis, oliguria, and bleeding diatheses.
- **Abdominal signs:** Abdominal distension, tenderness, bloody stools, vomiting. Management includes:
  - Supplemental $O_2$ and mechanical ventilation may be needed.
  - **Antibiotics:** Vancomycin, piperacillin/tazobactam, gentamycin, metronidazole.
  - Bowel resection in case of perforation.

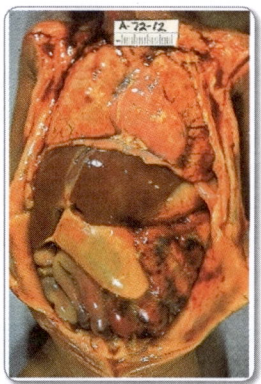

**Fig. 9:** Necrotizing enterocolitis

## Umbilicus

It further includes three complications which are as follows:

### *Umbilical Sepsis (Omphalitis)*

The infection is manifested by serous or seropurulent umbilical discharge which may be offensive (Fig. 10). The base of the cord stump looks moist and the periumbilical skin becomes red and swollen. There is delay in falling off of the cord. Systemic infections incude pyrexia and features of toxemia or jaundice in severe infection. Management includes antibiotic therapy with nafcillin and gentamycin or oxacillin may be used. The wound is dressed with spirit and antiseptic powder.

### *Umbilical Hernia*

It is often seen in preterm baby and needs no treatment. Herniation arises from just above the true navel and in such cases surgical intervention may be required at a later stage (Figs 11A and B).

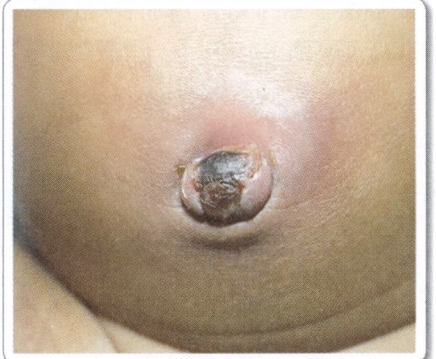

**Fig. 10:** Omphalitis

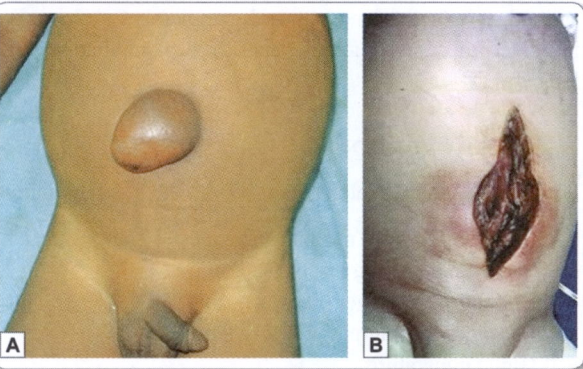

**Figs 11A and B: A.** Umbilical hernia; **B.** Extensive myonecrosis

### Cutis Navel

In this, abdominal skin is reflected to cover the proximal ½–1 inch of cord. It is a normal variation and gradually flattens after separation of the cord stump.

## NEONATAL INFECTIONS

**Neonatal infections** are infections of the neonate (newborn) during the neonatal period or first four weeks after birth. Neonatal infection can be acquired:

- *In utero* transplacentally or through ruptured membranes
- In the birth canal during delivery (intrapartum)
- From external sources after birth (postpartum)

**In utero infection:** It can occur any time before birth, and results from overt or subclinical maternal infection. Consequences depend on the agent and timing of infection in gestation and include spontaneous abortion, intrauterine growth restriction, premature birth, stillbirth, congenital malformation (e.g. rubella), and symptomatic (e.g. cytomegalovirus [CMV], toxoplasmosis, syphilis) or asymptomatic (e.g., CMV) neonatal infection.

Common infectious agents transmitted transplacentally include rubella, toxoplasma, CMV, and syphilis. HIV and hepatitis B are less commonly transmitted transplacentally.

**Intrapartum infection:** When the baby passes through an infected birth canal neonatal infections such as herpes simplex viruses, HIV, hepatitis B, group B streptococci, enteric gram-negative organisms (primarily *Escherichia coli*), *Listeria monocytogenes*, gonococci, and chlamydiae usually occur. If there is prolonged rupture of membranes, ascending infection can occur.

**Postpartum infections:** These are acquired when infant comes in direct contact with an infected mother (e.g., tuberculosis) or through breastfeeding (e.g., HIV, CMV) or from contact with family members, visitors, health care practitioners or the hospital environment.

### Risk Factors

Risk of contracting intrapartum and postpartum infection is inversely proportional to gestational age. Neonates are immunologically immature, with decreased polymorphonuclear leukocyte, monocyte, and cell-mediated immune function; premature infants are particularly so.

Maternal IgG antibodies are actively transported across the placenta, but its effective levels are not achieved until near term. IgM antibodies do not cross the placenta. Premature infants have decreased intrinsic antibody production and reduced complement activity. Premature infants are also more likely to require invasive procedures such as endotracheal intubation, prolonged IV access, etc. that predispose them to infection.

### Signs and Symptoms

When a baby first develops an infection, the baby might have the following signs and symptoms:

- Irritable, and does not settle down even after feeding
- Sleepy, not waking up for feeding
- Breathlessness (over 60 breaths/min)
- Improper feeding/not properly fed
- High temperature

Many healthy newborns have these symptoms at times. However, if a baby keeps having these symptoms, it needs to be checked.

As the infection gets worse, a baby might have:

- Pale or greyish skin.
- Breathlessness.
- Bluish discoloration around the lips and mouth.
- Hypothermia or hyperthermia.

Some newborns may have an infection in only one part of their body. In these cases, symptoms include:

- Blisters on the skin.
- Redness or swelling of skin (umbilical cord or circumcision).
- Redness, swelling, or yellowish discharge from the eyes.

Many congenital infections acquired before birth can cause various symptoms or abnormalities such as growth restriction, deafness, microcephaly, anomalies, failure to thrive, hepatosplenomegaly and neurologic abnormalities.

## Diagnosis

Certain lab tests will show if a baby has an infection and where it is located:

- **Blood test:** A sample of the baby's blood is taken for blood count (CBC) and blood culture. A complete blood count identifies different types of cells in the blood and blood culture is a test to see bacterial growth in the blood.
- **Urine test:** A sample of the baby's urine is tested for signs of infection.
- **Secretion test:** If there is an obvious site of infection, a sample of secretions (for example, pus from around the umbilical cord or eye) may be cultured.
- **Chest X-ray:** If a baby is suffering from breathlessness, a chest X-ray may be performed to look for signs of pneumonia.
- **Spinal tap:** It is a test in which lumbar puncture is performed to get a sample of spinal fluid, commonly to diagnose meningitis.

## Management

- Observe for signs and risks.
- 'Universal precautions'—prevention.
- Minimize risk of infection.
- Septic screen if infection suspected—full or partial.
- **The special care nursery (SCN):** If a baby has signs of infection, she is taken to the special care nursery (SCN) for evaluation and treatment. The baby is placed on a warming bed. She is attached to a monitor that continuously measures heart rate and breathing. If the baby has troubled breathing, she may also be attached to a pulse oximeter that records the amount of oxygen in her skin.
- **Medicine: Antibiotic therapy:** It should be administered considering the common causative organism. A combination of ampicillin and gentamycin/amikacin is recommended for treatment of sepsis and pneumonia. In case of suspected meningitis, chloramphenicol should be added. Duration of antibiotic therapy should be individualized. In general antibiotic should be given 0–14 days in septicemia and pneumonia, 14 days for UTI and 21 days for meningitis.

- **Another drug therapy:** Anticonvulsant can be administered in the cases of convulsions and corticosteroids in severely sick neonates with endotoxic shock, sclerema and adrenal insufficiency. Dopamine is used to treat shock and mannitol can be used in raised ICP (Intracranial pressure).
- Phototherapy and exchange transfusion may be necessary in hyperbilirubinemia. Blood transfusion may be required in anemia and bleeding disorders.
- Administer immunoglobulin preparations containing type-specific antibodies to group-'b' streptococci
- Treatment of superficial infections, like umbilical sepsis, pyoderma, oral thrush, conjunctivitis should be done appropriately.
- **Supportive care:** If the baby is breathing too fast and not eating, he is given fluids through the IV so he won't get dehydrated. If he is too sleepy and not eating, he may be given IV fluids or he may be fed by dripping milk through a tube that passes through his mouth and into the stomach. If the baby needs extra oxygen, it is given extra oxygen.

Some babies are not very sick and the only treatment they need is antibiotics. These babies can be breast fed or they can be fed with bottle.

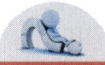

# ASSESS YOURSELF

## FREQUENTLY ASKED QUESTIONS IN EXAMS

1. Write down the minor disorders of newborn and their management.
2. Explain in detail about the immediate care of newborn.
3. Describe nursing management of newborn with ophthalmic neonatorum.
4. As a nurse, how you will care for a baby with oral thrush?
5. Describe in detail about Apgar score.
6. Write short notes on:
   - Breastfeeding
   - Bonding and rooming in
   - Baby-friendly hospital initiative (BFHI)

## MULTIPLE CHOICE QUESTIONS

1. **The neonate is:**
   a. Birth to first 28 days of life
   b. Immediately after birth
   c. Birth to 12-month
   d. None of the above

2. **Average head circumference of newborn at term birth is:**
   a. 31–33 cm
   b. 33–35 cm
   c. 32–33 cm
   d. 35–38 cm

3. **A term baby's average length is:**
   a. 46–56 cm
   b. 41–56 cm
   c. >40 cm
   d. <50 cm

4. **Anterior fontanels ossify at:**
   a. 18 months
   b. 8 months
   c. 12 months
   d. 9 months

5. **The shape of posterior fontanel is:**
   a. Triangular
   b. Diamond
   c. Globular
   d. Oval

6. **Normal respiratory rate of newborn is:**
   a. 80–110 breaths/min
   b. 120–160 breaths/min
   c. 110–180 breaths/min
   d. 140–160 breaths/min

7. **Umbilical cord contains:**
   a. 1 artery and 1 vein
   b. 2 arteries and 1 vein
   c. Two arteries only
   d. 2 veins and 1 artery

8. **Extra digits (finger) in hand and feet is called:**
   a. Polydactyly
   b. Syndactyly
   c. Adactyly
   d. None of the above

9. **When heat is transferred from body to cooler objects in the environment, it is called:**
   a. Evaporation
   b. Radiation
   c. Convection
   d. Conduction

10. **When the Apgar score is 8–10:**
    a. Mild depression
    b. No depression
    c. Severe depression
    d. Moderate depression

11. **When heat is lost from the surface of the body to the objects in direct contact with the skin is:**
    a. Evaporation
    b. Conduction
    c. Radiation
    d. Convection

12. **Apgar score criteria include:**
    a. Respiration
    b. Heart rate
    c. Muscle tone
    d. All of the above

13. **Baby-friendly hospital initiative was launched by WHO and UNICEF in:**
    a. 2006
    b. 2001
    c. 1991
    d. 1992

14. **The goals of BFHI are:**
    a. Promote breastfeeding
    b. Immunization services
    c. Baby's growth and development surveillance
    d. All of the above

15. **Average chest circumference of newborn is:**
    a. 35 cm
    b. 31 cm
    c. 36 cm
    d. 32 cm

16. **The meconium of baby during 2–3 days after birth contains:**
    a. Bile
    b. Mucus
    c. Fatty acids
    d. All of the above

17. **The amount of protein in colostrum as compared to natural milk is:**
    a. Same
    b. Two times
    c. Three times
    d. Four times

18. **Duration of feeding a newborn during first day is:**
    a. 2–3 minutes
    b. 5 minutes
    c. 10 minutes
    d. 15 minutes

19. **Exclusive breast feed is for:**
    a. First 3 months
    b. Up to 6 months
    c. Up to 9 months
    d. For one year

20. **With sudden jerking/loud noise, a newborn extends his forelimbs, the reflex is:**
    a. Babinski's reflex
    b. Moro's reflex
    c. Tonic neck reflex
    d. Rooting reflex

## Answer Key

| 1. a | 2. b | 3. a | 4. a | 5. a | 6. b | 7. b |
|------|------|------|------|------|------|------|
| 8. a | 9. b | 10. b | 11. b | 12. d | 13. d | 14. d |
| 15. a | 16. d | 17. c | 18. a | 19. b | 20. b | |

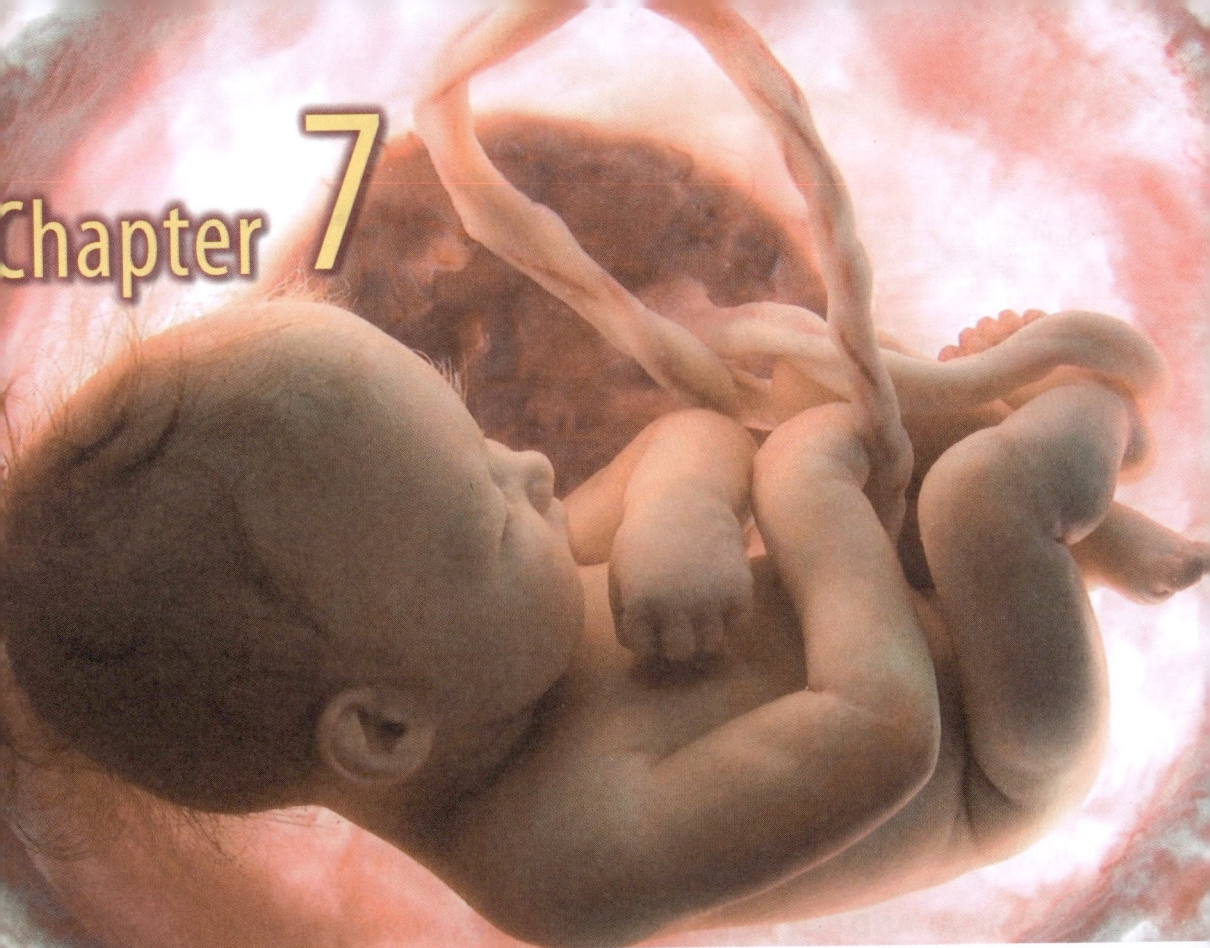

# Chapter 7

# Management of Normal Puerperium

## Learning Objectives

**Upon completing this chapter, the learner will be able to:**

- Describe the physiological changes during puerperium
- Discuss the care during puerperium
- Explain the minor ailments during puerperium and its management
- Describe in detail about various family planning methods

## Chapter Outline

- Introduction
- Duration of Puerperium
- Objectives
- Anatomical and Physiological Changes during Puerperium
- Postnatal Counseling

- Lactation and its Management
- Care during Puerperium
- Minor Ailments and Management
- Postnatal Exercises
- Family Planning

# INTRODUCTION

**Definition:** Puerperium is a period of 6 weeks following delivery when the major reproductive organs revert approximately to pregravid state both anatomically and physiologically.

# DURATION OF PUERPERIUM

Approximately 6 weeks. The postpartum period is divided into:

- **Immediate puerperium:** The first 24 hours
- **Early puerperium:** Up to 7 days
- **Remote puerperium:** Up to 6 weeks

# OBJECTIVES

- To assess the health status of mother
- To restore the health of the mother
- To prevent infection
- To take care of the breast, including promotion of breastfeeding
- To impart family planning guidance
- To note the growth and development of baby (including immunization schedule for the newborn)
- To promote and maintain lactation
- To help the mother to take care of the baby

# ANATOMICAL AND PHYSIOLOGICAL CHANGES DURING PUERPERIUM

## Changes Related to Reproductive Organs

### Anatomical Consideration

- **Uterus:** Immediately after delivery, uterus weighs about 1 kg after approximately 20 weeks of pregnancy. Height of fundus is about 5″ from symphysis pubis. The height of uterus comes down by ½ inch every day. By 12th day, the fundus is at the level of symphysis pubis. Uterine involution is complete by 6 weeks at which time the organ weighs less than 100 g slightly larger following pregnancy. The placental site contracts rapidly to a size less than half the diameter of placenta. This contraction causes constriction and permits occlusion of underlying blood vessels. The resulting hemostasis leads to endometrial necrosis. Endometrial regeneration is completed by 6–8 weeks.
- **Lower uterine segment:** Immediately following delivery the lower segment becomes a thin, flabby, collapsed structure. It reverts to normal size and shape in few weeks.
- **Cervix:**
  - Takes 6 weeks to regain contour = a slit-like opening on the OS.
  - One finger can be admitted even after one week of delivery
  - External OS never reverts to prepregnant state
- **Breasts:**
  - Lactation starts immediately after delivery on sucking by the baby as the hormone prolactin stimulates milk production.
  - During 3–4 days of puerperium, breast becomes heavy and engorged. To relieve breast engorgement, provide breastfeeding, massage the breast or give hot compression.

## Physiological Consideration

The physiological changes are most marked in the body of the uterus. During involution, the reproductive organs revert to their prepregnant state. Changes occur in the following components:

- **Muscles:**
  - During puerperium, the number of muscle fibers remains the same but there is reduction of the myometrial cell size.
  - Withdrawal of the steroid hormones, estrogen and progesterone, increases the activity of the uterine collagenase and the release of the proteolytic enzyme.
- **Blood vessels:**
  - The arteries are constricted by contraction of their walls and thickening of the intima followed by thrombosis
  - New blood vessels grow inside thrombi
  - Fibrous tissue on the wall undergoes hyaline degeneration and the products are removed by macrophages
  - Degeneration of elastic tissues also takes place
- **Endometrium:**
  - The superficial layer becomes necrotic and is sloughed in the lochia
  - The basal layer remains intact and is the source of new endometrium
  - The endometrium arises from proliferation of the endometrial glandular remnants and the stroma of the inter glandular connective tissue

    **Endometrium regenerates:**
    - **By the 10th day:** Regeneration of the epithelium is completed.
    - **By the day 16:** The endometrium is restored.
    - **At about 6 weeks:** The endometrium of placental site is restored.

    **Placental site involution**
    - Complete extrusion of the placental site takes up to 6 weeks
    - When this process is defective, there is late-onset puerperal hemorrhage.
    - Immediately after delivery, the size of placental site is approximately same as the size of the palm, but it rapidly decreases thereafter.
    - **Within hours of delivery:** Normally consists of many thrombosed vessels
    - **By the end of the 2nd week:** 3–4 cm in diameter

    **Abdominal wall**
    - Because of prolonged distension of the gravid uterus and ruptured elastic fibers in the skin, the abdominal wall remains soft and flaccid.
    - These structures require several weeks to return to normal.
- **Vagina**
  - Takes 4–8 weeks to involute.
  - It regains its tone but never to the virginal state.
  - For the first few weeks the mucosa remains delicate but submucosal venous congestion persists even longer.
  - At third week, rugae partially reappear.
  - Introitus remains permanently larger than the virginal state.
    **Lochia:** It is the vaginal discharge for 15–21 days maximum. It has peculiar offensive, fishy smell and is alkaline in nature.

It has three types (Based on the color of the vaginal discharge).

i. **Lochia rubra** (red color) 3–4 days. Constituents are blood, decidual and trophoblastic debris.

ii. **Lochia serosa** (brown) 5 days. It consists of the old blood, serum, leukocytes and tissue debris

iii. **Lochia alba** (white) 10–15 days. Contains old leukocytes deciduas, epithelial cells, mucus, serum and bacteria

**Amount:** The average amount of lochia for first 5–6 days is estimated to be 250 mL.

○ Excessive lochia discharge following cesarean, twin delivery and hydramnios

○ Scanty following premature labor

○ Persistent red bleeding beyond normal limit indicates subinvolution or retained products of conception

## General Physiological Changes during Puerperium

The woman in labor goes through a tremendous amount of stress and strain. And it takes some time for her to settle down to a normal state again. Immediately following labor, the general condition of the mother is one of physical fatigue.

### Vital Signs

#### Temperature

The temperature rises slightly 0.5 degrees for the first 24 hours. The temperature rises due to the absorption of waste products of muscular contractions of labor.

*Transient rise in temperature later on is due to:*

• Milk engorgement (by the 4th day postpartum):

   ▪ Constipation.

   ▪ Nervous excitation.

   ▪ Infection.

### The Pulse

Pulse rate is about 60–70 beats/minute for 24–48 hours after labor and is known as physiological bradycardia. It is due to:

• The rest period after labor:

   ▪ The increase in the circulating blood volume on account of the elimination of the placental pool.

   ▪ Normally, pulse remains below 100 beats/minute but pulse rate may rise due to after pains, visitors, excitement, exhaustion, the nursing infant, hemorrhage or infection.

### Respiration

This is in the usual relation with pulse and temperature. Because of relaxation of the abdominal wall and reduction in the size of the uterus, respiration is more abdominal in character. Abnormal respiration may develop in case of pneumonia or embolism.

### Blood Pressure

Normally there is no change in blood pressure, but if hypotension is present, postpartum hemorrhage may occur. If hypertension is present (over 140/90 mm Hg) postpartum toxemia may be suspected.

## Skin

Excessive sweating (diaphoresis), particularly in patients who were subjected to edema in late pregnancy, in order to get rid of excess fluids that were retained in the tissues. This gradually ceases within the 1st week and the skin reacts as usual. Skin pigmentation gradually disappears.

## Kidneys and Urinary Output

- There is usually physiological diuresis (polyuria).
- Painful, difficult micturition due to tears, lacerations or episiotomy may result in reflex retention of urine.
- Traces of albumin and peptone may be present as a result of muscle involution.
- Lactosuria is common with milk engorgement on the 4th day at the start of lactation.
- The parturient may experience some retention of urine in the first few days after labor due to: Laxity of the abdominal muscles.
- Inability to micturate in the recumbent position.
- Reflex inhibition due to stitched perineum or bruised urethra.
- Atony of the bladder.
- Compression of the urethra by edema or hematoma.

## Bowel Function and Intestinal Elimination

- Due to the marked fluid loss through sweat and urine, patient becomes thirsty.
- Tendency to atony of the gastrointestinal tract, with flatulence and constipation.
- Constipation may be present as a result of:
  - Intestinal atony
  - Hemorrhoids
  - Reflex inhibition
  - Loss of body fluids
  - Laxity of the abdominal wall
  - Enema in labor
  - Anorexia after labor

## Blood Picture

- Slight decrease in total blood volume due to dehydration and blood loss. This comes back to normal in 7 days.
- With proper antenatal care, the amount of blood loss during the 3rd stage of labor does not cause anemia.
- Blood volume decreases, Hb% also diminishes, but not proportionately, hydremia of pregnancy disappears and stabilizes by the 5th day.
- A moderate increase at around the 4th to the 10th day after delivery in the leukocyte count, fibrinogen and sedimentation rate occurs during the first then gradually gets back to normal values.
- In the absence of complications and with proper diet and hygiene, RBC count and content, and the blood constituents, usually return to the nonpregnant levels in 4–6 weeks.

## Body Weight

- A weight loss of about 4.0 kg takes place at the time of delivery of the baby, placenta, membranes and liquor amnii. A further loss of about 3 kg takes place during the puerperium due to the elimination of water and decreased size of the uterus.
- So, in a woman with a standard weight gain of 10 kg during pregnancy, there is a weight loss of 7 kg after delivery. She will thus have a net weight gain of 3 kg due to pregnancy.

## After-pains

- It is a spasmodic colicky pain in the lower abdomen during the early postpartum days due to the vigorous contractions of the uterus.

- It is more common and more severe in multiparas, multiple pregnancy, polyhydramnios, large-sized infant in diabetic mothers.
- After-pains can be precipitated due to the presence of piece of membrane, placental tissue or blood clots.
- After-pains increase during breastfeeding because the infant's sucking stimulates further milk production, which in turn stimulates the posterior pituitary gland to secrete Oxytocin that results in more uterine contractions, resulting in increase of after-pains.

### Return of Menstruation

- In nonlactating mothers, menstruation reappear within 6–8 weeks. It may be delayed for a longer period without any abnormal condition being present.
- In lactating mothers, menstruation usually reappears within 4–5 months, and sometimes as late as 24 months.
- The first period is generally profuse and prolonged.
- Sometime ovulation commences even in the absence of menstruation, and another pregnancy can occur.

### Neurologic System

Postpartum headaches may be caused by pregnancy-induced hypertension (PIH), stress or leakage of cerebrospinal fluid (CSF) into extradural space during placement of needle for spinal anesthesia in case of cesarean.

### Musculoskeletal System

Stabilization of joints takes 6–8 weeks following delivery.

### Integumentary System

Chloasma usually disappears after delivery.

## POSTNATAL COUNSELING

Counseling is the interaction process where one person referred to as counselor has taken the responsibility to make changes in other person's personality development. The counseling is done to facilitate development of self-actualization in client.

In postnatal counseling, the counselor advices the **postnatal mother** regarding the do's and don'ts for mother and the baby as described respectively in Tables 1 and 2.

**TABLE 1:** Do's and don'ts for mother

| Do's | Don't |
|---|---|
| • Adequate sleep and rest | • Lift heavy weight |
| • Balanced diet | • Long journey |
| • Plenty of fluids | • Cross legs |
| • Personal hygiene | • Abstinence from sexual intercourse for 6–8 weeks |
| • Care of episiotomy wound | • Avoid strain on sutures for constipation |
| • Adopt small family norms | • Conceive immediately after delivery |
| • Frequent urination | |
| • Postnatal exercises | |
| • Attend postnatal clinics after 6 weeks of puerperium | |

**TABLE 2: Do's and don'ts for baby**

| Do's | Don't |
|---|---|
| • Keep dry, clean and warm | • Tap feeds/solid feed up to 8 months |
| • Immunization | • Pull cord before falling itself |
| • Care for eyes | |
| • Weaning diet after 6 months | |
| • Expose to sunlight for 10–15 minutes | |
| • Exclusive breastfeeding | |

## LACTATION AND ITS MANAGEMENT

Lactation is a physiological process in which mother starts breastfeeding the baby after delivery. The breast becomes larger and fuller with prominent veins for milk secretion. In the first 2 days following delivery, no further anatomical changes occur in the breast. The secretion of colostrum which starts during pregnancy becomes more abundant during postpartum period.

### Colostrum

Colostrum is a thin serous fluid secreted from breast during first 24–48 hours following delivery. It is deep yellow in color, alkaline in reaction. On microscopic examination, it consists of fat globules, watery fluid, acinar cells and colostrum corpuscles (Table 3).

**TABLE 3: Composition of colostrum**

| Sl. no. | Constituents | Colostrum | Breast milk |
|---|---|---|---|
| 1. | Water component (%) | 86 | 87 |
| 2. | Carbohydrates (%) | 3.2 | 7.5 |
| 3. | Fats (%) | 2.3 | 3.2 |
| 4. | Proteins (%) | 8.6 | 1.2 |

**Benefits of Colostrum**

- Having nutritive value.
- Having laxative action due to large fat globules.
- Antibodies and humoral factors protect against infection.

### Physiology of Lactation

The preparation of lactation starts early during pregnancy although lactation starts following delivery. Lactation is divided into the following stages:

#### Preparation of the Breast (Mammogenesis)

Hormones responsible are:

- For ductal growth → estrogen
- For alveolar growth → progesterone.
- Cortisol and growth hormone also help in ductal alveolar growth.

During pregnancy, there is remarkable growth of both ductal and lobuloalveolar system. From pregnancy till 48 hours postpartum, the growth of duct and alveolar tissues takes place.

### Synthesis and Secretion from the Breast Alveoli (Lactogenesis)

Main hormone responsible for this is: Prolactin.

The milk synthesis starts during pregnancy but its secretion starts following delivery. Although prolactin level remains high during pregnancy because of circulating estrogen-progesterone, it makes the breast tissue unresponsive to prolactin. As a result, milk secretion does not take place. Following delivery, estrogen and progesterone level falls and prolactin begins its milk secretory activity.

Other hormones responsible for milk secretion are: Growth hormones, thyroxine, glucocorticoids and insulin.

### Ejection of Milk (Galactokinesis)

Main hormone responsible for this is prolactin.

Milk is discharged from the mammary glands by the contractile mechanism which expresses the milk from the alveoli into the duct. Ejection of milk from the duct occurs due to suction exerted by the baby during suckling.

Let down reflex/milk ejection process is as follows:

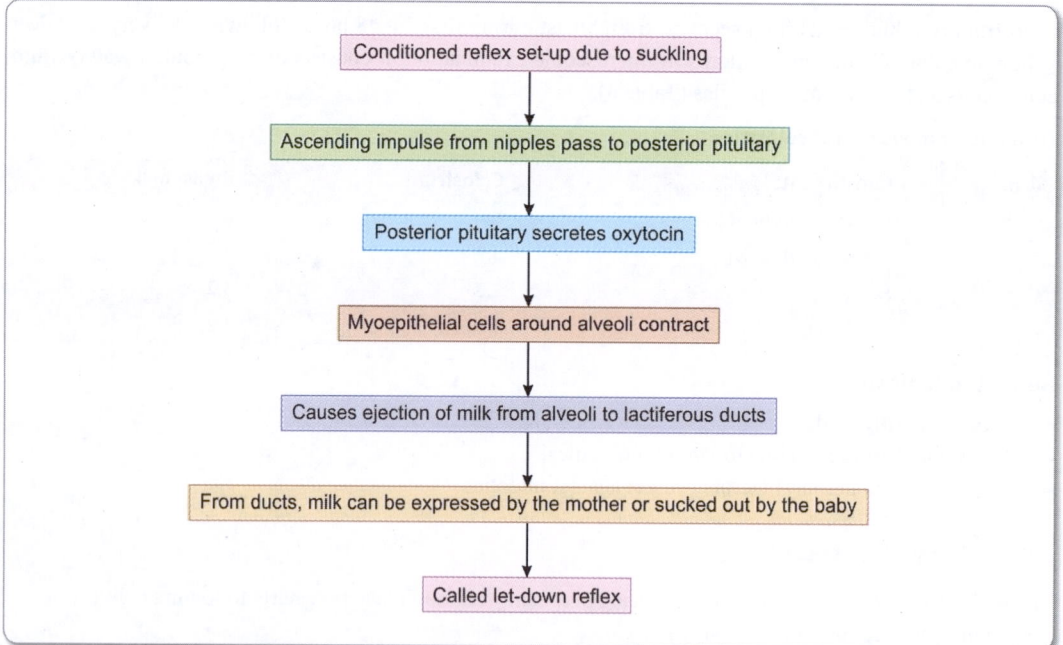

### Maintenance of Lactation (Galactopoiesis)

Hormones responsible for this are: Prolactin, oxytocin, growth hormone, thyroxine, cortisol and insulin.

Sucking by the baby is important for effective and continuous lactation. Suckling is essential for the removal of milk from the gland and also causes release of the prolactin from breast. Mother should feed the baby periodically so as to relieve milk pressure as full breast inhibits milk production (Fig. 1).

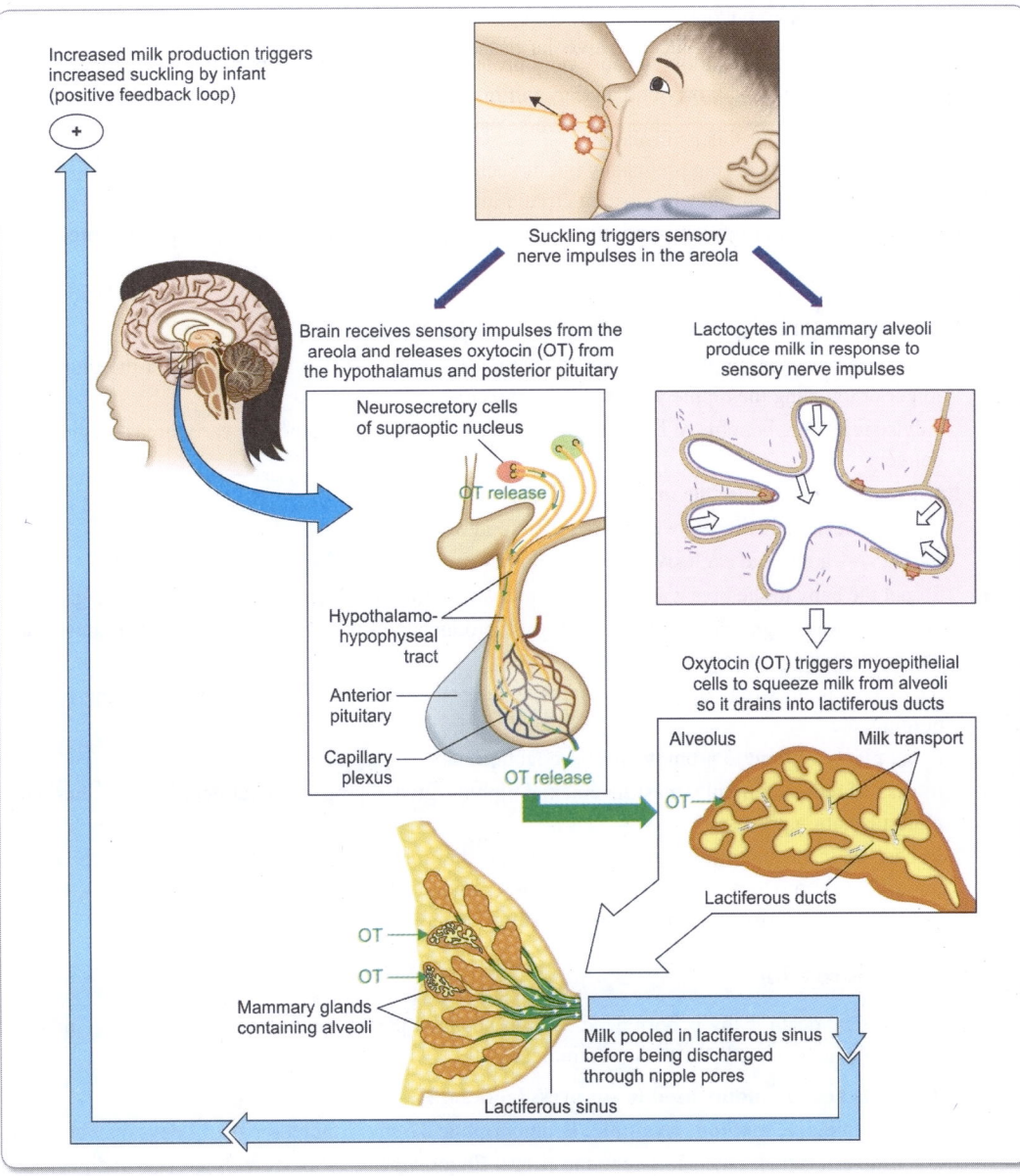

Suckling triggers sensory nerve impulses in the areola

Increased milk production triggers increased suckling by infant (positive feedback loop)

+

Brain receives sensory impulses from the areola and releases oxytocin (OT) from the hypothalamus and posterior pituitary

Lactocytes in mammary alveoli produce milk in response to sensory nerve impulses

Neurosecretory cells of supraoptic nucleus

OT release

Hypothalamo-hypophyseal tract

Anterior pituitary

Capillary plexus

OT release

Oxytocin (OT) triggers myoepithelial cells to squeeze milk from alveoli so it drains into lactiferous ducts

Alveolus

Milk transport

OT

Lactiferous ducts

OT

OT

Mammary glands containing alveoli

Milk pooled in lactiferous sinus before being discharged through nipple pores

Lactiferous sinus

**Fig. 1:** Physiology of lactation

## Causes of Lactation Failure

- Infrequent sucking
- Depression or anxiety state
- Reluctance to breastfeeding
- Retracted nipples/poor development of nipples
- Painful breast lesions
- Endogenous suppression of prolactin
- Prolactin inhibition

## Factors that Inhibit the Maintenance of Lactation

Sleeplessness, mental stress and smoking cause poor prolactin reflex, and frequent sucking is associated with high prolactin secretion. Stress, worry and anxiety inhibit oxytocin release. Milk ejection reflex is inhibited by factors such as pain, breast engorgement or adverse psychic conditions.

## Lactation Management

- **During pregnancy:** To manage lactation, since early pregnancy, advise the mother regarding breast care such as:
  - Wear supportive bra.
  - Clean the nipples if any crust formation so as to open the ducts.
  - If there is retracted nipple, then how to formulate. Gently roll the nipple between the thumb and finger or touching the nipple with a cold, damp cloth.
  - Advise regarding benefits of breastfeeding so as to prepare the mother for early breastfeeding after delivery.
- **Following delivery:** Advise the mother regarding:
  - No prelacteal feeds (honey, water) are given to newborn.
  - Early (½–1 hour) and exclusive breastfeeding in correct position are encouraged.
  - To put the baby to the breast at 2–3 hours interval for the first day, then on demand feeding.
  - To avoid breast engorgement as it inhibits milk production as well as secretion. It also produces pain among women during breastfeeding.
  - Advise the mother regarding proper breastfeeding, like feeding schedule, position during feeding, burping, etc.
  - Drink plenty of fluid to promote milk production.
  - In case of retracted nipple, mastitis cracked nipples, give appropriate treatment because these also inhibit lactation process.
  - In case of inadequate milk production, consult the doctor as certain drugs are also available to improve milk production. Example: Metoclopramide (10 mg thrice daily) increases milk volume (60–100%) by increasing prolactin levels, sulpiride has also been effective.

## Lactation Suppression

- Intrauterine fetal death, baby is born dead, dies in neonatal period, premature baby, are some medical conditions in which breastfeeding is contraindicated.

  **Two methods are commonly used to suppress lactation:**
  1. **Pharmacological method: Example:** Bromocriptine 2.5 mg, 1 tablet for 10–14 days may be given.
     - **Side effects:** Hypotension, rebound Breast Engorgement, Myocardial Infarction and puerperal stroke.
  2. **Mechanical method:** It is used in the cases where the lactation is to be suppressed after the establishment of milk secretion.
     - Instruct the patient to stop breastfeeding
     - She should not express or pump out the milk from the breast
     - A tight compression bandage is applied for about 2–3 days
     - Analgesic tablets containing aspirin and ice packs are given to relieve pain and breast engorgement.

# CARE DURING PUERPERIUM

- **Immediate attention:** Immediately after delivery:
  - Monitor mother's general condition, temperature, pulse and blood pressure
  - Give hot drinks if she is hungry.
  - Measure to promote sleep must be instituted.
- **Rest and sleep:** Eight hours night sleep and two hours day rest is required.
- **Early ambulation:** Within first 48 hours of delivery, it must be done to prevent complications.
- **Hygiene:**
  - Perineal care (4–6 hours)
  - Vulval pad change (frequently)
  - Breast care (while taking bath and before and after each feed)
  - Hand washing (before handling baby)
- **Care of bowel and bladder:**
  - Sufficient roughage and fluids
  - Encourage to pass urine every 2–3 hours
  - In case of constipation, administer mild laxative
- **Diet:**
  - Diet must contain additional 400–500 kcal to meet the lactation needs.
  - Diet should include plenty of proteins, meat, fish, fresh fruits and green leafy vegetables.
- **Rooming in:** It builds up mother-child relationship by cuddling, fondling, kissing and gazing
- **Postnatal exercises:** It must be started after 24 hours of normal vaginal delivery and 48 hours of cesarean section. Always start with light exercises on bed itself.
- **Contraception:**
  - Explain various methods of contraception, like temporary [intrauterine contraceptive devices (IUCD), pills, condom, etc.] and permanent methods (tubectomy and vasectomy) to postnatal mother
  - **Aim is to:** Maintain birth spacing and restore the health of the mother.
- **Education:** Guide mother for self-care and baby care.
  Baby care involves:
  - Baby bath
  - Baby clothing
  - Breastfeeding
  - Care of buttocks and umbilicus
- Immunization
- Weight gain of baby
- Physiological jaundice
- **Immunization of mother:**
  - Anti D gamma globulin to Rh-negative mother bearing Rh-positive baby
  - Rubella vaccine for mother who is not immunized for rubella in postpartum period.
- **Emotional needs:**
  - Encourage parents (mother and father) for the baby care.
  - Show confidence in mother's ability.
  - Observe for symptoms of postpartum blues and depression.
  - Observe for need of counseling.
- **Breastfeeding and breast care:**
  - Wear well-fitting bra
  - Keep breast and nipples clean/dry and wash with plain water only
  - Allow demand feeding on crying of baby
  - Maintain exclusive breastfeeding for first 6 months.

# MINOR AILMENTS AND MANAGEMENT

- **After pains:** The pain is felt 2–4 days after delivery due to contraction and relaxation of the uterus because of certain reasons such as presence of blood clots, increased parity or breast-fed woman.
  **Management:**
  - Advise for frequent urination to empty bladder, full bladder can cause discomfort.
  - Massage the uterus to expel the clot.
  - Analgesics and antispasmodic should be given to relieve pain.
- **Perineal pain:** Perineum has to be inspected for normal pain or presence of hematoma or infection
  **Management:**
  - Cold and hot application on perineal area. For example, ice packs, sitz bath, infrared lamp therapy.
  - Topical anesthetic spray or ointment may be used.
- **Constipation:**
  **Management:**
  - Take plenty of fluid
  - Sufficient roughage in diet
  - Administer mild laxatives/stool softeners
- **Anemia:** Majority of woman in tropics remains anemic following delivery.
  **Treatment:** Iron therapy (ferrous sulfate 200 mg) is to be given for a minimum period of 4–6 weeks
- **Hypertension:** For a few hours after normal vaginal delivery, the blood pressure is likely to be raised, which settles down to normal during the second day.
  **Management:** Blood pressure comes to normal spontaneously but consult physician if proteinuria occurs.
- **Breast engorgement:** Due to improper sucking by infant and increased hormonal level, sometimes breast becomes engorged.
  **Management:**
  - Wear supportive bra.
  - Provide warm compress.
  - Massage the breast.
  - Encourage for breastfeeding or removal of milk from breast by suction pump.
- **Lactation suppression:** Refers to the act of suppressing lactation by medication or other nonpharmaceutical means. There are many ways in which suppression of lactation is needed.
  - Woman who cannot breast-fed for personal reasons.
  - When the baby is born dead or dies in the neonatal period.
  - In medical conditions, e.g., human immunodeficiency virus (HIV) infection.
    **Methods for lactation suppression:**
    - To stop breastfeeding
    - To avoid pumping or milk expression
    - To wear breast support
    - Ice packs to prevent engorgement
    - Tight compression bandage is applied for 2–3 days.
- **Postnatal diuresis:** The postpartum body removes excess fluid accumulated during pregnancy by diuresis. During the early postpartum period there is a loss of plasma volume (3 L/day) that is greater than that of red blood cells.
  **Management:** Encourage the mother for spontaneous bladder emptying by early ambulation, running water, warm perineal cascades; catheterization may be necessary if above measures are unsuccessful and distension increases.

# POSTNATAL EXERCISES

**Definition:** A series of physical exercises that are performed by the postnatal mother to bring about optimal functioning of all systems and prevent complications.

## Purposes

- To educate about correct posture and body mechanics.
- To prevent genital prolapse.
- To prevent stress incontinence of urine.
- To improve muscle tone, especially perineal and abdominal muscle that are stretched during pregnancy and labor.
- To minimize the risk of deep vein thrombosis (DVT).
- To reduce in aches and pains after delivery, e.g., backache and cramps.
- To improve posture and body awareness.
- To reduce constipation by accelerating movements in the intestine.
- To help postnatal recovery.
- To help sleep better by relieving stress and anxiety that might make the mother restless at night.
- To increase blood flow to the skin, and give a healthy growth (glow).
- To give mother an emotional lift from the release of internal hormones, like endorphins.
- To make mother feel more contented, as the release of tranquilizer hormones that follows exercise, aids relaxation.
- To help mother regain the shape more quickly after delivery.

## Articles

- Mat/Dari to do laying exercises comfortably
- Chair to sit in a comfortable position

## Points to be Taken Care

- Warm up and cool down at every exercise session
- If woman feels faintness and dizziness, slow down or stop exercising
- Drink plenty of fluids
- Do not over heat the body as overheating of body has been linked to some birth defects
- Maintain good posture
- Wear a well fitted and supported brassiere
- From midway throughout pregnancy, avoid exercising on the back as it places too much pressure on major veins and reduces $O_2$ supply to placenta and baby

## Warning Sign to Stop Exercise

- Vaginal bleeding
- Dizziness or feeling pain
- Breathlessness
- Chest pain
- Headache
- Muscle weakness
- Calf pain/swelling
- Uterine contractions
- Decreased fetal movements
- Fluid leaking from vagina

## Procedure

| Nursing action | Rationale |
|---|---|
| **Preprocedural steps:**<br>(Same as for antenatal exercise)<br>**Intraprocedural steps:**<br>**Exercise 1: Abdominal exercises**<br>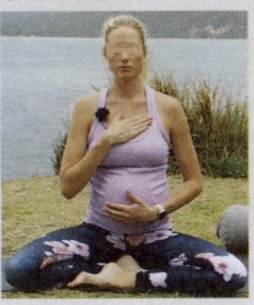 | • It strengthens the diaphragmatic muscles and improves oxygenation of the blood |
| • **Abdominal breathing:**<br> ▪ Instruct the woman to sit comfortably<br> ▪ Instruct her to inhale through nose, keep the ribcage as stationary as possible and allow the abdomen to expand and then contract the abdominal muscles as she exhales slowly through the mouth<br> ▪ Instruct her to place one hand on the chest and one on the abdomen when inhaling. The hand on the abdomen should rise and the hand on the chest should remain stationary<br> ▪ Repeat for five times | |
| • **Head lift:**<br> ▪ This exercise can be started within few days after childbirth<br> ▪ Instruct the mother to lie in supine position with knees bent and arms out-stretched at her side<br> ▪ Instruct her to inhale deeply at first and then exhale while lifting the head slowly, to hold the position for a few seconds and relax | • This exercise strengthens the abdominal muscles |
| • **Head and shoulder raising:**<br>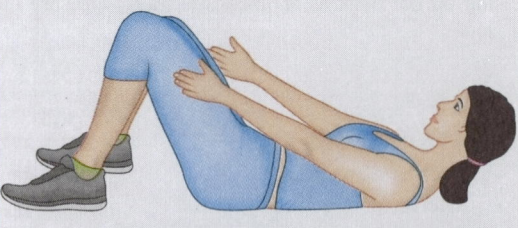<br>On 2<sup>nd</sup> postpartum day, instruct the mother to:<br> ▪ Lie flat without pillow and raise head until the chin touches the chest | • It strengthens the abdominal and diaphragmatic muscles |

*Contd...*

| Nursing action | Rationale |
|---|---|
| <ul><li>On 3<sup>rd</sup> postpartum day, raise both head and shoulders off the bed and lower them slowly</li><li>Repeat for 10 times</li></ul> | |
| <ul><li>**Leg raising:**</li></ul> 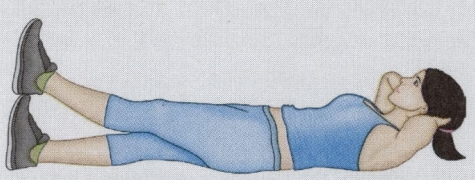 <ul><li>Instruct the mother to start this exercise on 7th postpartum day</li><li>Instruct her to lie flat on the floor with no pillows under the head, point toes and slowly raise one leg, keeping the knee straight</li><li>Lower the leg slowly</li><li>Gradually, increase the frequency to ten times with each leg</li></ul> | <ul><li>This exercise strengthens the abdominal muscles and helps in involutions of reproductive organs</li></ul> |
| <ul><li>**Knee and leg rolling:**</li></ul> 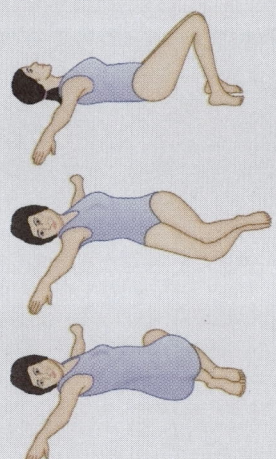 <ul><li>Instruct the mother to lie on the bed/floor with knee bent and feet flat on floor</li><li>Keep the shoulders and feet stationary and roll the knees to side to touch one side of the bed first and then other</li><li>Repeat it five times</li><li>Later, as flexibility increases, the exercise can be varied by the rolling of one knee only (the mother rolls her left knee to touch the right side of the bed, returns to center and rolls the right knee to touch the left side of the bed</li></ul> | <ul><li>This exercise will strengthen the oblique abdominal muscles</li></ul> |

*Contd...*

| Nursing action | Rationale |
|---|---|
| • **Pelvic tilting/rocking** (same as in antenatal exercises) | |
| • **Hip hitching:**<br>  ▪ Instruct the mother to lie on her back with one knee bent and another knee straight<br>  ▪ Slide the heel of the straight leg downwards, thus lengthening the leg<br>  ▪ Shorten the same leg by drawing the hip up toward the ribs on the same side<br>  ▪ Repeat up to 10 times keeping the abdomen pulled in<br>  ▪ Change to the opposite side and repeat | • It strengthens the deep transverse muscles which are the main support for the spine and thus prevents backache problem in the future |
| • **Abdominal tightening:**<br>  ▪ Instruct the woman to sit comfortably or kneel on all fours<br>  ▪ Breathe in and out, then pull the lower part of the abdomen below the umbilicus while continuing to breathe normally<br>  ▪ Hold for 10 seconds<br>  ▪ Repeat up to 10 times | • It strengthens the abdominal muscles and helps in involution of uterus after delivery |
| **2. Circulatory exercises:** Foot and leg exercise (same as in antenatal exercise)<br>**3. Pelvic floor exercises:** Kegel exercise (same as in antenatal exercise)<br>**4. Chest exercises:**<br>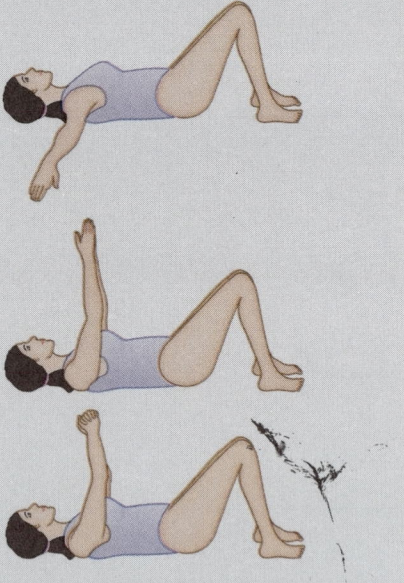<br>  ▪ Instruct the mother to lie flat on the floor mat with arms extended straight out to the side, bring both hands together above the chest, while keeping the arms straight, hold for a few seconds and return to the starting position | • To strengthen the diaphragmatic muscles |

*Contd...*

| Nursing action | Rationale |
|---|---|
| ▪ Repeat the exercise five times initially and follow the advice of the health care provider for increasing the number of repetitions<br>▪ Instruct the mother to bend her elbows, clasp her hands together above her chest, and press her hands together for a few seconds<br>▪ Repeat up to five times | |
| **Postprocedural steps** (same as in antenatal exercise) | |

# FAMILY PLANNING

Family planning is the practice of controlling the number of children one has and the interval between their births, particularly by means of contraception or voluntary sterilization.

## Objectives

- **Conception control:**
  - To bring down the birth rate to a realistic minimum during a given period.
  - To bring about certain special changes such as:
    - To educate and motivate couples to accept small family norms
    - To increase the literacy rate-woman in rural areas
    - To raise marriage age of both boys and girls
    - To maximize the access of good quality family planning services
- **Maternity and child health services:**
  - To extend maternity services through antenatal, intranatal and postnatal care with immunization against tetanus, and prevention and correction of anemia
  - To offer protection to children through immunization schedule and vitamins supplement program.
- **Other services:**
  - To provide sex education and marriage guidance
  - To promote research on normal reproduction, investigation and treatment of infertility and recurrent abortion.
- Birth control, contraception and family planning.

## Modern Concept of Family Planning

Family planning is not synonymous with birth control. A WHO expert committee in 1970 included the following:

- The proper spacing and limitation of birth
- Advice on sterility
- Education for parenthood
- Sex education
- Screening for pathological conditions related to reproductive system (Example: cervical cancer)
- Genetic counseling
- Premarital consultation and examination
- Carrying out pregnancy tests
- Marital counseling
- Preparation of couple for parenthood
- Providing adoption services
- Providing services for unmarried mothers
- Teaching home economics and nutrition.

## Methods of Contraception

Figure 2 shows the various methods of contraception:

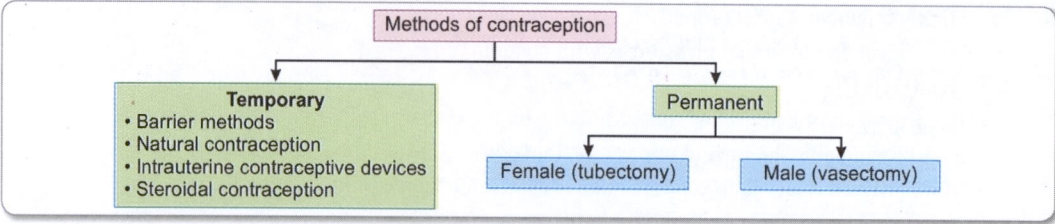

**Fig. 2:** Methods of contraception

### *Temporary Methods*

#### Barrier Methods

It includes:

- **Condom:** Condoms are made of polyurethane or latex. It is most widely used by males. A widely marketed brand in India is 'Nirodh' (Fig. 3).

  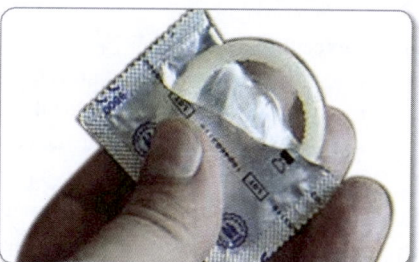

  **Fig. 3:** Condom

  **Instructions for use:**
  - Condom is unrolled over the erect penis
  - Rim of condom should be held against the base of penis
  - During withdrawal, make sure condom does not become dislodged from the penis.
  - After use, it should be checked for tears.
  - If found torn, spermicidal jelly should be put into vagina immediately
  - Throw away after single use.

  **Advantages:**
  - Easily available and inexpensive.
  - No side effects/no contraindications (except allergy).
  - Easy to carry, simple to use and disposable.
  - Protection against sexually transmitted infection (STIs).
  - Protection against pelvic inflammatory diseases.
  - Useful where sexual intercourse is infrequent and irregular.
  - Suitable to use during lactation.

  **Disadvantages:**
  - May accidentally break or slip off during coitus.
  - Inadequate sexual pleasure
  - Allergic reaction
  - Discard after one coital act
  - **Failure rate:** 15/Hundred women years (HWY) (When used correctly and consistently)

- **Diaphragm:** It is an intravaginal device made up of rubber with flexible metal or spring ring at the margin. Diameter varies from 5 cm to 10 cm (Fig. 4).

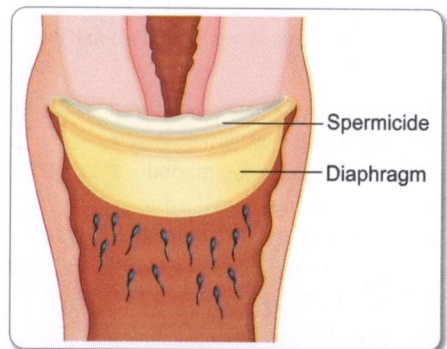

**Fig. 4:** Diaphragm

**Advantages:**

- Inexpensive
- It can be used repeatedly for long time
- Highly effective if used properly
- No interruption in sexual pleasure as with condom

**Disadvantages:**

- Requires help of a physician to measure the required size
- Risk of vaginal irritation and urinary tract infection (UTI)
- More difficult to use than condom and requires high degree of motivation for the user
- Not suitable for woman with uterine prolapse.

- **Vaginal contraceptives:** Spermicides are available as vaginal foams, gels, creams, tablets and suppositories. They contain surfactant, like nonxynol-9 and octoxynol. These agents mostly cause sperm immobilization. The cream or jelly is introduced high in vagina with the help of applicator before coitus.
  **Side effects:** Local allergic reactions.

## Natural Contraception

It includes:

- **Rhythm method:** The rhythm method is the only birth control method (beside total abstinence), which is approved by Roman Catholic Church. It is also referred to as "Safe period" or "temporary abstinence". The method is based on the identification of the fertile period of a cycle and to abstain from sexual intercourse during that period.
  The method to determine the approximate time of ovulation and the fertile period include:
  - Recording the previous menstrual cycle (calendar rhythm)
  - Recording the basal body temperature (temperature rhythm)
  - Taking note of the excessive mucoid vaginal discharge (mucus rhythm)
    - The user of calendar method obtains the period of abstinence from calculations based on the previous twelve menstrual cycle records. The first unsafe day is obtained by subtracting 20 days from the length of the shortest cycle and last unsafe day by deducting 10 days from the longest cycle.
    - User of temperature rhythm requires abstinence until the third day of rise of temperature.
    - User of mucus rhythm requires abstinence on all days of noticeable mucus and for 3 days thereafter.
- **Coitus interruptus (withdrawal):** It is the oldest and probably the most widely accepted contraceptive method used by man. It necessitates withdrawal of penis shortly before ejaculation. It requires sufficient self-control by man so that the withdrawal of penis precedes ejaculation.
  - **Advantages:**
    - No cost
    - No appliance is required
  - **Disadvantages:**
    - Requires sufficient self-control by man
    - The woman may develop anxiety, nervousness, vaginismus or pelvic congestion
    - Chances of pregnancy is more
    - Precoital secretion may contain sperm
    - Accidental chances of sperm deposition into the vagina

- **Breastfeeding/lactational amenorrhea:** Prolonged and sustained breastfeeding offers a natural protection of pregnancy. This is more effective in woman who are amenorrheic than those who are menstruating. The risk of pregnancy to a woman who is breastfeeding and amenorrheic is less than 2% in the first 6 months. Failure rate is 1–10%. Thus, additional contraceptives are required to provide complete contraception.

  When the mother is fully breastfeeding, a contraceptive method should be used in the 3rd postpartum month and with partial or no breastfeeding, she should use it in the 3rd postpartum week.

### Intrauterine Contraceptive Devices

Intrauterine contraceptive devices (IUCDs) are widely acceptable reversible method of contraception for spacing of births.

There are two main types (Fig. 5):

1. Medicated IUCD
2. Nonmedicated IUCD

Both are made of polyethylene or other polymer. Medicated IUCDs release either metal ions (Copper) or hormones (Progestogens).

The nonmedicated IUCDs are often referred to as first generation IUCDs. The copper IUCDs comprise the second and hormone releasing IUCDs comprise the third generation IUCDs. The medicated IUCDs were developed to reduce the incidence of side effects and to increase the contraceptive effectiveness.

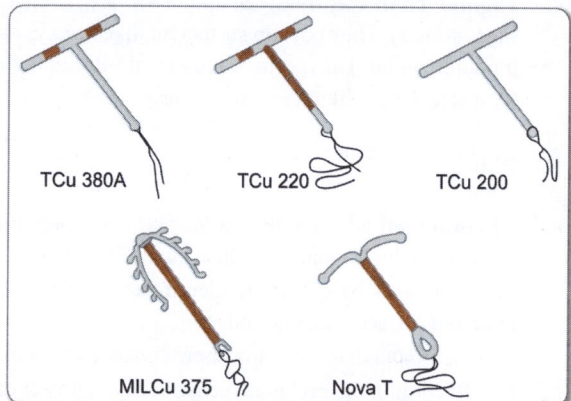

**Fig. 5:** Different types of intrauterine devices

- First generation IUCDs include Lippes loop, Saf-T-coil, Dana super and Margulies spiral.
- Second generation IUCDs include metallic copper devices such as:
  - Early devices
    - Cu T
    - Cu T-200
  - Newer devices: Variant of the T-devices such as:
    - Cu T-200C
    - Cu T-380A or Ag (Fig. 6)

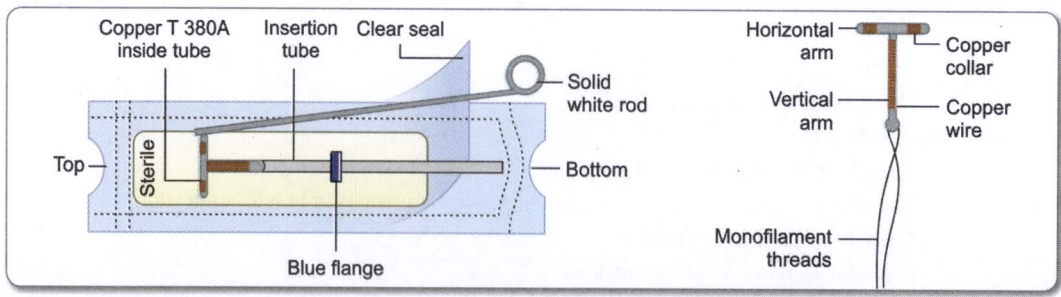

**Fig. 6:** Parts of Cu-T

- Nova T
- Multiload devices
  - Multi load Cu T-250 (ML Cu-250)
  - ML Cu T-375
- Third generation IUCDs include:
  - Progestasert
  - Levonorgestrel intrauterine system

## Description of devices

- **Copper T-200:** Carries 200 mm² surface area of wire containing 120 mg of copper and is removed after 3 years.
- **Copper T-380A:** Carries 380 mm² surface area of copper wire around the stem (175 mg) and sleeves and the horizontal arms (66.5 mg). Replacement is done after 10 years. Copper is lost at the rate of 50 mg per 24 hours during a period of 1 year.
- **Multiload Cu T-250:** Device emits 60–100 mg/day of copper during the period of one year. Replacement is done at an interval of every 3 years.
- **Multiload-375:** It has 375 mm² surface area of copper wire around its vertical stem. The device is to be replaced in every 5 years.
- **Progestasert:** It is a progesterone (38 mg) containing IUCD. Progestasert is no longer manufactured.
- **Lippes loop:** It is nonmedicated open IUCD. It is no longer manufactured in India
- **Levonorgestrel intrauterine system:** It is T-shaped device, with a polymethylsiloxane membrane around the stem, which contains levonorgestrel. It releases the hormone at the rate of 20 mg/day. The device is replaced in every 5 years. Its efficacy is comparable to sterilization.

## Mechanism mode of action of IUCDs

Figures 7A and B shows the mechanism of action of IUCDs.

- Biochemical and histological changes in the endometrium
- Increased tubal motility which prevent fertilization of ovum
- Endometrial inflammatory response decrease sperm transport.

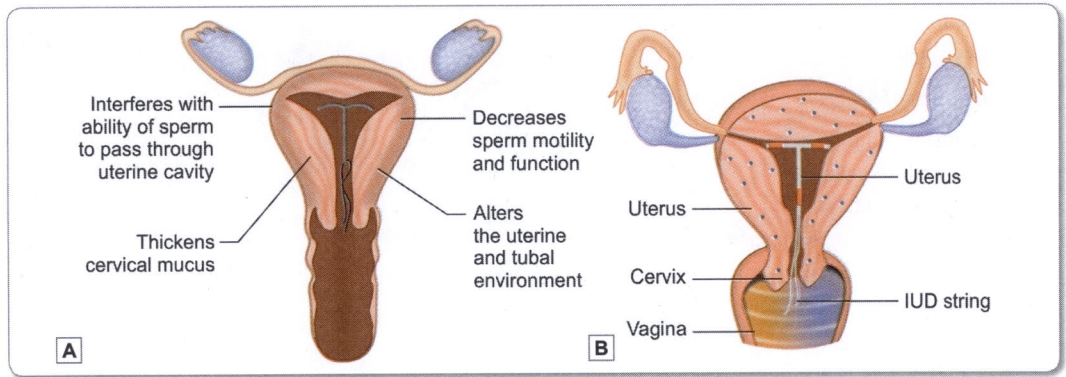

**Figs 7A and B:** Mechanism of action of IUCDs

## Time of insertion

- During menstruation or within 10 days of beginning of a menstrual period. During this period, diameter of cervical canal is greater than secretary phase and uterus is relaxed, thus the expulsion rate is less.

Chapter 7 ● Management of Normal Puerperium

- Postpartum insertion is done at 6–8 weeks after delivery. It has several advantages. It can be combined with the follow-up examination of the woman and her child.
- Post-abortion insertion can be taken up immediately after a legally induced first trimester abortion.
- Immediate postpartum insertions can be done during 1st week after delivery, before discharge from hospital. However, the disadvantages are high expulsion rate and greater risk of perforation.

### Contraindications for insertion of IUCD

- Presence of pelvic infection
- Suspected pregnancy
- Congenital uterine malformation
- Uterine fibroid
- Severe dysmenorrhea
- Past history of ectopic pregnancy
- Within 6 weeks of cesarean section
- History of sexually transmitted infections (STIs)
- Immunosuppressive client

### Follow-up

The objectives of follow-up are:

- To provide motivation and emotional support to the woman
- To confirm the presence of IUCD
- To diagnose and treat any side effect or complications

### Client instruction

- She should regularly check the threads or 'tail' to be sure that IUCD is in the uterus. If she fails to locate the thread, she must consult the gynecologist (Fig. 8).
- She should visit the clinic if she has fever, pelvic pain or bleeding.
- If she misses a period, she must consult the gynecologist.

### Complications of IUCDs

- Immediate complications:
  - Cramp-like pain
  - Syncopal attack
  - Partial or complete perforation
- Remote complications:
  - Pain
  - Abnormal menstrual bleeding
  - Pelvic infection
  - Spontaneous expulsion
  - Perforation of the uterus
  - Pregnancy
  - Ectopic pregnancy

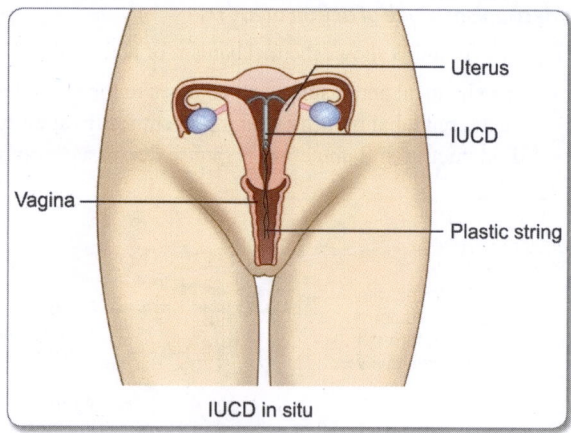

**Fig. 8:** IUCD in place

### Indications for removal of IUCD

- Persistent excessive regular or irregular bleeding and/or severe cramp-like pain in the lower abdomen
- Flaring up of salpingitis
- Perforation of uterus
- Partial expulsion
- Pregnancy occurring with the device in situ
- Woman desirous of baby
- Missing thread
- 1 year after menopause
- When effective life span of the device is over.

### Steroidal Contraceptives

Steroidal contraceptives (Fig. 9) when properly used are the most effective spacing methods of contraception. Oral contraceptives of the combined type are almost 100% effective in preventing pregnancy. About 10 million people in India use this contraceptive method.

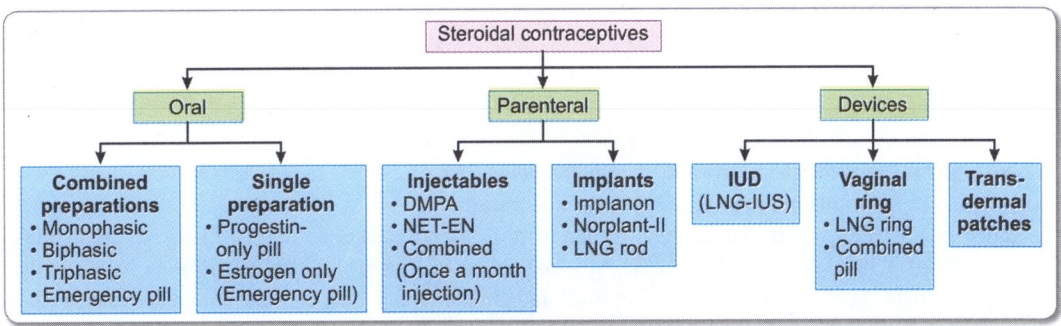

**Fig. 9:** Steroidal contraceptives

*Abbreviations:* DMPA, depomedroxyprogesterone acetate; IUD; intrauterine device; IUS, intrauterine system; LNG, levonorgestrel; NET-EN, norethisterone enanthate

### Oral contraceptives

- **Combined oral pills:** This is the most effective reversible method of contraception. In the combined pill, the commonly used progestins are either levonorgestrel/norethisterone/desogestrel and estrogens are either ethinyl estradiol/mestranol. Some of the preparations available in the market are given in Table 4.

**TABLE 4:** Composition of oral pills

| Trade name | Composition | | No. of tablets |
|---|---|---|---|
| | Progestins (mg) | Estrogen (mg) | |
| Mala D (Fig. 10A) | Levonorgestrel (0.15) | Ethinyl estradiol (30) | 21 + 7 iron tablets |
| Mala N (Govt of India) (Fig. 10B) | Levonorgestrel (0.15) | Ethinyl estradiol (30) | 21 + 7 Iron tablets |
| Loette (Wyeth) | Desogestrel (0.15) | Ethinyl estradiol (20) | 21 |
| Yasmin (Schering) | Desogestrel (0.15) | Ethinyl estradiol (30) | 21 |

Chapter 7 ♦ Management of Normal Puerperium

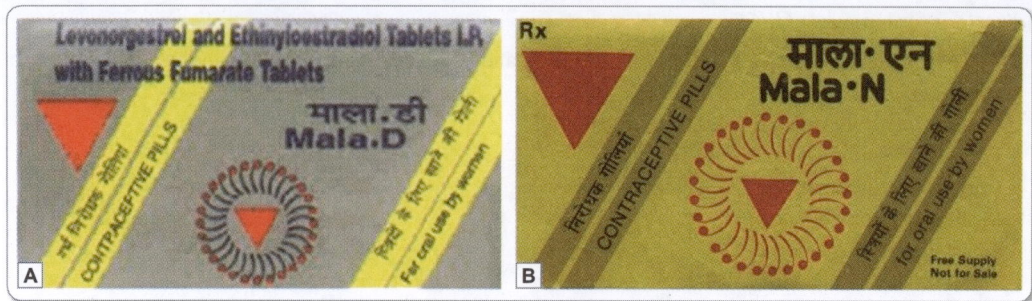

**Figs 10A and B:** Mala D and Mala N

- Types of pills:
    - **1st generation pills:** With estrogen 50 mg or more
    - **2nd generation pills:** With estrogen 20–35 mg and progesterone as norgestimate or levonorgestrel
    - **3rd generation pills:** With estrogen 20–30 mg and progesterone as desogestrel or gestodene
    - **4th generation pills:** Estrogen as 3rd generation, with progesterone as drospirenone, dienogest or nomegestrol
- Mode of action:
    - Inhibition of ovulation
    - Producing static endometrial hyperplasia
    - Alteration of the character of the cervical mucus
    - Interferes with tubal motility and alters tubal transport.
- **How to prescribe a pill:** Instruct the woman to start her pill packet on day 1 of her cycle. One tablet is to be taken daily preferably at bed time for consecutive 21 days. It is continued for 21 days and then 7-days break. Seven of the pills are dummies and contain either iron or vitamin preparations. Thus, a simple regime of "3 weeks on and 1 week off" is to be followed (Fig. 11).

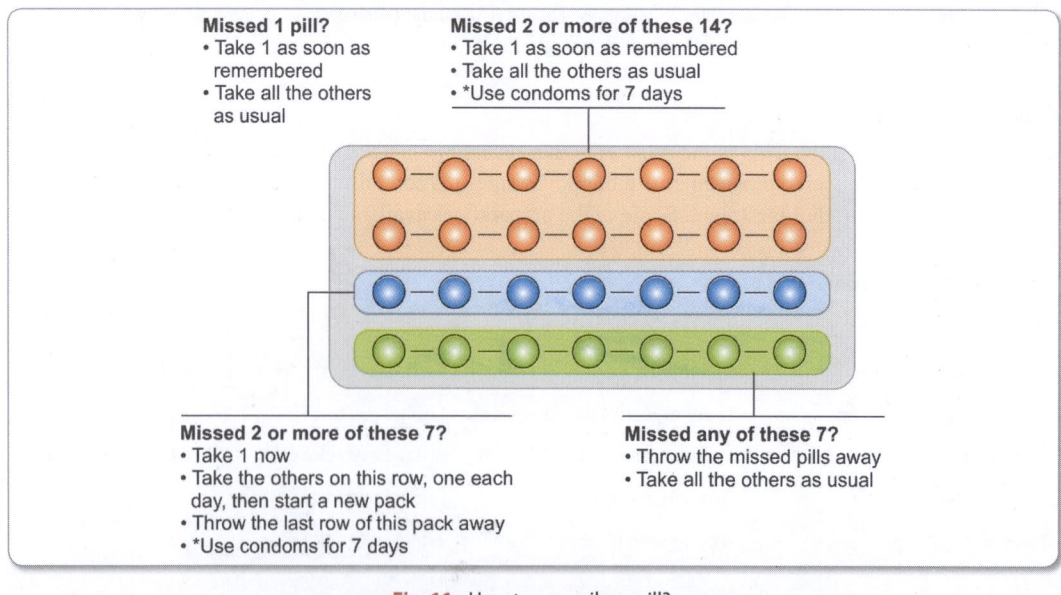

**Fig. 11:** How to prescribe a pill?

- Contraindications (Table 5)

**TABLE 5:** Absolute and relative contraindications of combined oral pills

| Absolute | | | Relative |
| --- | --- | --- | --- |
| Circulatory diseases | Diseases of the liver | Others | |
| • Arterial or venous thrombosis<br>• Severe hypertension, stroke<br>• Valvular heart disease, Ischemic heart disease, angina<br>• Diabetes with vascular complications<br>• Focal migraine, severe hypercholesterolemia<br>• Smokers over 35 years | • Acute liver disease<br>• Liver adenoma<br>• Carcinoma<br>• Liver tumors | • Pregnancy<br>• Genital tract lesions<br>• Estrogen dependent tumors<br>• Breastfeeding<br>• Major surgery or prolonged immobilization | • Age >40 years<br>• Smoker, <35 years<br>• History of jaundice<br>• Diabetes<br>• Gallbladder disease<br>• Hyperlipidemia<br>• Post breast cancer<br>• Breastfeeding<br>• Sickle cell disease |

- **Follow-up:** The woman should be examined after 3 months, 6 months and then once a year. Woman above 35 years should be checked more frequently. Any adverse symptoms are to be noted at each visit. Examination of breasts, weight, blood pressure and pelvic examination including cytology are to be done and compared with previous record.
- **Length of pill use:** For spacing of birth, use of 3–5 years is considered adequate and safe. However, with careful monitoring, pill use may continue until the age of 40 years. Beyond 40 years, pills may not be continued because of the risk of cardiovascular complications.
- **Beneficial effects:** The most important benefit is prevention of unwanted pregnancy. The noncontraceptive benefits are:
  - Relief of:
    - Menorrhagia (<50%)
    - Dysmenorrhea (<40%)
    - Premenstrual syndrome
    - Mittelschmerz syndrome
  - Improvement of:
    - Iron deficiency anemia
    - Endometriosis
    - Hirsutism
    - Rheumatoid arthritis
  - Reduction in risk of:
    - Pelvic inflammatory disease
    - Benign breast disease
    - Fibroid uterus
    - Functional ovarian cysts
    - Carcinoma of cervix and ovary
    - Osteoporosis
- **Adverse effects:**
  - Nausea, vomiting, headache and leg cramps
  - Mastalgia
  - Weight gain
  - Chloasma and acne
  - Menstrual abnormalities
  - Reduced libido
  - Leukorrhea
- **Complications:**
  - Depression, change of mood and sleep disturbances
  - Hypertension
  - Vascular complications
  - Cholestatic jaundice

### Progestogen-only pill

Progestogen-only pill is commonly referred to as minipill or micropill. It contains only progestogen, which is given in small doses throughout the cycle. The commonly used progestogens are norethisterone (350 mg) and levonorgestrel (30 mg).

- **Mechanism of action:** It works mainly by making cervical mucus thick and viscous, thereby prevents sperm penetration. Endometrium becomes atrophic. In about 2% of cases, ovulation is inhibited.
- **Advantages:**
  - No adverse effects on lactation and hence, can be suitably given to lactating woman and as such is known as lactation pill.
  - It can be given to woman having hypertension, fibroid, diabetes or epilepsy.
- **Drawbacks:**
  - There may be breakthrough bleeding (the bleeding between the cycle) or at times amenorrhea in about 20–30% of cases
  - Simple cysts in ovary may be seen
  - Failure rate is about 0.5–2 per hundred woman years (when used correctly and consistently)

### Postcoital pill (emergency pill)

Postcoital (or 'morning after') contraception is recommended within 48 hours of unprotected intercourse. Two methods are available:

- IUCD, especially a copper device.
- **Hormonal:** A hormonal method may be preferable (Fig. 12).

The method is to give a double dose of standard combined pill. The recommended regimen is to take two pills immediately, followed by another two pills 12 hours later, if pills containing 50 µg of estrogen are used. If pills containing 30–35 µg estrogen are available, four of these must be taken at one time rather than two in each dose.

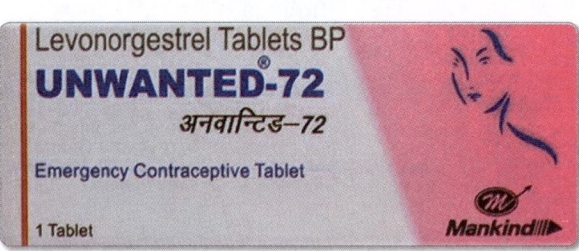
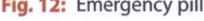

**Fig. 12:** Emergency pill

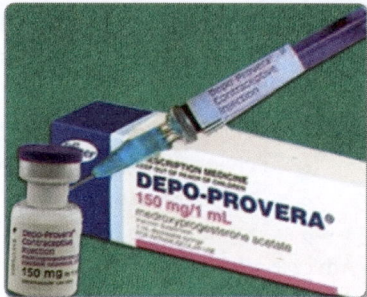

**Fig. 13:** Injection DMPA

### Injectable contraceptives

There are two types of injectable contraceptives:

- Depomedroxyprogesterone acetate (DMPA) (Fig. 13):
  - It is an artificial progestin preparation that resembles the naturally occurring female hormone, progesterone. It is given in dose of 150 mg and provides contraception for 3 months after infection.

- It prevents pregnancy in the following ways:
  - Inhibition of ovulation
  - Thickening of cervical mucus
  - Thinning of endometrium to make it unfavorable for implantation of fertilized eggs
  - Showing of sperm and ovum transport through reduced fallopian tubes peristalsis
- It is a very effective mode of contraception and has an advantage of being a long-acting method
- It is suitable for breastfeeding women as it does not have any side-effects of estrogen
- Disadvantages:
  - Disturbance of menstrual cycle
  - Delayed return of delivery
  - Weight gain
  - No protection against STIs
- It can be started:
  - In the first 7 days after the menstrual bleeding starts
  - 6 weeks after childbirth
  - Immediately or on the 7th day after childbirth if the woman is not breastfeeding
  - Immediately or on the 7th day after a miscarriage or abortion
  - Immediately after stopping another method

- **Norethisterone enanthate (NET-EN):** It is given in dose of 200 mg and provide protection for 2 months. Mechanisms, effectiveness, advantages and disadvantages of NET-EN one similar of DMPA.
- **Implants**
  - **Subdermal:** It contains six silicon rubber capsules containing 35 µg (each) of levonorgestrel (Fig. 14A). It initially releases 80 µg and later on it is reduced to 30 µg levonorgestrel per day over 5 years. Norplant capsules measures 34 mm × 24 mm and provide effective contraception for 5 years.
    - **Insertion:** The capsules are inserted subdermally, in the inner aspect of nondominant arm, 6–8 cm above the elbow fold. It is done under local anesthetic. It is ideally inserted on day 1 of menstrual cycle, immediately after abortion or 3 weeks after delivery.
    - **Removal:** Norplant should be removed within 5 years of insertion. Loss of contraceptive action is immediate.
    - **Advantages**
      - Improvement of anemia due to control of menorrhagia
      - Suitable for woman who have completed their family and do not desire permanent sterilization.

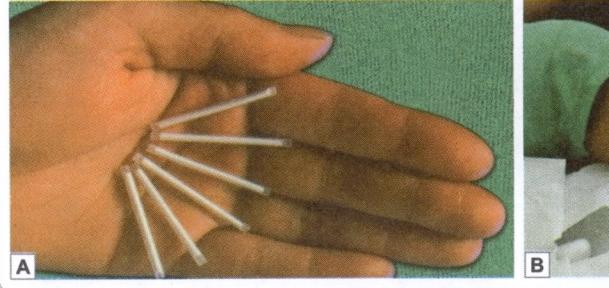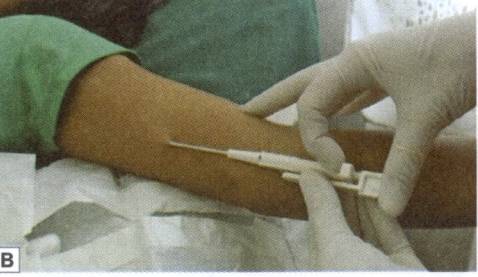

**Figs 14A and B: A.** Norplant; **B.** Implanon

- o **Disadvantages**
  - ◆ Frequent irregular, menstrual bleeding, spotting especially in the first year
  - ◆ Surgical procedure necessary to insert and remove implants.
- ■ **Implanon:** Single implant rod of 4 cm long, containing 60 mg of keto desogestrel is used (Fig. 14B). It releases the hormone about 60 µg per day over 3 years. Use of single rod makes implanon easier for insertion and removal. Efficacy and side effects are same as Norplant.
- • **Other steroidal contraceptive devices**
  - ■ **Vaginal ring (Nova-ring):** A ring-shaped device that contains the hormone estradiol and etonogestrel (a progestin) can be placed in the vagina. It remains in place for 3 weeks continuously and releases low levels of hormone into the bloodstream. Then it is removed for a week to allow for menstrual flow.

### Permanent Methods (Sterilization)

Permanent surgical contraception, also called voluntary sterilization, is a surgical method whereby the reproductive function of an individual male or female is purposefully and permanently destroyed. The operation performed on males is vasectomy and that on female is tubectomy.

### Vasectomy

Vasectomy (Fig. 15) is a permanent sterilization operation done in the males where a segment of vas deferens of both the sides are resected and the cut ends are ligated.

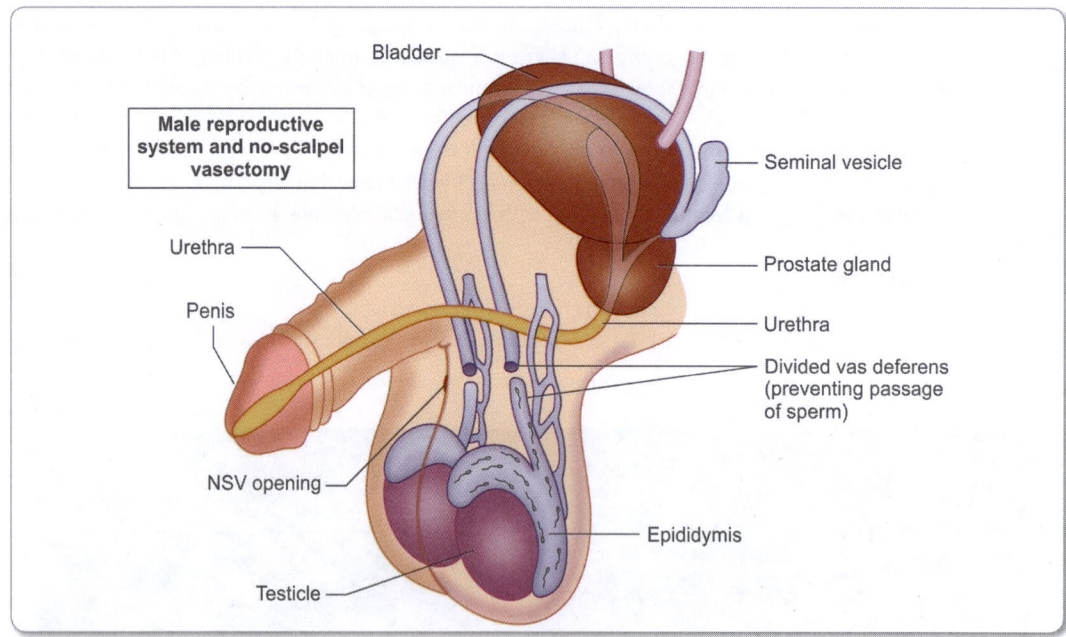

**Fig. 15:** Vasectomy

- • **Advantages:**
  - ■ Easily performed
  - ■ Outdoor procedure

- ▪ Failure rate 1/2000
- ▪ Fair chance of reversal anastomosis operation (70–80%)
- ▪ Free of cost operation
- • **Drawbacks:**
  - ▪ Additional contraceptive protection is needed for 2–3 months following operation or until the semen is declared to be free of sperms.
  - ▪ Frigidity or impotency when occurs is mostly psychological.
- • **Selection of person:**
  - ▪ Sexually active and psychologically adjusted husband having the desired number of children is an ideal one.
- • **Postoperative advices:**
  - ▪ Antibiotic injection (penidure intramuscularly) is administered as a routine and an analgesic is also prescribed.
  - ▪ Weight lifting, heavy work and cycling are restricted for about 2 weeks.
  - ▪ Wearing a scrotal support for 15 days is advised
  - ▪ The patient should report for checkup after 1 week or earlier, if complications arise.
  - ▪ Stitches should be removed on 5th day
  - ▪ Semen should be examined once a month and if two consecutive semen analysis show absence of spermatozoa, the man is considered sterile, until then additional contraceptives should be advised.
- • **Complications:**
  - ▪ *Immediate*
    - ○ Wound sepsis
    - ○ Scrotal cellulitis
    - ○ Abscess in scrotum
    - ○ Scrotal hematoma
  - ▪ *Remote*
    - ○ Frigidity or impotency
    - ○ Sperm granuloma
    - ○ Chronic intrascrotal pain and discomfort
    - ○ Autoimmune response
    - ○ Chances of recanalization is rare

## Tubectomy

Tubectomy (Figs 16A and B) is a surgical procedure in which the fallopian tubes are severed and sealed in order to prevent fertilization.

- • **Indications:**
  - ▪ Family planning
  - ▪ **Socioeconomic:** Individuals accept the method after having desired number of children
  - ▪ **Medicosurgical indications:** Medical conditions, like heart disease, diabetes, renal diseases likely to worsen if repeated pregnancies occur.
- • **Time of operation:**
  - ▪ **During puerperium:** 24–48 hours following delivery.
  - ▪ **Cesarean ligation:** Following cesarean childbirth for woman who has completed her families.
  - ▪ **Interval tubal ligation:** The operation is done beyond 3 months following delivery or abortion. Ideal time is: Proliferative phase of menstrual period.
  - ▪ Concurrent medical termination of pregnancy.
- • **Approaches for tubectomy:**
  - ▪ Abdominal conventional and mini laparotomy
  - ▪ Vaginal

- **Advantages of tubectomy:**
  - Very effective method of contraception
  - Gives permanent or lifelong protection
  - No interference with sex
  - Nothing to remember and no repeated visits to clinic are required
  - No side effect or health risks
- **Disadvantages:**
  - Pain for few days after surgery
  - Infection or bleeding at incision site
  - Injury to internal organs
  - Anesthesia risks
  - Reversal surgery is difficult and expensive.

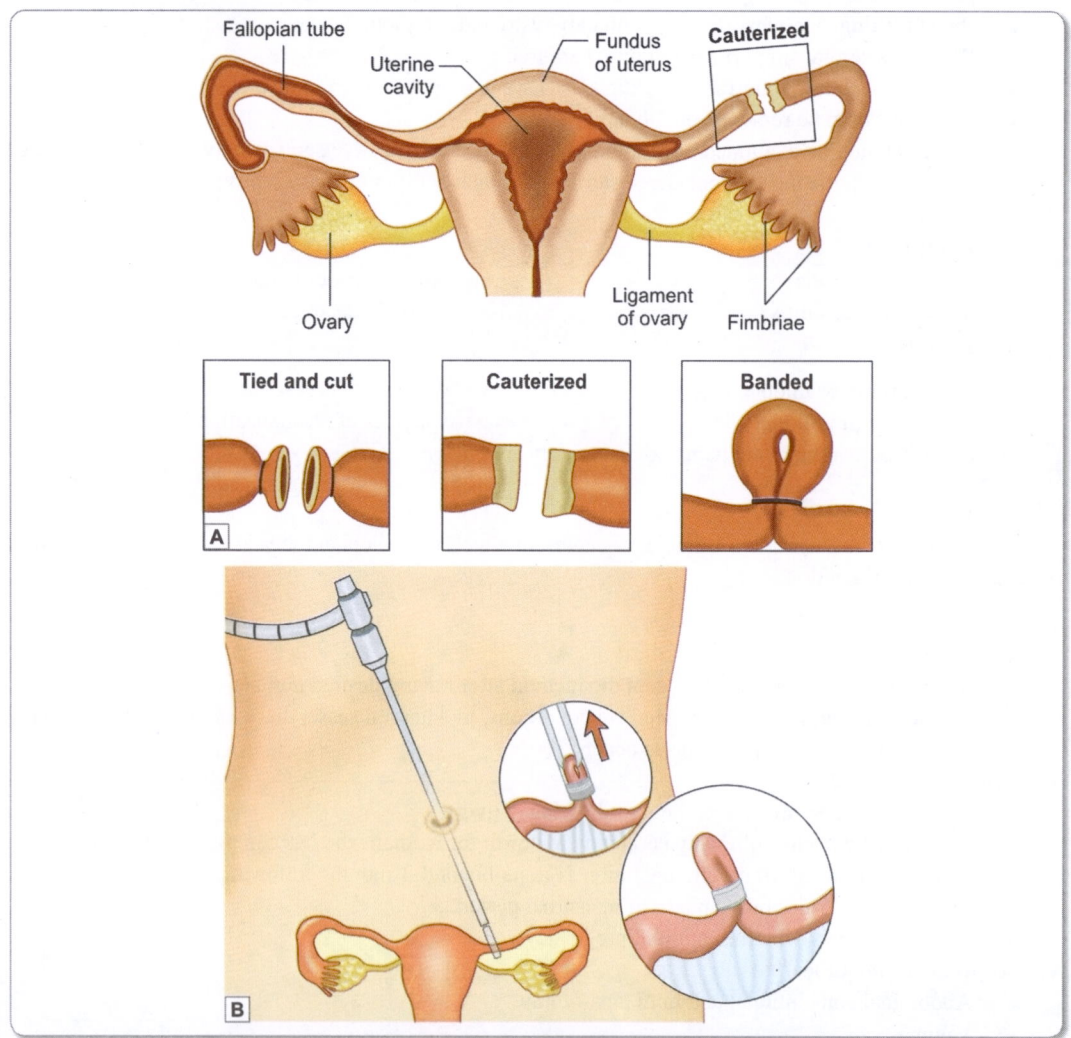

**Fig. 16A and B:** **A.** Procedures in tubectomy; **B.** Tying the fallopian tubes

## ASSESS YOURSELF

### FREQUENTLY ASKED QUESTIONS IN EXAMS

1. Define puerperium.
2. What are the objectives of care during puerperium?
3. Describe the physiological changes occurring during puerperium.
4. Explain the physiology of lactation.
5. Describe the nursing management of normal puerperium.
6. Write short notes on:
   - Postnatal exercises
   - Breastfeeding
   - Cu-T
   - Oral pills
   - Permanent sterilization
   - Lochia

### MULTIPLE CHOICE QUESTIONS

1. **Puerperium period is up to:**
   a. 4 weeks
   b. 6 weeks
   c. 8 weeks
   d. 12 weeks

2. **Lochial discharge is for:**
   a. 1–4 days
   b. 4–5 days
   c. 10–14 days
   d. 14–21 days

3. **Color of lochia rubra is:**
   a. Red
   b. Yellow
   c. Pink
   d. Orange

4. **The uterus becomes pelvic organ within:**
   a. 10–12 days
   b. 12–14 days
   c. 16–18 days
   d. 18–20 days

5. **Content of lochia are:**
   a. Blood
   b. Decidual membrane
   c. Bits of fetal membranes
   d. All of the above

6. **Female sterilization is called:**
   a. Tubectomy
   b. Vasectomy
   c. Laparotomy
   d. None of the above

7. **Oral pill of government supply:**
   a. Mala D
   b. Mala N
   c. Progestin only pill
   d. Postcoital pill

8. **Ideal time for Cu-T insertion is:**
   a. 2–3 days following menstruation
   b. 7 days after menstruation
   c. During menstruation
   d. 2–3 days prior to menstruation

9. **Adverse effects of combined oral contraceptives are the following except:**
   a. Nausea and vomiting
   b. Weight gain
   c. Mastalgia
   d. Normal menstruation

10. **At least how many ejaculations are required for a man to become sterile?**
    a. 20 ejaculations
    b. 5 ejaculations
    c. 40 ejaculations
    d. Nothing required

11. **Immediately following delivery, fundal height is:**
    a. 13.5 cm, above the symphysis pubis
    b. 12 cm, at the level of umbilicus
    c. 13 cm, in between umbilicus and symphysis pubis
    d. 10 cm, below symphysis pubis

12. **Duration of lochia serosa is:**
    a. 5–9 days
    b. 1–4 days
    c. 10–15 days
    d. 4–6 days

13. **Normal involution per day is:**
    a. 1.25 cm/day
    b. 1.5 cm/day
    c. 0.5 cm/day
    d. 2 cm/day

14. **Ejection of milk is:**
    a. Mammogenesis
    b. Lactogenesis
    c. Galactokinesis
    d. Galactopoiesis

15. **Suppression of milk production is done by:**
    a. Bromocriptine
    b. Metoclopramide
    c. Sulpiride
    d. None of the above

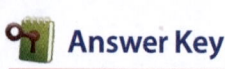 **Answer Key**

| 1. b | 2. d | 3. a | 4. b | 5. d | 6. a | 7. b |
| 8. a | 9. d | 10. a | 11. a | 12. a | 13. a | 14. c |
| 15. a | | | | | | |

# Chapter 8

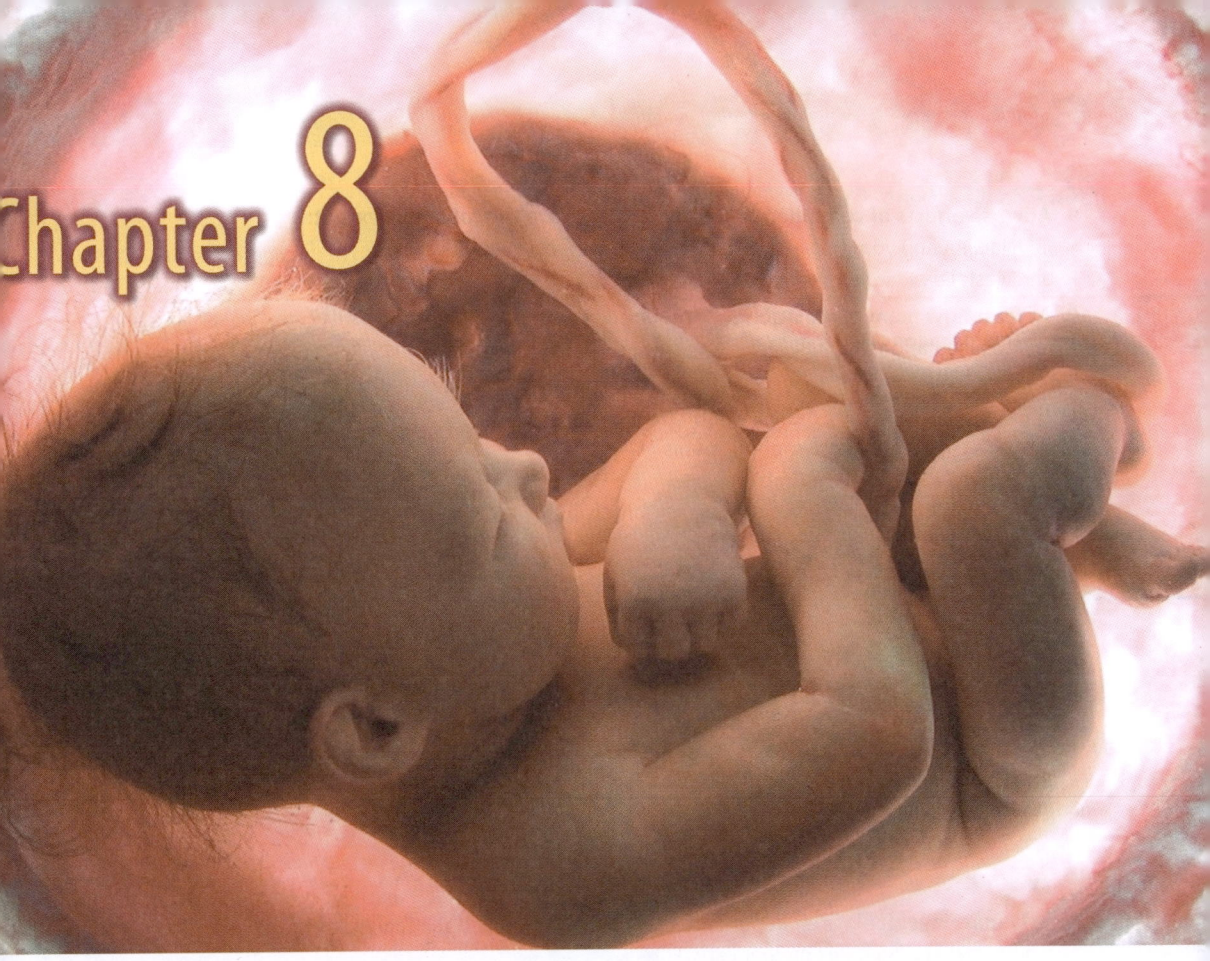

# Management of Complications during Pregnancy

## Learning Objectives

**Upon completing this chapter, the learner will be able to:**

➡ Discuss the varieties of ectopic gestation, their presentation, outcome and management

➡ Discuss the types of spontaneous and induced abortions and the medical and nursing management of patients

➡ Describe the clinical presentation and management of clients who suffer hyperemesis in pregnancy

➡ Define antepartum hemorrhage and explain its causes and effect on mother and fetus

➡ Discuss the classification, signs and symptoms, complications and nursing care for client with hypertensive disorders

➡ Explain post maturity, its causes, signs and symptoms and management of post-term baby

➡ Outline common medical disorders and management of women with different medical conditions during pregnancy

➡ Outline multiple pregnancy, clinical presentation, complications and its management

# TEENAGE PREGNANCY

**Definition:** It is defined as pregnancy occurring in under age or teenage girls (between 13 and 19 years).

In this case, the pregnant teen mother and the child born are likely to suffer with health problems, social, emotional and economic problems.

## Causes

- **Early marriage:** It plays an important in teenage pregnancy. If the female gets married early, it becomes obvious that she becomes mother early.
- **Early dating behavior:** Dating of teenage children has become common nowadays. In extreme cases, this can also lead to early pregnancy.
- **Rape on minor:** Rising incidence of rape on minor has also increased the rate of teenage pregnancy.
- **Lack of family bonding:** Children who do not show close relationships with their family members are more likely to go out and indulge in such activities because of unhealthy environment.
- **Intake of drugs:** Intake of drugs and alcohol is also one of the causes. Under intoxication, children can get into such activities.
- **Financial factors:** One of the important factors is the financial constraints and poverty. Sometimes, girls indulge in such activities because of lack of money that results in pregnancy.
- **Lack of contraceptives:** If marriage is done early and no contraceptive methods are used, it can lead to teen pregnancy and can have adverse effect on baby as well as the mother.
- **Traditional beliefs:** According to some societal norms, it is considered as good thing if girls become pregnant early after marriage. It is considered as a proof of her fertility.

## Effects of Teenage Pregnancy

- **High drop-out from school:** Teenage mothers are likely to drop out of school which leads to lack of proper education of the girl.
- **Premature birth:** Teenage pregnancy can lead to premature birth of babies. The child can also be low-birth weight.

- **Inadequate nutrition:** Teenage mothers are likely to get inadequate nutrition during pregnancy, this can give rise to further problems.
- **Maternal and infant mortality:** Teenage pregnancy results in many complications which can cause maternal deaths. Underdeveloped pelvis at this age can give rise to birth difficulties and can lead to infant mortality also.
- **Unfulfilled needs:** There are many needs of infants of teenage mothers, which remain unfulfilled. If there is poverty, she cannot meet the financial needs of her child. Medical aid is also not provided sometimes. She herself is not mature enough to understand the emotional needs of child.
- **Health risk:** Teenage mother is more likely to have anemia, pregnancy induced hypertension, lower genital tract infection, etc.

## Prevention of Teenage Pregnancy

One of the most effective ways of reducing rate of teenage pregnancy is to have open talks to teens.

A strong, emotional bond should be developed in the family members and such children are less likely to indulge in such activities. Emotional attachment of parents with their children is a strong force helping the teens to avoid such activities and the knowledge of contraception should be provided.

# HYPEREMESIS GRAVIDARUM

**Definition:** Excessive condition of nausea and vomiting during pregnancy, which has got serious effect on the health of the mother and incapacitate her in day-to-day activities. Because of excessive vomiting mother may have dehydration, metabolic acidosis, alkalosis electrolyte imbalance and weight loss.

## Etiology

Exact cause is unknown but the following factors are expected to cause hyperemesis gravidarum:
- High levels of human chorionic gonadotropin (hCG) as in twin pregnancy or hydatidiform mole.
- Previous history of hyperemesis
- Young age
- First pregnancy (more common)
- Low body mass index (<18.5)
- Family history of hyperemesis gravidarum

## Signs and Symptoms

- Pernicious vomiting (anything taken orally is rejected)
- Poor appetite and poor nutritional intake
- Loss of more than 25% of body weight
- Dehydration and electrolyte imbalance
- Acidosis due to starvation
- Alkalosis resulting from loss of hydrochloric acid (HC1) in vomitus
- Jaundice develops in severe cases
- Low urine output
- Rapid pulse and low blood pressure
- Hemoconcentration with rising blood urea nitrogen and falling serum levels of sodium, potassium and chloride.

The condition is said to be mild when there is loss of weight, but no dehydration. Moderate cases are those, characterized by dehydration and circulatory changes. Severe cases have biochemical changes with complications (metabolic acidosis).

## Investigations

- **Urinalysis:**
  - Quantity small
  - Dark color
  - High specific gravity with acid reaction
  - Presence of acetone, protein or bile pigments
  - Diminishes absence of chloride
- **Biochemical/circulatory changes:** Changes in the levels of serum electrolyte (sodium, potassium and chloride)
- Serum thyroid stimulating hormone (TSH), tri-iodo thyronine ($T_3$) and free thyroxine ($T_4$)
- **Ophthalmoscopic examination** in severe cases to detect retinal hemorrhage or detachment of retina
- **Electrocardiogram (ECG)** in case of abnormal serum potassium level

## Complications

- Circulatory changes
- Jaundice due to liver involvement
- Retinal hemorrhage
- Wernicke's encephalopathy
- Korsakoff's syndrome (disorientation and loss of memory)
- Renal insufficiency, renal failure
- Polyneuritis
- Delirium, coma, death

## Management

- Woman with hyperemesis gravidarum is admitted to hospital.
- Initially nothing is given through mouth (at least 24 hours after the cessation of vomiting).
- Hypovolemia and electrolyte imbalance are corrected by administering intravenous fluid. Approximately, 3 L of fluid is to be infused in 24 hours, out of which half is 5% dextrose and half is ringer solution. Extra amount of crystalloids equal to the amount of vomitus and urine in 24 hours, is to be added.
- Enteral nutrition through nasogastric tube is also helpful to manage the condition.
- Mother should be encouraged to rest and should be cared in a single room.
- Some women are prescribed a mild sedative, if they are agitated.
- Supportive psychotherapy and counseling may help.
- Before the intravenous fluid is omitted, the foods are given orally. At first, dry carbohydrate foods, like biscuits, bread and toast are given. Small palatable meals at regular interval may help the mother to regain her appetite. Gradually, full diet is restored.
- Instruct the mother for dietary recommendations, e.g., avoid taking fatty, spicy and preserved food items.
- Antiemetic (phenergan 25 mg, stemetil 5 mg twice daily) is helpful to treat nausea and vomiting.
- Hydrocortisone 100 mg IV in the drip is given in case with hypotension or in intractable vomiting. Oral prednisolone is also used in severe cases.

- Nutritional supplements (vitamins $B_1$, $B_6$, $B_{12}$ and vitamin C) are helpful to treat this condition.
- To monitor the recovery, check and record temperature, pulse, blood pressure at least twice daily.
- Maintain intake-output chart. Note the presence of acetone, protein and bile in the urine.
- Monitor blood biochemistry level and ECG report, if serum potassium level is abnormal.
- Termination of pregnancy is recommended in severe cases with jaundice, persistent albuminuria, poly neuritis to reverse the condition and to prevent maternal mortality.

## Nursing Process for Client with Hyperemesis Gravidarum

### Assessment

- Intractable vomiting
- Weight loss
- Ketosis, ketonuria
- Dehydration
- Epigastric pain
- Drowsiness and confusion
- Uncoordinated movements, jerking
- Urine output and total intake

### Goals and Objectives

**Ensure that the woman**
- Is well hydrated
- Has normal electrolyte values
- Verbalizes feelings and has ability to cope with the pregnancy
- Verbalizes knowledge of need for fluids

### Nursing Diagnosis

- Risk for fetal injury
- Risk for infection
- Ineffective airway clearance
- Risk for aspiration
- Anxiety related to pregnancy outcome
- Anticipatory grieving
- Altered family coping

### Planning

- Provide IV/oral fluids to re-establish fluid and electrolyte balance.
- Create opportunities for the woman to explore out the feelings about pregnancy and her coping abilities.
- Provide teaching related to need for fluids and the dietary changes

### Implementation

- Administer parenteral fluids, vitamins and sedatives as prescribed.
- Monitor intake, output and daily weight.
- Assess state of hydration.
- Begin oral feedings slowly with fluids, progress to six small feedings a day.
- Obtain psychiatric consultation, if indicated.

## ABORTION

Abortion is the expulsion or extraction of the product of conception (the fetus, fetal membranes and placenta) weighing 500 g or less when it is not capable of independent survival (World Health Organization [WHO]). The fetus gains weight of 500 g approximately at 22 weeks.

## Classification of Abortion

Figure 1 shows the classification of abortion.

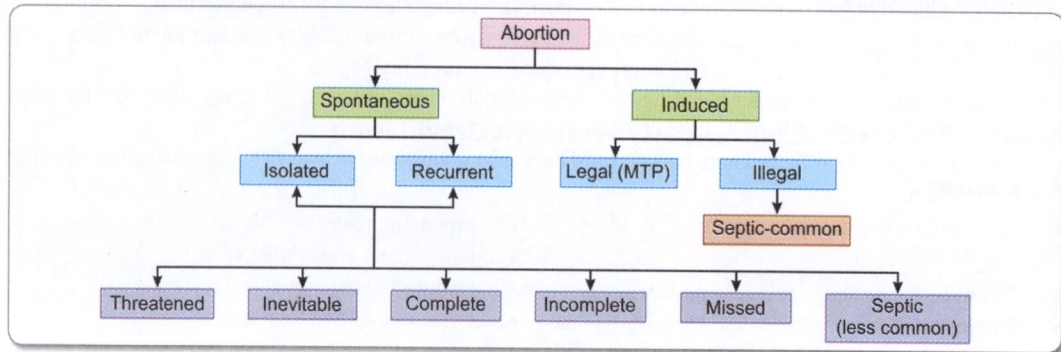

**Fig. 1:** Classification of abortion
*Abbreviation:* MTP, medical termination of pregnancy

## Causes

- **Genetic:** Majority (50%) of abortions are due to chromosomal abnormality in the conceptus. For example, trisomy, polyploidy, monosomy, structural chromosomal abnormalities, etc.
- **Endocrine and metabolic factors**
  - Luteal phase defect
  - Deficient progesterone
  - Thyroid abnormalities (hypothyroidism)
  - Diabetes mellitus.
- **Anatomical abnormalities**
  - Cervical incompetence
  - Congenital malformation of the uterus
  - Uterine fibroids
  - Intrauterine adhesion
- **Infections,** e.g., viral, bacterial and parasites
- **Immunological disorders:**
  - Antiphospholipid antibody syndrome
  - Immune factors, e.g., cytokines
- **Autoimmunity,** e.g., natural killer cells present in uterus and peripheral blood provide immunity
- **Maternal medical illnesses,** e.g., cyanotic heart disease, hemoglobinopathies are associated with early miscarriage.
- **Premature rupture of membranes** inevitably lead to abortion.
- **Inherited thrombophilia and protein C resistance** cause both early and late miscarriages.
- **Environmental factors:**
  - Smoking
  - Alcohol
  - Contraceptive agents
  - Drugs, chemicals, noxious agents
- **Unexplained (40–60%)** of abortion cause is unknown

## Threatened Abortion

**Definition:** It means when the process of miscarriage has started but has not progressed to stage from which recovery is impossible.

### Signs and Symptoms

- **Bleeding per vagina:** Slight bleeding may be brownish or bright red in color. Bleeding usually stops spontaneously.
- **Pain:** Bleeding is painless. There may be mild backache or dull pain in lower abdomen usually following hemorrhage.

### Investigations

- **Blood test:** For hemoglobin, hematocrit, ABO and Rh grouping.
- **Urine test:** For immunological test of pregnancy.
- Ultrasonography (transvaginal)
- Serum progesterone, serum hCG values are helpful to assess fetal well-being.

### Management

- **Rest:** Patient should be on bed until bleeding stops.
- **Drugs:** Diazepam 5 mg tablet twice daily for relief of pain.
- Advice patient to avoid heavy work load.
- Avoid intercourse.
- Advise patient for follow-up with repeat ultrasonography after 3–4 weeks.

## Inevitable Abortion

**Definition:** It is the state of abortion from where continuation of pregnancy is impossible.

### Signs and Symptoms

- Increased vaginal bleeding
- Lower abdominal pain—colicky in nature
- Dilated internal OS

### Management

- Administration of methergine 0.2 mg to control bleeding.
- Start intravenous (IV) fluid therapy or in severe cases and blood transfusion is required.
- If gestation is less than 12 weeks, dilatation and evacuation followed by curettage of the uterine cavity under general anesthesia. Suction evacuation followed by curettage is done.
- If gestation is after 12 weeks, uterine contractions are accelerated, by oxytocin drip (10 units in 500 mL of normal saline at rate of 40–60 drops/min). If fetus is expelled and lying separated but placenta is retained, it is removed by ovum forceps. If not separated, digital separation followed by its evacuation is done under general anesthesia.

## Complete Miscarriage

**Definition:** When all the products of conception are expelled out it is called complete abortion.

### Signs and Symptoms

- History of expulsion of fleshy mass per vagina
- Subsidence of abdominal pain followed by expulsion
- Vaginal bleeding become trace or absent
- Uterus is smaller than period of amenorrhea
- On vaginal examination, cervical os is found to be closed
- On examination, the expelled fleshy mass is found intact

### Management

- If there is doubt about complete expulsion of the products, transvaginal sonography is helpful, or uterine curettage should be done.
- The Rh-negative women with gestation more than 12 weeks anti-D gamma globulin 50 microgram or 100 microgram intramuscularly within 72 hours of abortion.

## Incomplete Abortion

**Definition:** When all the products of conception are not expelled out and some parts remain inside the uterine cavity, it is called incomplete abortion.

### Signs and Symptoms

- Continuous, colicky lower abdominal pain
- Persistent vaginal bleeding
- Uterus is smaller than the period of amenorrhea
- Patulous cervical os admit tip of the finger
- Expelled mass found in incomplete abortion on examination

### Management

- If the patient is in shock due to blood loss, she should be resuscitated before any active treatment is undertaken.
- In case of early abortion (before 12 weeks), dilatation and evacuation under general anesthesia are to be done.
- In late abortion (after 12 weeks), uterus is evacuated under general anesthesia and the products are removed by ovum forceps or by blunt curette. The removed products are subjected to a histological examination.

## Missed Abortion (Silent Miscarriage)

**Definition:** If the fetus is dead and remains inside the uterine cavity, it is called missed abortion.

### Signs and Symptoms

- Persistence of brownish vaginal discharge
- Subsidence of pregnancy symptoms
- Retrogression of breast changes
- Uterus is smaller than period of amenorrhea
- Absent fetal heart sound

- Firm cervix
- Immunological test of pregnancy becomes negative

## Complications

- Psychological upset
- Infection
- Blood coagulation disorders such as disseminated intravascular coagulation (DIC)
- **During labor:** Uterine inertia, retained placenta and postpartum hemorrhage (PPH)

## Management

- **Early abortion:** Suction evacuation or slow dilatation of the cervix by laminaria tent followed by dilatation and evacuation of the uterus under general anesthesia.
- **Late abortion:** Two methods can be used:
  - **Oxytocin:** Start 10–20 units of oxytocin in 500 mL normal saline at 30 drops per minute. If uterine contraction is not effective, maximum of 200 mIU/min, may be used.
  - Prostaglandin $E_1$ (misoprostol 200 ug tablet) is inserted into posterior fornix every 4 hours for a maximum of 5 such. Intramuscular administration of 15 methyl PGE1 (carboprost 250 mg) at three hourly intervals for a maximum of 10 such.

## Septic Abortion

**Definition:** Any abortion associated with clinical evidences of infection of the uterus and its contents is called septic abortion. It is characterized by:
- Rise of temperature of at least 100.4°F for 24 hours or more.
- Offensive or purulent vaginal discharge
- Evidence of pelvic infection such as lower abdominal pain and tenderness.

### Signs and Symptoms

Depends on severity of infection and extent of spread of infection. The signs of early pelvic infection include the following:
- Pain in lower abdomen and pelvis
- Fever with chills
- Foul smelling vaginal discharge
- Persistent tachycardia ≥90 bpm
- Tachypnea (respiratory rate >20/min)
- Impaired mental status
- Diarrhea and vomiting
- Ill health, lethargy and weakness
- **Pelvic examination:** Offensive, purulent vaginal discharge, uterine tenderness, pelvic abscess.

### Clinical Grading

| | |
|---|---|
| Grade I | Infection is localized in the uterus |
| Grade II | Infection spread beyond the uterus to the parametrium, tubes and ovaries or pelvic peritoneum |
| Grade III | Generalized peritonitis, endotoxic shock, jaundice or acute renal failure |

## Investigations

- Cervical or high vaginal swab for culture or sensitivity
- Urine analysis
- Blood test for hemoglobin, total and differential count of white cells, ABO and Rh grouping
- Kidney and liver function test
- Coagulation profile
- Upright X-ray abdomen and pelvis to detect uterine and gut perforation and peritonitis
- Pelvic imaging studies include pelvic ultrasound for retained products of conception, foreign body in uterus, pelvic abscess peritonitis with pyoperitoneum, computed tomography (CT) scan and magnetic resonance imaging (MRI) are also helpful

## Complications

### Immediate

- Hemorrhage due to abortion or injury
- Injury to uterus or adjacent structures, e.g., bowel or bladder
- Spread of infection leads to
  - Generalized peritonitis
  - Endotoxic shock
  - Acute renal failure
  - Thrombophlebitis

### Remote

- Chronic debility
- Chronic pelvic pain and backache
- Dyspareunia
- Ectopic pregnancy
- Secondary infertility due to tubal blockage
- Depression

## Management

The treatment of septic abortion depends on grade of infection. The most serious complication is septic shock, i.e. acute circulatory failure with sepsis. The management calls for the following:
- Large doses of broad-spectrum antibiotics to control infection
- Monitoring and correcting blood volume and electrolyte imbalance
- Early removal of septic foci

### Antibiotics

- If infection is mild and limited to the uterus and no evidence of tissue remains in the uterus, oral antibiotics are given and after 2–3 days patient is sent to home with advice to rest.
- If the symptoms persist or get worse and the uterus is bulky and tender, dilatation and curettage or suction evacuation should be done.
- Moderate to severe infection requires prompt and adequate use of antibiotics. Selected antibiotic should cover aerobic and anaerobic gram positive and negative organisms. Antibiotic should be given parenterally in high doses and the patient is observed for 24–48 hours.

- Commonly used medicines are:
  - Gentamycin (3–5 mg/kg single dose)
  - Piperacillin-tazobactam
  - Vancomycin
  - Clindamycin
- If the woman is not immunized for tetanus anti-tetanus serum 3,000 IU intramuscularly may be given. Also prophylactic antigas gangrene serum 8000 units should be given.

### Replacement of blood loss

Heavy blood loss may occur due to:

- Abortion or delivery process
- Retained pregnancy tissue
- Trauma to cervix, vagina and uterus
- Secondary hemorrhage may persist after 3–4 weeks. It is irregular and often heavier than normal menses
- Hemorrhage may be caused by disruption of clotting mechanism. DIC can occur with severe sepsis, curettage for missed abortion or removal of dead fetus from the uterus.

### Surgical therapy (removal of septic foci)

Retained products of conception are common after illegal abortion due to septic technique. As abortion is often incomplete, evacuation should be performed at a convenient time within 24 hours following antibiotic therapy. Excessive bleeding is, of course, an urgent indication for evacuation. Early emptying not only minimizes the risk of hemorrhage but also removes the nidus of infection. But if infection is not localized and spread to other organs, evacuation should be withheld for at least 48 hours after antibiotic therapy. Posterior colpotomy is to be done, if the infection is localized in the pouch of Douglas, pelvic abscess is formed.

### Role of Nurse in Prevention of Sepsis

- Provide women with basic health education on human reproduction
- Improve the socioeconomic condition and take steps to correct malnutrition and anemia
- Provide essential obstetric care to all pregnant women
- Guide women for safe legal abortion, especially in peripheral and rural areas
- Train the traditional dais and midwives for aseptic precautions
- Diagnose early a case of septic abortion and send them to appropriate centers for prompt management
- Provide intensive, multidisciplinary medical care to patients suffering from septic shock and its complications
- Boost up family planning acceptance in order to curb the unwanted pregnancies

## Recurrent Abortion

**Definition:** It is defined as a sequence of three or more spontaneous consecutive abortions

### Causes

- Genetic factors
- Endocrine and metabolic disorders
  - Diabetic mother
  - Thyroid disorder

- Luteal phase defect (LPD)
- Polycystic ovary syndrome (PCOS)
- **Infection:** Chlamydia, syphilis, Mycoplasma
- Inherited thrombophilia
- **Immunological factors:** Antiphospholipid antibodies, lack of cross-reacting antibodies
- Cervicouterine factors
  - Cervical incompetence
  - Intrauterine synechiae
  - Myoma uterus
  - Bicornuate uterus
  - Didelphys uterus
  - Septate uterus

## Investigations

- Blood glucose, venereal disease research laboratory (VDRL), thyroid function test, ABO and Rh groupings, toxoplasmosis, other infections rubella, cytomegalovirus, herpes simplex infection (TORCH) test
- Autoimmune screening: Lupus anticoagulant and anticardiolipin antibodies
- Serum luteinizing hormone (LH) on $D_2/D_3$ of cycle
- Ultrasonography to detect congenital malformation of uterus, polycystic ovaries, uterine fibroid
- Hysterosalpingography to detect cervical incompetence, uterine synechiae and uterine malformations
- Karyotyping (husband and wife)
- Endocervical swab to detect Chlamydia, Mycoplasma and bacterial vaginosis

## Management

- The mother is given reassurance, adequate counseling and support in addition to treatment.
- The mother should take adequate rest, and strenuous activities, intercourse and travelling should be avoided.
- All of these cases should receive careful antenatal supervision.
- Depending on the cause, the management is as follows:
  - **Genetic causes:** They should receive genetic counseling about donor sperm/donor eggs and gene therapy.
  - **Antiphospholipid antibody:** If mother has less antiphospholipid antibody, low dose aspirin 75 mg/day is given. If high level antibodies are there, then along with lose dose aspirin, prednisolone, 40–60 mg/day and heparin 5000–10,000 IU subcutaneously twice a day are there are required up to 34 weeks
  - **Luteal phase defect:** In this natural progesterone suppositories 100–400 mg orally/vaginally and injection hCG 2,000–5,000 IV, I/M every 2–5 days till 12 weeks
  - **Syphilis:** Benzathine penicillin 2.4 million units I/M weekly for 3 weeks. If allergic to penicillin, erythromycin or tetracycline can be used.
  - **Cervical incompetence:** History of repeated mid-trimester abortions without apparent cause, starting with escape of liquor amnii followed by painless expulsion of products of conception is suggestive of the cervical incompetence.

**Treatment for Cervical Incompetence**

**Cerclage operation:** These are performed around 14 weeks of pregnancy or at least 2 weeks earlier than lowest period of previous abortion.

**Procedure:** A nonabsorbable encircling suture is placed around the cervix at the level of internal OS. It acts by interfering with the uterine polarity, preventing the internal OS and adjacent segment from being taken up.

*Two types of operations are done:*

o **Shirodkar's operation:** In this, patient is put under general anesthesia and cervix exposed and lip of cervix pulled down by sponge holding or Allis forceps, a transverse incision is given anteriorly below the base of bladder on the vaginal wall and bladder is pushed up to expose the level of internal os. A vertical incision is given posteriorly on cervicovaginal junction. The nonabsorbable suture material no. 4 braided nylon is passed submucosally with the help of aneurysm needle to bring suture ends through the posterior incision. The anterior and posterior incisions are repaired by interrupted stitches using chromic catgut.

o **McDonald's operation:** In this, the nonabsorbable suture material is placed as a purse string suture as high as possible at the junction of rugose vaginal epithelium and the smooth vaginal part of cervix below bladder level. The suture starts at the anterior wall and taking successive bites, it is carried around the lateral and posterior walls back to the anterior wall where the two ends of suture are tied.

♦ Postoperative patient should be on bed rest for 5–7 days
♦ Natural progesterone and isoxsuprine injection and tablets are given
♦ The stitch is removed at 38th week or earlier if pains start

- **Contraindications of cerclage operation:**
  ▪ Intrauterine infection
  ▪ Ruptured membranes
  ▪ History of vaginal bleeding
  ▪ Severe uterine irritability
- **Complications of cerclage operation:**
  ▪ Chorioamnionitis
  ▪ Rupture of membranes
  ▪ Abortion/preterm labor

## Nursing Responsibilities in Abortion

- Check patient vital signs, blood test, bleeding and vaginal secretion (character, color and volume)
- Maintain strict aseptic technique
- Strengthen the perineal care and maintain the vulval cleanliness
- Psychological care: Sympathizing, understanding and caring
- To check ultrasound result
- Empty the bladder
- Comfort the bladder

## Postoperative Care after Abortion

- Monitor vital signs to identify any internal bleeding or infection. Blood pressure and pulse.
- Assess the client conscious level, the presence of malaise, cold clammy skin, pale or dizziness to rule out possibility of hypovolemic shock.
- Assess for severity of pain and provide analgesic as required.
- Check vaginal bleeding by weighing perineal pads (vaginal bleeding stops normally within 3–5 days).
- Assess the IV line and drip to make sure no kinking, obstruction and in accurate rate flow.
- Encourage fluid intake to prevent dehydration due to blood loss during abortion.
- Monitor and strict intake and output.
- Maintain strict aseptic technique while providing care to the patient to prevent cross infection.
- Maintain healthy diet to provide the body with enough nutrition for fast recovery.
- Provide emotional support, encourage family support due to pregnancy loss.
- Allow grieving and expression of her concerns over the loss of pregnancy.
- Refer the client to social support groups.

# MEDICAL TERMINATION OF PREGNANCY (MTP)

Legal abortion is the deliberate induction of abortion prior to 20 weeks gestation by a registered medical practitioner in the interest of maternal health and life.

## Provision for MTP Under MTP Act

- Continuation of pregnancy would involve serious risk of life or grave injury to the physical and mental health of the pregnant women
- There is substantial risk of the child being born with serious physical and mental abnormalities so as to be handicapped in life
- Pregnancy as a result of rape
- Pregnancy is caused as a result of failure of contraceptive method (tubectomy or vasectomy)
- Where there are actual or reasonably foreseeable environments (social or economic) which could lead to risk of injury to the health of the mother.

## Indications for MTP

- **Therapeutic:**
  - Deteriorating health due to pulmonary tuberculosis
  - Cardiac diseases grade III and IV with history of decompensation
  - Chronic glomerulonephritis
  - Malignant hypertension
  - Intractable hyperemesis gravidarum
  - Cervical/breast malignancy
  - Diabetes mellitus with retinopathy
  - Psychiatric illness.

- **Social:**
  - Parous women having unplanned pregnancy with low socioeconomic status
  - Pregnancy caused by rape
  - Pregnancy due to failure of contraceptive
- **Eugenic:**
  Risk of baby being born with various physical and mental abnormalities and include:
  - Inherited chromosomal and gene disorders
  - Exposure to teratogenicity drugs or disorders
  - Rubella infection in first trimester
  - One or both parents being mentally defective
  - Congenital malformations of siblings

## Prerequisites for MTP

- Only a registered medical practitioner having experience in gynecology and obstetrics to perform abortion where the length of pregnancy does not exceed 12 weeks. If pregnancy is more than 20 weeks, the opinions of two registered medical practitioners are necessary.
- The procedure can be only performed in hospitals established or maintained by government or places approved by the government for MTP.
- A pregnancy can be terminated only with the written consent of the woman.
- Pregnancy in a minor (below the age of 18 years) or lunatic can only be terminated with the written consent of parents or legal guardians.
- Each and every MTP has to be reported to the directorate of health services of the state.

## Methods of Termination of the Pregnancy

| First trimester (up to 12 weeks) | Second trimester (13–20 weeks) |
| --- | --- |
| **Medical**<br>• Mifepristone<br>• Mifepristone and misoprostol<br>• Methotrexate and misoprostol<br>• Tamoxifen and misoprostol<br>**Surgical**<br>• Menstrual regulation<br>• Vacuum aspiration<br>• Suction evacuation/curettage<br>• Dilatation and evacuation<br>  ▪ Rapid method<br>  ▪ Slow method | • Prostaglandins: PGE1 (misoprostol) 15-methyl-PGF2$\alpha$ (carboprost), PGE2 (dinoprostone) and their analogs (used intra vaginally, intramuscularly or intra-amniotically)<br>• Dilatation and evacuation<br>• Intrauterine instillation of hyperosmotic solutions<br>  ▪ Extra-amniotic: Ethacridine lactate, prostaglandins<br>  ▪ Extra-amniotic saline infusion (isotonic) with a transcervical catheter balloon<br>  ▪ Intra-amniotic hypertonic urea (30%), saline (20%)<br>• Oxytocin infusion: High dose used along with either of the above two methods<br>• Hysterotomy ([abdominal] less commonly done) |

# ECTOPIC PREGNANCY

An ectopic pregnancy is one where implantation occurs at a site other than the uterine cavity (Fig. 2).

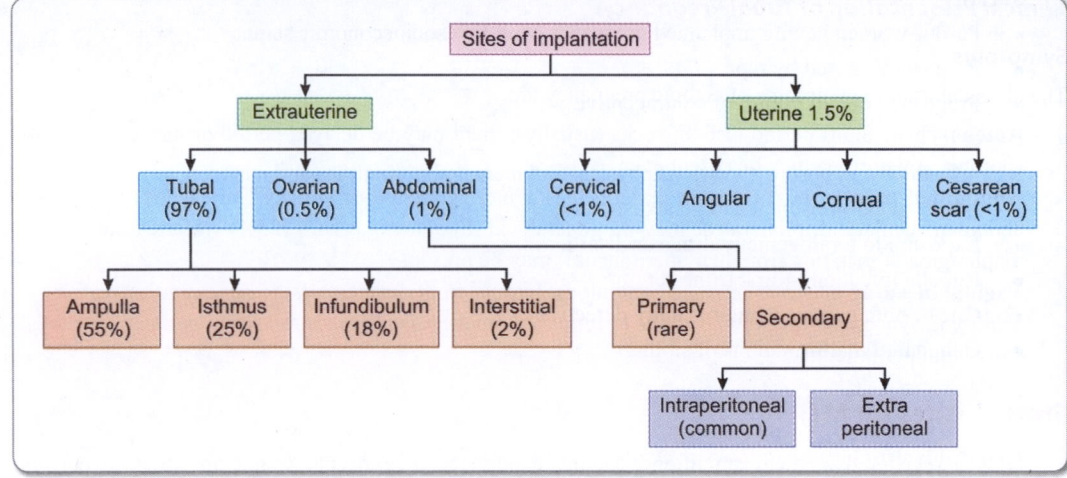

**Fig. 2:** Sites of implantation in ectopic pregnancy

## Tubal Pregnancy

**Definition:** When the pregnancy occurs in the fallopian tubes, it is called tubal pregnancy.

### Causes of Tubal Pregnancy

- **Salpingitis and pelvic inflammatory disease (PID):** It increases the risk of ectopic pregnancy. Chlamydia trachomatis infection is the most common cause.
- **Contraceptive failure:** There are less chances of ectopic with the use of contraceptive devices but the following contraception increases the incidence of ectopic pregnancy.
- **IUD:** There is relative increase in tubal pregnancy (7 times more) if pregnancy occurs with IUD in situ. CUT 380 A and levonorgestrel devices have the lowest rate of ectopic pregnancies whereas progestasert has got the highest one.
- **Sterilization operation:** There is highest incidence of being ectopic following laparoscopic bipolar coagulation.
- Use of progestin only pill or postcoital estrogen pills cause impaired tubal motility hence causes ectopic.

**Here are other reasons for tubal pregnancy:**

- **Tubal surgery:** Tubal reconstructive surgery, preexisting tubal pathology, kinking of the tube or terminal stricture cause ectopic pregnancy.
- **Intrapelvic adhesion:** Following pelvic surgery the chances of being ectopic increase.
- **Assisted reproductive techniques:** Like IVF, Embryo transfer increases the risk of ectopic pregnancy by 5–7%.
- **Developmental defect of the tube:** Such as hypoplasia, undue tortuosity and tubal diverticula.
- **Prior Induced abortion:** Increases the risk.
- **Previous ectopic pregnancy:** Increases the chances of ectopic by 10–15%.

## Clinical Presentation of Tubal Pregnancy

### Symptoms

The classical triad of symptoms of ectopic pregnancy are:

- **Amenorrhea:** Short period of 6–8 weeks (usually); there may be delayed period or history of vaginal spotting, amenorrhea may be absent even.
- **Abdominal pain** is most constant feature. It is acute, agonizing or colicky. Pain is located at lower abdomen: Unilateral, bilateral or may be generalized. Shoulder tip pain (25%) (referred pain due to diaphragmatic irritation from hemoperitoneum) may be present.
- **Vaginal bleeding** may be slight and continuous. Expulsion of decidual cast (5%) may be there.
- Vomiting, syncopal attack (10%) is due to reflex vasomotor disturbances following peritoneal irritation from hemoperitoneum.

### Signs

- **General look:** The patient looks quiet and conscious, perspires and looks blanched
- **Pallor:** Severe and proportionate to the amount of internal hemorrhage
- **Feature of shock:** Pulse– rapid and feeble, hypotension, cold clammy extremities
- **Abdominal Examination:** Lower Abdomen–Tense, tumid, tender. No mass is usually felt, shifting dullness present, bowels may be distended
- **Pelvic examination:** The findings are:
  - Vaginal mucosa-blanched white
  - Uterus seems normal in size or slightly bulky
  - Extreme tenderness on fornix palpation or on movement of the cervix
  - No mass is usually felt through the fornix
  - The uterus floats as in water

### Diagnosis of Tubal Pregnancy

- **Blood examination:** It includes hemoglobin (Hb), ABO and Rh grouping, total white cell count and differential count, erythrocyte sedimentation rate (ESR)
- **Culdocentesis:** It is simple and safe procedure to diagnose ectopic pregnancy. In this, through an 18- gauge lumbar puncture needle fitted with a syringe, the posterior fornix is punctured to gain access to the pouch of Douglas. Aspiration of nonclotting blood with hematocrit greater than 15% signifies ruptured ectopic pregnancy.
- **Estimation of β-hCG:** The suspicious findings are:
  - Lower concentration of β-hCG compared to normal intrauterine pregnancy
  - Doubling time in plasma fails to occur in 2 days
- **Sonography:** Transvaginal sonography is more informative. Combination of quantitative β-hCG values and sonography
- **Laparoscopy:** Offers benefit in cases of confusion with other pelvic lesions. It should be employed only when the patient is hemodynamically stable.
- **Dilatation and curettage:** Identification of decidua without villi structure is very much suggestive. Chorionic villi that float in normal saline as lacy fronds are diagnostic of intrauterine pregnancy.
- **Serum progesterone:** Level greater than 25 µg/mL is suggestive of viable intrauterine pregnancy whereas level less than 5 ng/mL suggests an ectopic or abnormal intrauterine pregnancy.
- **Laparotomy:** Offers benefits when in doubt.

## Management of Tubal Ectopic Pregnancy (Fig. 3)

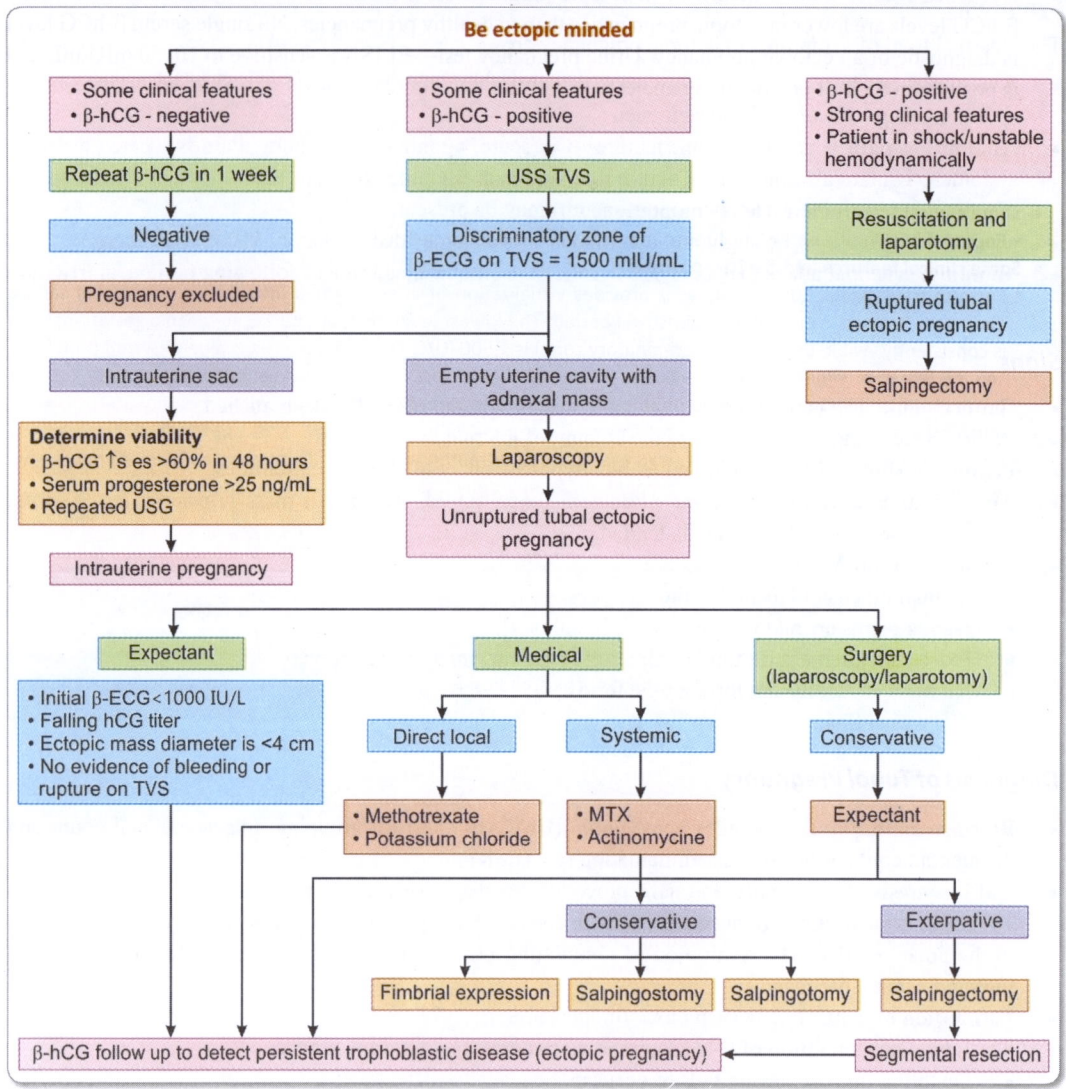

**Fig. 3:** Management of ectopic pregnancy

*Abbreviations:* β-hCG, beta human chorionic gonadotropin; MTX, methotrexate; TVs, transvaginal sonography; USG, ultrasonography

- **Detailed history, evaluation of risk factors and examination**
- **Ultrasound scan:** Transvaginal sonography provides visualization of a well-formed intrauterine gestational sac as early as 4–5 weeks from the last menstrual period.
- **Serum progesterone:** Level >25 ng/mL is suggestive of viable intrauterine pregnancy whereas level less than 5 ng/mL suggests an ectopic or abnormal intrauterine pregnancy.

- **Urine β-hCG/serum β-hCG:** In normal pregnancy, the β-hCG level doubles every 48–72 hours until it reaches 10,000–20,000 mIU/mL. In ectopic pregnancies, β-hCG levels usually increase less. Mean β-hCG levels are lower in ectopic pregnancies than in healthy pregnancies. No single serum β-hCG level is diagnostic of an ectopic pregnancy. Urine pregnancy test—ELISA is sensitive to 10–50 mIU/mL and is positive in 95% of ectopic pregnancies.

> **Know it**
>
> ### Be ectopic minded
>
> - **Some clinical features and β hCG—negative**
>   - Repeat β-hCG in one week, if values found negative exclude pregnancy.
> - **Some clinical features and β hCG—positive**
>   - Perform transvaginal sonography as it provides visualization of a well-formed intrauterine gestational sac as early as 4–5 weeks from the last menstrual period. The lowest level of serum β-hCG at which a gestational sac is consistently visible using TVS (discriminatory zone) is 1,500 IU/L. The corresponding value of serum β-hCG for TAS is 6,000 IU/L. When the β-hCG value is greater than 1500 IU/L and there is an empty uterine cavity, ectopic pregnancy is more likely. Failure to double the value of β-hCG by 48 hours along with an empty uterus is very much suggestive.
>   - If transvaginal sonography findings show well-formed intrauterine sac, β-hCG increase >60% in 48 hours and serum progesterone >25 ng/mL, then repeat ultrasonography to confirm intrauterine pregnancy.
>   - If transvaginal sonography findings show empty uterine cavity with adnexal mass, then perform laparoscopy. If there is unruptured tubal ectopic pregnancy, then manage the case as:
>     - **Expectant management:** Where only observation is done hoping spontaneous resolution. The indications are: (i) Initial β-hCG <1000 IU/L; (ii) Falling hCG titer; (iii) Ectopic mass diameter is <4 cm; (iv) No evidence of bleeding or rupture on TVS.
>     - **Medical management:** A number of chemotherapeutic agents have been used either systemic or direct local (under sonographic or laparoscopic guidance) as medical management of ectopic pregnancy. The commonly used drugs are: methotrexate, potassium chloride, prostaglandins, hyperosmolar glucose or actinomycin. The patient must be:
>       - Hemodynamically stable
>       - Serum hCG level <3000 IU/L
>       - Tubal diameter <4 cm and no fetal cardiac activity
>       - No intraabdominal hemorrhage
>     - **Surgical management:** It includes conservative and extirpative management. Conservative management means avoidance of major surgical intervention usually with the intent to preserve function or body parts. *In conservative treatment*, procedure can be done either through laparoscopically or by microsurgical laparotomy. In unruptured tubal ectopic pregnancy, commonly used conservative approaches are: salpingostomy, salpingotomy and fimbrial expression.
>       - **Salpingostomy:** A longitudinal incision is made on the antimesenteric border directly over the site of ectopic pregnancy. After removal of products of conception, the incision line is kept open to be healed later on by secondary intention. Hemostasis is achieved by electrocautery or laser.
>       - **Salpingotomy:** The procedure is same as that of salpingostomy. But the incision line is closed in two layers with 7–0 interrupted vicryl sutures. This is not commonly done.
>       - **Fimbrial expression:** This is ideal in cases of distal ampullary (fimbrial) pregnancy and is done digitally.
>         *Extirpation* means complete removal or eradication of an organ or tissue. In ectopic pregnancy, extirpative management includes segmental resection or salpingectomy.
>       - **Segmental resection:** This is a choice in isthmic pregnancy. End-to-end anastomosis can be done immediately or at a later date after appropriate counseling of the patient
>         Following conservative medical or surgical treatment, estimation of β-hCG should be done weekly till the value becomes less than 5.0 mIU/mL. Additional monitoring by TVS is preferred.
> - **Strong clinical features and β hCG-positive**
>   - In this case patient is in shock/hemodynamically unstable, antishock measures are to be taken energetically with simultaneous preparation for urgent laparotomy. If ruptured tubal ectopic pregnancy, salpingectomy is to be done.

## Abdominal Pregnancy

Abdominal pregnancy is rare. A primary abdominal ectopic pregnancy is the result of implantation of the fertilized ovum on the peritoneal surface. A secondary abdominal pregnancy forms when an embryo extruded through rupture or abortion of a tubal pregnancy. The embryo does not die because of its chorionic attachments to the uterine tube and grows by forming attachments to the pelvic peritoneum, omentum, intestines, etc. The fetus grows in the peritoneal cavity but the majority of these pregnancies do not survive. If these pregnancies occur, the fetus dies early in pregnancy, it maybe reabsorbed or calcification occurs.

### Signs and Symptoms

If pregnancy continues, the woman complains of persistent lower abdominal pain, nausea, vomiting, constipation, diarrhea, abdominal distention and increased urinary frequency. There may be vaginal spotting or hemorrhage. Fetal movements are painful. On abdominal examination, there is tenderness and fetal parts are superficial. Abnormal fetal lie and loud fetal heart sounds. Ultrasound confirms the diagnosis.

### Management

Delivery is by laparotomy. Separation of placenta may be followed by major hemorrhage. If the placenta is attached to the intestines, it may be left in situ. When the placenta is left inside, the risk of infection is high, but is considered a safer option. Fetal mortality is very high. The fetus is growth retarded and deformed in 20–40% of cases due to oligohydramnios. The fetus usually dies when the membranes rupture or in immediate neonatal period from respiratory distress.

## Cervical Pregnancy

Cervical pregnancy occurs due to implantation in the cervical canal. It may be due to rapid passage of the fertilized ovum or fertilization of the ovum after it reaches the cervical canal. It is rare and seldom lasts beyond the 20th week.

### Signs and Symptoms

- Painless bleeding soon after the time of implantation.
- Palpation of the cervical mass with distention and thinning of the cervical wall.
- Partial dilatation of the external os and a slightly enlarged uterine fundus.

### Management

Management is done by removal of products of conception by curettage and packing of the cervical canal or total abdominal hysterectomy.

## Nursing Responsibilities in Ectopic Pregnancy

- Upon arrival at the emergency room, place the woman flat in bed.
- Assess the vital signs to establish baseline data and determine if the patient is under shock.
- A woman who has a ruptured ectopic pregnancy might present signs of shock such as rapid, thread pulse, rapid respirations, and decreased blood pressure.
- There would be a decreased progesterone levels that would indicate that the pregnancy has ended.
- It is vital that midwives and nurses have an awareness of the emotional trauma of ectopic pregnancy when taking a history from a woman.

- Monitor maternal vital signs to determine the presence of hypotension and tachycardia caused by rupture or hemorrhage. Vital signs, especially the blood pressure and pulse rate, should be stable and within the normal range.
- Patient must exhibit moist mucous membranes, good skin turgor, and adequate capillary refill.
- Monitor intake and output. Maintain accurate intake and output to establish the patient's renal function. The patient must maintain adequate fluid volume at a functional level as evidenced by normal urine output at 30–60 mL/hr and a normal specific gravity between the ranges of 1.010 and 1.021.
- Monitor for presence and amount of vaginal bleeding to further assess the present situation indicating hemorrhage.
- Monitor for increase and pain and abdominal distention and rigidity since increased pain and abdominal distention indicates rupture and possible intra-abdominal hemorrhage.
- Monitor complete blood count (CBC) to determine the amount of blood loss.
- Provide comfort measures, like back rubs, deep breathing. Instruct in relaxation or visualization exercises.
- Administer analgesics as indicated to maintain acceptable level of pain.
- Provide diversional activities since these promote relaxation and may enhance patient's coping abilities by refocusing attention. Diversional activities aid in refocusing attention and enhancing coping with limitations.
- The loss of a baby and emergency surgery can have an enormous impact on a woman's psychological health and on her relationships. In addition, the surgery to treat ectopic pregnancy has an impact on the woman's fertility, usually decreasing it by 50% or more. Many women also exhibiting symptoms of posttraumatic stress disorder, experiencing flashbacks, nightmares, hypervigilance and depression after ectopic pregnancy.

## ANTEPARTUM HEMORRHAGE

**Definition:** Antepartum hemorrhage (APH) is defined as bleeding from the genital tract after 28th week of pregnancy and before the birth of the baby.

## Types

Figure 4 shows the various types of antepartum hemorrhage.

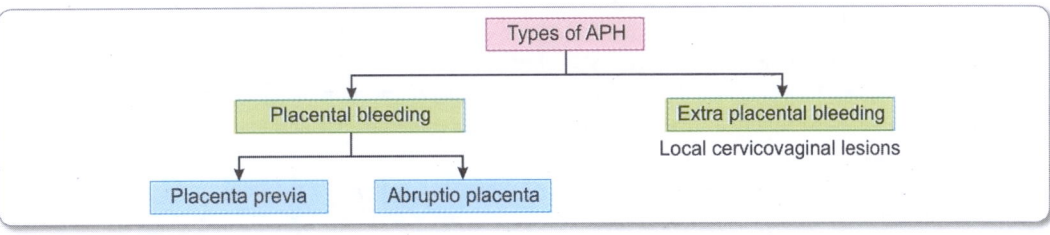

**Fig. 4:** Types of antepartum hemorrhage

*Abbreviation:* APH, antepartum hemorrhage

## Placenta Previa

**Definition:** Complete or partial implantation of placenta over the lower uterine segment is called placenta previa.

## Incidence

The incidence in India is 1 in 250. One-third of all APH occur due to placenta previa.

## Causes

Exact cause is unknown. The following theories are postulated.

- **Dropping down theory:** Due to poor decidual reaction, the fertilized ovum drops down to the lower uterine segment.
- **Multiple pregnancies:** Big surface area of placenta as in twins may encroach onto the lower segment.
- **Defective decidua:** Causes spreading of the chorionic villi over a wide area in the uterine wall.

## High Risk Factor of Placenta Previa

- Increased maternal age (>35 years)
- Multiparity
- Previous cesarean section or scar on the uterus
- Smoking
- Prior curettage

## Types or Degrees of Placenta Previa

- **Type I (low lying/lateral):** The lower margin of the placenta lies into the lower segment.
- **Type II (anterior):** It means placenta is implanted at the anterior wall of the uterus. The anterior placenta previa gets pulled up above the symphysis pubis during labor and does not compromise the fetal oxygenation to the same extent as the posterior placenta previa.
- **Type II (posterior):** It means placenta is implanted at the posterior or back wall of the uterus. The posterior placenta previa can be compressed by the presenting part and cause severe fetal asphyxia and cause fetal death. It is also called "Dangerous placenta previa" placenta reaches the internal os when closed, but does not cover it.
- **Type III (incomplete or partial or central):** The placenta covers the internal os when closed, but not when fully dilated.
- **Type IV (central/complete):** The placenta completely covers the internal os even when the cervix is fully dilated.

## Signs and Symptoms

- Painless vaginal bleeding in the 3rd trimester of pregnancy
- Bright red vaginal bleeding and the amount varies with the proportion of separation of placenta
- The bleeding may be scanty at first, and then it becomes more profuse and gradually increases with the placental separation
- There is no way that the bleeding can be stopped other than delivering the fetus and complete removal of the placenta.

## Diagnosis

- Ultrasonography
- Magnetic resonance imaging (MRI)
- Per vaginal examination
- Direct visualization during cesarean section
- Examination of placenta following vaginal delivery

## Complications

| Maternal | Fetal |
|---|---|
| **During pregnancy**<br>• APH with varying degree of shock<br>• Increased incidence of malpresentation<br>• Premature labor<br>• Death due to massive hemorrhage<br><br>**During labor**<br>• Early rupture of membranes<br>• Cord prolapses<br>• Slow dilatation<br>• Intrapartum hemorrhage<br>• Increased incidence of operative interference<br>• Postpartum hemorrhage<br>• Retained placenta<br><br>**Puerperium**<br>• Sepsis<br>• Increased operative interference<br>• Anemia and poor general condition of the patient<br>• Subinvolution<br>• Embolism | • Low-birth-weight babies<br>• Asphyxia<br>• Intrauterine death<br>• Birth injuries<br>• Congenital malformations<br>• Fetal morbidity and mortality |

## Management

### Prevention

- To improve the health status of women and correction of anemia, adequate antenatal care is required
- Antenatal diagnosis of low-lying placenta with repeat ultrasound
- Significance of "warning hemorrhage" should not be ignored or underestimated
- Family planning and limitation of birth reduce the incidence of placenta previa

### Home Management

- Put the patient to bed rest (strict bed rest)
- Assess the blood loss
- Quick but gentle abdominal examination
- Vaginal examination must not be done

### Management of Placenta Previa at Hospital

- If the gestational age is early, an attempt is made to prolong the pregnancy with the intention of optimizing the neonatal outcome. The woman is hospitalized to try and avoid preterm labor or hemorrhage
- The hemoglobin and hematocrit values are monitored
- Blood replacement therapy or iron therapy is instituted if anemia is present
- The pulmonary maturity of the fetus is monitored at appropriate intervals
- Unless emergency situation arises, delivery is planned for some point after the fetus has reached 37 weeks gestation and lung maturity is assessed

A vaginal delivery would be considered only, if the placenta previa is of first degree or very marginal, the fetal head has descended low enough to act as a tampon placing pressure against the placenta, active labor has begun and no other complications are evident. Vaginal delivery would also be considered, if the fetus is dead. In most situation however, surgical intervention (cesarean section) is the delivery method of choice.

### Nursing Role in Placenta Previa

- If woman is experiencing no bleeding or very light bleeding, instruct the mother for bed rest, no strenuous exercise or sexual intercourse for the rest of the pregnancy until baby is ready for delivery
- No vaginal exams, douching throughout the rest of the pregnancy (To prevent injury to the vulnerable placenta presenting at the cervical opening)
- If woman is experiencing bleed... hospitalized to monitor baby and mother.
- Assess baseline vital signs especially the blood pressure every 5–15 minutes.
- Assess fetal heart sounds to monitor the wellbeing of the fetus.
- Monitor uterine contractions to establish the progress of labor of the mother.
- Weigh perineal pads used during bleeding to calculate the amount of blood lost.
- Assist the woman in a side lying position when occurs.
- No abdominal manipulation
- IV access (pick 18 gauge or bigger) for transfusion of blood products and fluids, monitoring CBC, clotting levels
- Start blood transfusion (type and cross match, depend upon patient condition.

Figure 5 shows the scheme of management of placenta previa in hospital

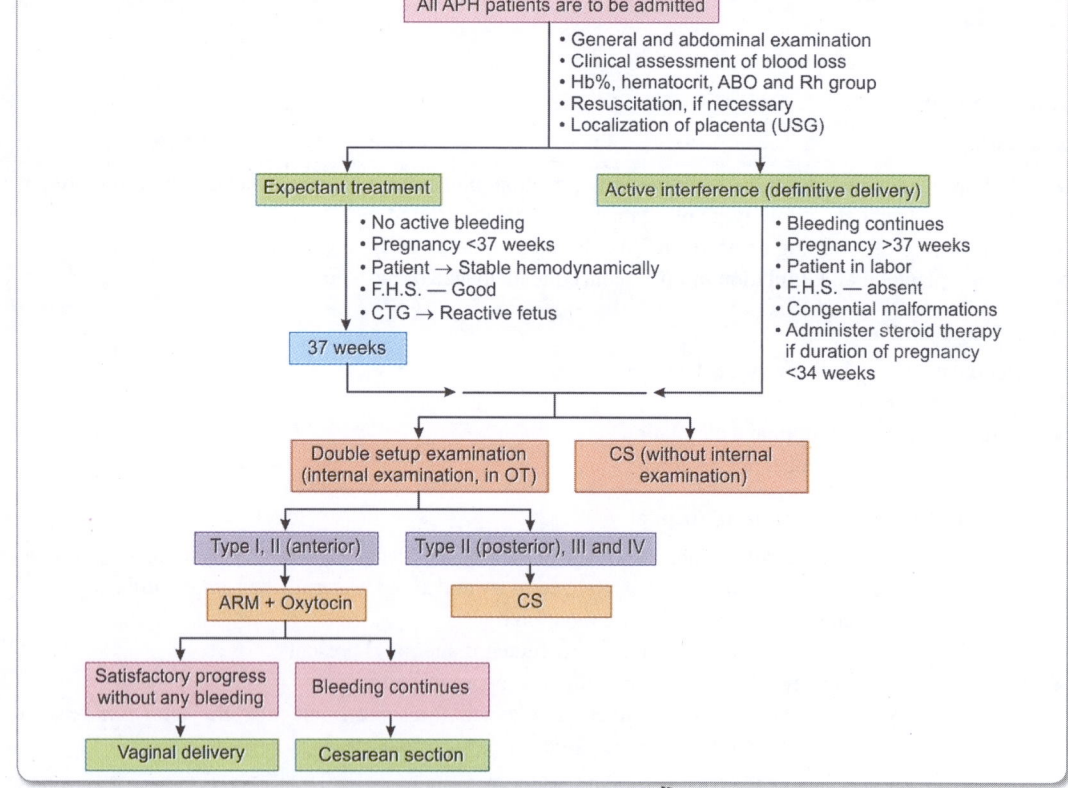

**Fig. 5:** Scheme of management of placenta previa in hospital
*Abbreviations:* APH, antepartum hemorrhage; ARM, artificial rupture of membranes; CTG, cardiotocography; FHS, fetal heart sound; OT, operation theater

- Rh-negative mother need, Anti-D gammaglobulin to prevent Rh isoimmunization.
- Contractions causing bleed: may be ordered to give tocolytics (drugs to stop contractions)
- Amniocentesis to assess lung maturity of baby and steroids may be given to help baby's lung mature
- If bleeding cannot be stopped will need c-section. C-section is usually ordered for a partial or complete previa. In some cases, women with a marginal previa (low lying) may be allowed to have baby vaginally.

## Abruptio Placenta

### Definition

The premature separation of a normally situated placenta after 28 weeks of gestation and before birth of baby is called abruptio placenta.

### Types/Varieties

- **Revealed:** It is the most common type. In this, following separation of the placenta, the blood escape downwards between the membranes and decidua. Ultimately, blood comes out of the cervical canal to be visible externally.
- **Concealed:** This type is rare. The blood collects behind the separated placenta or between the membranes and decidua. As a result, the blood cannot come out of the cervical canal and cannot be visible externally.
- **Mixed:** In this type, some portion of the blood collects inside (concealed) and a portion is expelled out (revealed).

### Causes of Abruptio Placenta

The exact cause is unknown, but several factors have been considered as causes:

- Spasm of the uterine vessels followed by pooling of blood into the choriodecidual space
- Malnutrition
- Folic acid deficiency
- Traction of short cord
- Trauma from external cephalic version (ECV)
- High birth order i.e. gravida >5
- Advancing age of mother
- Poor socioeconomic condition
- Smoking
- Major congenital malformations
- Abruption in previous pregnancy
- Pregnancy-induced hypertension (PIH)

### Clinical Classification/Grading of Abruptio Placenta

Depending upon the degree of placental abruption and its clinical effects, the cases are graded as follows:

- **Grade 0:** Clinical features are absent. The diagnosis is made after inspection of placenta following delivery.
- **Grade 1: External bleeding is slight. Uterus** → irritable, tenderness may or may not be present. Shock is absent. Fetal heart sound (FHS) is good.

- **Grade 2: External bleeding** → Mild to moderate uterine tenderness is always present. **Shock** → absent fetal distress or fetal death occurs.
- **Grade 3: Bleeding** → Moderate to severe. Uterine tenderness → marked. Shock → pronounced fetal death is inevitable. Coagulation defect/anuria may complicate.

## Signs and Symptoms

- Small to moderate amount of bright or dark red vaginal bleeding
- Acute abdominal pain associated with vaginal bleeding
- Uterine tenderness and high uterine tonicity often described as 'board-like abdomen"
- Increased size of uterus in case of concealed hemorrhage
- Failure of uterus to relax between contractions
- Fetal heart sound absent with concealed/mixed type
- Urine output is usually diminished

## Diagnosis

- **Ultrasonography:** To visualize the location of the placenta and presence of clots or hematoma
- **Coagulation profile:** To rule out disseminated intravascular coagulopathy (DIC)
  - Clotting time
  - Bleeding time
  - Fibrinogen level
  - Platelet count
  - Prothrombin (PT) and partial prothrombin time (aPTT)
  - Fibrin degradation products
- **Urine test:** For albumin
- **Renal function test**

## Management

### Prevention

The following guidelines may be helpful in prevention of abruptio placenta:

- Prevention, early detection and effective therapy of preeclampsia and other hypertensive disorders of pregnancy.
- Needle puncture during amniocentesis should be done under ultrasound guidance.
- **Avoidance of trauma:** Especially forceful external cephalic version under anesthesia.
- To avoid sudden decompression of the uterus: In acute or chronic hydramnios, amniocentesis is preferable to artificial rupture of membranes.
- To avoid supine hypotension, the patient is advised to lie in the left lateral position in the later months of pregnancy to avoid vena caval compression.
- Routine administration of folic acid from early pregnancy of doubtful value.

## Home

In case of abruptio placenta, it is not possible to treat the patient at home, so arrangement is made to shift the patient to an equipped maternity unit as early as possible.

## *In hospital*

### Assessment of the case is to be done to note:

- Maturity of the fetus
- Amount of blood loss
- Patient is in labor or not
- Presence of any complication
- Grade of abruptio placenta

### Emergency Measures

- Collect blood sample to note Hb%, hematocrit level, coagulation profile, ABO and Rh grouping.
- Check urine for the presence of protein.
- Administer Ringer solution using a wide bore hole cannula.
- Arrange blood transfusion for resuscitation.
- Close monitoring of fetal and maternal health condition.

### In Revealed Case

*Patient is in labor*

Most patient are in labor following a term pregnancy. The labor is accelerated by low rupture of membranes and it increases the uterine tone also. Oxytocin drip may be started to accelerate labor when needed. Conduct vaginal delivery.

> **Note:**
> - Delivery process is to be completed within 4–6 hours to reduce blood loss.

*Patient not in labor*

- If pregnancy >37 weeks, start oxytocin drip to accelerate labor and perform low rupture of membranes, then conduct vaginal delivery.
- If pregnancy <37 weeks, but bleeding continuous per vagina. Start oxytocin drip to accelerate labor and perform low ruptured of membranes. Conduct vaginal delivery. On the other hand, if bleeding stops, cardiotocography shows reactive fetus. Try to continue pregnancy up to 37 weeks then conduct delivery.

### In Concealed Case

- Start blood transfusion, at least one liter should be minimum when the diagnosis of concealed accidental hemorrhage is made.
- Collect blood sample to note Hb%, hematocrit level, coagulation profile, ABO and Rh grouping.
- Check urine for the presence of protein and oliguria.
- Close monitoring of fetal and maternal health condition.
- Start oxytocin drip to accelerate labor and perform low ruptured of membranes.
- If no progress in labor, fetal distress, oliguria and abnormal coagulation profile then cesarean section is the best option.

## Management of Abruptio Placenta in the Hospital

Figure 6 shows the management of abruptio placenta in the hospital:

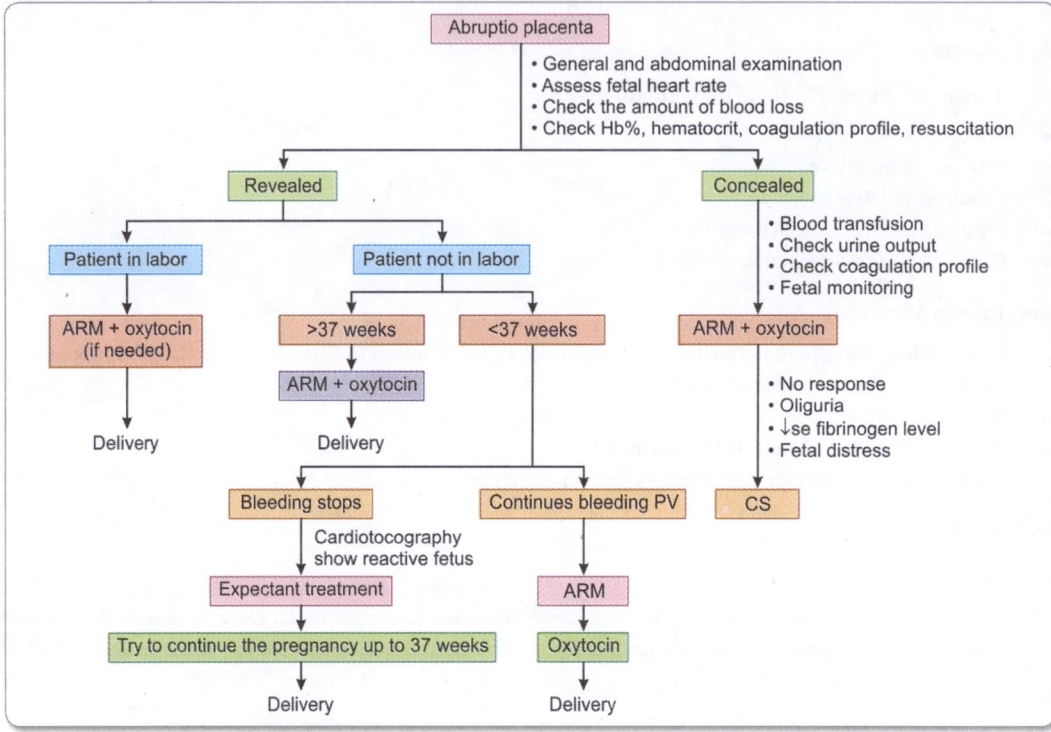

**Fig. 6:** Management of abruptio placenta in the hospital

*Abbreviations:* ARM, artificial rupture of membrane; PV, per vaginal examination

## Nursing Role in Abruptio Placenta

- Continuous evaluate maternal and fetal physiologic status, particularly:
  - Vital signs
  - Bleeding
  - Electronic fetal and maternal monitoring tracings
  - Signs of shock – rapid pulse, cold and moist skin, decrease in blood pressure
  - Decreasing urine output
  - Never perform a vaginal or rectal examination or take any action that would stimulate uterine activity.
- Assess the need for immediate delivery. If the client is in active labor and bleeding cannot be stopped with bed rest, emergency cesarean delivery may be indicated.
- Provide appropriate management.
  - On admission, place the woman on bed rest in a lateral position to prevent pressure on the vena cava.
  - Insert a large gauge intravenous catheter into a large vein for fluid replacement. Obtain a blood sample for fibrinogen level.

- Monitor the fetal heart rate (FHR) externally and measure maternal vital signs every 5–15 minutes. Administer oxygen to the mother by mask.
- Prepare for cesarean section, which is the method of choice for the birth
- Provide client and family teaching.
- Address emotional and psychosocial needs. Outcome for the mother and fetus depends on the extent of the separation, amount of fetal hypoxia and amount of bleeding.

# HYDATIDIFORM MOLE/GESTATIONAL TROPHOBLASTIC DISEASE

**Types of Gestational Trophoblastic Disease**
- Hydatidiform mole
- Invasive mole
- Choriocarcinoma
- Placental-site trophoblastic tumor
- Epithelioid trophoblastic tumors

**Definition:** Hydatidiform mole is the abnormal condition of the placenta where there are partly degenerative and partly proliferative changes occur in the young chorionic villi.

**Incidence:** Incidence is high at the beginning and end of child bearing period (<20 and >40 years of age)

## Causes

The exact cause is unknown but the following are the risk factors
- Prevalent in teenage pregnancies
- Faculty nutrition: Inadequate intake of protein, animal fat, low dietary intake of carotene
- Disturbed maternal immune system suggested by:
  - Rise in gamma globulin level as in hepatic diseases
  - Increased association of AB blood group which possesses no ABO antibody
- Genetic predisposition: In general, complete moles have 46, XX karyotype (85%), the molar chromosomes are derived entirely from the father. Infrequently, the chromosomal pattern may be 46 XY or 45 X.
- History of prior hydatidiform mole increases the chances of recurrence.

## Signs and Symptoms

### Symptoms

- Uterine bleeding: Browning or watery discharge per-vagina. The blood may be mixed with fluid from ruptured cyst and give appearance as "White currant in red currant juice"
- Varying degree of lower abdominal pain
- Expulsion of grape-like vesicles per vagina
- No quickening even at 20 weeks
- Constitutional symptoms:
  - Persistent nausea and vomiting (hyperemesis up to second trimester)
  - Breathlessness
  - Thyrotoxic features, like tremors/tachycardia

### Signs

- The patient becomes sick without apparent reason.
- Patient shows early signs of pregnancy.
- Anemia: Often it is out of proportion to the amount of blood loss due to rapidly growing tumor.
- Pregnancy induced hypertension, preeclampsia and features of eclampsia → present.

## Diagnosis

- Per abdominal findings
- Vaginal examination
- Investigations

### Per Abdomen Findings

- **Uterus size:** A large for date uterus, which is clearly out of proportion to the presumed gestational age in about 50% of cases
- **On palpation:** Uterus feels 'doughy' or elastic
- **Fetal parts:** Not felt
- No fetal movements
- Absence of fetal heart sound

### Vaginal Examination

- No internal ballottement is seen
- Often enlarged, tender ovaries
- Grape-like vesicles (per vaginum)
- Cervical os open

### Investigations

- **Blood test:** Hb%, Hematocrit, ABO and Rh grouping.
- Liver function test, renal and thyroid function test.
- **Urine pregnancy test:** Due to large amount of human chorionic gonadotropin (hCG), produced by the tumor, and test is positive in a dilution 1:2, 000 or more after 14 weeks of gestation.
- Serum level of hCG is high.
- **Uterus sonography:** Shows characteristics pattern and a snowstorm appearance.
- **Straight X-ray abdomen:** Carried out as a routine for evidence of pulmonary embolization.

## Possible Complications

- **Immediate:**
  - Hemorrhage and shock
  - Sepsis
  - Perforation of the uterus
  - Preeclampsia
  - Acute pulmonary insufficiency
  - Coagulation failure
- **Late:** Development of choriocarcinoma.

## Management

Figure 7 shows the management system of hydatidiform mole:

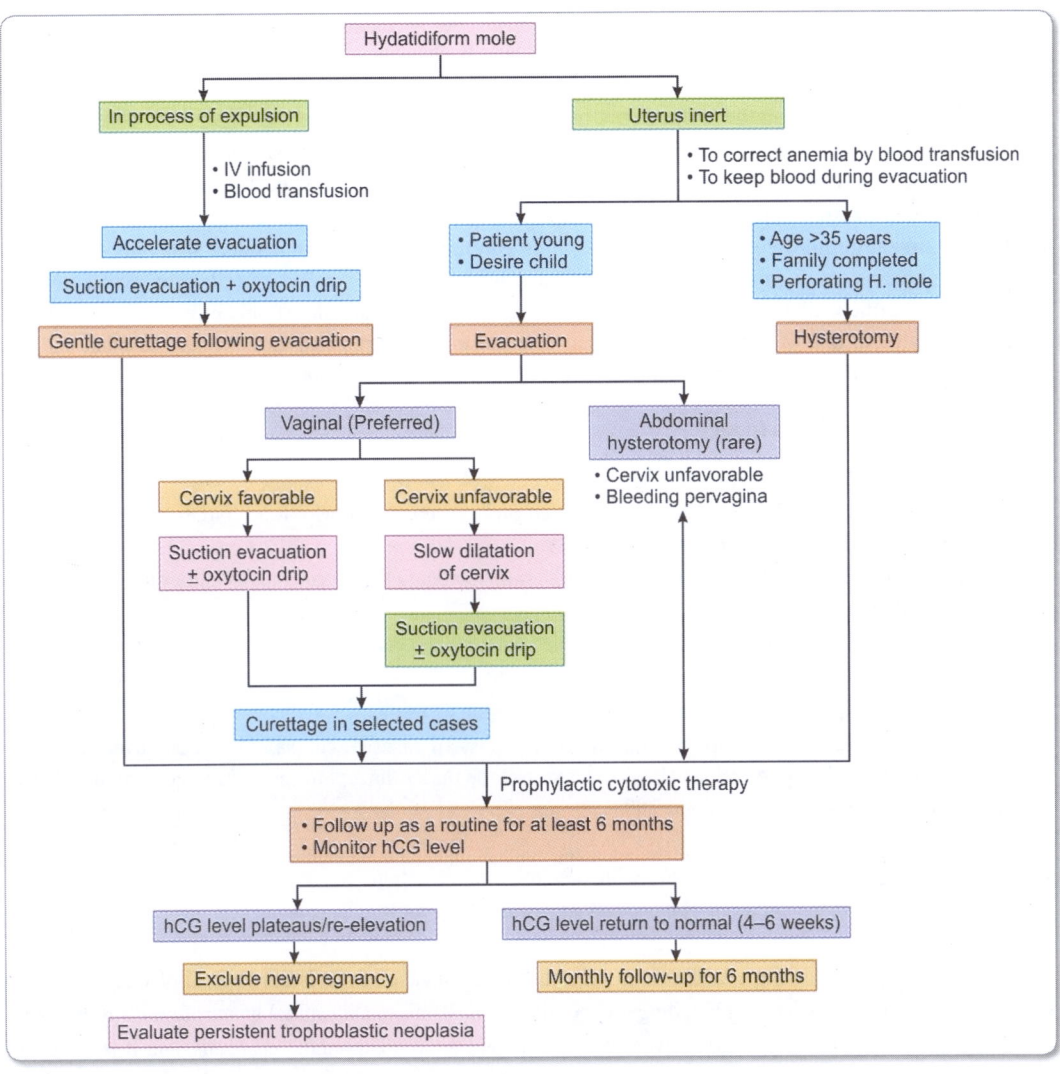

**Fig. 7:** Management of hydatidiform mole
*Abbreviation:* hCG, human chorionic gonadotropin

The principles of management:

- To restore the blood loss and to prevent infection → provide supportive therapy
- To evacuate the uterus as soon as the diagnosis is made
- Regular follow-up for early detection of hydatidiform mole

The patient is grouped into two:

## Group A: Mole is in Process of Expulsion

- **Provide supportive therapy:** It includes: Start IV infusion with ringer's solution.
  - If patient is anemic, start blood transfusion.

- Parenteral antibiotic is given if there is associated infection.
- Blood is kept reserved as during evacuation, there is chances of hemorrhage.
- **Administer oxytocin:** Use of oxytocin helps the expulsion of moles and reduces blood loss but its routine use is not recommended due to the risk of embolization.
- **Suction evacuation:** It is safe, effective and rapid in almost all cases. It can safely be done even when the uterus is of 28 weeks of gestation. The procedure is done under diazepam sedation or general anesthesia. A negative pressure is applied up to 200–250 mm Hg.
- **Gentle curettage following evacuation:** Routine curettage is not recommended. It is only performed in case of persistent vaginal bleeding. Gentle curettage may be done 5–7 days following evacuation. At this time, uterine wall gets thicker, firmer and the cavity becomes smaller so that effective curettage can be done without risk of damaging the uterus. The purpose is to remove the necrosed decidua and the attached vesicles so as to accelerate involution and to reduce the irregular bleeding.

## Group B: Uterus Remains Inert

- **Provide supportive therapy:** Same as in group A.
- If the patient age is >35 years, family completed and presence of perforating hydatidiform mole. The best option in this case is to perform hysterectomy.
- On the other hand, if patient is young and desire child, evacuate the uterine cavity either through vaginal or abdominal route.
- To perform evacuation through vaginal route, see whether the cervix is favorable or unfavorable.

*If the cervix is favorable:*

- Start oxytocin drip to accelerate the process of expulsion of mole.
- Suction evacuation is safe, effective and rapid in almost all cases. It can safely be done even when the uterus is of 28 weeks of gestation. The procedure is done under diazepam sedation or general anesthesia. A negative pressure is applied up to 200–250 mm Hg.

*If the cervix is unfavorable:*

- Slow dilatation of the cervix is done by introducing laminaria tent.
- Start oxytocin drip to accelerate the process of expulsion of mole.
- Perform suction evacuation.
- Gentle curettage following evacuation is only performed in case of persistent vaginal bleeding.
- If there is continuous vaginal bleeding and cervix is unfavorable, abdominal hysterotomy is to be done.
- **Prophylactic cytotoxic therapy:** About 80% of patient undergo spontaneous remission. It is indicated in the following circumstances:
  - If the hCG level fails to become normal within 10–12 weeks or there is re-elevation at 4–8 weeks.
  - Post evacuation hemorrhage (presence of trophoblastic activity)
  - Where follow-up facilities are not adequate.

**Regimes:** Methotrexate 1 mg/kg/day IV or IM is given on day 1, 3, 5 and 7 with folinic acid 0.1 mg/kg IM on day 2, 4, 6, and 8. It is to be repeated every 7th day. Total three courses are given. Serum hCG level should decrease by at least 15%, 4–7 days after methotrexate. Alternatively, IV Actinomycin D daily for 5 days may be given.

- **Follow-up:** Initially, the checkup should be at interval of one week till the serum hCG level becomes negative. This usually happens by 4–8 weeks. Once negative within 56 days, the patient is followed up at every one-month interval for 6 months. The women who undergo chemotherapy should be followed up for 1 year after hCG has been normal. The patient must not become pregnant during the period of follow-up.

# PREGNANCY INDUCED HYPERTENSION (PIH)

The hypertension develops as a direct result of the gravid state. The woman does not have a history of previous hypertension or evidence of it. The clinical types of PIH are:
- Preeclampsia
- Eclampsia
- Gestational hypertension

## Preeclampsia

### Definition

It is a multisystem disorder characterized by development of hypertension to 140/90 mm Hg or above with proteinuria after 20-weeks in a previously normotensive and nonproteinuric patient.

### Causes

The exact cause is unknown. The following are thought to be the cause of preeclampsia:
- There is a relative or absolute deficiency of vasodilator prostaglandins I2 (PGI2), synthesized in vascular endothelium and increased synthesis of thromboxane A2, a potent vasoconstrictor.
- There is an increased vascular sensitivity to the vasopressor agent angiotensin II. The sensitizing substances are yet to be explored
- Nitric oxide, which relaxes vascular smooth muscles, inhibits platelet aggregation and prevents intervillous thrombosis, is found deficient in preeclamptic clients. Hence, preeclampsia is characterized by complex endothelial cell dysfunction
- In preeclampsia, trophoblastic invasion of the spiral arteries is thought to be inhibited by some immunological mechanism.
- Excessive accumulation of fluids in the extracellular space is not clear. Excessive retention of sodium is due to increased aldosterone, diminished renal blood flow, decreased glomerular filtration rate and increased tubal reabsorption. The proteinuria is due to spasm of the afferent glomerular arterioles, anoxic damage to the endothelium of the glomerular tuft, increased capillary permeability and increased leakage of proteins.

### Diagnostic Criteria of Preeclampsia

- **Hypertension:** An absolute rise of blood pressure of at least 140 diastolic pressure 90 mm Hg or rise in systolic pressure of at least 30 mm Hg, diastolic pressure of at least 15 mm Hg over the previously known is blood pressure called PIH.
Calculation based on mean arterial pressure is done as following:

$$MAP = \frac{Systolic\ pressure + (diastolic\ pressure \times 2)}{3}$$

A rise of 20 mm Hg over the previous reading, or when MAP is 105 mm Hg or more should be considered significant.

- **Edema:** Demonstration of rapid gain in weight of more than 1 lb a week or more than 5 lb in a month in later month of pregnancy is the evidence of preeclampsia.
- **Proteinuria:** Presence of total protein in 24 hours urine of more than 0.3 g or $\geq 2 + (1$ g/L) on at least two random clean catch urine samples tested $\geq 4$ hours apart in absence of urinary tract infection (UTI) is considered significant.

Test for protein in urine by dipstick is as following:

| | | |
|---|---|---|
| Trace = 0.1 g/L; | 1 ± = 0.3 g/L; | 2 + = 1.0 g/L; |
| 3+ = 3.0 g/L; | 4 + = 10 g/L | |

## Signs and Symptoms

### Mild Symptoms

- On rising from the bed in morning → Slight swelling over the ankles, tightness of ring finger.
- Gradually, swelling may extend to face, abdominal wall, vulva and whole body.

### Alarming Symptoms

- **Headache:** Over occipital/frontal region
- Disturbed sleep
- **Diminished urine output:** (Less than 500 mL in 24 hours)
- **Epigastric pain:** Associated with vomiting, at times coffee colored due to hemorrhagic gastritis or subcapsular hemorrhage in liver
- **Eye symptoms:** Blurring or dimness of vision or at times complete blindness

### Signs

- **Abnormal weight gain:** A rapid gain in weight of more than 5 lb a month or more than 1 lb a week in later months of pregnancy is significant
- Rise of blood pressure $\geq 140/90$ mm Hg
- **Edema:** Over ankles, face, abdominal wall and whole body
- **Pulmonary edema:** Due to leaky capillaries and low oncotic pressure
- Abdominal examination reveals scanty liquor or intrauterine growth restriction (IUGR) due to placental insufficiency.

## Investigations

- **Urine:** 24 hours urine collection for protein measurement is done.
- **Ophthalmoscopic examination:** In severe cases, there may be retinal edema, constriction of arterioles, alteration in vein: arteriole diameter ratio, nicking of veins.
- **Blood values:** Biochemical marker of preeclampsia i.e. **Uric acid** more than 4.5 mg/dL. Blood urea remains normal or slightly raised. Serum creatinine level more than 1 mg/dL. Thrombocytopenia or abnormal coagulation profile. Hepatic enzymes may be increased.
- **Antenatal fetal monitoring:** By clinical examination, daily fetal kick count, ultrasonography for fetal growth and liquor pockets, cardiotocography, umbilical artery flow velocimetry and biophysical profile.

## Complications

| Immediate complications | |
|---|---|
| **Maternal** | **Fetal** |
| • During pregnancy:<br>  ▪ Eclampsia<br>  ▪ Accidental hemorrhage<br>  ▪ Oliguria and anuria<br>  ▪ Dimness of vision and even blindness<br>  ▪ Preterm labor<br>  ▪ Hemolysis, elevated liver enzymes and low platelet count (HELLP) syndrome<br>• During labor<br>  ▪ Eclampsia<br>  ▪ Postpartum hemorrhage<br>• Puerperium<br>  ▪ Eclampsia<br>  ▪ Shock<br>  ▪ Sepsis | • Intrauterine death<br>• Intrauterine growth restriction<br>• Asphyxia<br>• Prematurity |
| **Remote complications** | |
| • Residual hypertension<br>• Recurrent preeclampsia<br>• Chronic renal disease | |

## Management of Preeclampsia

### Preventive Measures

- Regular antenatal check-up at frequent interval from the beginning of pregnancy to detect at the earliest, the rapid gain in weight or a tendency of rising BP especially the diastolic pressure.
- Advise to take adequate rest in bed on her left side at least for 2 hours in the afternoon from the 20 weeks of pregnancy onwards.
- Antioxidants, vitamin C and E from 16–22 weeks onwards.
- Well-balanced diet, rich in protein, iron and calcium also helps to reduce the risk of preeclampsia.

### Hospital Management of Preeclamptic Patient

- **Rest:** Admission in hospital and rest is helpful for preeclamptic patient because it increases the renal blood flow → diuresis, increases uterine blood flow → improves placental profusion, reduces blood pressure.
- **Diet:** Contain adequate amount of protein (about 100 g/day).
- **Antihypertensives:** The commonly used oral drugs are:

| Drug | Mode of action | Dose |
|---|---|---|
| • Methyldopa | Central and peripheral anti adrenergic acid | 250–50 mg tid/qid |
| • Labetalol | Adrenoceptor antagonist | 250 mg tid or qid |
| • Nifedipine | Calcium channel blocker | 10–20 mg bid |
| • Hydralazine | Vascular smooth muscle relaxant | 10–25 mg bid |

Figure 8 shows the management of preeclampsia

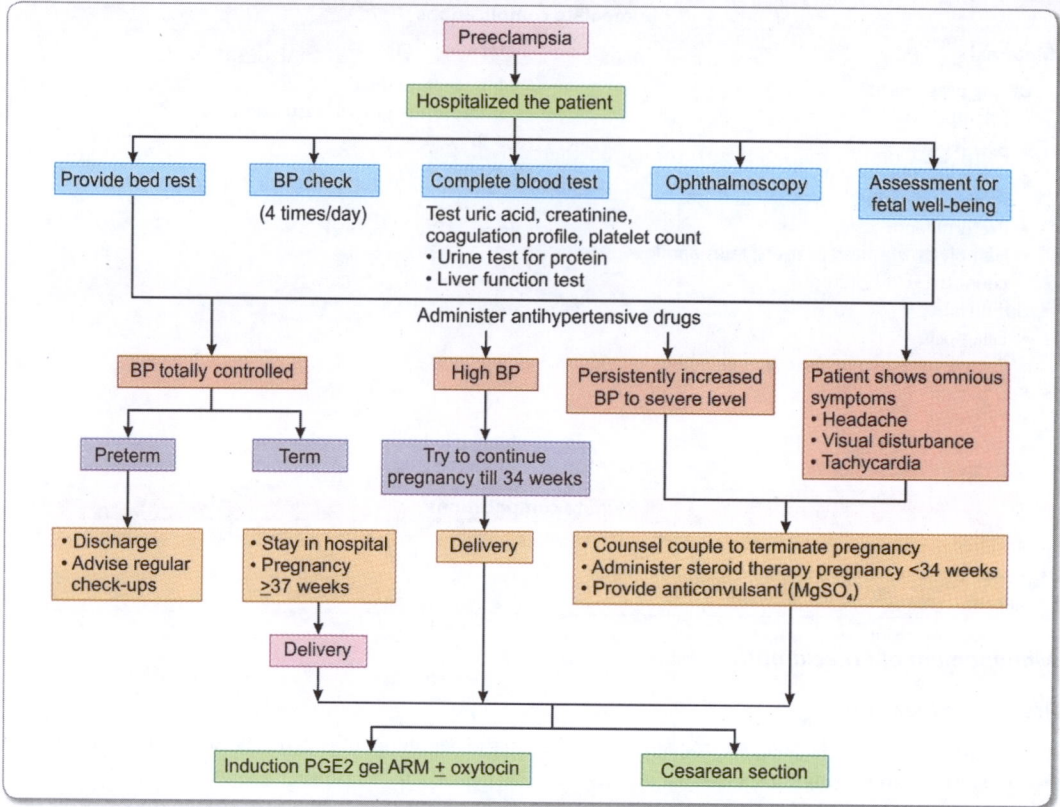

**Fig. 8:** Management of preeclampsia

*Abbreviations:* ARM, artificial rupture of membranes; BP, blood pressure; PGE2, prostaglandins E2

- **Sedatives:** Mild sedatives are given to reduce the emotional factor that contributes to elevation of blood pressure, e.g., phenobarbitone 60 mg or diazepam 5 mg at bedtime.
- **Laxatives:** If woman is constipated, mild laxative like milk of magnesia four teaspoons at bedtime may be given.
- **Diuretics:** The most patent diuretic commonly used is furosemide (Lasix) 40 mg, given orally after breakfast for 5 days in a week.
- **Recording and reporting:**
  - State of edema and daily weight record
  - Evaluation of symptoms, such as headache, right upper quadrant or epigastric pain, visual disturbances, oliguria.
  - Fluid intake and urinary output
- For assessing proteins (albumin) urine examination:
  - Blood test for hematocrit, platelet count, uric acid, creatinine, liver enzymes, coagulation profile at least once a week
  - Ophthalmoscopic examination
  - Assessment of fetal well being

**Depending upon the response to the treatment, the patients are grouped into the following:**

- **Group A:** If the pregnancy is less than 37 weeks, discharge the patient and instruct her to attend antenatal clinic weekly. If pregnancy is near term, try to continue the pregnancy till completion of 37 weeks thereafter, termination of pregnancy.
- **Group B:** If pregnancy is less than 37 weeks, expectant treatment may be extended judiciously at least up to 34 weeks.
- **Group C:** Counsel the couple. Termination of pregnancy is safe irrespective of period of gestation. If gestation is less than 34 weeks, administer steroid therapy for fetal lung maturity, prevent neonatal respiratory distress syndrome (RDS), intraventricular hemorrhage (IVH) and maternal thrombocytopenia. Anticonvulsant magnesium sulfate should be started.

## Method of Delivery

- **Induction of labor:** It is indicated in case of:
  - Persistent hypertension
  - Aggravation of preeclamptic features.
  - Post maturity.
    **Method:** If the cervix is unripe, prostaglandin gel is useful to make the cervix ripe then low rupture of membrane. If cervix is ripe, then surgical induction by low rupture of membranes.
- **Cesarean section:** It is performed by experienced surgeon and anesthetist in case of:
  - Urgent termination is indicated and cervix is unfavorable
  - Severe preeclampsia
  - Associated complicating factors such as elderly primigravida, contracted pelvis, malpresentation twins or polyhydramnios.

## Nursing Responsibility for Preeclamptic Patient

### Primary Goals

- Prevent convulsions through the use of magnesium sulfate
- Ensure adequate kidney function
- Monitor fetal status—assure moderate variability prior to initiating magnesium sulfate
- Stabilize the woman so that delivery can be accomplished
- The definitive treatment for preeclampsia is delivery

### Nursing Management

- Intense maternal monitoring. Assess vital signs, especially blood pressure. An elevated blood pressure of 140/90 mm Hg and above would indicate hypertension.
- Presence of protein could be determined through urine tests.
- Assess patient for the presence of edema on the face, fingers, and upper extremities.
- Magnesium sulfate administration as ordered.
- Antihypertensive medications as ordered.
- Depending on the condition of mother and fetus, select the mode of delivery.
- Regular Electronic fetal monitoring is indicated.
- 1:1 nurse to patient ratio is required for the management of eclampsia.
- Assess vital signs based on status to determine worsening of the disease and response to therapy.
- Obtain blood pressure with consistent methods.

- Record hourly intake and output using a Foley catheter with a urometer.
- Reduce stimulation from noise and light.
- Maintain patient on strict bed rest.
- Maintain IV access (D5W or LR at nor more than 150 mL/hr).
- Lab work as ordered including: type and cross match and platelets.
- Test urine for protein.
- Assess deep tendon reflexes.
- Ask patient to tell if she develops a headache, blurred vision, dizziness, or epigastric pain, or if she feels uncomfortable or different.
- Observe the patient for restlessness or apprehension.

## Eclampsia

**Definition:** Preeclampsia (hypertension, proteinuria and edema) when complicated with convulsions/coma is called eclampsia.

It is derived from a Greek word meaning "like a flash of lightening". It may occur quite abruptly, without any warning manifestations. In majority (over 80%), the disease is preceded by features of severe preeclampsia. Thus, it may occur in women with preeclampsia or in women who have preeclampsia superimposed on essential hypertension or chronic nephritis.

### Onset of Fits

Fits mostly occur beyond 36 weeks but on rare occasions, it may occur in early months

- **Antepartum (50%):** Fits occur before the onset of labor. More often, labor starts soon after and at times, it is impossible to differentiate it from intrapartum ones.
- **Intrapartum (30%):** Fits occur for the first time during labor.
- **Postpartum (20%):** Fits occur for the first time in puerperium usually within 48 hours of delivery.

### Signs and Symptoms

The fits are epileptiform and consists of four stages:

1. **Premonitory stage:** The patient becomes unconscious. There is twitching of the muscles of face, tongue and limbs. Eye balls roll and turned to one side and become fixed. This stage lasts for about 30 seconds.
2. **Tonic stage:** The whole body goes into a tonic spasm. The trunk–opisthotonos, limbs are flexed hands clenched. Respiration ceases and the tongue protrudes between the teeth. This stage lasts for about 30 seconds.
3. **Clonic stage:** All the voluntary muscles undergo alternate contraction and relaxation. Twitching starts in the face and then involves one side of the extremities and ultimately the whole body gets involved in the convulsion. Biting of the tongue occurs. Breathing is stertorous and blood stained frothy secretions fill the mouth; cyanosis gradually disappears. This stage lasts for 1–4 minutes.
4. **Stage of coma:** Following the fits, the patient goes into the state of coma. It may last for a brief period or may persist until another convulsion. At times, patient appears to be in a confused state following the fits and fails to remember the happening. Rarely, coma occurs without convulsion.

   The fits are usually multiple, occurring at varying interval. When it occurs frequently, it is called status eclampticus. Following fits, temperature rises, pulse, respiration and blood pressure also increase. Urinary output decreases, proteinuria occurs and serum uric acid is also raised.

## Complications

- **Injuries:** Tongue bite, patient falls out of bed
- **Cardiovascular:** Vasospasm, pulmonary embolism
- **Renal:** Oliguria, renal failure
- **Hematological:** Hypovolemia, hemoconcentration, thrombocytopenia, DIC
- **Neurological:** Cerebral edema, cerebral hemorrhage
- **Hepatic:** Hepatic necrosis, subcapsular hematoma
- **Respiratory:** Pneumonia
- **Sensory:** Disturbed vision due to retinal detachment
- **Others:** Puerperal sepsis, psychosis
- **Fetal complications:**
  - IUGR
  - Intrauterine death (IUD)
  - Fetal distress

## Management

### Preventive Measures

- Early detection and effective institutional management with judicious termination of pregnancy
- Adequate sedation is helpful
- In case of preeclampsia, prophylactic anticonvulsant therapy soon after delivery of the baby
- Close observation for 24–48 hours is necessary to prevent postpartum eclampsia

### Actual Management

The patient, if at home or in the peripheral health centers, should be shifted urgently to the referral hospitals. The patient must be heavily sedated before transferring to hospital.

The principles of management in hospital are:

- Maintain clear airway
- Oxygen administration
- Control convulsion
- Prevent hypoxia
- Prevent injury
- Hemodynamic stabilization
- Delivery by 6–8 hours
- Postpartum care

The midwife must remain with the mother constantly. In the first instance, all efforts are devoted to the preservation of mother's life.

- The patient should be placed in railed cot bed in an isolated room to prevent from noxious stimuli which provoke further fits. The patient should be side-lying, head slightly raised and on one side to facilitate drainage of saliva and prevent vena caval compression. Maintain airway and administer oxygen to prevent hypoxia. If patient is unconscious, change position frequently to prevent hypostatic pneumonia and bedsore.
- Detailed history is to be taken from relatives relevant of eclampsia, i.e. duration of pregnancy, numbers of fits and the medications administered outside.
- After the patient is properly sedated, thorough, but quick general, abdominal and vaginal examinations should be done. A self-retaining catheter is introduced and the urine is tested for protein. Continuous drainage is established for measurement of urinary output, periodic urinary analysis and for prevention of soiling of bed.
- Check the vital signs (Pulse, respiration and blood pressure) every 10 minutes and record. Urinary output noted every hourly. Note the progress of labor and fetal heart rate (FHR).

- **Fluid balance:** Ringer lactate is started as a first choice. Total fluid should not exceed the previous hours urinary output plus 1000 mL (insensible loss) skin and lungs. Normally, fluid intake should not exceed 2 L in 24 hours.
- **Fetal assessment:** Assessment of the fetal wellbeing must be done by use of kick charts, cardiotocograph monitoring and ultrasonography
- **Anticonvulsant therapy:** To control and prevent its recurrence. Magnesium sulfate ($MgSO_4$) is the drug of choice (Table 1). It reduces motor and plate sensitivity to acetylcholine and thereby reduces neuromuscular irritability. $MgSO_4$ induces cerebral vasodilation, dilates uterine arteries and inhibits platelet aggregation.

**TABLE 1:** Regimens of $MgSO_4$

| Regimen | Route | Loading dose | Maintenance dose |
|---|---|---|---|
| Pritchard | IM | 4 g IV over 3–5 minutes followed by 10 g deep IM (5 g in each buttock) | 5 g IM 4 hourly in alternate buttock |
| Zuspan | IV | 4 g IV over 5–10 minutes | 2 g/hr |
| Sibai | IV | 6 g IV over 20 minutes | 2 g/hr |

Repeated injections are given only if knee jerks are present, urine output exceeds 30 mL/hr and respiration rate is more than 12 per minute. Therapeutic level of serum Magnesium is 4–7 mEq/L. $MgSO_4$ is continued for 24 hours after the last seizure. For reoccurrence of fits, further 2 g IV bolus is given over 5 minutes in the above regimens.

Nurses' role during $MgSO_4$ therapy

- Check patellar reflex and respiratory rate regularly
- Through pulse oximetry, check oxygen saturation level at frequent interval
- In women with oliguria, regular monitoring of serum magnesium level is necessary
- Calcium gluconate is the antidote for magnesium toxicity and should be readily available

- **Antihypertensives:** These are used to control BP and development of severe preeclampsia, especially when the diastolic pressure is over 110 mm Hg, associated with proteinuria. The commonly used oral drugs are: methyldopa 0.5–2 g/day, labetalol 200 mg 6–8 hourly. If blood pressure is not under control, a calcium channel blocker 10–20 mg twice a day or hydralazine 25 mg twice daily are added.
- **Sedatives:** Mild sedatives are given to reduce emotional factor that contributes to elevation of blood pressure Phenobarbitone 60 mg or diazepam 5 mg at bedtime or more frequently are given
- **Laxatives:** Mild laxative such as milk of magnesia four teaspoons at bedtime is helpful to treat constipation.

## Obstetrical Management

### During Pregnancy

In majority of cases with antepartum eclampsia, labor start soon after convulsions. But if labor fails to start, the management depends on:

- Whether fits are controlled or not
- The maturity of the fetus

### Fits controlled

- **Baby mature:** Terminate the pregnancy
  - If cervix favorable: Low rupture of membrane → start oxytocin drip
  - If cervix unfavorable → Cervical ripening with $PGE_2$ gel
  - Artificial rupture of membranes (ARM)

- If cervix unfavorable or any obstetrical contraindications of vaginal delivery → Cesarean section is to be done
- **Baby premature:** Terminate the pregnancy either by induction of labor pain by PGE$_2$ gel/ARM and start oxytocin drip → for vaginal delivery. Otherwise, cesarean section is to be done in unfavorable conditions. Rarely continuation of pregnancy under strict supervision for few days in hospital may be considered.
- **Baby dead:** Wait for spontaneous expulsion.

*Fits not controlled*

If fits are not controlled with antihypertensive for a period of 6–8 hours, terminate the pregnancy. Before termination, check the induction score. If it is favorable, induction of labor, by ARM along with oxytocin drip. If unfavorable score, cesarean section is to be done.

- **During labor:** If there is not any contraindication to vaginal delivery, low rupture of membranes is to be done to induce labor pains and to cut short the second stage of labor, delivery is conducted by forceps/ventouse. Ergometrine during the delivery of anterior shoulder not to be given as it further raises the BP. If patient is unconscious, fits are not controlled in spite of therapy or any obstetrical indication → cesarean section is to be done.
- **Puerperium:** Check the maternal condition every 4 hourly for next 48 hours, period during which convulsions usually occurs. To sedate the mother phenobarbitone 60 mg in repeated doses is given. Administer antihypertensive drugs. If diastolic pressure is above 100 mm Hg. Mother should remain in hospital until BP is controlled and proteinuria disappears.
- Scheme of management of eclampsia in hospital is given in Figure 9.

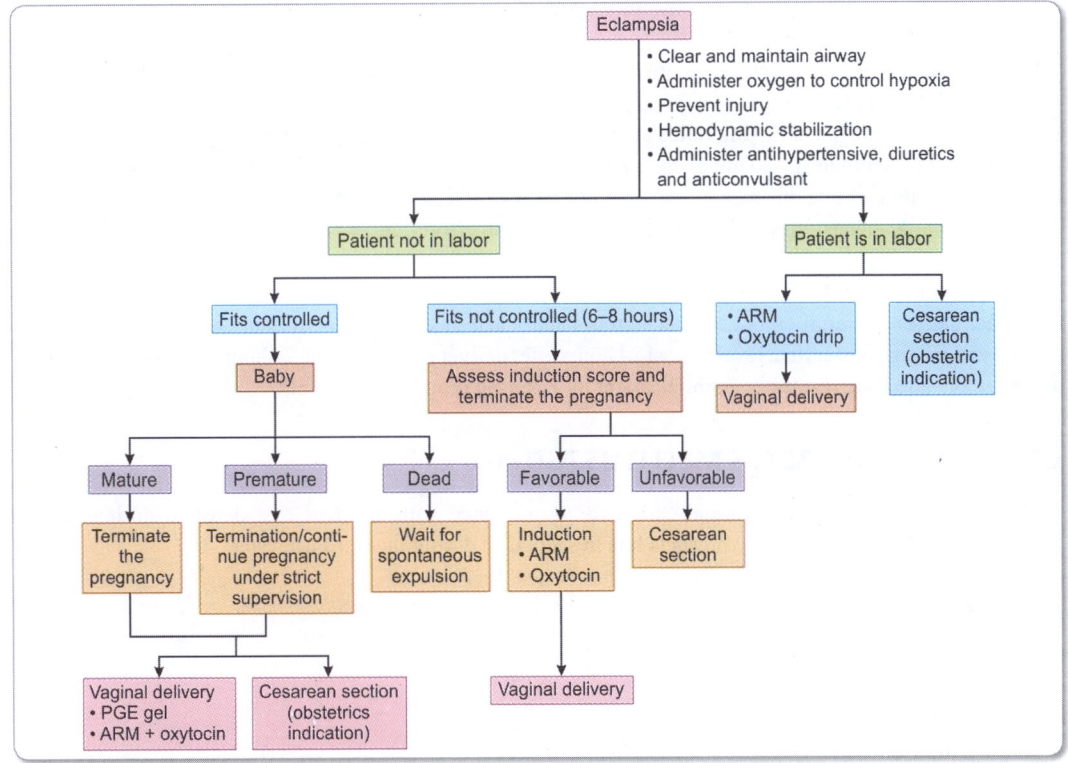

**Fig. 9:** Scheme of management of eclampsia in hospital

*Abbreviations:* ARM, artificial rupture of membranes; PGE, prostaglandin

### Nursing Interventions of Eclamptic Patient

- Insert large bore hole cannula for fluid administration as order.
- Indwelling Foley's catheter to monitor urine output and magnesium excreted through the urine.
- If Oliguria present, inform doctor and increase fluid intake and reduce the dose of magnesium sulfate.
- Keep the patient NPO to prevent aspiration.
- Provide lateral position to the patient to avoid aspiration of vomits and secretions.
- To remove oral secretion and vomiting gently perform suctioning.
- To avoid tongue bite and open the airway properly, insert padded tongue blade or airway tube in the mouth.
- Avoid inducing gag reflex of eclampsia patient.
- Maintain oxygenation 8–10 L/min through face mask to avoid hypoxia and metabolic acidosis.
- Monitor Arterial Blood Gas (ABG) at regular interval. (not less than 92%).
- Keep bed side rails up to prevent fall of eclampsia patient.
- Use of physical restraints as needed.
- Check vital sign every 15 minutes during critical time (first 1–4 hours).
- Administer injection magnesium sulfate loading dose of 6 g over 15–20 minutes as ordered.
- Carefully administer maintenance dose of 2 g/hr as a continuous intravenous solution as ordered.
- If repeatedly convulsion occurs, give inj. Sodium Amobarbital 250 mg intravenous over 3–5 minutes as doctor order.
- If respiratory arrest occurs start CPR.
- Closely observe the patient for magnesium toxicity like flushing, a feeling of warmth, nausea, vomiting, double vision and slurred speech.
- Try to keep systolic blood pressure between 140 and 160 mm Hg and diastolic blood pressure 90 and 110 mm Hg.
- Give inj. Hydralazine 5–10 mg bolus or inj. labetalol 20–40 mg every 15 minute.
- Give oral Nifedipine 10–20 mg every 30 minutes as ordered if patient is conscious.
- Assess fetal heart rate during and immediately following a convulsion.
- If bradycardia persists beyond 10–15 minutes despite all efforts, check the eclamptic patient for abruption placenta.
- Prepare the patient for delivery.
- After delivery carefully monitor vital sign of patient and evaluate risk of further convulsion.
- Ensure magnesium sulfate level at least 24 hours after delivery or for at least 24 hours after last convulsion.
- Promote adequate rest for eclamptic patient by ensuring quite environment.

## GESTATIONAL DIABETES MELLITUS (GDM)

**Definition:** It is defined as abnormal carbohydrate tolerance with onset or first detected during present pregnancy. This condition usually presents late in second or during the third trimester.

### Risk Factors

- Diabetes in a first degree relative (parents/sibling)
- Recurrent abortion
- Unexplained stillbirth
- Congenital abnormality
- A baby whose birth weight was 4 kg or more at 40 weeks

- Previous gestational diabetes or impaired glucose tolerance
- Persistent glycosuria
- Age over 30 years
- Obesity

## Screening

Women considered to be at risk of gestational diabetes undergo a glucose tolerance test. This will indicate whether they have normal or impaired glucose tolerance, or have developed diabetes. Before proceeding to a full glucose tolerance test, a fasting blood sample may be examined for glucose.

**Glucose tolerance test (GTT):** The method is employed by using 50 g oral glucose challenge test without regard to time of day or last meal, between 24 and 28 weeks of pregnancy. A plasma glucose value of 140 mg% or that whole blood of 130 mg% at 1 hour is considered as cut of 6 points for consideration of a 100 g (WHO–75) glucose tolerance test.

## Effects of Diabetes

- **On pregnancy:**
  - Infertility
  - Increase chances of spontaneous abortion and stillbirth
  - Increase incidence of macrosomia and birth trauma
  - Increase perinatal mortality
  - Women more prone to urinary tract infection (UTI)
  - Increase incidence of preeclampsia and polyhydramnios
- **On fetus:**
  - Intrauterine fetal death
  - Increased chances of neural tube, heart and kidney defects
  - Intrauterine growth restriction (IUGR)
  - Increased incidence of macrosomia
  - Neonatal complications include
    - Hypoglycemia
    - Respiratory distress syndrome
    - Hyperbilirubinemia
    - Polycythemia
    - Hypocalcemia
    - Hypomagnesemia
    - Cardiomyopathy

## Management

- Antenatal supervision should be done at monthly intervals up to 20th week and thereafter at 2 weeks interval up to 30th week
- **Diet:** Diet with 2,000–2500 Kcal/day for normal weight woman and restriction to 1,200–1,800 Kcal/day for overweight woman is recommended. Complex carbohydrates are preferred because simple carbohydrates produce significant postprandial hyperglycemia.
- The control of high blood glucose is done by restriction of diet, exercise with or without insulin. Human insulin should be started if fasting plasma glucose level exceeds 90 mg/dL and 2 hours post prandial value is greater than 120 mg/dL even on diet control.
- Exercise (aerobic, brisk walking) are safe in pregnancy and may obviate the need of insulin therapy.

- Frequent blood glucose estimation is required. Estimation of glycosylated hemoglobin should be done at the end of first trimester and 3 months thereafter.
- Sonographic evaluation is helpful to detect fetal macrosomia, growth retardation and other congenital malformations.
- Assessment of fetal wellbeing is to be made from 32 weeks onwards.
- The midwife should alert the women of her predisposition to UTI and vaginal infections so that she will seek treatment as soon as possible if symptoms develop. It is important to teach the women about maintenance of hygiene.
- Check maternal weight and abdomen to detect polyhydramnios.
- In uncomplicated cases, the woman is admitted in hospital at 34th to 36th week. Early hospitalization facilitates.
    - Stabilization of diabetes
    - Minimizes incidence of polyhydramnios, preeclampsia, preterm labor
    - Selection of appropriate time for hospitalization

### Obstetric Management

- Women with good glycemic control and who do not require insulin may wait for spontaneous onset of labor. However elective delivery (induction or cesarean section) is considered in patients requiring insulin or with complications at around 38 weeks.

### Follow-up

- Nearly 50% of women with gestational diabetes mellitus would develop overt diabetes over a follow-up period of 5–20 years. Women with fasting hyperglycemia have got worse prognosis to develop type 2 diabetes and cardiovascular complications. Recurrence risk in subsequent pregnancy is more than 50%.

## Nursing Management for Gestational Diabetes Mellitus

1. **Nursing diagnosis:** Fluid volume deficit related to osmotic diuresis.
   **Goal:** Demonstrate adequate hydration evidenced by stable vital signs, palpable peripheral pulse, skin turgor and capillary refill well, individually appropriate urinary output, and electrolyte levels within normal limits.

   **Nursing interventions have been tabulated as follows:**

   | Nursing interventions | Rationale |
   | --- | --- |
   | Monitor vital signs | Hypovolemia can be manifested by hypotension and tachycardia |
   | Assess peripheral pulses, capillary refill, skin turgor, and mucous membranes | This is an indicator of the level of dehydration, or an adequate circulating volume |
   | Monitor input and output, record the specific gravity of urine | To provide estimates of the need for fluid replacement, renal function, and effectiveness of the therapy given |
   | Measure weight every day | To provide the best assessment of fluid status of ongoing and further to provide a replacement fluid |
   | Provide fluid therapy as indicated | The type and amount of liquid depends on the degree of lack of fluids and the response of individual patients |

2. **Nursing diagnosis:** Imbalanced nutrition less than body requirement related to insufficiency of insulin, decreased oral input.

*Goal:*
- Digest right amount of calories/nutrients.
- Shows the energy level, i.e. usually high
- Stable or increasing weight.

**Nursing interventions have been tabulated as follows:**

| Nursing interventions | Rationale |
|---|---|
| Determine the patient's diet and eating patterns and compared with food that can be spent by the patient | Identify deficiencies and deviations from the therapeutic needs |
| Check weight daily | Assessing an adequate food intake (including absorption and utilization |
| **Identification of preferred food:** Include ethnic/cultural need | If the patient's food preferences can be included in meal planning, this cooperation can be pursued after discharge |
| Involve patients in planning the family meal as indicated | Increase the sense of involvement; provide information on the family to understand the patient's nutrition |
| Give regular insulin treatment as indicated | Regular insulin has a rapid onset therefore it can help move glucose into cells |

3. **Nursing diagnosis:** Risk for infection related to hyperglycemia.

   **Goal:** Identify interventions to prevent/reduce the risk of infection. Demonstrate techniques, lifestyle changes to prevent infection.

   **Nursing interventions have been tabulated as follows:**

| Nursing interventions | Rationale |
|---|---|
| Observe signs of infection and inflammation | Patients entered with an infection that usually has sparked a state of ketoacidosis or may have nosocomial infections |
| Improve efforts to prevent infection by good hand washing. All the people who come in contact with patients including the patients themselves should follow this. | Prevents cross infection |
| Maintain aseptic technique in invasive procedures | High glucose levels in blood would be the best medium for the growth of germs |
| Provide skin with regular care and earnest | The peripheral circulation may be disturbed that puts patients at increased risk of damage to the skin/skin irritation and infection |
| Make changes to the position, effective coughing and encourage deep breathing | To mobilize pulmonary secretions |

# POLYHYDRAMNIOS

**Definition:** Polyhydramnios is an excessive amount of amniotic fluid, which exceeds 1,500 mL. It occurs in 0.9% pregnancies. Polyhydramnios is diagnosed if the deepest vertical pool is more than 8 cm or amniotic fluid index (AFI) is more than 95th percentile for the corresponding gestational age.

## Causes

- **Fetal anomalies:** Congenital malformations increases the incidence of polyhydramnios in about 20% cases
    - Anencephaly
    - Open spina bifida
    - Esophageal/duodenal atresia
    - Hydrops fetalis
    - Aneuploidy
- **Placenta:** Chorioangioma of the placenta
- **Multiple pregnancy:** Increases the chances of polyhydramnios about 10%. It is more common is monozygotic twins, usually affecting second sac
- **Maternal:**
    - Diabetes
    - Cardiac diseases
    - Renal diseases
- **Idiopathic:** 50–60%

## Types

- **Chronic polyhydramnios:** It is gradual in onset, usually from about 30 weeks of pregnancy. This is the common type.
- **Acute polyhydramnios:** It is rare. It occurs at about 20th week and comes on very suddenly. The uterus reaches the xiphisternum in about 3–4 days. It is often associated with monozygotic twins/severe fetal abnormalities.

## Signs and Symptoms

- Uterine enlargement, abdominal girth and fundal height are far beyond that expected for gestational age.
- Tenseness of the uterine wall making it difficult or impossible to:
    - Auscultate fetal heart rate (FHR)
    - Palpate fetal parts
- Elicitation of uterine fluid thrill (fluid thrill may be elicited by placing hand on one side of the abdomen and tapping the other side with the fingers)
- Mechanical problems such as:
    - Severe dyspnea
    - Pedal and vulval edema
    - Pressure pains in the back, abdomen and thighs
    - Nausea and vomiting
- Frequent change in fetal lie (unstable lie)
- Auscultation of fetal heart is difficult because the quantity of fluid allows the fetus to move away from the stethoscope.

## Investigations

- **Ultrasonography:** To confirm the diagnosis and identify any coexisting conditions or complications
- **Blood:**
    - **ABO and Rh grouping:** May cause hydrops fetalis and fetal ascites
    - **Post-prandial sugar/glucose tolerance test**
- **Amniotic fluid:** $\alpha$ feto protein level increases the risk of open neural tube defect.

# Complications

## Maternal Complications

- **During pregnancy:**
  - Preeclampsia
  - Malpresentation
  - Premature rupture of membranes (PROM)
  - Preterm labor
  - Accidental hemorrhage
- **During labor:**
  - Early rupture of membranes
  - Cord prolapse
  - Uterine Inertia
  - Increased operative interference
  - Retained placenta
  - Postpartum hemorrhage (PPH) and shock
- **During puerperium:**
  - Subinvolution
  - Increased puerperal morbidity

## Fetal Complications

- Cord prolapse
- Hydrops fetalis
- Increased chances of operative delivery
- Accidental hemorrhage
- Fetal death

# Management

- **Mild asymptomatic polyhydramnios:**
  - Treated at home
  - Instruct mother to get adequate rest
  - Instruct her for immediate admission in hospital if membrane is ruptured.
- **Symptomatic polyhydramnios:**
  - Admission to hospital is required
  - Care depends on condition of woman and fetus, the cause and degree of hydramnios and the stage of pregnancy
  - Provide upright position to mother for relief of dyspnea
  - Administer antacid to relieve heartburn and nausea
  - If because of excessive accumulation of fluid mother feels discomfort, amniocentesis/ amnioreduction is useful.

  **Amnioreduction:** It is the procedure in which amniotic fluid is withdrawn from the amniotic sac. Slow decompression is done at the rate of about 500 mL/hour and the amount of fluid to be removed should be sufficient enough to relieve mechanical distress. Normally amniodrainage is stopped when AFI is less than 25 cm. Because of slow decompression, chance of accidental hemorrhage is less but liquor amni may again accumulate, for which the procedure may have to be repeated. Amniotic fluid is tested for fetal lung maturity.
- Labor should be induced, if the symptoms become worse or gross abnormality is diagnosed.
- **For induction:**
  - Lie must be corrected (longitudinal)
  - Membranes should be ruptured → to avoid altering the lie and to prevent cord prolapse or abruption placenta

- Labor will be usually normal, but (PPH) is a possibility
- Examine the baby for abnormalities

## Nursing Management

### Assessment

- Maternal respiratory condition
- Fetal condition by electronic fetal monitoring
- Abdominal girth to assess uterine height and compare with previous measurement
- Abdominal pain, edema, varicosities of vulva and lower extremities

### Nursing Diagnosis

- Fluid volume excess related to decrease urine output and retention of sodium and water
- Ineffective breathing pattern related to pressure on the diaphragm
- Impaired physical mobility related to edema and discomfort from the enlarged uterus
- Anxiety related to fetal outcome
- Risk for injury at delivery related to prolonged over distention of uterus

### Nursing Interventions

- **To assess the excess fluid volume:**
  - Assess patient general condition
  - Discuss the causative factors of excess fluid volume
  - Monitor intake output every 4 hourly
  - Take weight of patient daily and compare to previous weight
  - Auscultate breath sounds for the presence of crackles and monitor frothy sputum production
  - Follow low sodium diet or fluid restriction
  - Encourage oral care
  - Monitor for distended neck veins and ascites
- **Facilitate effective breathing by:**
  - Using fowler's bed and propped up position to increase the vital capacity of lungs to inhale more air.
  - Administer oxygen (8–10 L/min)
  - Provide comfort and rest
- **Early ambulation:** When the general condition of the mother improves, assist her in changing position and sitting on the bed and help to ambulate
- Encourage for diversional activities
- Educate the mother regarding personal hygiene including the dress and the footwear she should wear
- Provide psychological support to decrease anxiety and prepare for delivery
- Administer medications to prevent hemorrhage during labor and postpartum period

## OLIGOHYDRAMNIOS

**Definition:** When the liquor amnii is deficient in amount to the extent of less than 200 mL at term it is called oligohydramnios. It is typically diagnosed by ultrasonography and can be described qualitatively (e.g., normal, reduced) or quantitatively (e.g., amniotic fluid index <5).

## Causes

- **Maternal:**
  - Hypertensive disorders
  - Uteroplacental insufficiency
  - Dehydration
  - Idiopathic
- **Fetal:**
  - Fetal chromosomal or structural anomalies
  - Renal agenesis
  - Obstructive uropathy
  - Spontaneous rupture of membranes
  - Intrauterine infection
  - **Drugs:** Prostaglandin inhibitors, angiotensin converting enzyme inhibitors
  - Post maturity
  - IUGR
  - Amnion nodosum

## Signs and Symptoms

- Uterus appears smaller than expected for the period of gestation
- Reduced fetal movements compared to previous normal pregnancies
- Uterus small and compact and fetal parts easily felt
- Fetus is nonballotable
- Auscultation is normal

## Diagnosis

Amniotic fluid volume detection is done by ultrasonography. Diagnosis is made when largest pocket is less than 5 cm.

### Amniotic Fluid index (AFI)

- AFI = sum of 4 quadrants
- Normal = 9–10 cm
- Borderline = 5.8 cm
- Oligohydramnios ≤5 cm
- Polyhydramnios ≥25 cm

## Complications

### Maternal

- Prolonged labor
- Increased operative interference

### Fetal

- Abortion
- Increased chances of deformities
- Fetal pulmonary hypoplasia
- Cord compression
- High fetal mortality

## Management

- Admit the mother to hospital.
- If ultrasound scan demonstrates renal agenesis, baby will not survive, if agenesis not present, placental function tests are performed.
- If fetal anomalies are not considered lethal, amnioinfusion with normal saline or ringer's lactate may be performed in order to prevent compression deformities and hypoplastic lung disease.
- In case of oligohydramnios, labor may intervene or it may be induced because the possibility of placental insufficiency.
- Epidural anesthesia is indicated because uterine contractions are painful.
- Continuous fetal monitoring is essential because of possibility of cord compression or placental insufficiency and resultant hypoxia. There are chances of development of constriction ring or membranes may adhere to fetus.
- Aspiration of amniotic fluid (more concentrated with meconium), may add danger to an asphyxiated baby when born.

## Nursing Interventions in Oligohydramnios

- Monitor maternal and fetal status closely, including vital signs and fetal heart rate patterns.
- Monitor maternal weight gain pattern, notifying the health care provider if weight loss occurs.
- Provide emotional support before, during, and after ultrasonography.
- Inform the patient about coping measures if fetal anomalies are suspected.
- Instruct her about signs and symptoms of labor, including those she'll need to report immediately.
- Reinforce the need for close supervision and follow-up.
- Assist with amnioinfusion as indicated.
- Encourage the patient to lie on her left side.
- Ensure that amnioinfusion solution is warmed to body temperature.
- Continuously monitor maternal vital signs and fetal heart rate during the amnioinfusion procedure.
- Note the development of any uterine contractions, notify the health care provider, and continue to monitor closely.
- Maintain strict sterile technique during amnioinfusion.

## INTRAUTERINE GROWTH RESTRICTION/RETARDATION (IUGR)

*Syn: (Fetal growth restriction [FGR], small for dates, dysmaturity, chronic placental insufficiency)*
**Definition:** Intrauterine growth restriction (IUGR) is present in those babies whose birth weight is below the tenth percentile of average for the gestational age. Growth restriction can be present in preterm, term or post term babies.

Formula to calculate Ponderal Index: PI is calculated from measurement of body mass (M) and height (H).

$$PI = Weight\ (kg)/[Height\ (m)]^3$$

where body mass is in kilograms and height in meters.

## Types

Based on clinical evaluation and ultrasound examination, the small fetuses are divided into two types:

1. Fetuses that are small and healthy: the birth weight is less than 10th percentile for their gestational age. They have normal subcutaneous fat and usually have uneventful neonatal course.

2. Fetuses whose growth is restricted by pathological processes (True IUGR): Depending upon the relative size of their head, abdomen and femur, the fetuses are subdivided into (Table 2):
   ■ Symmetrical IUGR or type I
   ■ Asymmetrical IUGR or type II

TABLE 2: Differences between symmetrical and asymmetrical IUGR

| Symmetrical IUGR | Asymmetrical IUGR |
| --- | --- |
| • Uniformly small | • Head larger than abdomen |
| • Ponderal index (birth weight) crown-heel length → Normal | • Low |
| • HC: AC and FL: AC ratio → Normal | • Elevated |
| • Etiology: Genetic disease or infection | • Chronic placental insufficiency |
| • Total cell number-less cell size = normal | • Normal, smaller |
| • Neonatal course-Complicated with poor prognosis | • Uncomplicated having good prognosis |

*Abbreviations:* AC, abdominal circumference; FL, femur length; HC, head circumference

## Causes

- **Maternal:**
  - **Constitutional:** Small women, thin built, low body mass index (BMI), maternal genetic and racial background are associated with small babies
  - Maternal nutrition before and during pregnancy
  - **Maternal diseases:** Anemia, hypertension, thrombotic diseases, heart disease, chronic renal diseases, vascular diseases, etc. are the important causes
  - **Toxins:** Alcohol, smoking cocaine, heroin and other toxic drugs
- **Fetal:** There is enough substrate in maternal blood and also crosses the placenta but is not utilized by the fetus. The failure of nonutilization may be due to:
  - Structural anomaly
  - Chromosomal abnormality like Turner's syndrome
  - Syphilis toxoplasmosis, other infections, rubella, cytomegalovirus, herpes simplex (STORCH), infection
  - Multiple pregnancy
- **Placental:** Poor uterine blood flow to the placenta for longtime leads to chronic placental insufficiency with inadequate substrate transfer. This occurs in condition such as preeclampsia, essential hypertension, placental infarction, chronic placental abruption, circumvallate placenta, velamentous insertion of cord, etc.
- **Idiopathic:** 40% causes of IUGR are unknown.

## Clinical Features

- Weight deficit at birth about 600 mg
- **Length:** Unaffected
- Head circumference larger than body
- **Physical features:** Dry, wrinkled skin, scaphoid abdomen, thin meconium-stained vernix caseosa, thin umbilical cord, Pinna of ear has cartilaginous ridges and plantar creases well defined.
- Baby is alert, active, normal cry and eyes open
- **Reflexes:** Normal

## Diagnosis

- **Clinical:**
  - Clinical palpation of uterus helpful to diagnose IUGR
  - **Symphysis fundal height:** Correlates with gestational age after 24 weeks. A lag of 3 cm or more suggests IUGR
  - **Maternal weight gain:** Stationary/falling values
  - **Measurement of abdominal girth:** Stationary/falling values
- **Biophysical:**
  - **Head circumference and abdominal circumference:** In symmetrical babies: Normal, in asymmetrical: Elevated.
  - **Femur length:** Femur length (FL)/abdominal circumference (AC) is 22 at all gestational ages from 21 weeks to term. FL/AC ratio greater than 23.5 suggests IUGR.
  - **Amniotic fluid volume:** Reduced, often associated with asymmetrical IUGR.
- **Other tests:**
  - Ultrasonography
  - Doppler velocimetry
  - Uterine artery blood flow
  - Reduced/absent/reversed end diastolic velocity in umbilical artery.

## Complications

- **Maternal:** Growth restriction does not cause any harm to the mother.
- **Fetal:**
  - **Immediate complications:**
    - Asphyxia (Intrauterine/neonatal)
    - Respiratory distress syndrome (RDS)
    - Hypoglycemia
    - Meconium aspiration syndrome
    - Pulmonary hemorrhage
    - Polycythemia, anemia, thrombocytopenia
    - Necrotizing enterocolitis
    - Intraventricular hemorrhage (IVH)
    - Electrolyte abnormalities
    - Multiorgan failure
    - Increased perinatal morbidity/mortality
  - **Remote complications:**
    - Retarded neurological/intellectual development
    - Increased risk of metabolic syndrome in adult life
    - Renal vascular hypertension
    - Altered orexigenic mechanism → reduced appetite and satiety.

## Management

- When small for gestational age fetus is suspected prenatally: Careful search is made to determine the presence of growth retardation with the help of sonography.
- If it is present, the type of IUGR and possible causes are investigated.

- If fetus is symmetrically growth retarded, tests are done to detect fetal anomalies (to prevent unnecessary cesarean section)
- Hospitalize the patient, termination of pregnancy is done after 38th week in an equipped hospital where intensive care unit (ICU) facilities are available for newborn.
- Precautions during labor as same for preterm delivery
- During labor, provide left lateral position to mother → to improve uteroplacental blood flow.
- Any evidence of hypoxia should be immediately dealt with by cesarean section in the first stage and forceps in the second stage
- A pediatrician should be available at the time of delivery. All precautions as outlined for premature delivery are to be taken.
- Place the baby in neonatal intensive care unit (NICU), all protocols for preterm babies are to be followed.
- Special care is to be taken to prevent and treat hypoglycemia
- Early feeding within ½ hour is to be started with 5–10 mL of 10% dextrose
- Blood glucose is checked using dextrostix screening test 2 hourly after birth and before each feeding for 48 hours
- If blood glucose level falls below 30 mg%, 10% glucose is to be given intravenously

## Nursing Management

### Care before Pregnancy

- Providing care to women before and between pregnancies (interconception care) improves the chances of mothers and babies being healthy.
- Advocating healthy eating and physical activity to women in their daily routine to improve weight and cardiovascular status before pregnancy.
- Diagnosis and management of chronic diseases such as hypertension and diabetes before pregnancy.
- Correction of anemia/folic acid supplementation before pregnancy.

### Care during Pregnancy

- Educate the pregnant mother to take only those medicines which are prescribed by doctors.
- Healthy diet should be advised to pregnant women with behavior change to encourage healthier eating patterns during pregnancy. Foods fortified with nutrients can be provided to pregnant women.
- Pregnant women are advised to take enough rest with proper duration of sleep during night and an hour or two of rest in the afternoon.
- Instruct the expectant mothers to follow healthy lifestyle habits. Tobacco use, smoking and alcohol intake should be avoided during pregnancy.

### Care during Delivery

Delivery should be planned in health facilities having emergency obstetric care and neonatal care facilities.

## POST MATURITY

*Syn: (Prolonged and post-term pregnancy, post dated pregnancy)*
**Definition:** Post-term pregnancy is defined as one that exceeds 294 days calculating from the 1st day of the last menstrual period (LMP).

The pregnancy continues beyond 2 weeks of expected date of delivery. The terms 'Prolonged pregnancy' and 'Post-term pregnancy' are used synonymously and relate to duration of pregnancy. 'Post maturity' and 'postmature' are terms that relate to the neonate and refer to features and conditions of the baby.

## Etiology

Exact cause is not known, but certain factors are seen related.

- Wrong dates: Inaccurate LMP
- Hereditary factors
- High standard of living with sedentary habits tends to prolong pregnancy
- Elderly primigravida or elderly multiparae
- Fetal factors example congenital anomalies
- Placental factors: Sulfatase deficiency, low estrogen

## Diagnosis

- **Menstrual history:** If woman is sure about her date with previous history of regular cycles, it is reliable diagnostic aid in the calculation of period of gestation. However, in the cases of pregnancy occurring during lactational amenorrhea or soon following withdrawal of the pills, difficulty arises. In such cases, previously documented antenatal records of first visit may help.
- **Clinical findings:** Clinical findings, which are evident when an otherwise uncomplicated pregnancy overrun the expected date by 2 weeks are:
  - **Weight loss:** Regular periodic weight checking shows stationary or falling weight
  - **Girth of the abdomen:** Diminishes gradually because of diminishing liquor
  - **History of false pain:** Appearance of false pain followed by its subsidence is suggestive
  - **Abdominal palpation:** As liquor amnii diminishes, there may be changes in the height of the fundus, size of the fetus and hardness of the skull bones. The uterus 'full of fetus' is a feature usually associated with post-term pregnancy
  - **Internal examination:** Feeling of hard bones either through the cervix or through the fornix usually suggests maturity
  - **Straight X-ray abdomen:** Overall fetal shadow, thickness and density of the skull bone shadow, appearance and density of the ossification centers in the upper end of the tibia and lower end of the femur are taken together to assess the maturity.

## Clinical Features

In addition to the increased length of gestation at which the baby is delivered, the following criteria have been used to establish the diagnosis of post-term pregnancy retrospectively, i.e. after the birth of baby:

- **General appearance:** Baby looks thin and old, absence of vernix caseosa, body and cord are stained with greenish yellow color, head is hard and too much evidence of molding, nails are protruding beyond the nail buds.
- **Liquor amnii:** Scantly and may be saffron colored with meconium
- **Placenta:** Evidence of aging of the placenta manifested by excessive infarction and calcifications
- **Cord:** Diminished quantity of Wharton's jelly, which may precipitate cord compression
- **Macrosomia:** Birth weight of 4 kg or more in about 10% cases

# Complications

- **Maternal:** Post-maturity in majority of cases does not put the mother at risk. There may be increased chances/risk of instrumental delivery, operative delivery, morbidity, etc.
- **Fetal**
    - **During pregnancy:** Diminished placental function, oligohydrammios and meconium-stained liquor lead to fetal hypoxia and fetal death.
    - During labor:
- Fetal hypoxia/acidosis
- Labor dysfunction
- Meconium aspiration syndrome
- Risk of cord compression
- Shoulder dystocia
- Increased incidence of birth trauma
- Increased incidence of operative delivery

Following birth:
- Chemical pneumonitis atelectasis and pulmonary hypertension due to meconium aspiration syndrome
- Hypoxia
- Hypoglycemia and polycythemia
- Increased NICU admissions

# Management

Before formulating, the scheme of management, one should be sure about lung maturity of the fetus. Increased fetal surveillance is maintained (twice weekly), when conservative management is done. Induction of labor may be considered at or beyond 41 weeks. For the formulation of management, the cases are grouped into:

- Uncomplicated
- Complicated

## Uncomplicated

- **Selective induction:** In this, pregnancy may be allowed to continue till spontaneous onset of labor.
- **Routine induction:** Allow pregnancy to extend for 7–10 days past the expected date and thereafter labor is induced.
- **Induction:** If cervix is ripe, induction done by stripping of the membranes or by low rupture of the membranes. If liquor is clear, administer oxytocin to enhance uterine contraction. If cervix is unripe administer prostaglandin gel per vagina, followed by low rupture of membranes. Oxytocin infusion is added when required.

## Complicated Group

- **Elective cesarean:** In high-risk cases like elderly primigravida, preeclampsia, Rh incompatibility, etc.

## Care during Labor

Because of big baby and poor molding of head, there is an increased chance of prolonged labor. More analgesia is required for pain relief. There may be chances of shoulder dystocia. Adequate fetal monitoring is required. If fetal distress occurs, delivery is conducted by cesarean section/forceps ventouse.

# INTRAUTERINE FETAL DEATH

**Definition:** Antepartum death occurring beyond 28th week of gestation and usually resulting in the delivery of a macerated fetus is called intrauterine death (IUD) of fetus.

## Causes

Most of IUD occurs because of maternal and fetal complications that result in placental insufficiency. However, in 20–30% of cases, cause remains unknown.

- **Maternal causes:**
  - **Hypertensive disorders,** e.g., eclampsia, preeclampsia, chronic nephritis, chronic hypertension.
  - **Diabetes:** Long-term diabetes with atherosclerotic changes in the pelvic blood vessels may lead to chronic placental insufficiency and IUD.
  - **Antepartum hemorrhage (APH):** Both placenta previa and abruptio placenta causes placental insufficiency and finally IUD.
  - **Severe anemia:** Causes maternal hypoxemia: IUD
  - **Hyperpyrexia:** Temperature over 39.4°C can kill the fetus directly. In malaria, placental parasitization causes placental insufficiency and IUD.
  - **Maternal infections:** Toxoplasmosis, other infections, rubella, cytomegalovirus, herpes simplex infection (TORCH), hepatitis, malaria, poliomyelitis, mumps.
  - **Antiphospholipid syndrome:** Presence of lupus anticoagulant and anticardiolipin antibodies is associated with increased fetal loss.
- Hereditary thrombophilias.
- **Fetal causes:**
  - Congenital malformations
  - Fetal infection, example, rubella, cytomegalovirus, parvovirus-big and chorioamnionitis
  - Rh incompatibility: Excessive hemolysis of fetal RBC causes fetal anoxia → IUD
  - External version
  - Post-term pregnancy
  - Drugs (quinine overdose)

## Clinical Features

- Absence of fetal movements, which were previously experienced by the women.
- Retrogression of breast changes that occur during pregnancy.
- Gradual retrogression of the height of the uterus, so that it becomes smaller than the period of amenorrhea.
- Uterine tone is diminished and the uterus feels flaccid. Braxton-Hick contractions are not easily felt.
- Fetal movements are not felt during palpation.
- Fetal heart sound → absent.
- Eggshell crackling like feel of fetal head, if elicited is more indicative of the diagnosis.

## Investigations

- **Sonography:** Evidences of fetal death are lack of fetal movements over a period of 10 minutes, collapsed cranial bones and oligohydramnios.
- Straight X-ray abdomen may reveal the following features:

- **Spalding sign:** It mostly occurs 7 days after death. The irregular overlapping of the cranial bones one on another due to liquefaction of brain matter and softening of the ligamentous structures supporting the valut.
- Hyperflexion of spine and neck.
- Crowding of ribs shadow with loss of normal parallelism.
- Appearance of gas shadow (Robert sign) in the chambers of heart and great vessels may be seen as early as 12 hours after death.

## Complications

- Extreme psychological distress in women
- **Infection:** By gas forming bacteria, e.g., *Clostridium welchii* in case of ruptured membrane
- Blood coagulation disorder: due to gradual absorption of thromboplastin, liberated from dead placenta and decidua into the maternal circulation
- During labor:
  - Uterine inertia
  - Retained placenta
  - Postpartum hemorrhage

## Prevention

- **Regular antenatal checkups:** To prevent and detect early condition that contributes to IUD
- Screening of high-risk mothers for fetal well being
- In case of fetal compromise: Terminate the pregnancy at the earliest

## Management

Figure 10 shows the management of intrauterine death.

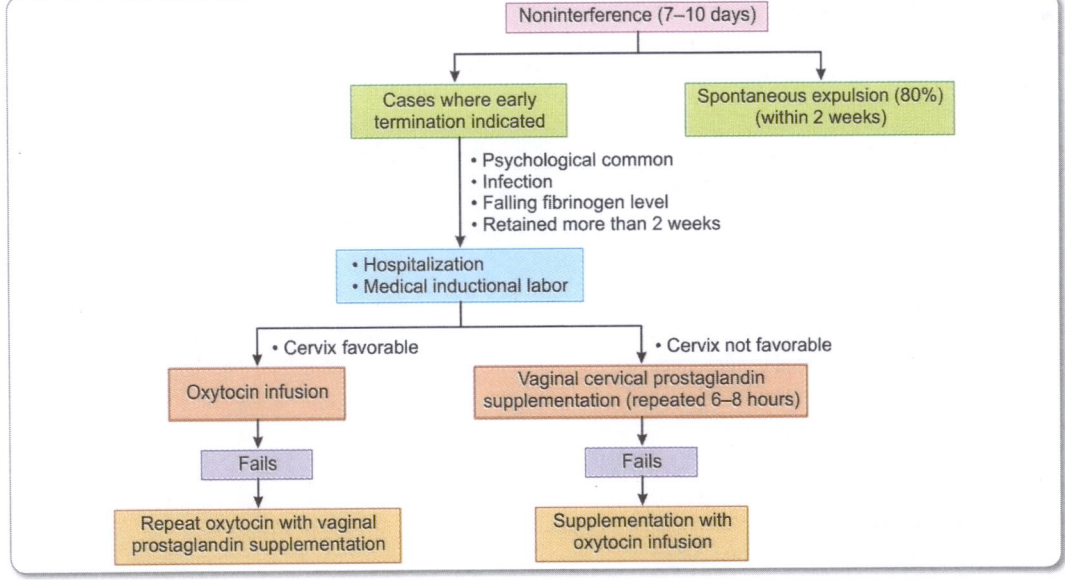

**Fig. 10:** Management of intrauterine death

# HIGH-RISK PREGNANCY

## Anemia

According to World Health Organization (WHO), when the hemoglobin concentration in peripheral blood is 11 g/100 mL or less is called anemia. It is responsible for 20% of maternal death in 3rd world countries.

It is the most common hematological disorder in pregnancy. It reduces the $O_2$ carrying capacity of blood, due to:

- Reduced number of RBCs
- A low concentration of hemoglobin
- A combination of both

### Incidence

The incidence is 40–80% in tropics as compared to 10–20% in the developed countries.

### Classification of Anemia

- Physiological anemia
- Pathological anemia
  - Iron deficiency
  - Folic acid deficiency
  - Vitamin $B_{12}$ deficiency
  - Protein deficiency
- Hemorrhagic anemia
  - **Acute:** Antepartum hemorrhage
  - **Chronic:** Hookworm infestation, bleeding piles, etc.
- Hemolytic anemia
  - **Familial:** Sickle cell anemia, Thalassemias, etc.
  - **Acquired:** Malaria, severe infections, etc.
- **Bone marrow insufficiency:** Hypoplasia/aplasia due to radiation, drugs or severe infection.
- Hemoglobinopathies

### Causes

- In tropical areas, the causes are:
  - Faulty dietary habits
  - Faulty absorption mechanism
  - Iron loss
    - Through sweat
    - Due to repeated pregnancies
    - Hookworm infestation
    - During menstruation
    - Chronic malaria
    - Bleeding piles and dysentery
- During pregnancy, the causes are:
  - Increased demand of iron (20%)
  - Diminished intake of iron

- Disturbed metabolism
- Prepregnant health status
- Excess demand:
  - Multiple pregnancy (increases 2 folds)
  - Repeated pregnancies
  - Teenage pregnancy

## Physiological Anemia

In physiological anemia of pregnancy, there is reduction in concentration that results from dilution because the plasma volume expands more than the erythrocyte volume. The hematocrit in pregnancy normally drops several points below its pregnancy level. In pathological anemia of pregnancy, the oxygen-carrying capacity of the blood is deficient because of disordered erythrocyte production or excessive loss of erythrocytes through destruction or bleeding.

## Pathological Anemia

Pathological anemia is a common complication of pregnancy, occurring in approximately half of all pregnancies. Disordered production of erythrocytes may result from nutritional deficiency of iron, folic acid, or vitamin $B_{12}$ or from sickle cell or another chronic disease, malignancy, chronic malnutrition, or exposure to toxins. The 4 main types of anemia occur due to the pathological conditions which are as follows:

### Iron deficiency anemia

Majority (95%) of pregnant women suffer from iron deficiency anemia. A pregnant woman is said to be anemic if the hemoglobin is less than 10 g%

*Causes*

- Reduced intake or absorption of iron → Dietary deficiency and gastrointestinal disturbances such as morning sickness.
- Excess demand such as multiple pregnancy, repeated pregnancy, urinary tract infection (UTI).
- Blood loss due to heavy menstruation, bleeding piles, antepartum hemorrhage (APH)/postpartum hemorrhage (PPH), hookworm infestation.
- Decreased absorption due to decreased gastric acidity and dietary imbalance causing formation of insoluble salts of iron.

*Signs and Symptoms*

- Pallor of mucous membranes
- Lassitude and feeling of weakness
- Giddiness
- Tachycardia and palpitations
- Dyspnea
- Anorexia and indigestion
- Swelling of the legs

*Complications of Anemia*

- **Maternal:**
  - Increase chances of preeclampsia
  - PPH

- Recurrent infection
- Preterm labor
- Heart failure
- Uterine inertia during labor
- Shock → even with minor traumatic delivery
- Puerperal sepsis
- Subinvolution
- Pulmonary embolism, disseminated intravascular coagulation (DIC)
- **Fetal:**
  - Low-birth-weight babies
  - Intrauterine death

## Investigation

- **Blood test:** Includes mean corpuscular hemoglobin concentration (MCHC), mean corpuscular volume (MCV), mean corpuscular hemoglobin (MCH), total red cells count and packed cell volume (PCV).
- **Urine test:** Presence of pus cells, sugar, proteins indicate infection.
- **Stool examination:** To detect helminthic infestation.
- **Bone marrow study:** Rare, for aplastic anemia.

## Management

### Prophylactic

- Avoidance of frequent childbirths.
- **Supplementary iron therapy:** Daily administration of 200 mg of ferrous sulfate along with 1 mg folic acid is effective.
- **Dietary prescription:** A realistic balanced diet, easily digestible and with the reach of the patient that is rich in iron and protein should be prescribed.
- Adequate treatment of hookworm infestation, dysentery, malaria, bleeding piles and UTI.
- Early detection of falling hemoglobin level is to be made. Hemoglobin should be estimated at the first antenatal visit, at the 30th and finally at 36th week.

### Curative

- **Hospitalization:** If hemoglobin level is 7 g/100 mL or less should be admitted for investigation and treatment.
- **Diet:** Well-balanced diet should be given to patient.
- To improve the appetite and facilitate digestion, pepsin may be given thrice daily after meals.
- To eradicate even a minimal septic focus by appropriate antibiotic therapy.
- Effective therapy to cure the disease that causes anemia.
- Iron therapy is given either in oral or parenteral forms.

### Oral iron

The daily dose of iron for treating anemia is between 120 g and 180 g in divided doses. Iron is best absorbed in the ferrous fumarate form and ferrous sulfate 200 mg tablets or ferrous gluconate 300 mg tablets are mostly used. Intolerance is evidenced by epigastric pain, nausea, vomiting, diarrhea or constipation. It is because of increased dose of iron or to some preparation. To avoid intolerance, instruct the mother to start the therapy with smaller dose and then increase the dose to a maximum of 3 tablets a day. Always take iron after meals and advise to take iron with a glass of lime juice.

The woman should be warned that her stools may turn black, but that does not mean that iron is not being absorbed.

### Parenteral iron

Parenteral iron is indicated for women who have intolerance to oral iron and those with severe anemia in advanced pregnancy. Parenteral iron is contraindicated for women who have liver or renal disorders.

### Intramuscular iron

It is given in form of dextran (Imferon), contains 50 mg of elemental iron in 1 mL and one ampule contains 2 mL. It is not given in conjunction with oral iron as this enhances headache, dizziness, nausea and vomiting. The injection should be given deep into muscle to prevent staining of the skin, formation of abscess and fat necrosis. After initial test of 1 mL, injections are given daily or on alternate days in doses of 2 mL I/M. It is given in 'Z' tract technique (pulling the skin and subcutaneous tissue to one side before inserting the needle).

### Blood transfusion

It is used rarely to treat anemia. It may be used to raise the hemoglobin level quickly if delivery is imminent (beyond 36 weeks). With transfusion improvement is seen in 3–4 days.

## Management during Labor

### First stage

- The patient should be in bed and should lie in position comfortable to her.
- Light analgesics are preferred for pain relief.
- Oxygen administration to increase the oxygenation of maternal blood and thus diminish the risk of fetal hypoxia.
- Strict asepsis to minimize puerperal infection.

### Second stage

Generally, there is no problem. IV Methergine 0.2 mg should be given following the delivery of anterior shoulder.

### Third stage

Close observation of patient during 3rd stage is required. Blood loss should be replenished by fresh packed cell transfusion. The volume of transfusion should not be more than the amount lost (to avoid overloading the heart).

## Puerperium

- Provide proper bed rest to the patient.
- Any sign of infection should be detected and treated promptly.
- Iron therapy should be continued for at least 3 months following delivery.
- Instruct patient to take adequate, easily digestible well-balanced diet.
- Patient should be warned of the danger of recurrence in subsequent pregnancies.

## Folic acid deficiency anemia (megaloblastic anemia)

The type of anemia is caused by lack of either vitamin $B_{12}$ or folate or both. Folic acid is needed for the increased cell growth of mother and fetus, but there is a physiological decrease in serum folate levels in pregnancy. Anemia is more likely to be found towards the end of pregnancy when the fetus is rapidly growing. In India, megaloblastic anemia is due to deficiency of folic acid.

*Etiology*

- Increase demand during pregnancy.
- Inadequate intake due to dietary insufficiency, nausea, vomiting and lack of appetite.
- Diminished absorption, e.g., intestinal malabsorption syndrome.
- Interference with utilization; drugs such as anticonvulsant, sulfonamides, alcohol are folate antagonists.
- Infections: They reduce the lifespan of RBCs and increase cell production requiring more folic acid.
- Decreased storage related to vitamin C deficiency and liver disease.

*Clinical Features*

- Pallor of varying degree
- Ulceration in the mouth and tongue
- Hemorrhagic patches under skin and conjunctiva
- Enlarged liver and spleen
- Anorexia and protracted vomiting.

*Diagnosis*

- Hemoglobin level below 10 g%
- Stained blood film shows: Hypersegmentation of the neutrophils, macrocytosis and anisocytosis, megaloblast
- Peripheral blood smears show deficiency of iron and folic acid
- Bone marrow shows both megaloblast and normoblasts
- MCV either normal or raised.

*Complications*

Deficiency of folic acid cause placental abruption, neural tube defects and congenital cardiac septal defects.

*Management*

Folic acid is administered orally in a dose of 5 mg 8 hourly. If time is short, treatment may be given with 30 mg I/M for 3 days or 90 mg I/V in 250 ml of normal saline to be followed by oral therapy. Instruct the patient to take diet rich in folic acid such as spinach and broccoli, but is destroyed easily by prolonged boiling or steaming. Other sources include peanuts, chick peas, bananas and citrus fruits.

## Vitamin B$_{12}$ deficiency megaloblastic anemia

Deficiency of vitamin B$_{12}$ also produces megaloblastic anemia. Vitamin B$_{12}$ level falls during pregnancy, but anemia is rare because body draws on its stores. Deficiency is most likely in vegetarians who do not eat any animal products, so vitamin B$_{12}$ supplements must be taken during pregnancy. Folic acid supplements should not be given in case of vitamin B$_{12}$ deficiency because it enhances degeneration of spinal cord.

### Protein deficiency

Decreased dietary intake of protein may lead to mild to moderate anemia. Protein deficiency may even develop in people with chronic liver disease, chronic kidney disease and low function thyroid.

### Hemolytic Anemia

It is a condition in which red blood cells are destroyed and removed from the bloodstream before their normal lifespan is over. Red blood cells are disc-shaped and look like doughnuts without holes in the center. These cells carry oxygen to the body.

## Sickle Cell Anemia

The sickle cell hemoglobinopathies are the hereditary disorders in which defective genes produce abnormal Hb β-chains; resulting Hb is called sickled hemoglobin (HbS). In sickle cell anemia, abnormal genes have been inherited from both parents whereas in sickle cell trait (HBAS) only one abnormal gene has been inherited.

- **Sickle cell trait:** Sickle Hb comprises 38–45%. The patients are usually asymptomatic. There is no anemia under the stress of pregnancy. Hematuria and urinary infection are common. If husband is carrier, there is 25% chances that infant will be homozygous sickle cell disease and 50% chances for sickle cell trait.
- **Sickle cell disease:** It is genetically inherited disease and transmitted equally in males and females. Sickle cells have increased fragility and shortened life span of 17 days resulting in chronic hemolytic anemia and causing episodes of ischemia and pain; known as sickle cell crisis.

### Clinical Features

- Anemia
- Episodes of pain
- Painful swelling of hands and feet
- Frequent infections
- Delayed growth
- Vision problems.

### Diagnosis

- Identification by sickling test
- Persistent reticulocytosis
- High fasting serum iron level
- Identification of type of hemoglobinopathies by electrophoresis

### Complications

- **Effects on pregnancy:**
  - Increased chances of abortion, prematurity, IUGR and fetal loss
  - Increased incidence of preeclampsia, PPH and infections
  - Increased maternal and fetal morbidity and mortality
- **Effects of pregnancy on the disease:**
  There are chances of sickle cell crisis, mostly occur in 3rd trimester. Two types of crises are generally found
  i. **Hemolytic crisis:** Due to hemolysis with rapidly developing anemia along with jaundice. There is associated leukocytosis and fever.
  ii. **Painful crisis:** Occurs due to vascular occlusion of various organs by capillary thrombosis resulting in infarction.

### Management

- **Preconceptional counseling:** Prenatal identification of homozygous state of the disorder is an indication for early termination of the pregnancy, if the parents desire.
- **During pregnancy:**
  - Careful antenatal supervision
  - Prophylactic folic acid 5 mg per oral daily
  - Iron supplementation in proven cases of deficiency
  - Regular blood transfusion at 6 weeks interval to raise Hb level

- Hospitalize the patient in case of any infection
- Air travel should be avoided
- **During labor:**
    - Adequate fluid infusion to avoid dehydration and acidosis
    - Continuous oxygen therapy by nasal cannula is helpful
    - Avoid anoxia during anesthesia. Epidural anesthesia is preferred
    - Fetus should be monitored closely for signs of distress
    - Cesarean section in case of obstetrical indications.
- **In puerperium:** Routine antibiotic to prevent infection
    - Neonatal testing of all babies at risk by cord blood testing
    - Barrier method of contraception is ideal, otherwise sterilization is to be done.

## Thalassemia Syndrome

Thalassemia syndrome is commonly found genetic disorders of blood. The basic defect is a reduced rate of globin chain synthesis. This leads to ineffective erythropoiesis, hemolysis and ultimately anemia. The syndromes are of two types: The $\alpha$ and $\beta$ thalassemia depending on the globin chain synthesis affected. $\alpha$- and, $\beta$-thalassemia exist in both homozygous (major) and heterozygous (minor) states.

### Clinical Features

- Hepatosplenomegaly
- Impaired growth
- Intercurrent infections
- Congestive cardiac failure
- Early childhood death

### Diagnosis

- Chorionic villus sampling
- Amniocentesis

### Management

Majority of the women tolerate pregnancy well with good maternal and fetal outcome. Oral folic acid supplementation is continued. Oral iron therapy is given only when the laboratory diagnosis of iron deficiency is established. Blood transfusion is rarely indicated.

## Hemoglobinopathies

Hemoglobinopathies are inherited specific biochemical disorders within the polypeptide chains of globin fraction. Hemoglobin is a conjugated protein which contains a globin fraction bound to 4 heme moieties. There are 4 polypeptide chains named alpha, beta, gamma and delta within the globin fraction. The position of amino acids in the protein chain determines the types of Hb produced. Adult Hb has two $\alpha$- and $\beta$-chains each, while the fetal Hb has two $\alpha$- and $\gamma$-chains each. By 6 months 96% babies Hb is HbA. The type of protein is genetically determined. Defective genes lead to formation of abnormal hemoglobin. Two common varieties are seen example sickle cell disease and thalassemia.

# JAUNDICE IN PREGNANCY

When the serum bilirubin level exceeds 2 mg%, visible yellow staining of the tissue appears. Overall incidence in India is 1–4 per 1000 deliveries.

## Causes

The causes of jaundice during pregnancy may be grouped as follows:

- **Jaundice due to pregnant state:**
  - Intrahepatic cholestasis
  - Preeclampsia, eclampsia, hemolysis, elevated liver enzymes and low platelet count (HELLP) syndrome
  - Fatty liver disease
  - Severe hyperemesis gravidarum
  - DIC
- **Jaundice unrelated to pregnant state:**
  - Viral hepatitis (A, E, G)
  - Obstructive Jaundice e.g., Due to gallstones
  - Drug induced, e.g., isoniazide
  - Hemolytic Jaundice, e.g., malaria, mismatched blood transfusion, *Clostridium welchii* infection, etc.
- **Jaundice when pregnancy superimposed on chronic liver disease:**
  - Chronic hepatitis
  - Cirrhosis, tumors
- **Obstetric cholestasis:**
  - Obstetric cholestasis the second most common cause of jaundice in pregnancy, the first one being viral hepatitis. In India, overall incidence is 1.2–1.5%. Due to excess circulating estrogen during pregnancy result in stasis of bile in the bile canaliculi with rise in conjugated bilirubin. Genetic, familial and abnormal progesterone metabolism have been also observed.

## Clinical Features and Diagnosis

- Generalized pruritis
- Weakness
- Nausea/vomiting
- Slight jaundice
- Rise aspartate aminotransferase (AST), alanine aminotransferase (ALT) and serum alkaline phosphates level
  - Liver biopsy shows features of intrahepatic cholestasis

## Complications

- Preterm labor
- Low-birth-weight babies
- Meconium-stained liquor
- IUD
- PPH

## Management

- Regularly monitored the prothrombin level.
- Features subside within two weeks postpartum, cholestyramine is effective for itching.
- Give vitamin K to reduce PPH and neonatal bleeding.
- Avoid combined oral contraceptives in women with history of obstetric cholestasis.
- To increase bile acid excretion and reduces pruritus, ursodeoxycholic acid is helpful.

# VIRAL INFECTIONS IN PREGNANCY

## Herpes Simplex Virus (HSV)

Herpes simplex is one of a family of herpes viruses, which includes varicella zoster, cytomegalovirus (CMV) and Epstein Barr virus (EBR). All within this family share the ability to establish lifelong, persistent infection in their last and to undergo periodic reactivation.

HSV type 1 is associated with infection of the lip and oropharynx and type 2 associated with genital infection. Neonatal infection is often associated with HSV type 2.

### Clinical Features

#### HSV-I

- Usually asymptomatic
- Gingivostomatitis
- Pharyngitis in young adults

#### HSV-II

- Painful genital ulcers after incubation period of less than 7 days.
- Skin lesions begin with erythema, progresses to vesicles and then ulcers and finally ends in crusting.
- Local lesions with viral shedding may last about 12 days with complete healing takes another week.

### Complications

- **Effects on pregnancy:**
  - Increased risk of miscarriage
  - Premature labor
  - Intrauterine growth restriction (IUGR)
- **Effects on fetus:**
  - Chorioretinitis
  - Microcephaly
  - Mental retardation
  - Seizures
  - Neonatal death

### Diagnosis

Diagnosis is made by detection of viral deoxyribonucleic acid (DNA) by polymerase chain reaction (PCR).

### Management

Because most genital herpes infection is unrecognized, it is important that a careful vulval inspection is done at the time of labor of all women. When the infection occurs in the first or second trimester of pregnancy the women are treated with oral or IV acyclovir.

When the first episode occurs in 3rd trimester there is increased risk of premature labor. If labor becomes established, the recommended management of IV administration of acyclovir and delivery by cesarean section, on the grounds of reducing maternal viremia and reducing exposure of the fetus to virus.

In case of women who have recovered from the first episode without going into labor, because of high risk of continued viral shedding, an elective cesarean section at 38 weeks may be done; especially if symptoms began within 6 weeks of the expected date of delivery

If following a first episode of infection in 3rd trimester, a vaginal delivery is unavoidable or if the membranes have been ruptured for more than 4 hours prior to cesarean section, then mother and baby must be treated with IV acyclovir to reduce the risk of neonatal infection.

## Rubella (German Measles)

The virus that causes rubella is particularly virulent during pregnancy. If the women contract rubella during 1st trimester, there is 20% chances that the baby will be born with congenital malformations. The figure may be 50% during the 1st month of pregnancy.

### Transmission

By respiratory droplet exposure.

### Manifestations

- Maternal infection is manifested by:
  - **Rash:** Pale or bright red on 1st and 2nd day, spreading rapidly over face over the entire body and fading rapidly.
  - Malaise, drowsiness
  - Fever, sore throat
  - Lymphadenopathy
  - Polyarthritis
- Congenital rubella syndrome includes:
  - Cochlear (sensorineural neural deafness) defects
  - Cardiac defects (septal defects, patent ductus arteriosus)
  - Hematologic (anemia, thrombocytopenia) disorders
  - Liver and spleen (enlargement, jaundice)
  - Ophthalmic (cataract, retinopathy, cloudy cornea) disorders
  - Bone (osteopathy)
  - Chromosomal abnormalities

### Complications

- Abortion
- Still birth
- IUGR
- Congenitally malformed baby.

### Diagnosis

Detection of viral ribonucleic acid (RNA) by PCR is possible. Prenatal diagnosis of rubella virus infection using PCR can be done from chorionic villi, fetal blood and amniotic fluid samples.

### Management

Active immunity can be conferred in nonimmune subjects by giving rubella vaccine. It is not recommended in pregnant women. When given during the child bearing period, pregnancy should be prevented within three months by contraceptive measures. However, if pregnancy occurs during the period, termination of pregnancy is not recommended.

## Cytomegalovirus (CMV)

Cytomegalovirus is another group of herpes viruses, which can be found in saliva, urine, breast milk, semen and cervical secretions.

### Transmission

- **In adults:** By direct contacts e.g., kissing and sexual contacts
- **In fetus:** By transplacental route

### Clinical Manifestations

- Fever
- Sore throat
- Headache
- Influenza
- Anorexia/malaise

### Diagnosis

By culture of specimens of urine, blood, saliva, or of a swab taken from the cervix. Serology is performed for antibody levels.

### Complications

- Abortion
- Chorioretinitis
- Mental retardation
- Sensorineural defects
- Nonimmune hydrops fetalis
- Stillbirth
- IUGR
- Microcephaly
- Intracranial calcification
- Hepatosplenomegaly
- Thrombocytopenia

### Management

Treatment is supportive only, and care should be taken to avoid infection of other babies and members of staff, particularly pregnant staff. The virus may continue to be shed by the infected infant for a prolonged period. It is estimated that 50% of women of child bearing age have been infected by CMV, but only 1% of their infants will be infected. A recombinant protein vaccine against CMV glycoprotein $\beta$ has been suggested to prevent maternal CMV infection.

## Hepatitis B Infection

Hepatitis B (HBV) virus is the most common cause of jaundice in pregnancy. Incubation period: 1–6 month.

### Transmission

- A parenteral route
- Sexual contact
- Vertical transmission (mother to baby through placenta)
- Rarely through breast milk

Neonatal transmission: Mainly at the time of delivery through mixing of maternal blood and genital secretions. Approximately 25% of the carrier neonate die from cirrhosis or hepatic carcinoma, between late childhood to early adulthood. HBV is not teratogenic.

## Clinical Features

- Malaise
- Anorexia
- Vomiting
- Arthralgia
- Skin rashes
- Fever or jaundice

## Diagnosis

HBV is confirmed by serological detection of hepatitis B viral surface antigen (HBsAg). HBsAg (donate high infectivity) and antibody to HBV core antigen. Chronic carriers are diagnosed by presence of HBsAg or hepatitis B e antigen (HBeAg) and anti HBc antibodies 6 months after initial infection. Liver enzymes are elevated during initial phase.

## Screening

All pregnant women should be screened for HBV infection at the first antenatal visit and it should be repeated during 3rd trimester for high-risk groups (IV drug abusers, sexually promiscuous individuals, hemophiliacs or woman with multiple sex partners).

## Management

Babies of mother who are chronic carriers or who have been infected with HBV during pregnancy should receive hepatitis B vaccine within 24 hours of birth and repeated at 1st and 6th month of age. In addition, the babies of mothers who had acute hepatitis B during pregnancy and those who do not have anti-HBe antibodies should receive 0.5 mL of hepatitis B immunoglobulin I/M, administered in different site from the vaccine, not later than 48 hours after birth to provide passive immunity.

Infection control measures should be instituted where the mother is considered infectious. The woman should be given information about the disease and advice regarding sexual behavior. Household contacts and husband should be tested for HBsAg and offered immunization.

## Chicken Pox (Varicella)

Varicella zoster virus (VZV), DNA virus does not cross the placenta and may cause congenital or neonatal chicken pox. Maternal mortality is high due to varicella pneumonia. Other maternal complications are: Encephalitis and bacterial super infection.

Congenital varicella syndrome is characterized by: Hypoplasia of limb, psychomotor retardation, IUGR, chorioretinal scarring, cataracts, microcephaly and cutaneous scarring. The risk of congenital malformations is nearly absent when maternal infection occurs after 20 weeks. Varicella (live attenuated virus) vaccine is not recommended in pregnancy. Varicella polymerase chain reaction (PCR) can identify (VZV) specific DNA from vesicular fluid. Enzyme linked immunosorbent assay (ELISA) can detect Varicella zoster virus (VZV) specific DNA from vesicular fluid. ELISA can detect VZV specific IgG and IgM. Varicella zoster immunoglobulin should be given to exposed nonimmune patient as it reduces the morbidity. Varicella-Zoster Immunoglobulins (VZIG) should also be given to newborn exposed within 5 days of delivery. Oral acyclovir, valacyclovir is safe in pregnancy and reduces the duration of illness when given within 24 hours of the rash.

## Measles

The virus (RNA) is not teratogenic. However, high fever may lead to miscarriage, fetal growth retardation (FGR), microcephaly and oligohydramnios, still birth or premature delivery. Nonimmunized women coming in contact with measles may be protected by I/M injection of immune serum globulin (5 mL). Diagnosis is made by assay of IgM and detection of viral RNA (RT-PCR). Mortality is high when complication like pneumonia and encephalitis develop. Management is supportive care. Antibiotics are given to prevent secondary bacterial infections. Ribavirin may be given for viral pneumonia. Active vaccination with live attenuated should not be given in pregnancy.

# HEART DISEASES IN PREGNANCY

The overall incidence of cardiac disease in pregnancy is falling in both the developed and developing part of the world. It is less than 1% in hospital deliveries. The commonest cardiac lesion is of Rheumatic origin followed by the congenital disorders. Adequate treatment for rheumatic fever with appropriate antibiotics with the advancement in cardiac surgery to rectify the congenital cardiac lesions, are responsible for change in profile over the past two decades.

Rheumatic valvular lesions predominately include mitral stenosis. Predominant congenital lesions include

- Patient ductus arteriosus (PDA)
- Atrial/ventricular septal defect (ASD/VSD)
- Pulmonary stenosis
- Coarctation of aorta
- Tetralogy of Fallot (TOF)

Rare causes are hypertension, syphilis or coronary heart disease (CHD)

## Changes in Cardiovascular Dynamics during Pregnancy and their Effects on Heart Lesions

In normal pregnancy, the cardiovascular dynamics alter in order to meet the increased demands of the utoplacental unit. This increases the workload of the heart quite significantly. The major cardiac changes are:

- An increase in cardiac output by 30–50%
- An increase in blood volume by 20–40%
- A rise in stroke volume by 20–40% in early pregnancy
- A fall in blood pressure in the second trimester

These changes start early in pregnancy and gradually reach a maximum by 30th week and maintained at term. Estrogen and prostaglandins are thought to be the reason for heart diseases during pregnancy. Cardiac failure occurs during pregnancy around 30 weeks, during labor and mostly soon following delivery. Additional factors responsible for deterioration of function of the damaged heart are:

- Advanced age
- Left ventricular hypertrophy (LVH)
- Appearance of risk factors, such as infection, anemia, preeclampsia, excessive weight gain, and multiple pregnancy
- History of previous heart failure
- Inadequate supervision

## Grading

According to classification of New York Heart Association, heart diseases are graded as:

**Grade I:** (Uncomplicated): Patient with cardiac disease, but no limitation of physical activity.

**Grade II:** (Slightly compromised): Patient with cardiac disease with slight limitation of physical activity. Comfortable at rest, but ordinary physical activity causes discomfort.

**Grade III:** (Markedly compromised): Patient with cardiac disease with marked limitation of activity. Comfortable at rest, but discomfort occurs with less than ordinary activity.

**Grade IV:** (Severely compromised): Patient has discomfort even at rest.

## Rheumatic Heart Disease

Valvular lesions predominate in rheumatic heart disease (RHD) and constitute approximately 50% of all heart disease seen in pregnancy.

- **Mitral and aortic valve incompetence:** Pregnancy can be helpful in case as it lowers the pressure in the arterial system, encouraging blood to flow the right away through the valves.
- **Mitral stenosis:** As the demand for cardiac output rises in pregnancy, pressure in the left atrium rises. This may lead to back pressure in the pulmonary system and pulmonary edema. The left atrium being unable to cope with the demands made upon it begins to fibrillate and heart failure may occur.

## Congenital Heart Disease

The most common congenital defects, which may remain uncorrected during the childbearing age are:
- Atrial septal defect
- Patient ductus arteriosus
- Ventricular septal defect

All of these are opening, which allow communication between the right and left sides of the heart or in case of patient ductus arteriosus between the pulmonary artery and the aorta. Problem arises when pulmonary vesicular resistance rises, as it does in preeclampsia and blood flows from right to the left side instead to passing through the lungs, leading to cyanosis. This may also happen in the third stage of labor when there is a sudden return of blood to the heart.

### Risk to Mother and Fetus

- Because of structural defect, a woman is proved to develop bacterial endocarditis and thromboembolism.
- In RHD, maternal mortality is low and during pregnancy no adverse effect on fetus.
- Maternal mortality is high in those conditions where pulmonary blood flow cannot be increased as in Eisenmenger's syndrome.

### Signs and Symptoms

- Breathlessness
- Nocturnal cough
- Syncope
- Check pain
- Chest murmur: Pan systolic, late systolic, loud ejection systolic or diastolic associated with thrill
- Cardiac enlargement, Arrhythmia
- Tachycardia, shift of ventricular apex
- Decrease exercise tolerance, fatigue
- Loud first sound with splitting

## Diagnosis

- **Chest radiography:** It shows cardiomegaly, increased pulmonary vascular marking, enlargement of pulmonary vein.
- **Electrocardiography:** T-wave inversion, biatrial enlargement, dysrhythmias.
- **Echocardiography:** Structural abnormalities (ASD, VSD), valve anatomy, valve area, left ventricular ejection fraction, pulmonary artery systolic pressure.
- Cardiac MRI can delineate complex (anatomy when it is not well evaluated by echocardiography).

## General Management

### Principles

- Early diagnosis and functional grading.
- Detection and institution of effective therapy for cardiac failure.
- Prevention and control of additional complications such as pulmonary hypertension.
- Mandatory hospital delivery.

### Preconception Care and Advice

- To reduce complications during pregnancy, women must consult the obstetrician and cardiologist before becoming pregnant.
- Initial valvotomy may be helpful in some cases.
- Advise the women to take well-balanced diet and control obesity.
- Limit the family size, as the risk increases with each pregnancy, use contraceptive devices.

### Place of Therapeutic Termination

Absolute indications are:

- Primary pulmonary hypertension
- Eisenmenger's syndrome
- Pulmonary veno-occlusive disease

Relative indications are:

- Parous women with grade IV and III Cardiac lesions.
- Grade I or II with previous history of cardiac lesions or in between pregnancy.

Termination should be done within 12 weeks by suction evacuation or by conventional D and E.

### Complications

The aim of management is to maintain or improve the physical and psychological well-being of mother and fetus. This involves keeping a steady hemodynamic state and preventing complications. The major maternal complications are:

- Bacterial endocarditis
- Thromboembolism
- Cyanosis
- Heart failure

The risk factors for heart failure include:

- Infections (UTI)
- Hypertension
- Anemia
- Multiple pregnancy
- Obesity
- Smoking

## Patient Advices

The following advices are given to mother:

- **Adequate rest:** For at least 10 hours at night and 2 hours nap during a day.
- **Avoid undue strain and excitement:** To prevent breathlessness
- Avoid caffeine, alcohol, β-mimetic drugs and high calorie or spicy diet. The diet should contain low salt, less carbohydrate, caffeine, alcohol and fat, but more protein.
- Anemia is to be corrected by appropriate therapy.
- Avoid cold and infections as it might precipitate heart failure. Injection penidure (benzathine penicillin) intramuscularly, given at 4-week interval throughout pregnancy and puerperium to prevent recurrence of rheumatic fever.
- Adequate dental care. Dental extraction, if necessary, should be carried out with antibiotic cover to eliminate sources of sepsis and reduce the risk of endocarditis.

## Hospitalization

Elective admission is necessary in case of:

- **Grade-I:** At least 2 weeks prior the expected date of delivery
- **Grade-II:** At 28-week especially in case of unfavorable social surroundings
- **Grade III and IV:** As soon as pregnancy is diagnosed, the women should be kept in hospital throughout pregnancy

## *Intrapartum Care*

### First Stage

- The women should be confined to bed and to be placed in lateral recumbent position to minimize aortocaval pressure by the gravid uterus.
- $O_2$ and resuscitation equipment must be ready and functioning. $O_2$ must be administered at 5–6 L/min rate when required.
- Analgesia in the majority is best given by epidural
- Prophylactic antibiotics against bacterial endocarditis
- Fluids should not be infused more than 75 mL/hour to prevent pulmonary edema
- Careful watch of pulse and respiratory rate. If pulse rate exceeds 110 per minute between uterine contractions, rapid digitalization is done by IV digoxin 0.5 mg.
- Cardiac monitoring and pulse oximetry can detect arrhythmias and hypoxemia early
- Prophylactic antibiotics are given during labor and for 48 hours after delivery, as these women are at risk of developing endocarditis. The recommended regimens include IV ampicillin 2 g and gentamycin 1.5 mg/kg (not more than 80 mg), at the onset, followed by repeated doses at 8 hours interval.

### Second Stage

- 2nd stage of labor should be short and no undue exertion by the mother
- To cut-short duration of 2nd stage, use forceps or ventouse, perineal block anesthesia
- Do not provide lithotomy position to patient because it may increase cardiac overload
- Avoid strong bearing down effort by the mother
- Do not administer methergine during delivery of anterior shoulder to prevent sudden overloading of heart

### Third Stage

- No ergot containing preparations should be used as it causes tonic contractions.
- Oxytocin is used as compared to methergine as it has effect on blood vessels.
- If oxytocin is given, it is to be administered by infusion accompanied by IV furosemide to prevent pulmonary edema.

### Cesarean Section

In general, there is no indication of cesarean section for heart disease. However, in correction of aorta, elective cesarean section is indicated to prevent rupture of the aorta or cerebral aneurysm. The anesthesia should be epidural (preferred) or general.

### *Puerperium*

- Provide absolute bed rest to mother and comfortable position to her.
- Methergine intramuscularly is given following delivery.
- Administer $O_2$ if required.
- Check pulse and respiration every hourly and temperature 4 hourly.
- Puerperal fever of any origin should be dealt seriously with appropriate use of antibiotics.
- Breastfeeding is not contraindicated but examine the baby for hereditary heart disease.
- Women should be kept in hospital for 2 weeks. In 1st week, allow the women to move her limbs and have breathing exercises during bed rest. In 2nd week if everything normal, she may be allowed to go out of bed.
- **Contraception:** Steroidal contraception is avoided as it may cause thromboembolic phenomenon. Intrauterine contraceptive devices (IUCDs) are avoided as they cause uterine infection progestin only pills or parenteral progestin are safe and effective. Barrier method (condom) is best. Sterilization at the end of first week following delivery is safe if family is complete.

## ACQUIRED IMMUNODEFICIENCY SYNDROME

Acquired immunodeficiency syndrome (AIDS) is caused by human immunodeficiency virus (HIV) which is a group of retrovirus, HIV-1 and HIV-2. The virus specifically reduces the CD-4 receptors molecule of the T-lymphocyte, monocytes, macrophages and other antigen-presenting cells leading to immunodeficiency. As a result, the individual is susceptible to infections by opportunistic microorganisms and specific tumors.

### Incubation Period

2 months to 4 years.

### Mode of Transmission

- Sexual contact
- Transplacental
- Exposure to infected blood or tissue fluids
- Through breast milk

## WHO Clinical Stages of HIV/AIDS

### WHO Clinical Stage I (APLAP)

- Asymptomatic infection
- Persistent generalized
- Lymphadenopathy (Lymph nodes ≥1.5 cm in ≥2 extrainguinal sites of ≥3 months duration) (Fig. 11)
- Acute retroviral infection
- **Performance scale I:** Asymptomatic, normal activity

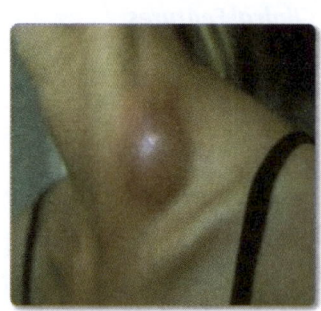

**Fig. 11:** Lymphadenopathy

### WHO Clinical Stage II (HUMR)

- Herpes zoster within previous 5 years.
- Unintentional weight loss <10%.
- Minor mucocutaneous manifestations.
- Recurrent upper respiratory tract infection.
- **Performance scale II:** Symptoms, but nearly fully ambulatory.

### WHO Clinical Stage III (COUPVCOSP)

- Chronic diarrhea >1 month
- Oral candidiasis
- Unintentional weight loss >10%
- Prolonged fever >1 month
- Vulvovaginal candidiasis >1 month
- Oral hairy leukoplakia
- Severe bacterial infections
- Pulmonary tuberculosis (within the last year)
- **Performance scale III:** In bed <50% of normal daytime, but more than during previous month.

### WHO Clinical Stage IV

WHO clinical stage IV has been given in table as follows:

| | | | |
|---|---|---|---|
| • Atypical mycobacteriosis <br> • Nontyphoid salmonella septicemia <br> • Extra-pulmonary TB | • Cytomegalovirus disease of an organ other than liver, spleen, or lymph node <br> • Herpes simplex virus infection | • Any disseminated endemic mycosis <br> • Candidiasis of the esophagus, trachea, bronchi and lungs | • Toxoplasma of the brain <br> • Cryptosporidiosis with diarrhea >1 month <br> • Isosporiasis with diarrhea <br> • Extrapulmonary cryptococcosis |
| • HIV wasting syndrome <br> • HIV encephalopathy | | • Lymphoma <br> • Kaposi's sarcoma | |
| **Performance scale IV:** In bed >50% of day, over the previous month. | | | |

## HIV Infection in Pregnancy

The transmission from mother to fetus is about 30%. Fetus may be affected through uteroplacental transfer, during delivery by contaminated secretions and blood of the birth canal and through breast milk in the neonatal period.

## Clinical Features

- Fever
- Malaise
- Headache
- Sore throat
- Lymphadenopathy
- Maculopapular rash
- Multiple opportunistic infections (e.g., candida, tuberculosis, *Pneumocystis carinii*)
- Neoplasms (Cervical carcinoma, lymphomas, Kaposi sarcoma)
- Constitutional symptoms (weight loss, lymphadenopathy, diarrhea)

## Diagnosis

Diagnosis of asymptomatic adult HIV infection is made on the basis of the presence in serum of antibodies to the virus. Most individuals will produce antibodies within 3 months after the exposure. During so called "Window of infectivity" (3 months), a negative result will require repeat test in order to account for the late seroconversion.

There are two commonly used tests for HIV:
1. Enzyme-linked immunosorbent assay (ELISA) is highly sensitive to the presence of antibodies
2. Western blot assay has a greater specificity for HIV, is used to confirm the presence of antibodies

## Management

### Prenatal

- All clients should be offered voluntary serologic testing for HIV infection.
- In seropositive cases, additional investigations should be done to test for other sexually transmitted infections (STIs). Husbands should be offered serologic testing for HIV.
- Counseling about the risk of HIV Transmission to the fetus and neonates should be made and termination of pregnancy offered.
- Tuberculin test is to be done. If it is positive, a chest X-ray should be performed. Even if chest X-ray is negative, chemoprophylaxis with Isoniazid 300 mg orally should be given.
- Check women have T-lymphocyte count in each trimester. If falls to less than 200 cells/uL, the woman should be treated with Zidovudine, she should receive prophylaxis against Pneumocystis carinii infection with Pneumocystis carinii infection with Trimethoprim 160 mg and sulfamethoxazole 800 mg orally thrice weekly. Nevirapine is found to reduce the viral transmission to breastfed infant.
- The progression of the disease is assessed by CD4 lymphocyte count (gradual fall), presence of P24 core antigen and decrease titer of P24 antibody.

### Intrapartum

- Women in labor, need to check recent viral load to plan mode of delivery.
- Zidovudine is given. IV infusion starting at the onset of labor (vaginal delivery) or 4 hours before cesarean section. Loading dose 2 mg/kg/hr, maintenance dose 1 mg/kg/hr until cord clamping is done.
- Women taking highly active antiretroviral therapy (HAART) can have planned vaginal delivery when plasma viral load is <50 copies/mL.
- If plasma load >50 copies/mL, elective cesarean section is recommended at 38 weeks for women taking HAART. Preoperative broad-spectrum antibiotics should be given as per hospital protocol. Cesarean section does not protect the baby from vertical transmission. It should only be for obstetric indications:

- Procedure that might result in break in the skin or mucous membrane of the baby such as amniotomy, attachment of scalp electrodes and fetal blood sampling should be avoided.
- Healthcare workers should be protected from contact with potentially infected body fluids.
- Caps, waterproof gowns, double gloves and goggles should be worn by physician and midwives.
- Disposable needles and syringes should be used and needles should be placed in puncture proof containers.
- Mechanical suctioning devices should be used to remove secretions from the neonate's air passages.
- Any blood contamination must be washed off the skin immediately.

## Postpartum Care

- Mother must be counseled about the risk and benefits of breastfeeding and helped to make an informed choice.
- Zidovudine syrup 2 mg/kg is given to the neonate 4 times daily for first 6 weeks.
- Mother should be encouraged to manage the baby care herself with the support of the midwife.
- Gloves must be worn for examination of perineum, lochia and cesarean wound.
- Disposal of sanitary pads and disinfection and clearing of any spilled blood must be done correctly.

## Contraception

Barrier method of contraception are effective in preventing the transmission of disease. Simultaneous use of spermicidal agents such as nonoxynol–9 is found to improve the efficacy. Disease could be prevented predominantly by health education and by practice of safer sex.

## Counseling

Prepregnant and early pregnancy counseling for HIV infected patient is essential which enables the patient to make an informed choice.

## Follow-up Care of Baby

Babies born to HIV or positive women will have passively acquired maternal antibodies to HIV and these may persist for as long as 18 months. Therefore, diagnosis of HIV cannot be achieved by antibody testing and confirmation of the infant's infection status may not occur for an extended period. Patient must be counseled with regard to this period of uncertainty and doubt.

# ELDERLY PRIMIGRAVIDA

**Definition:** Women having their first pregnancy at or above age of 30–35 years are called elderly primigravida.
**There are two types of patients:**
1. **Patient with high fecundity:** A woman married late but conceives soon after marriage
2. **Patient with low fecundity:** Woman married early but conceives long after marriage

## Complications

- **Maternal complications:**
  - **During pregnancy:**
    - Abortion
    - Preeclampsia
    - Abruptio placenta
    - Uterine fibroid
    - Pregnancy-induced hypertension (PIH), gestational diabetes, organic heart lesions, etc.

o Post maturity chances increases
o IUGR
- **During labor:**
  o Preterm labor
  o Prolonged labor
  o Maternal distress
  o Retained placenta
  o Increased chances of cesarean section
- **Fetal complications:**
  - Prematurity
  - Increased chances of congenital malformations
  - Operative interference increases
  - Increased perinatal morbidity/mortality

## Management

- Preconception counseling should be done.
- Patient is considered as "high risk". So, all steps followed for high risk mother, should be kept in mind while giving care at each step.
- Patient requires meticulous antenatal supervision and should have a mandatory hospital delivery.
- Vaginal delivery is possible in this case but if the induction score is unsatisfactory, cesarean section should be done.

## GRAND MULTIPARA

**Definition:** It is a term coined for a pregnant mother who has four or more viable children.

## Complications

**Maternal complications:**
- **During pregnancy:**
  - Abortion
  - Obstetric hazards as malpresentation, multiple pregnancy, placenta previa
  - Medical disorders (anemia, HIV, preeclampsia, cardiac disease)
  - Prematurity
- **During labor:**
  - Cord prolapse
  - Cephalopelvic disproportion (due to advancing age of mother and large sized baby)
  - Obstructed labor
  - Rupture uterus
  - Complications:
    o Postpartum hemorrhage
    o Shock
    o Operative interference
- **During puerperium:**
  - Increased morbidity due to sepsis, intranasal hazards
  - Subinvolution
  - Lactation failure

## Management

- Preconception counseling should be done.
- Patient is considered as "high risk" so all steps followed for high-risk mother should be kept in mind while giving care at each step.
- Patient requires meticulous antenatal supervision and should have a mandatory hospital delivery.
- During labor, the following guidelines are followed:
  - Pelvic assessment as routine
  - Check fetal position and presentation
  - Undue delay in progress should be viewed and cancelled. Use partograph carefully and record timely.
  - Take prophylactic measures against PPH.

## MULTIPLE PREGNANCY

**Definition:** When more than one fetuses simultaneously develop in the uterus, it is called multiple pregnancy. Two fetus growth and development in uterus (twins) is common although three (triplets), four (quadruplets), five (quintuplets) or six (sextuplets) can also occur.

### Classification of Twin Pregnancy

- **Dizygotic (binovular) twins:** Results from the fertilizing of two oval nest likely rupture from two distinct graafian follicles usually of the same or one from each ovary by two sperms during a single ovarian cycle. The body bears only fraternal resemblance to one another that of brothers and sisters, hence called fraternal/dizygotic twins.
- **Monozygotic (uniovular twins):** Results from fertilization of a single ovum. In this twinning may occur at different periods after fertilization and this influences the process of implantation and formation of fetal membranes.

### Determination of Zygosity

Table 3 shows how the zygosity of fetuses is determined:

**TABLE 3:** Determining the zygosity of fetuses

| Zygosity | Placenta | Communicating vessels | Intervening membranes | Sex | Genetic features | Skin grafting | Follow-up |
|---|---|---|---|---|---|---|---|
| Monozygotic | One | Present | 2 (amnions) | Always identical | Same | Acceptance | Usually identical |
| Dizygotic | Two | Absent | 4 (2 amnions 2 chorions) | May differ | Differ | Rejection | Not identical |

### Causes

The exact cause is unicorn. It may be due to national and environmental factors. Several risk factors include

- **Race:** Highest among Negroes, lowest among Mongols and intermediate among Caucasians.
- **Hereditary:** More transmitted through the female (maternal side)
- Advancing age of mother (maximum between 30 and 35 years)
- Increased parity (mostly from 5th gravida onward)
- **Iatrogenic:** Example drug (gonadotropin therapy)

## Signs and Symptoms

- Undue enlargement of uterus
- Increased nausea and vomiting
- Cardiorespiratory embarrassment
- Swelling of legs
- Increased chances of varicose veins/hemorrhoids
- Excessive fetal movements

## Diagnosis

- **History taking:**
  - History of ovulation induced drugs specially gonadotropins, for infertility or use of antiretroviral therapy (ART)
  - Family history of twinning
- **General examination:**
  - Increased prevalence of anemia
  - Unusual weight gain
  - More chances of preeclampsia
- **Abdominal examination:**
  - **Inspection:** It may reveal undue enlargement
  - **Palpation:** Height of uterus and girth is more than period of amenorrhea. On palpation, fetal parts are felt sometime two fetal heads can be palpated easily.
  - **Auscultation:** Simultaneous hearing of two distinct fetal heart sounds located at separate spots with a silent area in between.
- **Internal examination:** In some cases, one head is felt deep in the pelvis, while the other one is located by abdominal examination. On occasions, the clinical methods fail to detect twins prior to the delivery of first baby
- **Investigations:**
  - **Sonography:** It can detect two gestational sacs as early as 10th week. Repeated sonography is helpful.
  - Biochemical tests like serum human chorionic gonadotropin (hCG) α-fetoprotein, unacquainted estriol almost double than those of single for pregnancies.

## Complications

- **Maternal complications:**
  - During pregnancy:
    - Nausea/vomiting
    - Anemia
    - Hydramnios
    - Antepartum hemorrhage
    - Malpresentation
    - Preterm labor
    - Mechanical distress (Ex: Palpitation, dyspnea, etc.)
  - During labor:
    - PROM
    - Cord prolapse

- o Prolonged labor
- o Increased operative interference
- o Bleeding (following delivery of first baby and following separation of placenta)
- o PPH
  - ▪ During puerperium:
    - o Subinvolution
    - o Increased operative interference
    - o More chances of infection
    - o Lactation failure
- **Fetal complications:**
  - ▪ Miscarriage
  - ▪ Premature birth
  - ▪ Discordant twin growth
  - ▪ Intrauterine death of one fetus
  - ▪ Congenital malformations
  - ▪ Asphyxia

## Other Complications

- Twin to twin transfusion syndrome
- Dead fetus syndrome
- Twin reversed Arterial perfusion
- Monoamniotic
- Conjoined twins

# Management

## Antenatal Management

- Early diagnosis to detect chorionicity, amniocity, fetal growth pattern and congenital malformations.
- Careful antenatal supervision throughout pregnancy.
- **Diet:** Increased dietary supplement is needed for increased energy supply to the extent of 300 Kcal/day.
- **Increased rest:** At home and early cessation of work from 24 weeks onward is advised to provided pre-term labor and other complications.
- Supplement therapy, e.g., iron therapy, additional multivitamins are given.
- Serial sonography at every 3–4 weeks interval or earlier if needed. Assessment of fetal growth, AFI, nonstress test and Doppler velocimetry are correlated.
- Hospitalize the patient at term if no complication arises, if emergency occurs, admit the patient at earlier phases also.

## During the First Stage of Labor

- The woman should be kept in bed and the enema should be withheld to prevent early rupture of membranes.
- Skilled obstetrician should be present. An experienced anesthetist should be made available.
- Use of analgesics is limited as the babies are small and rapid delivery may occur. Epidural analgesia is preferred as it facilitates manipulation of second fetus if it would become necessary.
- Neonatologists should be present. Careful fetal monitoring of both babies should be done; continuous fetal monitoring using electronic fetal monitor is better.
- Vaginal examination should be done soon after the rupture of membranes to exclude cord prolapse.

- A line with ringer's lactate should be setup for any urgent IV therapy, if required.
- One IV unit of cross matched blood should be made readily available.
- Presence of neonatologists at the time of delivery is mandatory and if fetal distress occurs, delivery will need to be expedited, usually by cesarean section.
- In case of poor uterine contractions, start oxytocin drip once the membranes have been ruptured.
- Artificial rupture of membranes is helpful to induce uterine contraction but may need to be used in conjunction with IV syntocinon.
- Midwife should provide physical and emotional support to the mother throughout labor.

## During Second Stage (Management of Delivery)

- Delivery of first twin should be conducted in the same manner as in normal labor if it presents by vertex.
- Liberal episiotomy under local infiltration with 1% lignocaine is given to prevent intracranial damage to the fore coming or after coming head of the premature baby.
- Methergine should not be given after the delivery of first baby.
- Clamp the cord at two places and cut in between, to prevent exsanguination of second baby through communicating placental circulation in monozygotic twins.
- At least 8–10 cm of cord is left behind for administration of any drug or transfusion, if required.
- When the first twin is born, the time of delivery and the sex of fetus is noted.
- The baby must be labeled as "twin one" immediately.
- After delivery of first twin, abdominal palpation must be done to ascertain the lie, presentation and position of the second twin and to auscultate the fetal heart.
- A vaginal examination should be done to exclude cord prolapse, if any and to note the status of the membranes.
- If lie is not longitudinal, an attempt may be made to correct it by external cephalic version.
- If presenting part is not engaged, it should be pushed into the pelvis by fundal pressure before the second sac of membranes is ruptured.
- If uterine contractions are not effective, oxytocin drip should be started to stimulate contractions.
- When presenting part of second twin becomes visible, mother should be encouraged to push with contractions to deliver the second twin.
- Delivery will proceed as normal if the presentation is vertex.
- Delivery of second twin must be completed within 45-minutes of the birth of first twin as long as there are no signs of fetal distress.
- If there is delay, to cut short the duration of second stage of labor, forceps/ventouse should be used.
- If baby is in breech presentation, breech extraction is to be done.
- Following the delivery of anterior shoulder of second twin, methergine 0.2 mg is given intravenously.
- The baby is labeled as 'twin two' and the time of delivery and sex of baby is noted.

## Management of Third Stage

- The placenta is delivered by cord-controlled traction.
- Oxytocin drip should be continued for at least 1 hour following the delivery of second twin.
- Mother and baby should be carefully watched for 2 hours following delivery.
- If blood loss is more than average, it should be replaced by blood transfusion.
- Placental membranes and cord should be examined carefully for any abnormality.

## Indications for Cesarean Section

- **Obstetric causes:**
  - Contracted pelvis
  - Placenta previa
  - Severe preeclampsia
  - Previous history of cesarean section
  - Cord prolapse of first baby
  - Abnormal uterine contractions
- **Fetal causes:**
  - Both babies or first baby in transverse lie
  - Non/vertex twins with estimated weight 2 kg or less
  - Conjoined twins
  - Collision of both heads at brim preventing engagement of either head

## Management of Postnatal Period

- **Care of the babies:**
  - After the delivery of both twins, make sure that airway should be cleared and temperature must be maintained (Fig. 12).
  - Identification of the infants should be clear and parents must be given the opportunity to check the identity bracelets and cuddle their babies.
  - Until the mother's condition stabilizes after delivery, admit the infants directly to the neonatal unit from the labor room and later transfer to the postnatal ward to be with the mother.

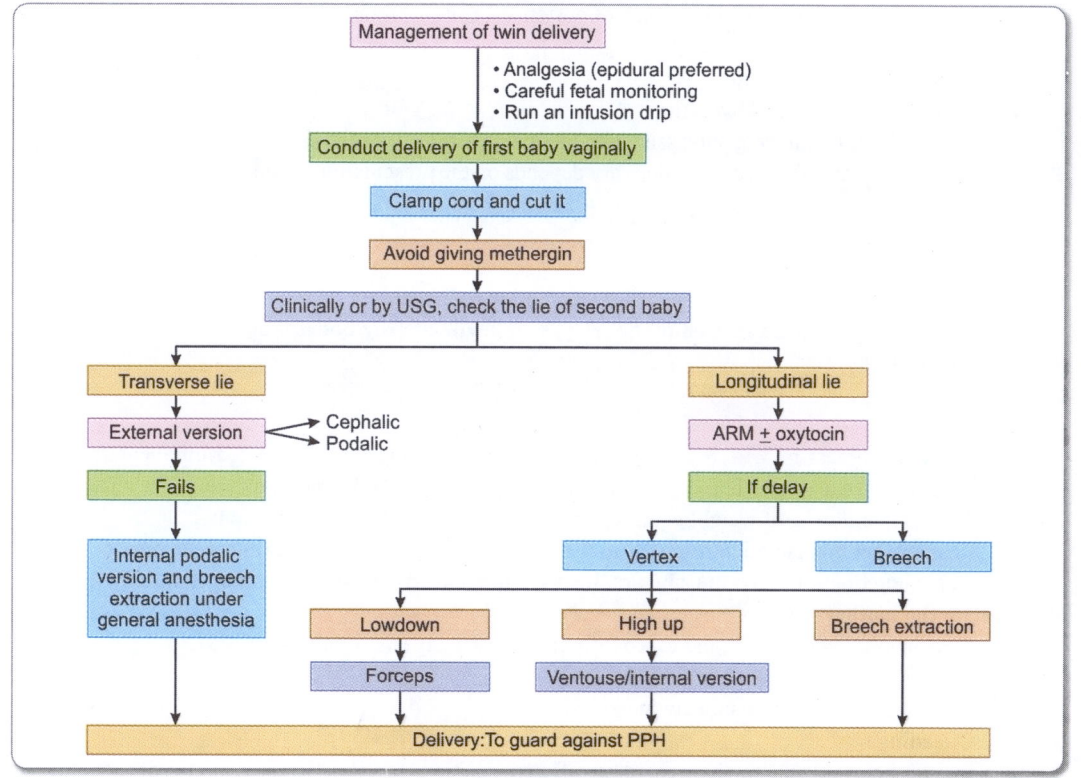

**Fig. 12:** Management of twin pregnancy
*Abbreviations:* ARM, artificial rupture of membranes; PPH, postpartum hemorrhage; USG, ultrasonography

- Advise the mother for breastfeeding either simultaneously or separately to both babies. Offer help during initial days.
- If babies are preterm, they may have to be fed with expressed breast milk.
- If infants are low-birth-weight, they are more susceptible to infection and hence the mother should be encouraged to wash her hands before and after handling her babies, particularly after changing their nappies.

- **Care of the mother:**
  - Involution of the uterus will be slower because of increased bulk.
  - After pains may be troublesome and analgesics must be given when she needs.
  - If mother is breastfeeding, a high calorie diet, high proteins are required.
  - Instruct the mother for postnatal exercises to improve the tone of the abdominal and pelvic floor muscles.
  - Provide reassurance to mother if babies are in nursery.
  - Provide appropriate support and assistance because mother of multiple twins is more susceptible to postpartum depression.

## *Nursing Interventions in Multiple Pregnancy*

*Antenatal management*
- Nutrition counseling
- Fetal evaluation
- Evaluate woman for signs and symptoms of obstetrical complications
- **PTL prevention:**
  - Explain for hospitalization
  - Encourage bed rest and hydration
  - Institute fetal monitoring and assist with tocolytic therapy, if ordered
- Explain to the woman that mode for delivery depends on the presentation of the twins, maternal and fetal status, and gestational age.

*Intrapartum management*
- **Establish IV access:**
  - Electronic fetal monitoring to assess the condition of the fetus
  - Double setup is recommended for delivery, so midwife prepare both set-ups
- **Emotional support**

*Postnatal period*
- **Nutrition:**
  - Expressed breast milk is best (for small babies), they may need to be fed intravenously or by nasogastric tube or cup-fed, depending on their size and general condition.
  - Careful monitoring of weight gain, regular capillary blood glucose estimations.
  - Reassure her that lactation responds to the demands made by babies sucking at the breast.
  - At feeding times, mother must be provided support and advised on positioning and fixing babies.
- **Care of the mother:**
  - Slow involution of uterus, increased 'after pains' so analgesia should be offered.
  - High calorie diet.
  - Teach extra support to handle twin babies.
- **Breastfeeding:**
  - Provide knowledge to mother regarding different positions for breastfeeding, along with advantages, attachment, positioning and timing.

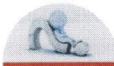

## ASSESS YOURSELF

### FREQUENTLY ASKED QUESTIONS IN EXAMS

1. Define ectopic pregnancy, sites of implementation of ectopic pregnancy, its causes and management of tubal ectopic pregnancy.

2. What do you mean by eclampsia, stages of convulsion, complications of eclampsia? As a nurse, how you manage a patient suffering from eclamptic fits?

3. Explain the nursing management of patient with hyperemesis gravidarum.

4. Define hydatidiform mole, its clinical manifestations, complications and obstetrical management.

5. Write short notes on:
   - Oligohydramnios
   - Teenage pregnancy
   - IUD
   - IUGR
   - AIDS
   - Elderly primigravida
   - Osteomalacia in pregnancy
   - Anemia in pregnancy

### MULTIPLE CHOICE QUESTIONS

1. Which hormone is mostly responsible for pernicious vomiting?
   - a. hCG
   - b. Prolactin
   - c. Estrogen
   - d. FSH

2. If a patient has chief complaints of intractable vomiting, dehydration, weight loss, epigastric pain, the condition is known as:
   - a. Eclampsia
   - b. Ectopic pregnancy
   - c. Hyperemesis gravidarum
   - d. Hydatidiform mole

3. A mother at 18-week gestation came to hospital with complaint of painless slight vaginal bleeding that is bright red in color and stops spontaneously, the condition is known as:
   - a. Inevitable abortion
   - b. Threatened abortion
   - c. Septic abortion
   - d. Complete abortion

4. If the fetus is dead and remains inside the uterine cavity, it is called:
   - a. Complete abortion
   - b. Missed abortion
   - c. Septic abortion
   - d. Incomplete abortion

5. According to clinical grading of septic abortion, if infection spread beyond the uterus to the parametrium, tubes and ovaries and pelvic peritoneum, then the patient is put in grade:
   - a. Grade I
   - b. Grade II
   - c. Grade III
   - d. None of the above

6. What is the cause of recurrent abortion?
   - a. Genetic factors
   - b. Endocrinal/metabolic factors
   - c. Cervical-uterine factors
   - d. All of the above

7. The classical symptoms of ectopic pregnancy are:
   - a. Abdominal pain
   - b. Amenorrhea
   - c. Vaginal bleeding
   - d. All of the above

8. Lower concentration of $\beta$-hCG compared to normal intrauterine pregnancy indicates:
   - a. Ectopic pregnancy
   - b. H. mole
   - c. Placenta previa
   - d. Multiple pregnancy

9. Bleeding from the genital tract after 28th week of pregnancy and before the birth of the baby is called:
   - a. Antepartum hemorrhage
   - b. Abortion
   - c. Ectopic pregnancy
   - d. Hydatidiform mole

10. When the placenta covers the internal os when closed, but not when fully dilated then it is:
   - a. Type-I placenta previa
   - b. Type-II Placenta previa
   - c. Type-III placenta previa
   - d. Type-IV placenta previa

11. A woman came to the hospital at 32-weeks gestation with chief complaints of painless, bright red vaginal bleeding, the condition is known as:
   - a. Placenta previa
   - b. Abruptio placenta
   - c. Ectopic pregnancy
   - d. Abortion

12. Following separation of placenta, the blood escapes downwards between the membranes and decidua, the type of abruptio placenta is:
   - a. Revealed
   - b. Concealed
   - c. Mixed
   - d. None of the above

13. Expulsion of grape-like vesicles per-vagina is the classical symptom of:
   - a. Complete abortion
   - b. Hydatidiform mole
   - c. Ectopic pregnancy
   - d. Placenta previa

14. If a previously normotensive and nonproteinuric patient after 20 weeks of gestation shows BP 140/90 mm Hg or more with proteinuria, the condition is known as:
   - a. Eclampsia
   - b. Epilepsy
   - c. Preeclampsia
   - d. Gestational hypertension

15. Which is the first choice of drug in case of eclampsia:
   - a. $MgSO_4$
   - b. Nifedipine
   - c. Methyldopa
   - d. Labetalol

16. The action of methyldopa is:
   - a. Anticonvulsant
   - b. Antihypertensive
   - c. Antispasmodic
   - d. Anti-inflammatory

17. When all the voluntary muscles undergo alternate contraction and relaxation, then it is:
   - a. Tonic stage
   - b. Clonic stage
   - c. Premonitory stage
   - d. Stage of coma

18. Abnormal carbohydrate tolerance with onset or first detected during present pregnancy, the condition is known as:
   - a. Gestational thyroidism
   - b. Gestational diabetes
   - c. Gestational anemia
   - d. None of the above

19. In case of glucose tolerance test, how much dose of oral glucose is given to pregnant women to diagnose gestational diabetes mellitus:
   - a. 100 g
   - b. 50 g
   - c. 80 g
   - d. 30 g

20. When the amount of amniotic fluid exceeds 1500 mL, the condition is known as:
    a. Polyhydramnios
    b. Oligohydramnios
    c. Hydrops fetalis
    d. None of the above

21. In case of intrauterine fetal death, appearance of gas shadow in the chambers of heart and great vessels is known as:
    a. Spalding sign
    b. Buddha sign
    c. Robert's sign
    d. Chadwick sign

22. Eggshell crackling-like feel of fetal head is the indication of:
    a. IUFD
    b. IUGR
    c. PROM
    d. None of the above

23. Megaloblastic anemia is also known as:
    a. Folic acid deficiency anemia
    b. Aplastic anemia
    c. Iron deficiency anemia
    d. Sickle cell anemia

24. German measles is also known as:
    a. Rubella
    b. Herpes simplex
    c. Mumps
    d. Pertussis

25. In case of dizygotic twins, genetic features of both twins are:
    a. Same
    b. Different
    c. Slightly identical
    d. None of the above

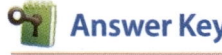 **Answer Key**

| 1. a | 2. c | 3. b | 4. b | 5. b | 6. d | 7. d |
|------|------|------|------|------|------|------|
| 8. a | 9. a | 10. c | 11. a | 12. a | 13. b | 14. c |
| 15. a | 16. b | 17. b | 18. b | 19. b | 20. a | 21. c |
| 22. a | 23. a | 24. a | 25. b | | | |

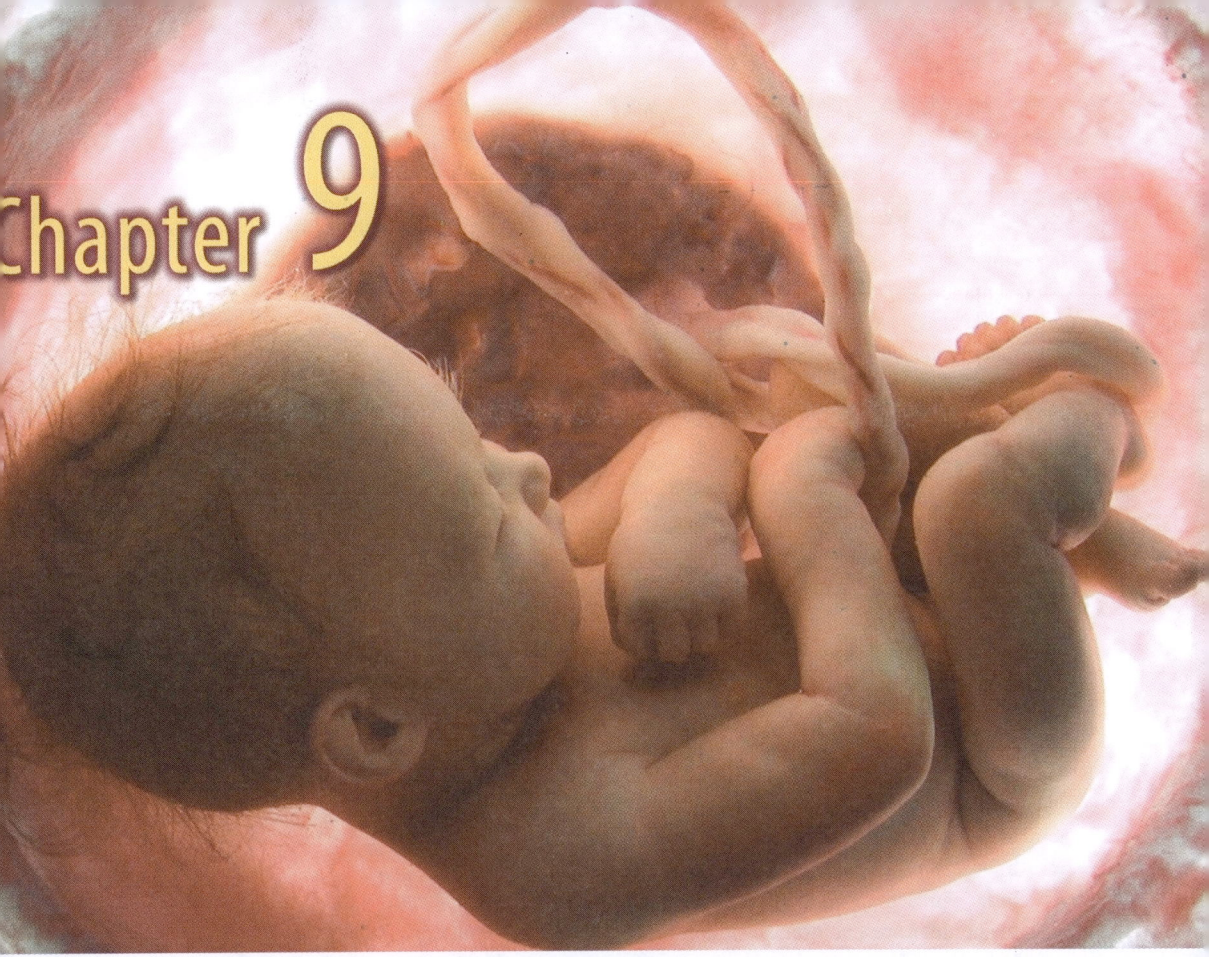

# Chapter 9

# Management of High-risk Labor

## MALPOSITIONS

- **Position:** Position is the relationship between the denominator of the presenting part with six points on the pelvic Brim
  - i. Right anterior
  - ii. Left anterior
  - iii. Right posterior
  - iv. Left posterior
  - v. Right lateral
  - vi. Left lateral
- **Denominator:** It is the part of presentation that indicates or determines the position. Each presentation has different denominator and these are as follows.
  - In vertex presentation, occiput is the denominator
  - In breech presentation sacrum is the denominator
  - In face presentation, mentum is the denominator
  - In shoulder presentation, acromion process is the denominator.
  - In brow presentation, no denominator is used.
- **Malposition:** When the denominator of the presenting part points on the pelvis other than the iliopectineal eminence, it is known as malposition. Factors favoring malposition are shown in Figure 1.

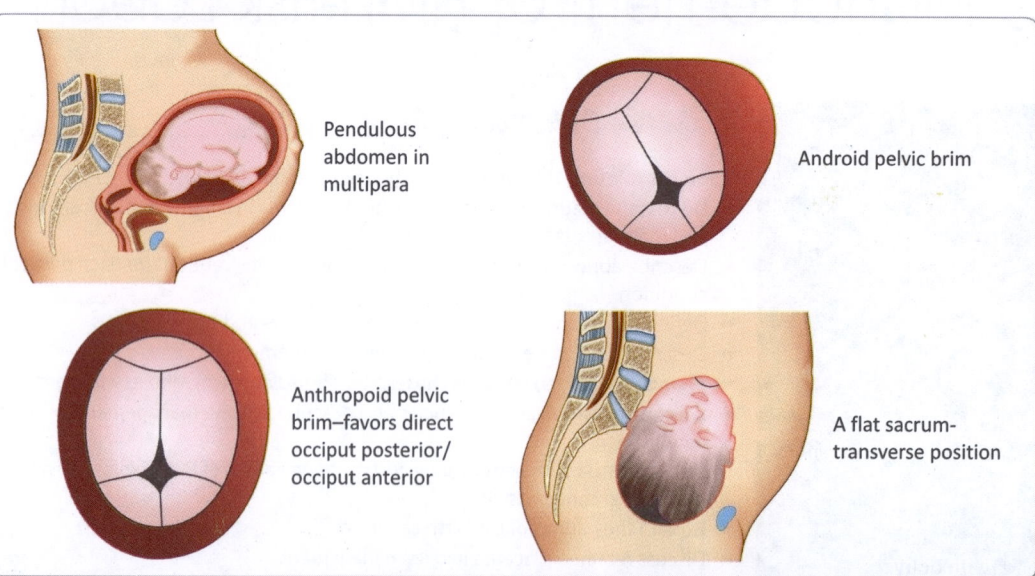

Pendulous abdomen in multipara

Android pelvic brim

Anthropoid pelvic brim—favors direct occiput posterior/occiput anterior

A flat sacrum-transverse position

**Fig. 1:** Factors favoring malposition

# Diagnosis of Malposition/Malpresentation

## Determine the Presenting Part

- The most common presentation is the vertex of the fetal head. If the **vertex is not the presenting part**, it means malpresentation.
- If the **vertex is the presenting part**, use landmarks of the fetal skull to determine the position of the fetal head (Fig. 2).

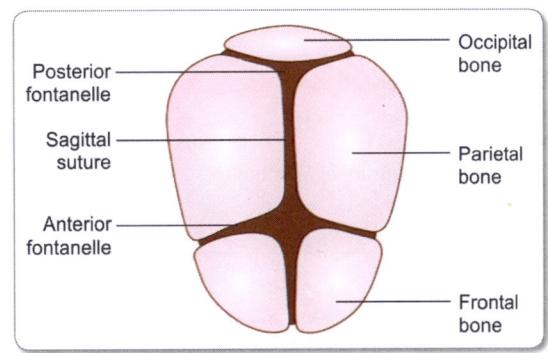

**Fig. 2:** Landmarks of the fetal skull

## Determine the Position of the Fetal Head

- The fetal head normally engages in the maternal pelvis in an occiput transverse position, with the fetal occiput transverse in the maternal pelvis (Figs 3A and B).
- With descent, the fetal head rotates so that the fetal occiput is anterior in the maternal pelvis (Figs 4A to C). Failure of an occiput transverse position to rotate to an occiput anterior position should be managed as an occiput posterior position.

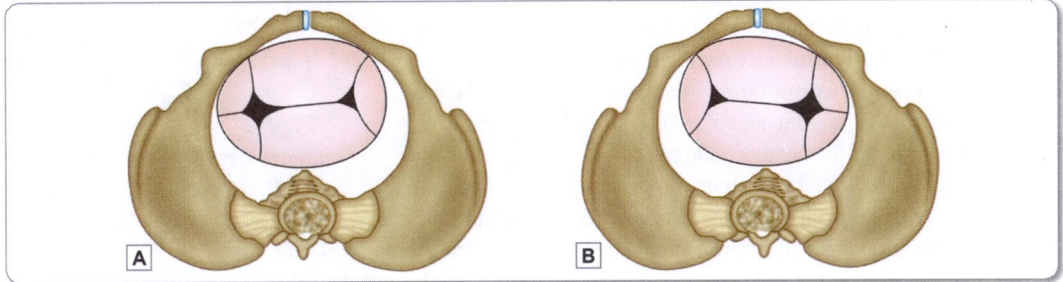

**Figs 3A and B:** Occiput transverse positions. **A.** Left occiput transverse; **B.** Right occiput transverse

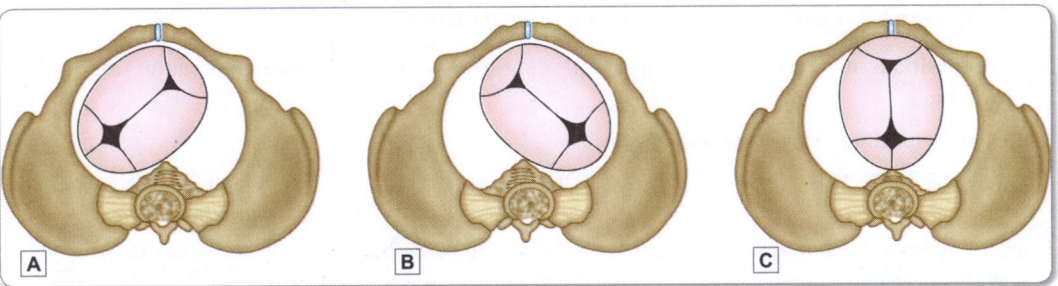

**Figs 4A to C:** Occiput anterior positions. **A.** Left occiput anterior; **B.** Right occiput anterior; **C.** Occiput anterior

- An additional feature of a normal presentation is a well-flexed vertex (Fig. 5), with the fetal occiput lower in the vagina than the sinciput.
- If the **fetal head is well-flexed** with **occiput anterior or occiput transverse** (in early labor), proceed with delivery.

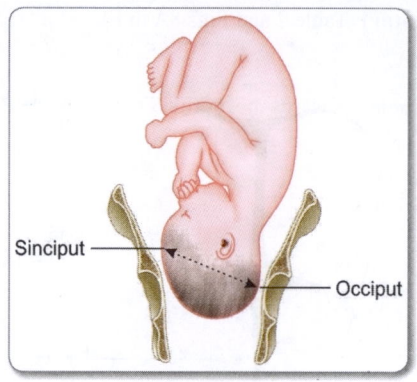

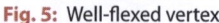

Sinciput

Occiput

**Fig. 5:** Well-flexed vertex

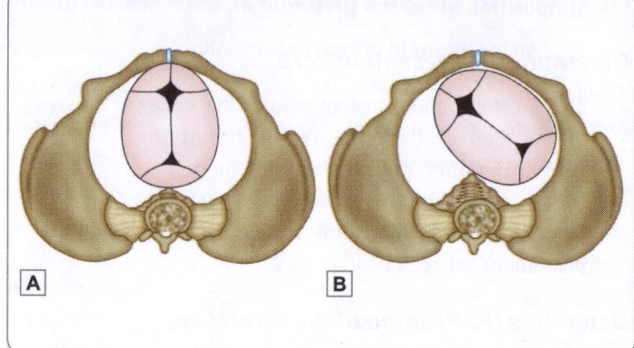

A          B

**Figs 6A and B:** Occiput transverse position. **A.** Occiput posterior; **B.** Left occiput posterior

- If the **fetal head is not occiput anterior**, identify and manage the malposition.
- **Occiput posterior position** occurs when the fetal occiput is posterior in relation to the maternal pelvis (Figs 6A and B).
  - On **abdominal examination**, the lower part of the abdomen is flattened, fetal limbs are palpable anteriorly and the fetal heartbeat may be heard in the flank.
  - On **vaginal examination**, the posterior fontanels are toward the sacrum and the anterior fontanels may be easily felt if the head is deflexed.

It occurs when the fetal occiput is transverse to the maternal pelvis (Fig. 7). If an occiput transverse position persists into the later part of the first stage of labor, it should be managed as an occiput posterior position.

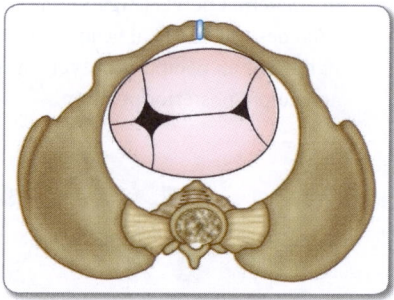

**Fig. 7:** Left occiput transverse

If the **fetal head is not the presenting part** or the **fetal head is not well-flexed**, identify and manage the malpresentation (given ahead in detail-malpresentation).

## Malpositions According to Different Presentations

- **Malpositions in vertex presentation** (In vertex presentation, occiput is the **Denominator**) are displayed in Table 1.

**TABLE 1:** Malpositions in vertex presentation

| Malposition | Occiput points towards | Sagittal suture of fetus in mother's pelvis |
|---|---|---|
| Left occipitolateral position (LOL) | Left iliopectineal line (midway between iliopectineal eminence and ileosacral joint | Transverse diameter |
| Right occipitolateral position (ROL) | Right iliopectineal line (midway between iliopectineal eminence and ileosacral joint) | Transverse diameter |
| Left occipitoposterior position (LOP) | Left sacroiliac joint | Left oblique diameter |
| Right occipitoposterior position (ROP) | Right sacroiliac joint | Right oblique diameter |
| Occipitoanterior position | Symphysis pubis | Anteroposterior diameter |
| Occipitoposterior position | Sacrum | Anteroposterior diameter |

- **Malposition in breech presentation** (sacrum is the **denominator**) (Table 2 and Figs 8A to F).

**TABLE 2:** Malpositions in breech presentation

| Malposition | Sacrum of fetus points towards the mother's pelvis on |
|---|---|
| Left sacrolateral position (LSL) | Left iliopectineal line |
| Right sacrolateral position (RSL) | Right iliopectineal line |
| Left sacroposterior position (LSP) | Left sacroiliac joint |
| Right sacroposterior position (RSP) | Right sacroiliac joint |
| Sacro-anterior position | Symphysis pubis |
| Sacro-posterior position | Sacrum |

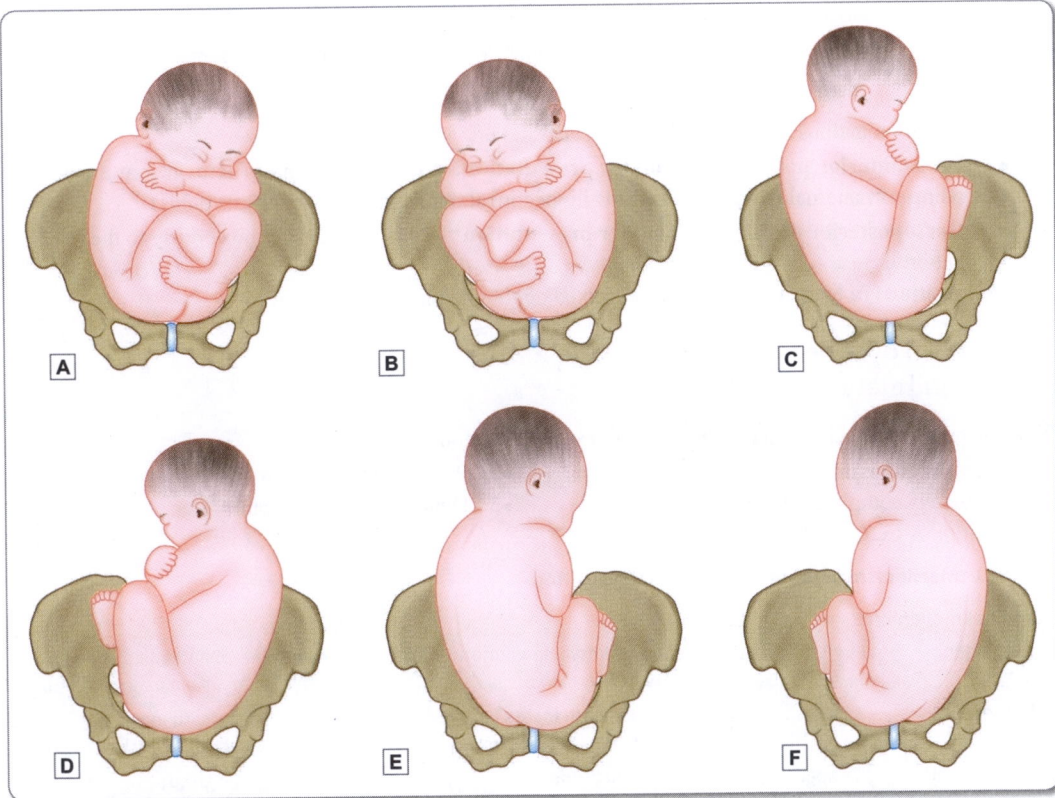

**Figs 8A to F:** Positions in breech presentation. **A.** Right sacroposterior; **B.** Left sacroposterior; **C.** Right sacrolateral; **D.** Left sacrolateral; **E.** Right sacroposterior and **F.** Left sacroposterior

- **Malpositions in face presentations** (in face presentation, mentum is the denominator).
  - Right mentoposterior (RMP)
  - Left mentoposterior (LMP)
  - Left mentoanterior (LMA)
  - Right mentoanterior (RMA)
  - Right mentotransverse (lateral)
  - Left mentotransverse (lateral)
  - Mentoposterior
  - Mentoanterior
- **Malpositions in shoulder presentations:** In shoulder presentation—acromion process is the denominator, but in practice, dorsum (fetal back) is used to describe the position (Figs 9A and B).

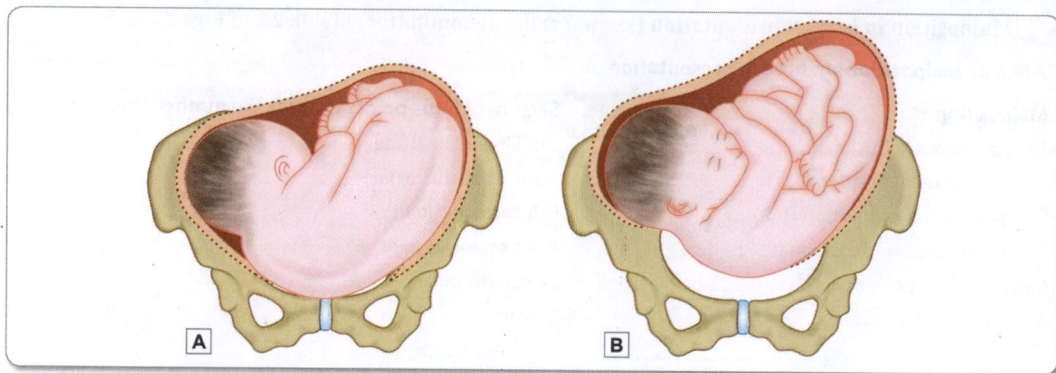

**Figs 9A and B:** Positions in shoulder presentation. **A.** Shoulder presentation, dorsoanterior and **B.** Shoulder presentation dorsoposterior

Two common malpositions in shoulder presentation are:

- **Dorsoanterior position in shoulder presentation:** When the dorsum of fetus lies in the anterior points of maternal pelvis (i.e. towards iliopectineal eminence and symphysis pubis)
- **Dorsoposterior position in shoulder presentation:** In this, dorsum lies posteriorly to the mother's pelvis.
- **Malpositions in brow presentation:** No fixed denominator.

## Mechanism of Labor in Left Occipitoposterior and Left Occipitolateral Position

Table 3 shows the mechanism of labor in LOL as LOP positions:

- Lie is longitudinal
- Attitude is complete flexion
- Position is LOL and LOP
- Presentation is vertex
- Denominator is occiput

**TABLE 3:** Mechanism of labor in LOL and LOP position

| Cardinal movements | LOL | LOP |
|---|---|---|
| Engagement | Occurs in left transverse diameter of the maternal pelvis | Occurs in left oblique diameter of pelvis |
| Flexion | Descend occurs with increasing flexion and occiput is the leading part | Descend occurs with increasing flexion and occiput is the leading part |
| Internal rotation of the head | **In well flexed attitude**<br>• Occiput reaches the pelvic floor first and rotates anteriorly 2/8th of the circle along the left side of the pelvis and comes under the symphysis pubis<br>• Shoulder moves 1/8th or the circle<br>• Twist occurs in the neck | **In well flexed attitude**<br>• Occiput reaches the pelvic floor first and rotates anteriorly 3/8th of the of the circle along left side and comes under symphysis pubis<br>• Shoulder moves 2/8th of the circle<br>• Twist occurs in the neck |
| Crowning: Further descends occur until occiput comes under the sub pubic arch and crowning takes place. After crowning, fetal head extends pivoting on suboccipital region around the pubis bone and the sinciput, face and chin sweep the perineum and head is born by movement of extension | | |
| Restitution | Occiput moves 1/8th of the circle to the left resulting in untwisting of the neck that occur during internal rotation of head | |

*Contd...*

| Cardinal movements | LOL | LOP |
|---|---|---|
| Internal rotation of shoulder | The shoulder also moves 1/8th of the circle to the left and anterior shoulder reaches under the symphysis pubis first. Rotation occurs in the same direction as restitution | |
| External rotation of the head | Simultaneous with internal rotation of shoulders, external rotation of head (1/8th of circle) takes places in the same direction | |
| Lateral Flexion of body | The anterior shoulder comes under the symphysis pubis first and escapes beneath the subpubic arch, posterior shoulder sweeps the perineum. With the birth of shoulder, the whole body is born by movement of lateral flexion | |

(**Note:** Other malpositions discussed side by side in malpresentations)

# MALPRESENTATION

Malpresentation means the fetus is present in the maternal pelvis other than vertex, longitudinal lie and well-flexed attitude. The common malpresentations are:

- Face presentation
- Brow presentation
- Shoulder presentation
- Breech presentation
- Compound presentation
- Cord presentation

## Face Presentation

When the attitude of the head is one of extension, the occiput of the fetus will be in contact with its spine and the face will present.

### Incidence

Incidence is 0.2%

### Causes

- Contracted pelvis
- Polyhydramnios
- Congenital abnormality for example, anencephaly, fetal goiter
- High maternal parity

### Diagnosis

- Generally diagnosed on vaginal examination in labor
- May be confused with breech

### Diagnosis (percentage-wise)

- 60% mentoanterior
- 15% mentotransverse
- 25% mentoposterior

### Mechanism of Labor in Mentoanterior Presentation

- Lie is longitudinal
- Attitude is flexed body with head deflexed fully
- Presentation is vertex

Figure 10 shows the mechanism of labor in mentoanterior presentation.

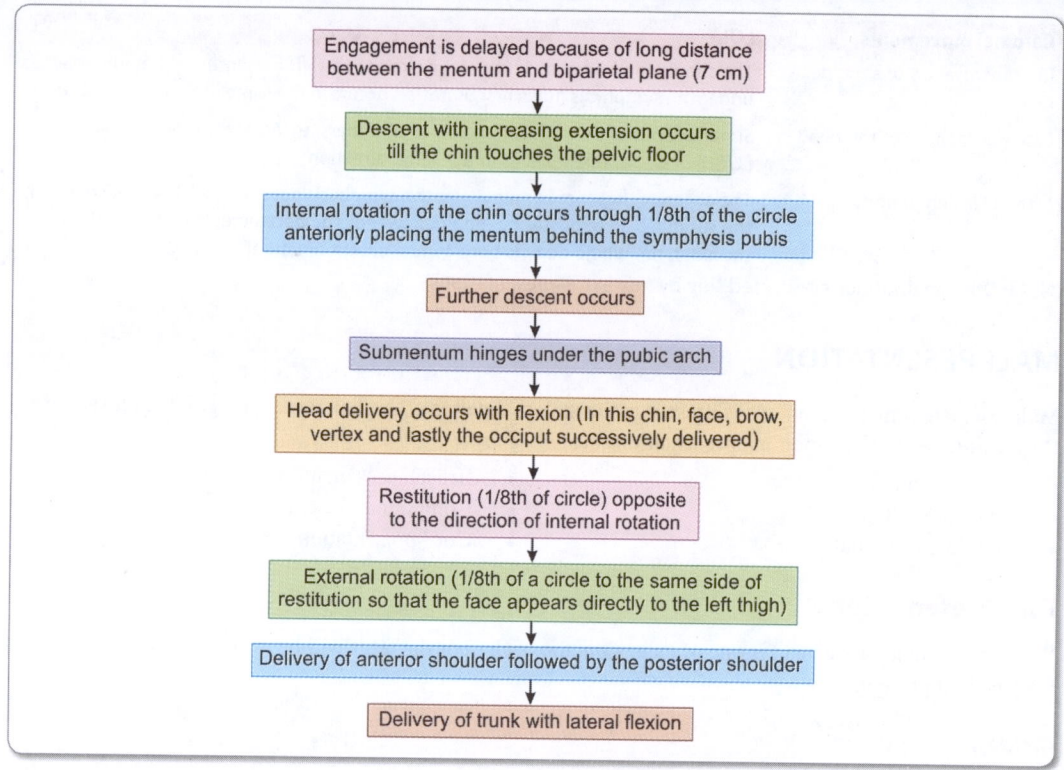

**Fig. 10:** Mechanism of labor in face presentation (Mentoanterior presentation)

- Position is left mentoanterior (LMA)
- Denominator is mentum in face
- Engaging diameter of fetal head is submentobregmatic (9.5 cm)
- **Presenting part:** Face of the fetus

## Mechanism of Labor in Mentoposterior Presentation

The cardinal movements in the mechanism of mentoposterior are like those of occiput posterior position. In 20–30% cases, anterior rotation of mentum occurs and in the rest (70–80%), incomplete anterior rotation, non-rotation or short posterior rotation of the mentum occur. There are more chances of arrest in this presentation.

## Complications

Complications of face presentation are shown in Figs 11A to E.

- **Obstructed labor:** Because face molding is difficult, a minor pelvic condition leads to obstructed labor.
- **Cord prolapse:** Common, because face is ill fitting presenting part.
- **Facial bruising:** Face is always brushed and swollen with edematous eyelids and lips.
- **Cerebral hemorrhage:** Lack of molding of facial bones leads to intracranial hemorrhage caused by excessive compression of fetal skull.
- **Maternal trauma:** For example, perineal laceration and increased chances of operative delivery (forceps/ventouse) may increase the chances of maternal morbidity.

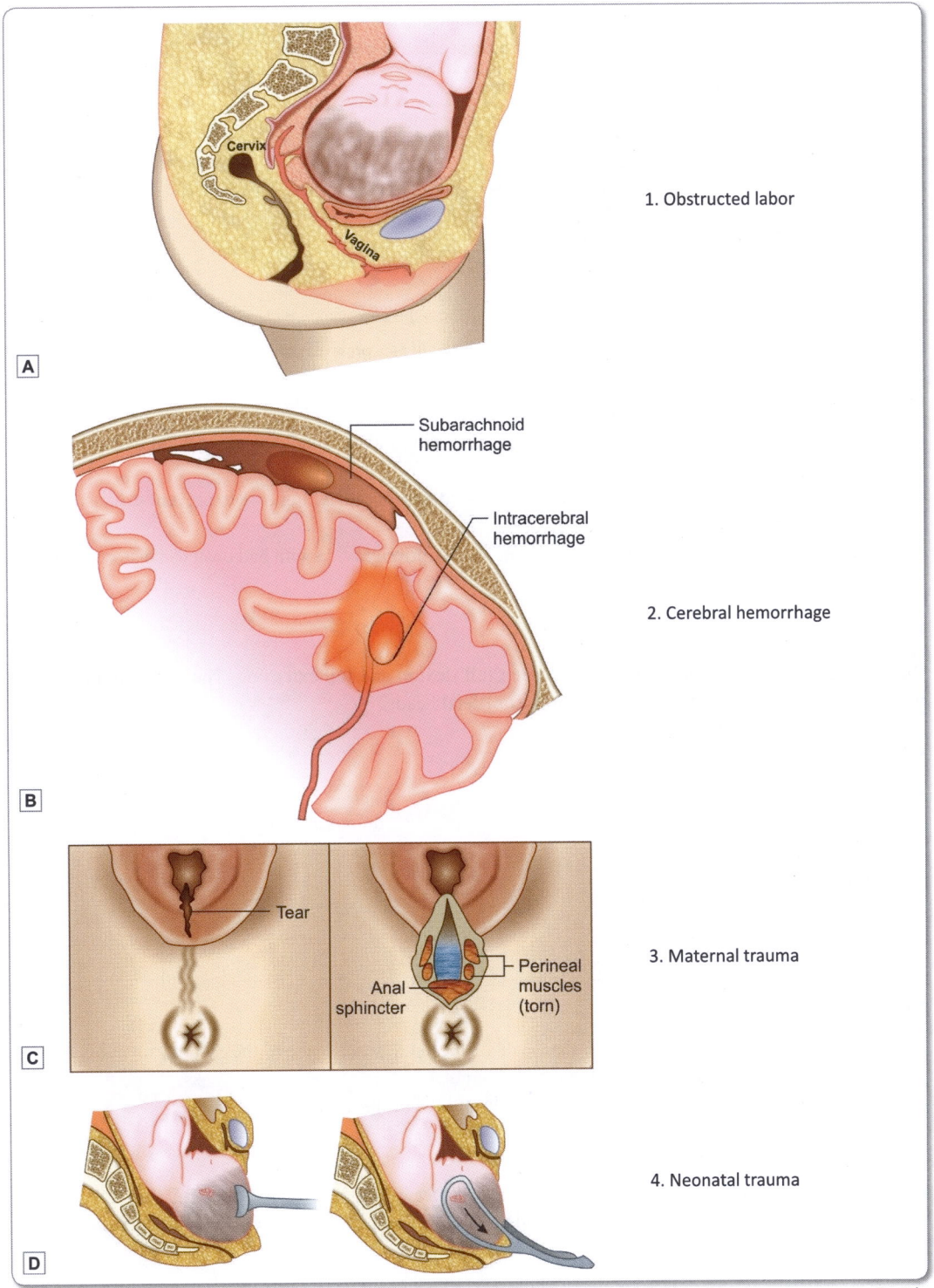

1. Obstructed labor

2. Cerebral hemorrhage

3. Maternal trauma

4. Neonatal trauma

**Figs 11A to D:**

*Contd...*

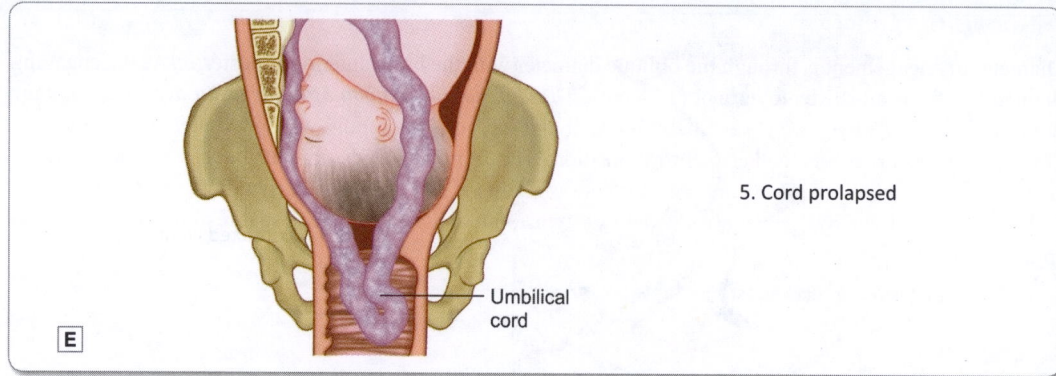

5. Cord prolapsed

Umbilical
cord

E

**Figs 11A to E:** Complications of face presentation

## Management of Face Presentation

- Ultrasonography should be done to confirm the diagnosis, to exclude bony, congenital malformation of the fetus and to note the size of the baby
- If the pelvis is normal and adequate, labor is allowed to proceed, taking care to prevent exhaustion from prolonged labor
- If the pelvis is contracted and the patient is an elderly primigravida with bad obstetric history, treatment is cesarean section

## Brow Presentation

Brow presents when the head is midway between full flexion and full extension. The engaging diameter is mentovertical 13.0 cm and is the largest diameter of fetal head.

### Causes

- **Fault in passage**
  - Contracted pelvis
  - Obliquity of uterus
  - Pendulous abdomen
  - Tumors of lower uterine segment
- **Fault in passenger**
  - Tumor on the neck of fetus
  - Cord round the neck
  - Anencephaly

### Diagnosis

- On **abdominal examination**, more than half of the fetal head is above the symphysis pubis and the occiput is palpable at a higher level than the sinciput.
- On **vaginal examination**, the anterior fontanele and the orbits are felt.

### Outcome of Labor

- If the position is unstable, it may get converted to either vertex or face presentation
- If no conversion occurs, there is no mechanism of labor for an average size baby with normal pelvis

## Mechanism of Labor

Diameter of engagement is through the oblique diameter with the brow anterior or posterior. As the engaging diameter of the head is Mentovertical (13.5 cm). *There is no mechanism of labor in an average size baby with normal pelvis.* However, if the baby is small and the pelvis is roomy with good uterine contractions, delivery can occur in mentoanterior brow position. The brow descends until it touches the pelvic floor. Internal rotation and descend occurs until the root of the nose hinges under the symphysis pubis. The brow and vertex are delivered by flexion followed by extension to deliver the face. Usual restitution and external rotation occur.

**Note:** There is no mechanism in posterior brow position.

## Management

- If brow presentation is diagnosed during pregnancy and there is no contraindication such as contracted pelvis and congenital malformation of the fetus, one may wait for spontaneous correction to occur until one week prior to the expected date of delivery (EDD).
- Elective cesarean section, if brow presentation with complicating factors such as elderly primigravida and contracted pelvis.
- If diagnosed during labor, with mother and baby in good condition, cesarean section is the best method
- If obstructed labor with dead baby, craniotomy may be choice for management.

## Shoulder/Transverse Presentation

When the long axis of the fetus lies perpendicular to the maternal spine, it is called transverse lie. The shoulder is most likely to present over the cervical opening during labor. Shoulder presentation is about five times greater in multigravida than in primigravida.

### Causes

- Contracted pelvis
- Uterine deformities
- Prematurity
- Lax abdomen in multigravida
- Polyhydramnios
- Multiple pregnancy
- Hydrocephalus and anencephaly
- Placenta previa

### Types of Shoulder Presentation

- *Dorsoanterior position in shoulder presentation:* When the dorsum of fetus lies in the anterior side of maternal pelvis, i.e. towards iliopectineal eminence and symphysis pubis
- *Dorsoposterior position in shoulder presentation:* In this, the dorsum lies posteriorly to the mother's pelvis.

### Diagnosis

- *Abdominal examination*
  - **Inspection:**
    - The uterus appears broader and asymmetrical with the height of fundus less than the period of amenorrhea
    - Transverse bulging of the abdomen with bulging flanks
  - **Palpation:**
    - Hard, ballotable, rounded head on one iliac fossa, at a lower level than breech
    - Soft, broad and irregular breech to one side of midline

- - The back is felt anteriorly across the long axis in dorsoanterior or irregular, small parts are felt anteriorly in dorsoposterior.
  - The lower pole of the uterus is found empty in the prenatal period (during labor, it may be occupied by the shoulder).
  - **Auscultation:**
    Fetal heart sounds are heard much below the umbilicus. It is quite distinct in dorsoanterior position and indistinct in dorsoposterior.
- *Vaginal examination (During labor)*
  Elongated bag of membranes can be felt if it does not rupture prematurely. Presenting part may be high up and floating after the rupture of membranes, the shoulder can be identified by palpating the following parts: The acromion process, the scapula, the clavicle and axilla. Palpating the ribs and intercostal space are the characteristic landmarks. Occasionally an arm is found prolapsed. Hand can be differentiated from a foot and an elbow from a knee.
- *Ultrasonography:* It can diagnose transverse lie and position of the placenta.

## Mechanism of Labor

There is no mechanism of labor in transverse lie and an average-size baby fails to pass through an average-size pelvis.

## Management of Shoulder Presentation

### Antenatal

External cephalic version should be done in all cases beyond 35 weeks if there is no contraindication. If the lie fails to stabilize even at 36th week, then the management is same as in case of unstable lie.

### If version fails or is contraindicated

- The patient is to be admitted at 37th week, because of risk of PROM and cord prolapse. Elective cesarean section is to be performed
- Vaginal delivery may be allowed in a dead or congenitally malformed (small size) fetus. Labor may be allowed to continue under supervision till full dilation of cervix then the baby can be delivered by internal podalic version

### Intrapartum Period

If the transverse lie is detected early in labor, when the membranes are still intact, the physician may attempt an external cephalic version followed by a controlled rupture of membranes. If the membranes have ruptured spontaneously, a vaginal examination must be performed immediately to detect possible cord prolapse.

### Immediate Cesarean Section should be Performed

- If the cord prolapses
- When the membranes have already ruptured
- When external cephalic version is unsuccessful
- When labor has already been in progress for some hours

## Complications of Shoulder Presentation

- Prolapse of cord when the membranes rupture
- Prolapse of arm when the shoulder has become impacted
- Obstructed labor and rupture of uterus
- Fetal death

# Breech Presentation

It is the presentation in which the lie of the fetus is longitudinal and the podalic pole presents at the pelvic brim.

## Types of Breech Presentation

There are two varieties of breech presentation (Figs 12A to D)

1. **Complete breech (flexed breech):** The normal attitude of full flexion is present. The thighs are flexed at the hips, legs are flexed at the knees and arms flexed over chest. The presenting part consists of two buttocks and external genitalia and two feet. It is commonly present in multipara.

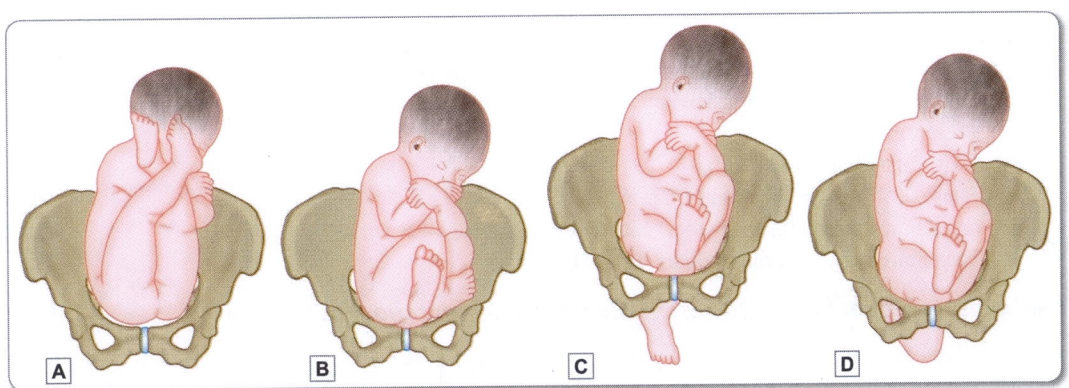

Figs 12A to D: Types of breech presentations. **A.** Frank breech; **B.** Complete breech; **C.** Footling presentation and **D.** Knee presentation

2. **Incomplete breech:** Occurs due to varying degree of extension of thighs or legs at the podalic pole. Three varieties are possible:
   i. **Breech with extended legs or frank breech:** In this condition, the thighs are flexed on the trunk and the legs are extended at the knee joints. The presenting part consists of two buttocks and external genitalia only. It is commonly present in primigravida.
   ii. **Footling presentation:** Both thighs and legs are partially extended bringing the legs to present at brim
   iii. **Knee presentation:** Thighs are extended but the knees are flexed, bringing the knees down to present at the brim.

## Causes of Breech Presentation

- **Prematurity:** Higher incidence of breech in earlier weeks of pregnancy. Smaller size of fetus and comparatively larger volume of amniotic fluid allow the fetus to undergo spontaneous version by kicking movements until 36th week when the position became stabilized.
- **Factors preventing spontaneous version such as:**
  - Breech with extended legs
  - Twins
  - Oligohydramnios
  - Congenital malformation of the uterus such as septate or bicornuate uterus
  - Short cord
  - Intrauterine death of fetus

Chapter 9 ◆ Management of High-risk Labor

- **Favorable adaptation in cases like:**
  - Hydrocephalus
  - Placenta previa
  - Contracted pelvis
  - Cornual-fundal insertion of placenta
- **Undue mobility of fetus:**
  - Polyhydramnios
  - Multipara with lax abdominal wall

## Diagnosis

- **Abdominal palpation** reveals the cephalic pole at the fundus and podalic pole in lower uterine segment
- **Auscultation:** Fetal heart sound is heard above the umbilicus
- **Ultrasonography:** Diagnosis can be confirmed by sonography
- **Vaginal examination:** In early labor, vaginal examination will reveal the following:
  - Presenting part is high up
  - Slow dilatation of the cervix
  - Sausage shaped, elongation of forewater
  - Sometimes presenting part (foot) can be felt in the bag of waters
  - Premature rupture of membranes (PROM)

## Mechanism of Labor in Breech Presentation (Left Sacroanterior Position)

- Lie is longitudinal
- Attitude is complete flexion
- Presentation in Breech
- Position is left sacroanterior
- Denominator is sacrum (left)
- Presenting part is anterior (left) buttock
- Bitrochanteric diameter, 10 cm enters the pelvis in left oblique diameter of the brim
- Sacrum points to the left iliopectineal eminence.

### Steps Involved in Mechanism

- **Compaction:** Descent takes place with increasing compaction, owing to increased flexion of the limbs.
- **Internal rotation of the buttocks:** The anterior buttock reaches the pelvic floor first and rotates 1/8 of a circle along the right side of the pelvis to lie underneath the symphysis pubis. The bitrochanteric diameter is now in the anteroposterior diameter of the outlet.
- **Lateral flexion of the body:** The anterior buttock escapes under the symphysis pubis, the posterior buttock sweeps the perineum and the buttocks are born by a movement of lateral flexion.
- **Restitution of the buttocks:** Anterior buttock turns slightly to the mother's right side.
- **Internal rotation of the shoulders:** The shoulders enter the pelvis in the same oblique diameter as the buttocks, the left oblique. The anterior shoulder rotates forwards 1/8 of a circle along the right side of the pelvis and escapes under the symphysis pubis; the posterior shoulder sweeps the perineum and the shoulders are born.
- **Internal rotation of the head:** The head enters the pelvis with the sagittal suture in the transverse diameter of the brim. The occiput rotates forward along the left side and the suboccipital region (the nape of the neck) impinges on the under surface of the symphysis pubis.

- **External rotation of the body:** At the same time, the body turns so that the back comes upwards.
- **Birth of the head:** The chin, face and sinciput sweep the perineum and the head is born in a flexed attitude.

## Types of Breech Delivery

- **Spontaneous breech delivery:** The delivery occurs with little assistance from the birth attendant
- **Assisted breech delivery:** The buttocks are born spontaneously, but some assistance is required for delivery of extended legs, arms and head.
- **Breech extraction:** In this manipulative delivery is performed by an obstetrician to hasten delivery in an emergency situation. For example, fetal distress and maternal cardiac diseases.

## Management of Vaginal Breech Delivery

### Preliminaries

- Complete dilatation of the cervix
- Adequate maternal pelvis
- Empty the bladder
- Ready resuscitative equipment for both mother and baby
- Instruct the mother regarding bearing down efforts
- Provide lithotomy position to the mother
- Delivery should be conducted in the presence of obstetrician, neonatologist and anesthesiologist so that if emergency situation arises, it can be handled properly.

### Delivery of the Trunk

- When the presenting part is completely engaged, shift mother to labor room and provide lithotomy position to the mother.
- Vulva and vagina should be swabbed and draped with sterile towels.
- Catheterize the bladder.
- Epidural anesthesia, pudendal block or local infiltration should be administered.
- Encourage the women to bear down during contractions and buttocks are delivered spontaneously.
- If the legs are flexed, the feet disengage at the vulva and the baby is born up to the umbilicus.
- Gently pull down the loop of cord to avoid traction on the umbilical cord.
- Feel for the elbows, which are usually on the chest. If so, the arms will escape with the next contraction.
- If the arms are not felt, they are extended. There is no need for facilitation of the progress of the mechanism of labor until the baby is born in 3–5 minutes to avoid any anoxia with resulting possible brain damage.
- Place a warm towel below the umbilicus of the baby to keep the baby warm and gives a nonslippery hold on the baby during fetal extraction.

### Delivery of the Shoulders

- Allow the baby to hang on its own weight and with uterine contractions, this brings shoulders down onto the pelvic floor where they rotate to the anteroposterior diameter of the outlet.
- Grasp the baby by the hips with thumbs on either sacroiliac region and fingers on the corresponding iliac crest.
- The baby is then tilted towards the maternal sacrum in order to free the anterior shoulder.
- When the anterior shoulder has escaped, the buttocks are lifted towards the mother's abdomen to enable the posterior shoulder and arm to pass over the perineum.

- If the arms are extended, they are delivered first by inserting the fingers of the hand in vagina to reach the elbow and sweeping it across the baby's chest downwards for delivery. In order to do this, the feet of the baby is grasped in one hand with the index finger between the legs, and the middle finger and thumbs each encircling a leg.
- Care must be taken in holding the baby at an angle so that head will enter the pelvis in transverse diameter and back must remain in lateral position.
- If ergometrine is being given, it should be administered intravenously with the crowing of the head.

### Delivery of the Head

- When the fetal back has been turned, allow the baby to hang on its own weight for 1–2 minutes, so that the head reaches the pelvic floor on which the occiput rotates forwards.
- Sagittal suture is now in the anteroposterior diameter of the outlet.
- Gradually, the neck elongates, the hairline appears and the suboccipital region can be felt.
- Controlled delivery of the head is vital to avoid any sudden change in intracranial pressure and subsequent cerebral hemorrhage.

### Methods of Delivering the after Coming Head of Breech

- **Forceps delivery:** The obstetrician usually applies forceps to the after coming head to achieve a controlled delivery.
- **Burns-Marshall method (Figs 13A to D):** Allow the baby to hang by its own weight for 1–2 minutes. The assistant is asked to give suprapubic pressure with the flat of hand in a downward and backward direction, the pressure is to be exerted more toward the sinciput to promote flexion of the head. When the nape of the neck comes under pubic arch, the baby is grasped by the ankles with a finger in between the two. The trunk is swung in upward and forward direction. Mean-while, the left hand to guard the perineum, slipping the perineum off successively the face and brow. When face and brow is delivered, mucus from the mouth and pharynx is cleared by mucus sucker. Depress the trunk to deliver the rest of the head.

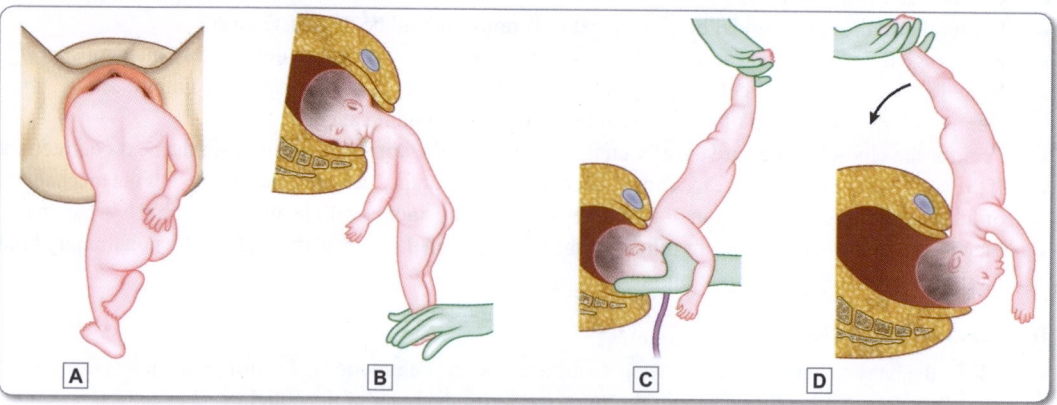

**Figs 13A to D:** Burns Marshall maneuver. **A.** Let the baby to hang by its own weight until nape of neck comes under pubic arch; **B.** Hold his feet; **C.** With delivery of face and mouth, suction mucus should be performed; **D.** Swing his head clear

- **Molar flexion and shoulder traction (Modified Mauriceau-Smellie-Veit Technique) (Fig. 14):** The baby is placed on the supinated left forearm with the limbs handing on either side. The middle and the index fingers of left hand are placed over the maxillary/molar bones on either side to maintain flexion of the head. The ring and little fingers of the pronated right hand are placed on the child's right shoulder, the index finger is placed on the left shoulder and the middle finger is placed on the suboccipital region. Traction is now given in downward and backward direction till the nape of the neck is visible under the pubic arch. The assistant gives suprapubic pressure during the period to maintain flexion. Thereafter, the fetus is carried in upward and forward direction toward the mother's abdomen releasing the face, brow and lastly the trunk is depressed to release the occiput and vertex.

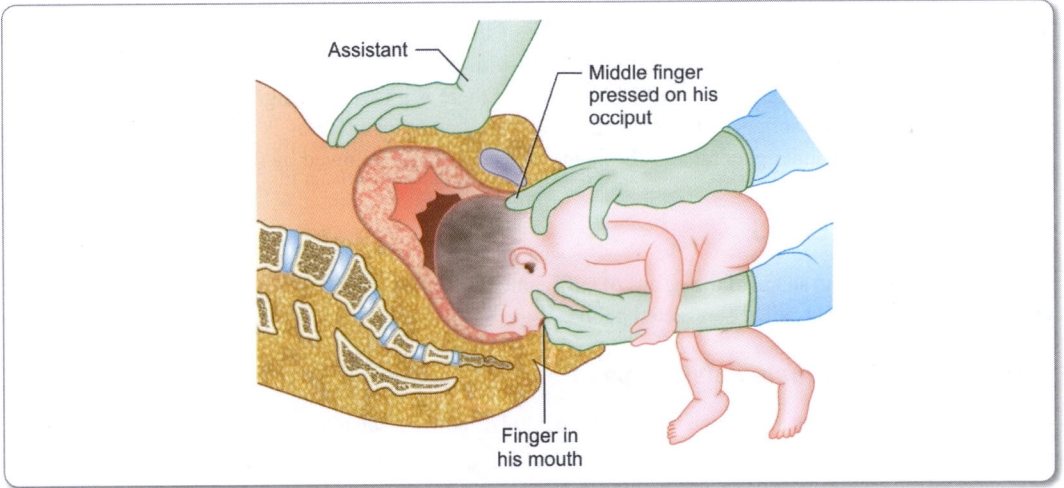

**Fig. 14:** Mauriceau-Smellie-Veit maneuver

### Delivery of the Placenta

The placenta is usually expelled out soon after delivery of the head.

### Care of the Newborn

The baby may be asphyxiated in breech delivery and need to be resuscitated. Otherwise care of newborn is same as that of vertex presentation.
(**Note:** Essential care of newborn already discussed in the Chapter 6: Management of a Newborn)

## Compound Presentation

Presence of a hand or foot or both alongside the head or both hands by the side of the breech is called compound presentation (Fig. 15).

- The most common compound presentation is head with the hand.
- The rarest is the head with a hand and foot.

### *Causes*

- Prematurity
- Pelvic tumors
- Contracted pelvis
- Multiple pregnancy

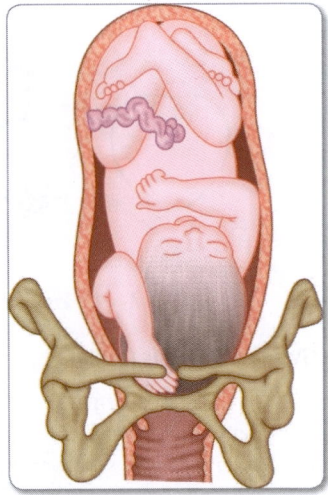

**Fig. 15:** Compound presentation

- Macerated fetus
- High head with early rupture of membranes
- Polyhydramnios

### Diagnosis

Feeling the limb alongside head when cervix is sufficiently dilated.

### Management

Management depends on the stage of labor, maturity of the fetus, number of fetuses, pelvis adequacy and associated cord prolapse. In cases of single, live fetus with contracted pelvis or cord prolapse, delivery by cesarean section is the choice. In uncomplicated cases, if there is a favorable sign of elevation of prolapsed limb during uterine contraction in the first stage and the condition of fetus is good, replacement of the prolapsed limb is done under general anesthesia in the second stage followed by forceps delivery.

## CONTRACTED PELVIS

Alteration in the size and shape of the pelvis of sufficient degree so as to alter the normal mechanism of labor in an average size baby is called contracted pelvis.

### Classification of Female Pelvic Types

Four types of female pelvis are shown in Figures 16A to D. Actually, the majority of pelvis is of mixed types. They are as follows:

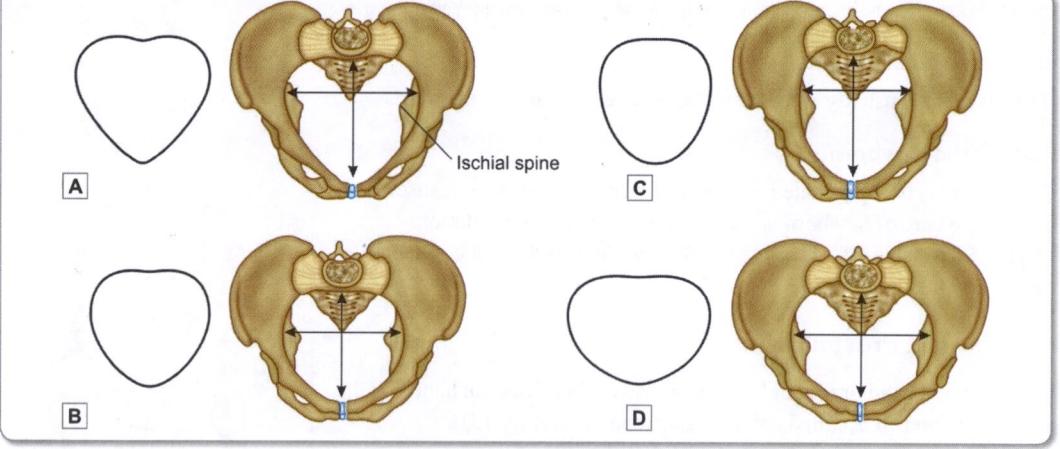

Figs 16A to D: Types of female pelvises. **A.** Android; **B.** Gynecoid; **C.** Anthropoid; **D.** Platypelloid

### Gynecoid Pelvis (50%)

- It is the normal female type.
- Inlet is slightly transverse oval.
- Sacrum is wide with average concavity and inclination.
- Side walls are straight with blunt ischial spines.

- Sacrosciatic notch is wide.
- Subpubic angle is 90°–100°.

### Anthropoid Pelvis (25%)

- It is ape-like type.
- All anteroposterior diameters are long.
- All transverse diameters are short.
- Sacrum is long and narrow.
- Sacrosciatic notch is wide.
- Subpubic angle is narrow.

### Android Pelvis (20%)

- It is a male type.
- Inlet is triangular or heart-shaped with anterior narrow apex.
- Side walls are converging (funnel pelvis) with projecting ischial spines.
- Sacrosciatic notch is narrow.
- Subpubic angle is narrow; <90°.

### Platypelloid Pelvis (5%)

- It is a flat female type.
- All anteroposterior diameters are short.
- All transverse diameters are long.
- Sacrosciatic notch is narrow.
- Subpubic angle is wide.

Figures 17A to F show the various causes of asymmetrical pelvises.

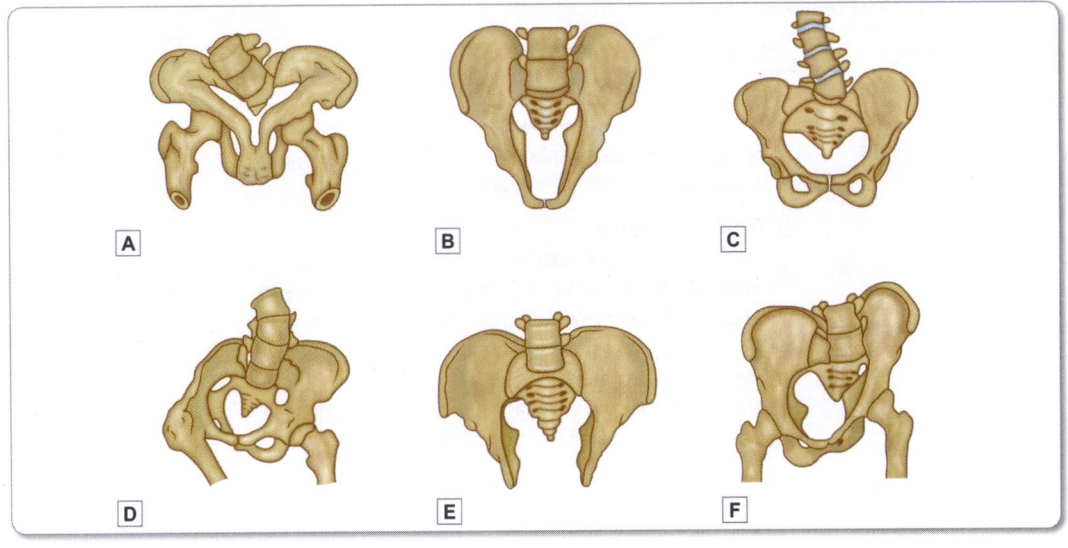

**Figs 17A to F:** Asymmetrical pelvises. **A.** Osteomalacic pelvis; **B.** Robert's pelvis; **C.** Scoliotic pelvis; **D.** Coxalgic pelvis; **E.** Split pelvis, **F.** Naegele's pelvis

## Causes of Contracted Pelvis

- **Nutritional and environmental defects:**
  - Deficiency of vitamin D during early childhood causes rickets, due to which bones become soft and unossified.
  - Deficiency of calcium and vitamin D can cause osteomalacic pelvis.
- **Diseases or injuries to pelvic bones:**
  - **Diseases:** Tumor, tubercular arthritis, poliomyelitis, scoliosis, spondylosis, kyphosis.
  - **Injury:** Fractures.
- **Developmental defect:** Naegele's pelvis, Robert pelvis, high or low assimilation pelvis
  - **Naegele's pelvis:** It is produced due to arrested development of one ala of the sacrum
  - **Robert's pelvis:** Ala of both the sides are absent and the sacrum is fused with the innominate bone.

## Signs and Symptoms

- Arresting of the head in the pelvic inlet
- Uterine contractions abnormality
- Positive **Vasten sign** (It means disproportion between fetal head and symphysis pubis is prominent)
- Signs of urinary bladder compression
- Edema of the cervix, and vaginal walls, production of fistula
- Danger of uterine rupture—over distension of lower uterine segment
- Pushing occurs in location of fetal head in inlet

## Diagnosis

Table 4 shows the diagnosis of contracted pelvis.

**TABLE 4: Diagnosis of contracted pelvis**

| Method/Technique | Diagnosis |
| --- | --- |
| History | **Rickets:** A history of delayed walking and dentition<br>**Trauma or disease:** Of the pelvis, spine or lower limbs<br>**Bad obstetric history:** For example, prolonged labor ended by: Difficult forceps and cesarean section |
| Examination | **General examination:**<br>• **Gait:** Abnormal gait suggesting abnormalities in the pelvis, spines of lower limbs<br>• **Stature:** Women with less than 150 cm height usually have contracted pelvis<br>• Spines and lower limbs may have a disease or lesion<br>• Manifestations of rickets as: Square head, pigeon chest and Bow legs<br>**Abdominal examination:**<br>• Nonengagement of the head: In the last 3–4 weeks in primigravida<br>• Malpresentations are more common |
| Investigations | **Pelvimetry:** Assessment of the pelvic diameters<br>**Imaging:** X-ray, CT scan, MRI |

## Effects of Contracted Pelvis on Pregnancy/Labor

Figure 18 shows the effects of contracted pelvis on pregnancy or labor.

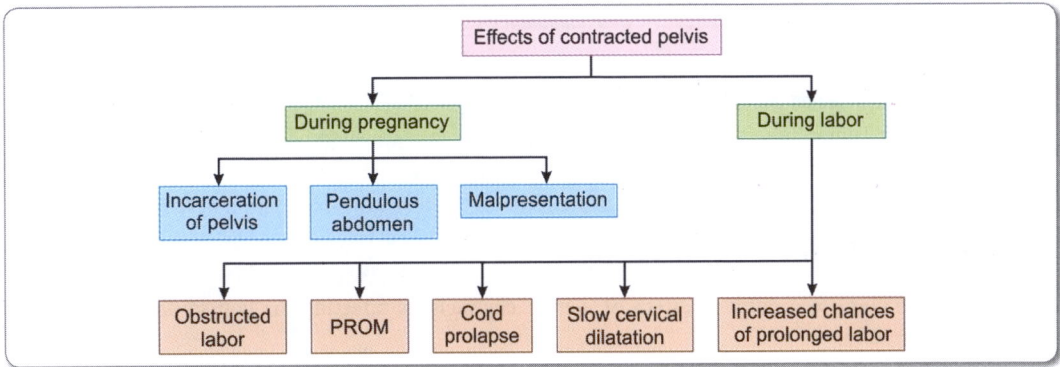

**Fig. 18:** Effects of contracted pelvis on pregnancy or labor

## Effects of Contracted Pelvis on Mother and Fetus

Figure 19 displays the effects of contracted pelvis on mother and fetus.

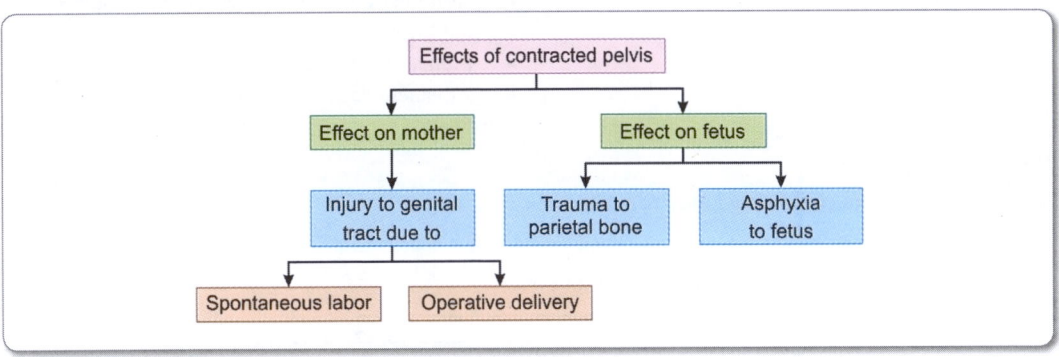

**Fig. 19:** Effects of contracted pelvis on mother and fetus

## Management of Contracted Pelvis

- Assess the degree of disproportion by clinical examination and supplemented by imaging pelvimetry.
- Minor degree of inlet contraction does not give rise to much problem and the cases are left to have a spontaneous vaginal delivery at term.
- The moderate and the severe degrees are to be dealt by any one of the following methods:
  - Induction of labor prior to estimated date of delivery (EDD) (especially 2–3 weeks)
  - Cesarean section:
    - **Elective cesarean section at term:** For major conjugate vera (CV <8 cm), major disproportion.
    - **Emergency cesarean section:** When trial labor has failed.
  - Trial labor (Fig. 20):
    **Indication:** Moderate contraction (CVS = 9 cm) with average sized baby (i.e. 1° inlet disproportion)

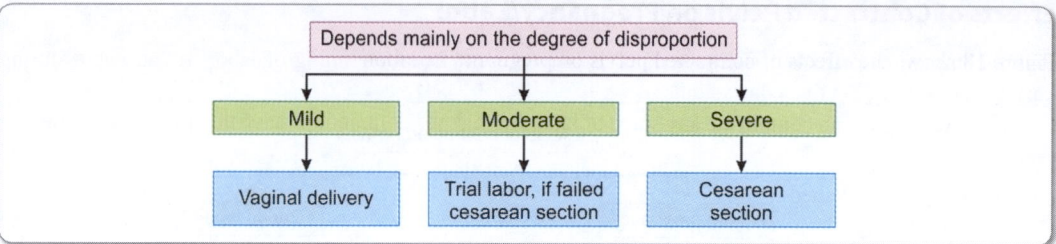

**Fig. 20:** Trial labor

## ABNORMAL UTERINE ACTION

**Definition:** Deviation from normal pattern of uterine contractions affecting the course of labor is called abnormal uterine action.

### Etiology of Abnormal Uterine Action

The exact cause of abnormal uterine action remains unknown but the following conditions are thought to be associated with this:

- Prolonged pregnancy
- Twin pregnancy
- Polyhydramnios
- Contracted pelvis
- Malpresentation

- Psychological factors
- Administration of drug: Sedatives, analgesics or oxytocics
- Premature attempt for delivery
- Advancing age of mother

### Types

Figure 21 shows types of abnormal uterine action.

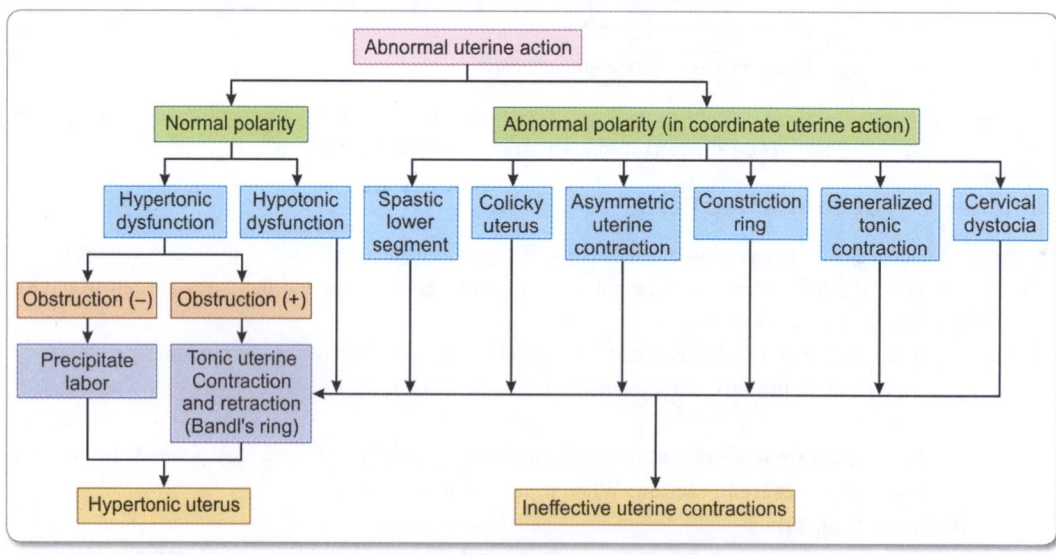

**Fig. 21:** Types of abnormal uterine action

# Hypotonic Uterine Dysfunction (Uterine Inertia)

It is a common disorder but is less serious. It may present from beginning of labor. It can occur during variable period of effective contractions.

Uterine inertia can complicate any stage of labor. In this, the contractions have the following distinctive features:

- **Intensity:** Diminished
- **Duration:** Short
- **Interval between contractions:** Increased relaxation between contractions
- **Intrauterine pressure during contractions:** Less and hourly rises to 25 mm Hg.

## Clinical Manifestations

- Less pain during contractions
- Less hardening of uterus
- Uterine wall indentable at the arrival of pain
- Poor dilatation of cervix

## Diagnosis

It is made from the clinical picture and associated presence of certain factors such as:

- Contracted pelvis
- Malposition
- Deflexed head
- Malpresentation

## Effects on Mother and Fetus

- On mother : Maternal exhaustion
- On fetus : Fetal distress

## Management

- Provide left lateral position to mother and avoid supine position
- Catheterize the patient
- Start intravenous fluid to maintain hydration
- Provide pain relief by IM pethidine 100 mg
- Accelerate uterine contractions by artificial rupture of membrane and start oxytocin drip
- Even on oxytocin drip, if progress in uterine contractions is not seen, then best alternative is to do cesarean section.

## Incoordinate Uterine Actions

Incoordinated uterine action means that the uterine action between upper segment and lower segment of uterus is not coordinated (Fig. 22).

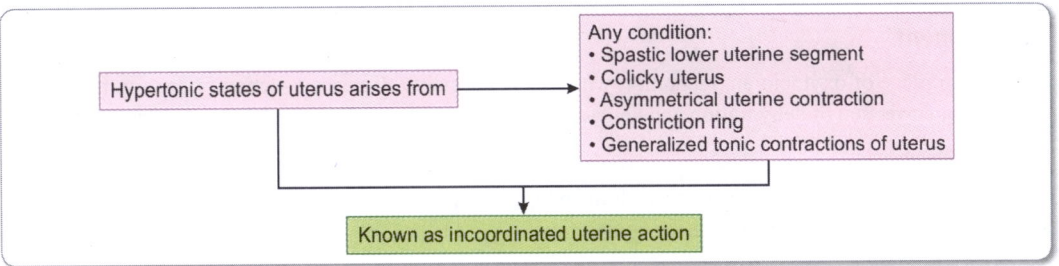

**Fig. 22:** Pathophysiology of incoordinated uterine action

### *Impact of Incoordinated Uterine Action (Fig. 23)*

Figure 23 shows the impact of incoordinated uterine action.

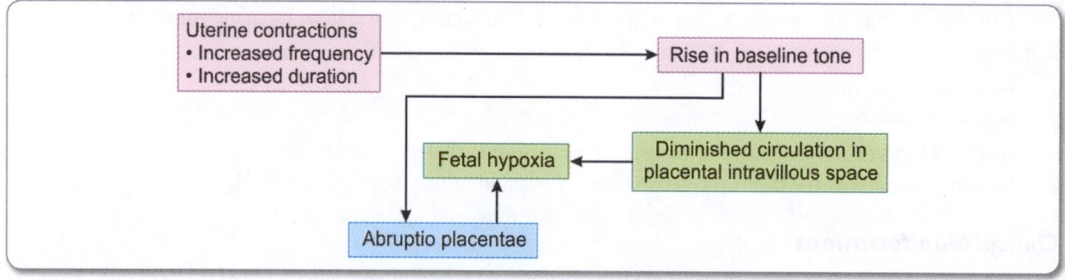

**Fig. 23:** Impact of incoordinated uterine action

## Spastic Lower Segment

It occurs when the fundal dominance is lacking, reversed polarity is there, relaxation between contractions is inadequate and basal tone is raised above 20 mm Hg.

### *Signs and Symptoms*

- Unbearable pain referred to back
- Dehydration due to exhaustion
- Distended bladder due to retention of urine
- Distended stomach and bowel
- Gentle manipulation of abdomen and excess hardening of uterus with pain which precedes and outlasts uterine contractions
- Uterus tender and tense even after passing off the contractions
- Cervix is thick and edematous and hangs like a curtain
- Varying degree of caput succedaneum
- Cervix not dilated appropriately

### *Diagnosis*

Diagnosis can be made from clinical signs and symptoms.

### *Effect on Mother and Fetus*

- **On mother:** Maternal exhaustion
- **On fetus:** Fetal distress

### *Management*

There is no place of oxytocin augmentation with this abnormality. Cesarean section is done in majority of cases. Prior correction of dehydration and ketoacidosis must be achieved by rapid infusion of ringer solution.

### Nursing Diagnosis

- Fluid deficit related to maternal exhaustion and inadequate intake
- Pain related to incoordinated uterine contractions
- Risk for injury

- Risk for infection related to retention of urine and poor septic techniques in vaginal examination
- Anxiety related to nonprogress of labor.

### Nursing Intervention

- Start IV line and correct dehydration and ketoacidosis by rapid infusion of ringer's solution
- Give drugs to relieve pain as prescribed
- Assess the maternal and fetal condition
- Avoid use of oxytocin
- Maintain records and reports
- Check fetal heart rate (FHR) and report if any change found.

## Constriction Ring

Constriction ring (Fig. 24) occurs due to localized annular spasm of uterine muscle and at junction of upper and lower uterine segment during 1st, 2nd, 3rd stage of labor.

Constriction ring is situated at the junction of upper and lower uterine segment around constricted part of fetus, i.e. neck in vertex presentation.

### Causes

Exact cause is unknown but it is associated with:
- Malpresentation
- Malposition
- Rough and repeated intrauterine manipulations
- Improper use of uterine stimulants such as oxytocics
- Premature rupture of membranes (PROM)
- Premature attempts of instrumental delivery under light anesthesia.

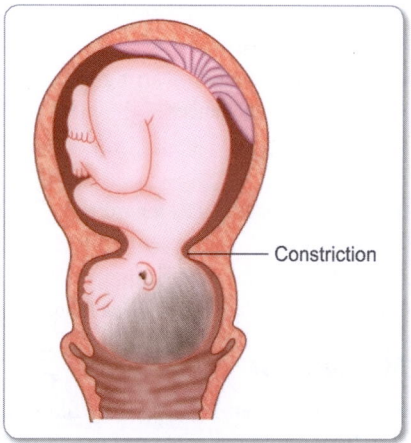

**Fig. 24:** Constricting ring

### Diagnosis

- It is revealed during cesarean section in first stage, during forceps application in the second stage and during manual removal in third stage.
- It is diagnosed by doing per vaginal examination and telling it with hand introduced inside the uterus.
- It is suspected when there is prolonged 2nd stage without any cause.
- In third stage, it may cause contraction of the uterus with retained placenta and postpartum hemorrhage (PPH).

### Management

- Assess for disproportion, malpresentation and malposition.
- Analgesics such as pethidine and antispasmodic. For example, hyoscine.
- In 2nd stage, give deep general anesthesia, a vertical incision of the lower segment is needed to cut ring.
- In 3rd stage, deep general anesthesia and amyl nitrite inhalation then remove placenta manually in cases of contraction of the uterus.

## Cervical Dystocia

Cervical dystocia is a condition in which there is difficulty in labor due to failure of cervical dilatation within a reasonable time in spite of presence of strong, regular uterine contractions, i.e. no abnormalities in the uterine expulsive power.

### Types

- **Primary dystocia:** It is commonly observed during the
  - First birth where the external OS fails to dilate
  - Rigid cervix
  - Inefficient uterine contractions
- **Secondary dystocia:** It occurs due to:
  - Excess scarring or rigidity of the cervix from previous operation or disease
  - Post delivery
  - Postoperative scarring
  - Cervical cancer

### Diagnosis

The external os is felt as a hard rim.

### Complications

Prolonged labor and obstructed labor.

### Management

- In case of cervix stenosis by fibrosis, cesarean section is the best method of delivery.
- In case of functional rigidity (i.e. in the absence of organic lesion in the cervix) → Give time to cervix to dilate with good uterine contractions.
- Analgesics: Pethidine and antispasmodics (hyoscine) may be given.
- If cervix is not fully dilated and head is not engaged, fetal distress occurs → Perform cesarean section.
- If head is sufficiently low down with only thin rim of cervix left behind, the rim may be pushed up manually during contraction or traction is given by ventouse.
- In case the cervix is very much thinned out but only half dilated, Duhrssen incision at 2 and 10'o clock position followed by forceps or ventouse extraction is quite safe and effective.

## Generalized Tonic Contraction

*(Syn: Uterine tetany)*

In this condition, pronounced retraction occurs involving whole of the uterus up to the level of internal os. Thus, there is no physiological differentiation of the active upper segment and the passive lower segment of the uterus. The whole uterus undergoes a sort of muscular spasm (tonic) holding the fetus inside uterus.

### Etiology

- Cephalopelvic disproportion (CPD)
- Obstruction in the birth canal
- Injudicious use of oxytocics

### Signs and Symptoms

- Severe and continuous pain
- Uterus tense, hard, somewhat smaller in size
- Not well-defined fetal parts
- Fetal heart sound not audible
- Jammed head observed on vaginal examination
- Caput succedaneum on fetal head
- Edematous vagina

### Treatment

- IV infusion to correct dehydration and ketoacidosis
- Antibiotics to control infection
- Analgesics to relieve pain
- If fetal distress occurs due to oxytocics, then stop oxytocin infusion
- If obstruction suspected, then cesarean section is done

## Precipitate Labor

A labor is called precipitate when the combined duration of first and second stage is less than 3 hours (Fig. 25).

In other words, precipitate labor is rapid expulsion of fetus due to combined effect of hyperactive uterine contractions associated with soft tissue resistance.

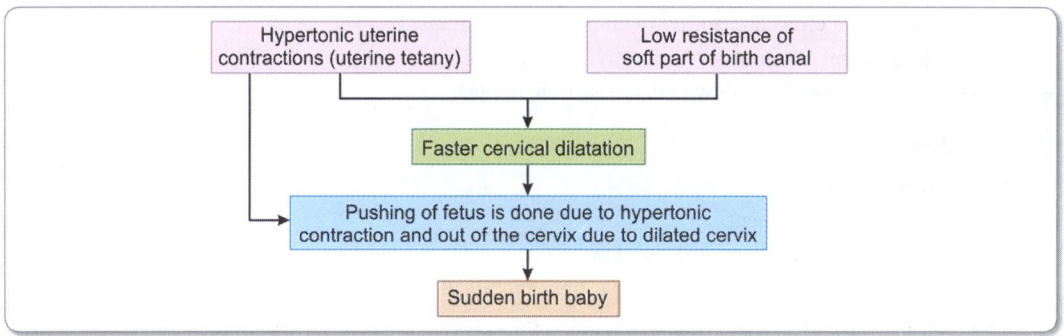

**Fig. 25:** Mechanism of precipitate labor

### Risk due to Precipitate Labor

#### Maternal Risks

- Extensive laceration of the cervix, vagina and perineum
- Postpartum hemorrhage (PPH) due to uterine hypotonia
- Inversion of uterus
- Uterine rupture
- Infection
- Amniotic fluid embolism

#### Fetal Risk

- Fetal hypoxia
- Intracranial hemorrhage

- Bleeding from torn cord
- Direct trauma to fetal skull

## Signs and Symptoms

- Intense pain more than normal
- Anxiety
- Restlessness
- Diaphoresis
- Increased heart rate, pulse and temperature
- Increased blood pressure
- Nasal flaring

## Management

- Management of precipitate labor largely depends on fetal condition.
- Stop oxytocin, if infusion is running.
- Give tocolytics such as subcutaneous Terbutaline or intravenous ritodine injection.
- Deliver the baby by instrument or cesarean, if severe hypoxia present.
- Perform vaginal examination prior to cesarean as cervix may dilate rapidly during time taken in transfer to theater.
- Assess for abruptio placenta as frequent uterine contractions can cause antepartum hemorrhage (APH).
- Assess the client's effect and ability to understand directions.
- Stay with the client all times.
- Advise woman to pant and blow to decrease urge to push.

### During Labor

- Don't prevent the birth of baby.
- Maintain sterile environment.
- Check for Nuchal cord, slip over-head if possible.
- Check around infant's neck for a possible tight umbilical cord and if present, clamp and cut it before delivery.
- Support perineum with a sterile towel as crowning occurs.
- Use gentle aspiration with bulb syringe to remove blood and mucus from nose and mouth.
- Hold baby in a head down position to facilitate drainage of secretions.
- Monitor for excessive bleeding.

### Surgical Management

Surgical management is done by episiotomy. An episiotomy is a surgical incision made in the perineum, the area between the vagina and anus. Episiotomies are done during the second stage of labor to expand the opening of the vagina to prevent tearing of the area during the delivery of the baby.

Episiotomy is usually done during the birthing process in order to deliver a baby without tearing the perineum and surrounding tissue. Reasons for an episiotomy include:

- Evidence of maternal or fetal distress
- Premature baby

- Malpresentation
- Large size baby
- Forceps delivery
- Mother becomes exhausted
- Less bearing down efforts
- Existing perineal trauma

## Procedure

During childbirth, the area called the perineum is often cut to facilitate delivery. First, a local anesthetic may be given. The perineum is cut on an angle with scissors. After delivery, the layers of muscle and skin are repaired (Figs 26A to C).

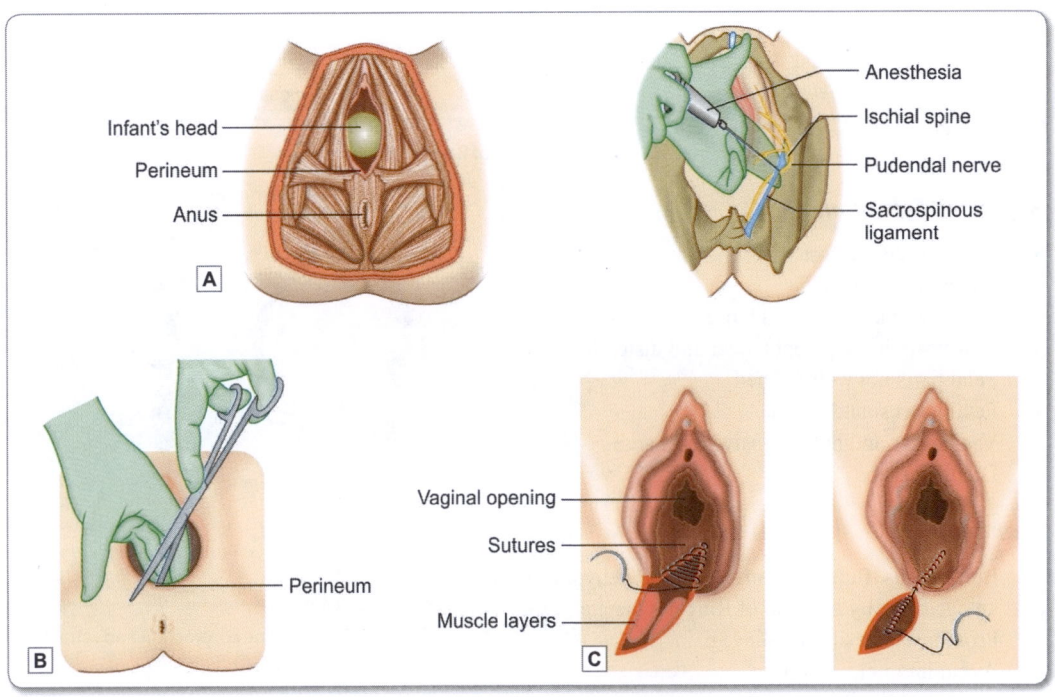

**Figs 26A to C:** Episiotomy procedure

## Nursing Management

A nurse assesses the mother and fetal conditions and manages the case in coordination with health team.

## Tonic Uterine Contraction and Retraction

*(Syn: Bandl's ring, Pathological Retraction ring)*
Tonic uterine contraction and retraction occur due to obstructed labors.
Figure 27 shows the mechanism of Bandl's ring. Tonic uterine contraction and retraction are exhibited in Figure 28.

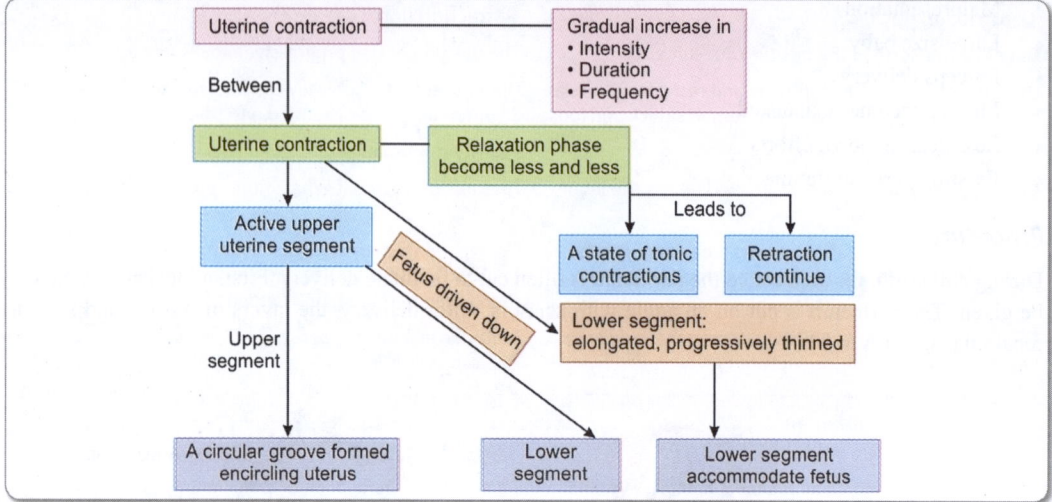

**Fig. 27:** Mechanism of Bandl's ring

## Signs and Symptoms

- Pain and discomfort
- Maternal exhaustion
- Upper segment hard and tense
- Lower uterine segment tender and distended
- Fetal parts not well defined
- Fetal heart sound absent
- Vagina-dry and hot, offensive discharge
- Dilated cervix

## Management

- Intravenous fluid for correction of dehydration and ketoacidosis by infusion of Ringer's lactate (RL).
- Provide analgesics to relieve pain.
- Avoid internal version.
- Provide antibiotics and prepare women for cesarean section.
- Exclude rupture of uterus before attempting destructive operation.

**Fig. 28:** Tonic uterine contraction and retraction

## Differences between Constriction Ring and Retraction Ring

Table 5 displays the differences between constriction and retraction ring

**TABLE 5:** Differences between constriction and retraction ring

| Constriction ring | Retraction ring |
|---|---|
| It is a manifestation of incoordinated uterine contraction | It is the end result of tonic uterine contraction and retraction |
| It occurs due to irritability of uterus | It occurs following obstructed labor |
| It is usually present at the junction of upper and lower segment but may occur in other places | Always situated at the junction of upper and lower segment |

*Contd...*

| Constriction ring | Retraction ring |
|---|---|
| Once the ring formed the position doesn't alter | The position of ring progressive moves upwards |
| Uterine upper segment contracts and retracts with relaxation in between; lower segment remains thick and loose | Upper segment is tonically contracted with no relaxation. Segment becomes distended and thinned out |
| Uterine polarity is abnormal | Polarity is normal |
| Maternal condition almost unaffected unless the labor is prolonged | Features of maternal exhaustion, sepsis appear early |
| On abdominal examination, uterus feels normal, fetal parts felt, Ring not felt, fetal heart sound (FHS) present. | On abdominal examination, uterus feels tense and tender, fetal parts not felt, ring felt as a groove placed obliquely, round ligaments are taut and tender, FHS absent |
| End Result: Maternal exhaustion and fetal anoxia appear late. No chance of uterine rupture | Maternal exhaustion, sepsis, fetal anoxia appear early, Rupture uterus in multigravida is common |
| Management: Relax the ring followed by delivery of the baby or to cut the ring during cesarean section | Cesarean delivery after excluding rupture uterus |

## Nursing Management of Abnormal Uterine Actions

Table 6 elaborates on the various steps of nursing management.

**TABLE 6: Steps of nursing management**

| Nursing interventions | Rationale |
|---|---|
| Review the history of labor, onset, and duration. | Helpful in identifying possible causes, needed diagnostic studies, and appropriate interventions. Uterine dysfunction may be caused by an atonic or a hypertonic state. Uterine atony is classified as primary when it occurs before the onset of labor (latent phase) or secondary when it occurs after well-established labor (active phase). |
| Note timing/type of medication(s). Avoid administration of narcotics or of epidural block anesthetics until the cervix is 4 cm dilated. | A hypertonic contractile pattern may occur in response to oxytocin stimulation; sedation/analgesia given too early (or in excess of needs) can inhibit or arrest labor. |
| Assess uterine contractile pattern manually (palpation) or electronically via external, or internal monitor with internal uterine pressure catheter (IUPC). | Dysfunctional contractions lengthen labor increasing the risk of maternal/fetal complications. A hypotonic pattern is reflected by frequent, mild contractions measuring less than 30 mm Hg via IUPC or "soft as chin" per palpation. A hypertonic pattern is reflected by increased frequency, an elevated resting tone per palpation or greater than 15 mm Hg via IUPC, and possibly decreased intensity of contractions. Note: Intensity of contractions cannot be measured by an external monitor. |
| Note the condition of cervix. Monitor for signs of amnionitis. Note elevated temperature or white blood cell count; odor and color of vaginal discharge. | A rigid or unripe cervix will not dilate, impending fetal descent/labor progresses. Development of amnionitis is directly related to length of labor, so that delivery should occur within 24 hours after rupture of membranes. |
| Evaluate the current level of fatigue, as well as activity and rest prior to onset of labor. | Excess maternal exhaustion contributes to secondary dysfunction, or may be the result of prolonged labor/false labor. |
| Note effacement, fetal station, and fetal presentation. | These indicators of labor progress may identify a contributing cause of prolonged labor. For example, breech presentation is not as effective a wedge for cervical dilation as in vertex presentation. |

*Contd...*

| Nursing interventions | Rationale |
| --- | --- |
| Evaluate degree of hydration. Note amount and type of intake. | Prolonged labor can result in a fluid-electrolyte imbalance as well as depletion of glucose reserves, resulting in exhaustion and prolonged labor with increased risk of uterine infection, postpartal hemorrhage, or precipitous delivery in the presence of hypertonic labor. |
| Graph cervical dilation and fetal descent against time (i.e., Friedman curve). | Used to record progress/prolongation of labor. |
| Review bowel habits and regularity of evacuation | Bowel fullness may hinder uterine activity and interfere with the fetal descent. |
| Encourage client to void every 1–2 hours. Assess for bladder fullness over symphysis pubis. | A full bladder may inhibit uterine activity and interfere with the fetal descent. |
| Place client in lateral recumbent position and encourage bed rest or sitting position/ ambulation, as tolerated. | Relaxation and increased uterine perfusion may correct a hypertonic pattern. Ambulation may assist gravitational forces in stimulating normal labor pattern and cervical dilation. |
| Have emergency delivery kit available. | May be needed in the event of a precipitous labor and delivery, which are associated with uterine hypertonicity. |
| Remain with the client, if possible, arrange for the presence of doula as appropriate; provide a quiet environment as indicated. | Decrease external stimuli may be important to allow sleep after administration of medication to a client in the hypertonic state. Also helpful in decreasing the level of anxiety, which can contribute to both primary and secondary uterine dysfunction. |
| Remain with the client, if possible, arrange for the presence of doula as appropriate; provide a quiet environment as indicated. | Decrease external stimuli may be important to allow sleep after administration of medication to a client in the hypertonic state. Also helpful in decreasing the level of anxiety, which can contribute to both primary and secondary uterine dysfunction. |
| Palpate the abdomen of thin client for the presence of pathological retraction ring between uterine segments. (These rings are not palpable through the vagina or through the abdomen, in the obese client). | In obstructed labor, a depressed pathological ring (Bandl's ring) may develop at the juncture of lower and upper uterine segments, indicating an impending uterine rupture. |
| Investigate reports of severe abdominal pain. Note signs of fetal distress, cessation of contractions, presence of vaginal bleeding. | May indicate developing uterine tear/acute rupture necessitating emergency surgery. Note: Hemorrhage is usually occult since it is intraperitoneal with hematomas of the broad ligament. |
| Prepare client for amniotomy, and assist with the procedure, when the cervix is 3–4 cm dilated. | Rupture of membranes relieves uterine over distension (a cause of both primary and secondary dysfunction) and allows presenting part to engage and labor to progress in the absence of cephalopelvic disproportion (CPD). Note: Active management of labor (AML) protocols may support amniotomy once presenting part is engaged to accelerate labor/help prevent dystocia. |
| Administer narcotic or sedative, such as morphine, pentobarbital (nembutal), or secobarbital (seconal), for sleep as indicated. | May help distinguish between true and false labor. With false labor, contractions cease; with true labor, a more effective pattern may happen following a rest. Morphine helps promote heavy sedation and eliminate hypertonic contractile pattern. A period of rest conserves energy and reduces utilization of glucose to relieve fatigue. |

*Contd...*

| Nursing interventions | Rationale |
|---|---|
| Use nipple stimulation to produce endogenous oxytocin or initiate infusion of exogenous oxytocin (Pitocin) or prostaglandins. | Oxytocin may be necessary to increase or institute myometrial activity for a hypotonic uterine pattern. It is usually contraindicated in hypertonic labor pattern because it can accentuate the hypertonicity, but may be tried with amniotomy if the latent phase is prolonged and if CPD and malpositions are ruled out. |
| Prepare for forceps delivery, as necessary. | Excessive maternal fatigue, resulting in ineffective bearing-down efforts in stage II labor, necessitates the use of forceps. |
| Assist with preparation for cesarean delivery, as indicated, e.g., malposition, CPD, or Bandl's ring. | Immediate cesarean birth is indicated for Bandl's ring or fetal distress due to CPD. Note: Once labor is diagnosed, if delivery has not occurred within 12 hours and amniotomy and oxytocin have been used appropriately, then a cesarean delivery is recommended by some protocols. |

## OBSTRUCTED LABOR

Labor is said to be obstructed when there is absence of progress of labor in spite of strong uterine contractions (Fig. 29). Absence of progress can be due to:

- Failure of the cervix to dilate.
- Failure of the presenting part of fetus to descent the birth canal.
- Fault in passage of baby, i.e. contracted pelvis.

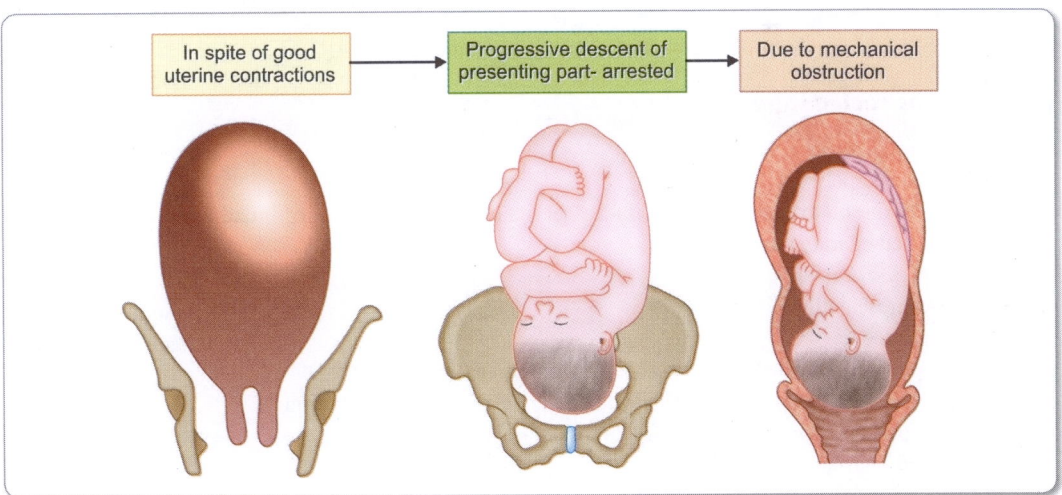

**Fig. 29:** Mechanism of obstructed labor

## Incidence

It is about 1–2% in the developing countries.

## Physiology of Obstructed Labor

Figure 30 shows the physiology of obstructed labor.

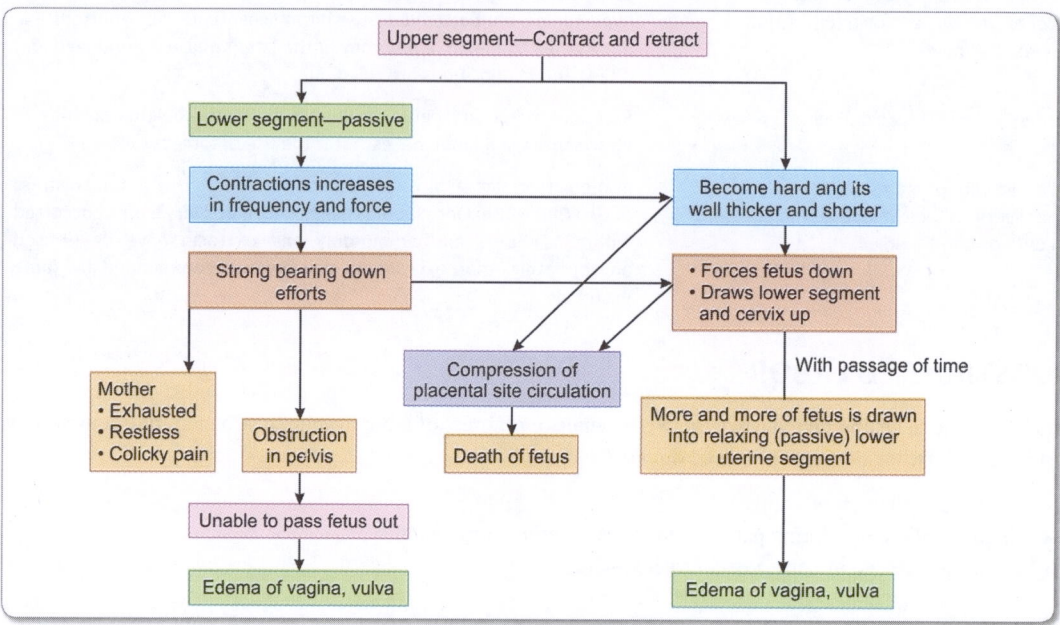

**Fig. 30:** Physiology of obstructed labor

## *Causes of Obstructed Labor*

- *Fault in the passage:*
  - Contracted pelvis (CPD common)
  - **Soft tissue obstruction:** This includes cervical dystocia, cervical or broad ligament fibroid, and impacted ovarian tumor.
- *Fault in the passenger:*
  - Brow presentation
  - Transverse lie
  - Congenital malformation as hydrocephalus, fetal ascites, etc.
  - Big baby associated with deflexed head and occipitoposterior position
  - Compound presentation
  - Locked twins (Figs 31A and B)

## Signs and Symptoms

- Patient becomes exhausted due to pain and uterine contractions
- Temperature may rise
- Upper part of uterus is hard
- Lower segment of uterus is tender and distended
- Presence of retraction ring
- Over thickening of upper part and over thinning of lower part of uterus
- Increased pulse rate
- Birth canal hot and dry
- Vulva edematous
- Large caput on fetal head

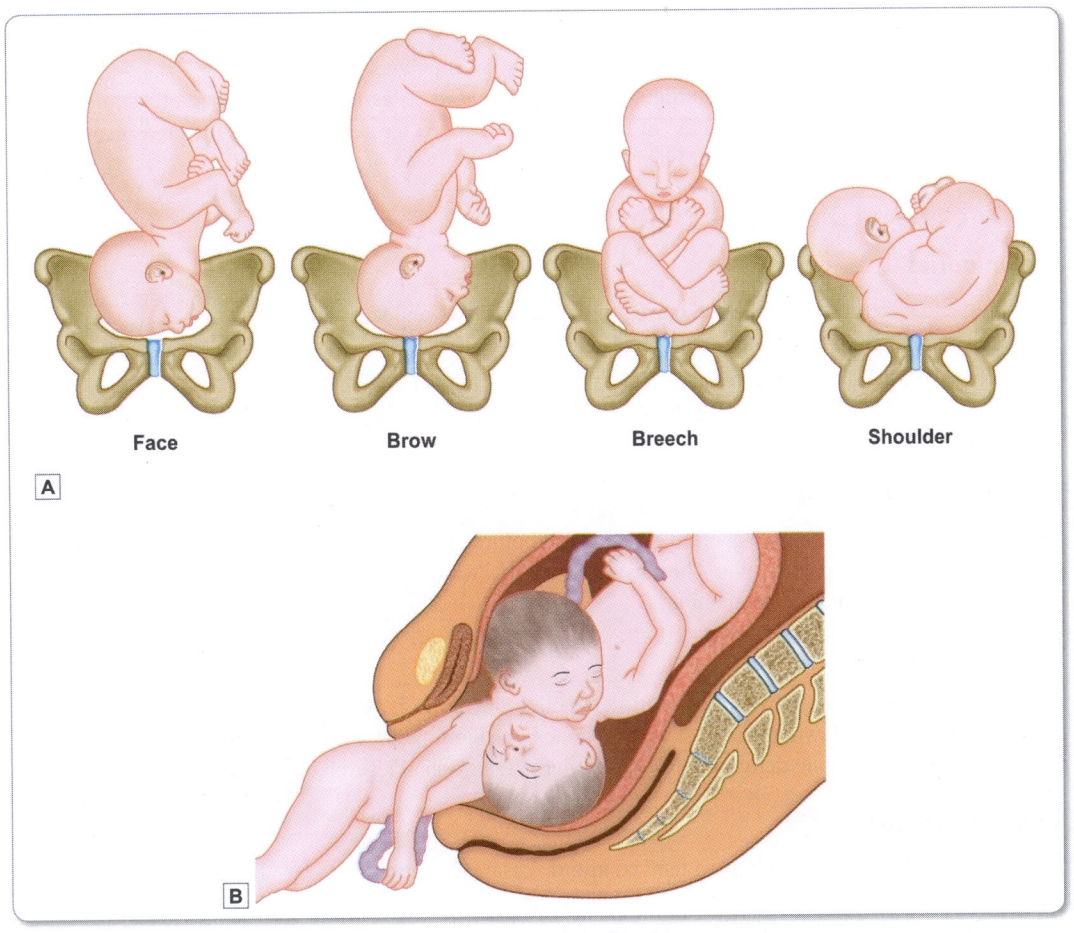

Face Brow Breech Shoulder

**Figs 31A and B:** Causes of obstructed labor. **A.** Abnormal presentations and **B.** Locked twins

## Complications

| Maternal complications | Fetal complications |
|---|---|
| • Immediate<br>• Remote<br>**Immediate maternal complications**<br>• Maternal exhaustion due to pain and anxiety<br>• Dehydration<br>• Metabolic acidosis<br>• Genital sepsis<br>• Injury to the genital tract (e.g., Rupture of uterus)<br>• PPH and shock<br>• Maternal death<br>**Maternal remote complications**<br>• Rectovaginal fistula (RVF) and vesicovaginal fistula (VVF)<br>• Vaginal atresia<br>• Secondary amenorrhea | • Asphyxia<br>• Acidosis<br>• Intracranial hemorrhage<br>• Infection<br>• Increased perinatal loss |

## Prevention of Effects of Obstructed Labor

- Identifying factors such as CPD, large size baby, tumor of pelvis, etc.
- During intranatal period, use partograph to keep a record so as to have vigilance of factors causing obstructed labor. Failure of progress of labor in spite of good uterine contractions for a reasonable period is an impending sign of obstructed labor.

## Management of Obstructed Labor

### Preliminaries

- Fluid and electrolyte balance and correction of dehydration and ketoacidosis
- High vaginal swab (HVS) for culture and sensitivity
- Blood sample for grouping and cross matching
- Antibiotic: Ceftriaxone 1 g I/V is administered
- IV infusion, Metronidazole is given for anaerobic infection.

### Obstetric Management

Before proceeding for definitive operative treatment, rupture of uterus must be excluded. A balanced decision is taken to relieve the obstruction. There is no place of "wait and watch", neither is any scope of using oxytocin to stimulate uterine contraction.

### Vaginal Delivery

In most of the cases, the baby is dead and destructive operation is best to relieve obstruction. If baby is alive, and head is low down, delivery should be done by using forceps. Internal version is contraindicated in obstructed labor. Following delivery, explore the uterovaginal canal to exclude uterine tear or rupture.

### Cesarean Section

If the case is detected early with good fetal condition, cesarean section gives best results.

# PREMATURE RUPTURE OF MEMBRANES

*(Syn: Prelabor rupture of membrane [PROM])*
Spontaneous rupture of the membranes any time beyond 28 weeks of pregnancy but before the onset-of labor is called premature rupture of membrane (PROM)

- When the membranes rupture beyond 37 weeks but before the onset of labor, it is called PROM.
- When it occurs before 37th completed weeks, it is called preterm PROM.
- Rupture of membranes for >24 hours before delivery is called prolonged rupture of membranes.

## Incidence

PROM occurs in approximately 10% of all pregnancies.

## Causes

In majority, the causes are not known. Possible causes are:
- Increased friability of membranes
- Decreased tensile strength of membranes

- Polyhydramnios
- Cervical Incompetence
- Multiple pregnancies
- Infection such as chorioamnionitis, urinary tract infection (UTI) and lower genital tract infection
- Certain congenital anomaly in the fetus

## Signs and Symptoms

Main symptom in case of PROM is the escape of watery discharge per vagina either in the form of gush or slow leak.

## Diagnosis

- Speculum examination: To inspect the liquor escaping out through the cervix
- Examination of the fluid collected from the posterior fornix for:
    - Detection of pH by litmus or nitrazine paper. The pH becomes 6–6.2 (normal pH during pregnancy is 4.5–5.5, whereas that of liquor amnii is 7–7.5).
    - **Fern test:** To note the characteristic ferning pattern when a smeared slide is examined under microscope.

## Complications

- Preterm labor or delivery (80–90%)
- Chorioamnionitis
- Cord prolapse
- Dry labor because of continuous escape of liquor
- Placental abruption
- Fetal pulmonary hypoplasia (Necrotizing enterocolitis)
- Neonatal sepsis, respiratory distress syndrome (RDS), intraventricular hemorrhage (IVH) and necrotizing enterocolitis (NEC) in preterm PROM
- Perinatal morbidity
- Retained placenta
- Endometritis
- Maternal sepsis and death

## Management

- Admit the mother to the hospital.
- Careful history collection.
- Sterile speculum examination is done to note the escape of liquor, state of cervix, to detect any cord prolapse.
- Patient is put to bed rest and sterile vulval pad is applied to look for leakage.
- Vaginal digital examination should be avoided because of risk of infection.
- Frequent checking of fetal heart rate to assess fetal condition.
- Check maternal pulse, temperature, uterine tenderness and vaginal discharge.

Once the diagnosis is made, management depends on:

- Gestational age of the fetus.
- Whether the woman is in labor or not.

- Any evidence of sepsis.
- Prospect of fetal survival if delivery occurs.

### Term PROM

Figure 32 shows the management system in case of term PROM, while Figure 33 displays the management system in the case of preterm PROM.

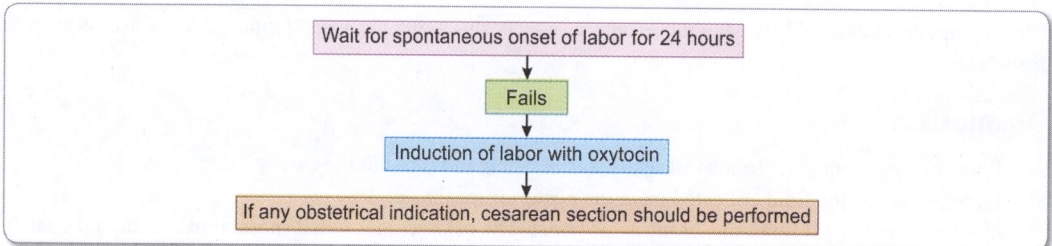

**Fig. 32:** Management in case of term PROM

### Preterm PROM

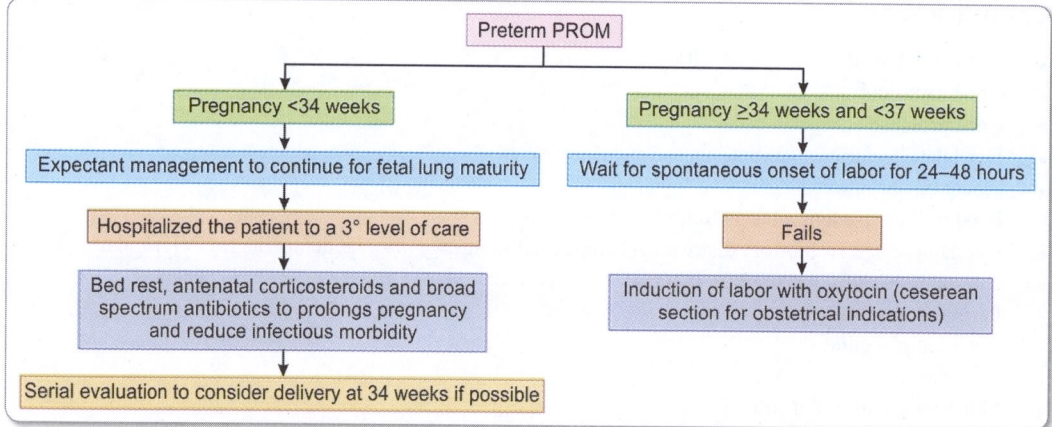

**Fig. 33:** Management in case of preterm PROM

### Nurse's Responsibility

- **Prevent infection and other potential complications:**
  - Make an early and accurate evaluation of membrane status, using sterile speculum examination and determination of ferning. Thereafter, keep vaginal examinations to a minimum to prevent infection.
  - Obtain smear specimens from vagina and rectum as prescribed to test for beta hemolytic streptococci, an organism that increases the risk to the fetus.
  - Determine maternal and fetal status, including estimated gestational age. Continually assess for signs of infection.
  - Maintain the client on bed rest if the fetal head is not engaged. This method may prevent cord prolapse if additional rupture and loss of fluid occur. Once the fetal head is engaged, ambulation can be encouraged.

- **Provide client and family education:**
  - Inform the client, if the fetus is at term, that the chances of spontaneous labor beginning are excellent; encourage the client and partner to prepare themselves for labor and birth.
  - If labor does not begin or the fetus is judged to be preterm or at risk for infection, explain treatments that are likely to be needed.

# PROLONGED LABOR

**Definition:** When the combined duration of first and second stage is more than the arbitrary time limit of 18 hours, the labor is said to be prolonged labor.

According to World Health Organization (WHO), labor is considered prolonged when for a period of 4 hours, observation shows:

- Cervical dilatation less than 1 cm/hr
- Descent of presenting part <1 cm/hr

## Causes of Prolonged Labor

- **First stage:** Failure to dilate the cervix:
  - **Fault in power** includes abnormal uterine contraction such as uterine inertia or uncoordinated uterine action
  - **Fault in the passage** includes contracted pelvis, cervical dystocia, pelvic tumor or even full bladder
  - **Fault in the passenger** includes malposition and malpresentation, congenital anomalies of the fetus such as hydrocephalus
  - **Others:** Injudicious early administration of sedatives and analgesics before the actual active labor begins.
- **Second stage:** Sluggish or non-descent of the presenting part due to:
  - **Fault in power:**
    - Uterine inertia
    - Inability to bear down
    - Epidural analgesia
    - Constriction ring
- **Fault in the passage:**
  - Contracted pelvis and CPD
  - Undue resistance of pelvic floor muscles due to old scarring/spasm
  - Soft tissue pelvic tumor
- **Fault in the passenger:**
  - Malposition
  - Malpresentation
  - Large size baby (more than 3.5 kg)
  - Congenital malformation of the baby

## Signs and Symptoms

- Mother looks exhausted and distressed.
- Dry mouth due to prolonged mouth breathing.
- Presence of dehydration.
- Pain more on back radiating to thighs rather than inside the abdomen.

- Initially pain may be severe, frequent and prolonged but later decrease and became very mild due to muscle fatigue.
- Uterus tender and does not feel relax fully between contractions.
- Fetal distress may be present.

## Diagnosis

Prolonged labor is a manifestation of an abnormality, the cause of which should be detected by a thorough abdominal and vaginal examination supplemented by partographic analysis of labor. Intranatal radiography is useful in determining the fetal station and position as well as pelvic shape and size.

### First Stage

If the first stage of labor lasts more than an arbitrary period of 12 hours or if the cervical dilatation arrests more than 2 hours, it is considered abnormal.

Rate of cervical dilation is sluggish to less than 1 cm/hr in nulliparous and less than 1.5 cm/hr in multipara. There may be slow descending of head (normal 1 cm/hr in primipara and less than 1.5 cm/hr in multipara).

The first stage of labor is divided into a latent and active phase. During latent phase, the uterus contracts regularly and the mother experiences discomfort and pain. The cervix effaces and dilatation occurs. The duration of latent phase varies according to each individual and with parity. The average duration of latent phase in multiparous women is 8.6 hours.

The active phase is distinguished by an increased rate of dilatation of cervix with descend of the presenting part. A prolonged active phase is caused by a combination of factors including the cervix, the uterus, the fetus and the mother's pelvis.

### Second Stage

The second stage is considered prolonged if it lasts for more than 2 hours in primigravida and 1 hour in multipara.

The diagnostic features are:
- Sluggish or non-descend of the presenting part even after full dilatation of the cervix (failure of the head to descend within 1 hour is called arrest)
- Variable degree of molding and caput formation in cephalic presentation.

## Dangers of Prolonged Labor

Figure 34 shows various sorts of dangers involved in prolonged labor

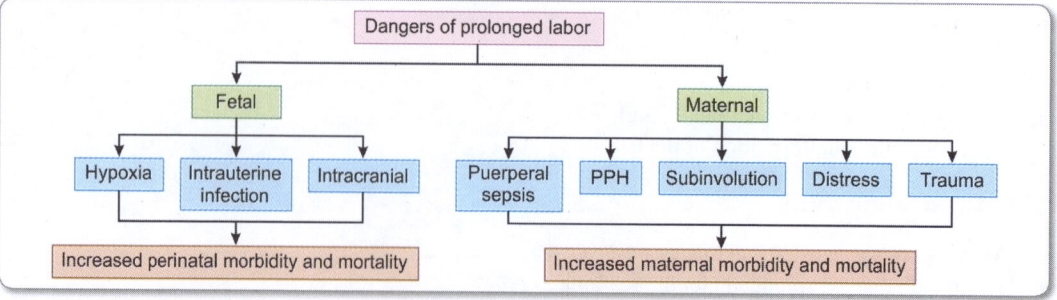

**Fig. 34:** Dangers of prolonged labor

*Abbreviation:* PPH, postpartum hemorrhage

## Prevention

- Detection of factors responsible for prolonged labor as early as possible. The factors such as good size baby, small pelvis, malpresentation and malposition, etc.
- Use partograph for early detection of prolonged labor.
- Induction of labor by low rupture of membrane followed by oxytocin drip.
- Position the woman in other than supine position to increase uterine contractions.
- Avoid dehydration by adequate fluid intake.
- Use analgesics for relieving pain.

## Management

- Early diagnosis and prompt management of prolonged labor is important.
- Careful evaluation to find out the cause of prolonged labor.
- Assess the effect of prolonged labor on mother and fetus and manage accordingly.

**In case of first stage delay:** Vaginal examination should be performed to note fetal presentation, position and station. If uterine activity is suboptimal.

- Amniotomy
- Epidural analgesia or IM Pethidine to relieve pain for management of secondary arrest, especially is multipara, administration of oxytocin very safely
- In case of malposition, malpresentation and CPD - cesarean section is to be done.

**Second stage delay:** Short period of expectant management is reasonably provided if the FHR is reassuring and vaginal delivery is imminent. Otherwise, forceps, ventouse or cesarean is to be done.

### Nursing Management of Prolonged Labor

| Nursing interventions | Rationale |
|---|---|
| Review the history of labor, onset, and duration. Note timing/type of medication(s). Avoid administration of narcotics or of epidural block anesthetics until the cervix is 4 cm dilated. | Helpful in identifying possible causes, needed diagnostic studies, and appropriate interventions. A hypertonic contractile pattern may occur in response to oxytocin stimulation; sedation/analgesia given too early (or in excess of needs) can inhibit or arrest labor. |
| Note the condition of cervix. Monitor for signs of amnionitis. Note elevated temperature or WBC; odor and color of vaginal discharge. | A rigid or unripe cervix will not dilate, impending fetal descent/labor progress. Development of amnionitis is directly related to length of labor, so that delivery should occur within 24 hours after rupture of membranes. |
| Assess uterine contractile pattern manually (palpation) or electronically via external, or internal monitor with internal uterine pressure catheter (IUPC). | Dysfunctional contractions lengthen labor increasing the risk of maternal/fetal complications. A hypotonic pattern is reflected by frequent, mild contractions measuring less than 30 mm Hg via IUPC or "soft as chin" per palpation. |
| Evaluate the current level of fatigue, as well as activity and rest prior to onset of labor. Note effacement, fetal station, and fetal presentation. | Excess maternal exhaustion contributes to secondary dysfunction, or may be the result of prolonged labor/false labor. These indicators of labor progress may identify a contributing cause of prolonged labor. For example, breech presentation is not as effective a wedge for cervical dilation as is vertex presentation. |

*Contd…*

| Nursing interventions | Rationale |
|---|---|
| Evaluate degree of hydration. Note amount and type of intake. | Prolonged labor can result in a fluid-electrolyte imbalance as well as depletion of glucose reserves, resulting in exhaustion and prolonged labor with increased risk of uterine infection, postpartal hemorrhage, or precipitous delivery in the presence of hypertonic labor. |
| Review bowel habits and regularity of evacuation. Encourage client to void every 1–2 hours. Assess for bladder fullness over symphysis pubis. Place client in lateral recumbent position and encourage bed rest or sitting position/ ambulation, as tolerated. | Bowel fullness may hinder uterine activity and interfere with the fetal descent. A full bladder may inhibit uterine activity and interfere with the fetal descent. Relaxation and increased uterine perfusion may correct a hypertonic pattern. Ambulation may assist gravitational forces in stimulating normal labor pattern and cervical dilation. |
| Assist with preparation for cesarean delivery, as indicated, e.g., malposition, cephalopelvic disproportion (CPD), or Bandl's ring. | Immediate cesarean birth is indicated for Bandl's ring or fetal distress due to CPD. Note: Once labor is diagnosed, if delivery has not occurred within 12 hours, and amniotomy and oxytocin have been used appropriately, then a cesarean delivery is recommended by some protocols. |

## INDUCTION OF LABOR

*Discussed in Chapter 12: Obstetric Operations*

## OBSTETRICAL EMERGENCIES

### Cord Prolapse

There are three clinical types of abnormal descends of the umbilical cord by the side of the presenting part. All these are included under the heading cord prolapse (Figs 35A to C)

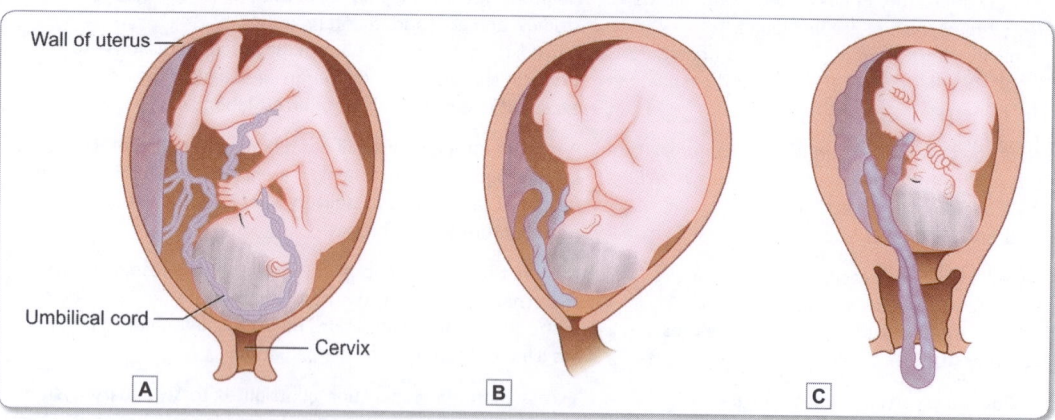

**Figs 35A to C:** Three clinical types of abnormal descends of cord

- **Occult prolapse:** The cord lies alongside, but not in front of the presenting part and is not felt by the fingers on internal examination.
- **Cord presentation:** The cord is slipped down below the presenting part and lies in front of it in the intact bag of membranes.

- **Cord prolapse:** The cord lies in front of the presenting part inside the vagina or outside the vulva following rupture of the membranes.

## Incidence

Cord prolapse is about 1 in 300 deliveries; mostly occurs in parous women.

## Causes

- Malpresentation
- Prematurity
- Multiple pregnancy
- Contracted pelvis
- Hydramnios
- High head
- Multiparity
- Placental factor, e.g., placenta previa
- Iatrogenic, e.g., low rupture of membranes, version.

## Diagnosis

- **Occult prolapse:** It is difficult to diagnose. The possibility should be suspected if there is:
  - Persistence of variable deceleration of fetal heart rate (FHR). Pattern detected on continuous fetal monitoring in an otherwise normal delivery.
  - Persistent fetal souffle with irregular fetal sound.
- **Cord presentation:** To diagnose cord presentation, feeling of pulsation of the cord through the intact membranes.
- **Cord prolapse:**
  - On vaginal examination, cord is felt below or beside the presenting part
  - In cases where the presenting part is high, cord may be felt at the cervical os
  - A loop of cord may be visible at the vulva
  - Pulsation of the cord can be felt between contractions if the fetus is alive

## Risk to Mother and Fetus

### Maternal Risks

The maternal risks are incidental due to emergency operative delivery, which involves the risk of anesthesia, blood loss and infection.

### Fetal Risks

Fetal anoxia occurs due to acute placental insufficiency or vasospasm. Danger is more in vertex presentation, especially when the prolapse is through the anterior segment of the pelvis or when the cervix is partially dilated.

## Management of Cord Presentation

The aim is to preserve the membranes and to expedite the delivery:

- Avoid unnecessary vaginal examination in order to reduce the risk of rupturing the membranes.
- Once the diagnosis is made; no attempt should be made to replace the cord.
- FHR should be auscultated as frequently as possible or obtained through continuous electronic monitoring.
- If immediate vaginal delivery is not possible or contraindicated, cesarean section is the best method of delivery.
- During the time of preparing the women for operative delivery, she is kept in exaggerated Sim's position to minimize cord compression.

## *Management of Cord Prolapse*

Figure 36 shows different positions of a mother during a cord prolapse and Figure 37 shows the management of cord prolapse

- Check whether baby is alive or dead
- Check the status of cervical dilatation.
- Assess the maturity of the baby

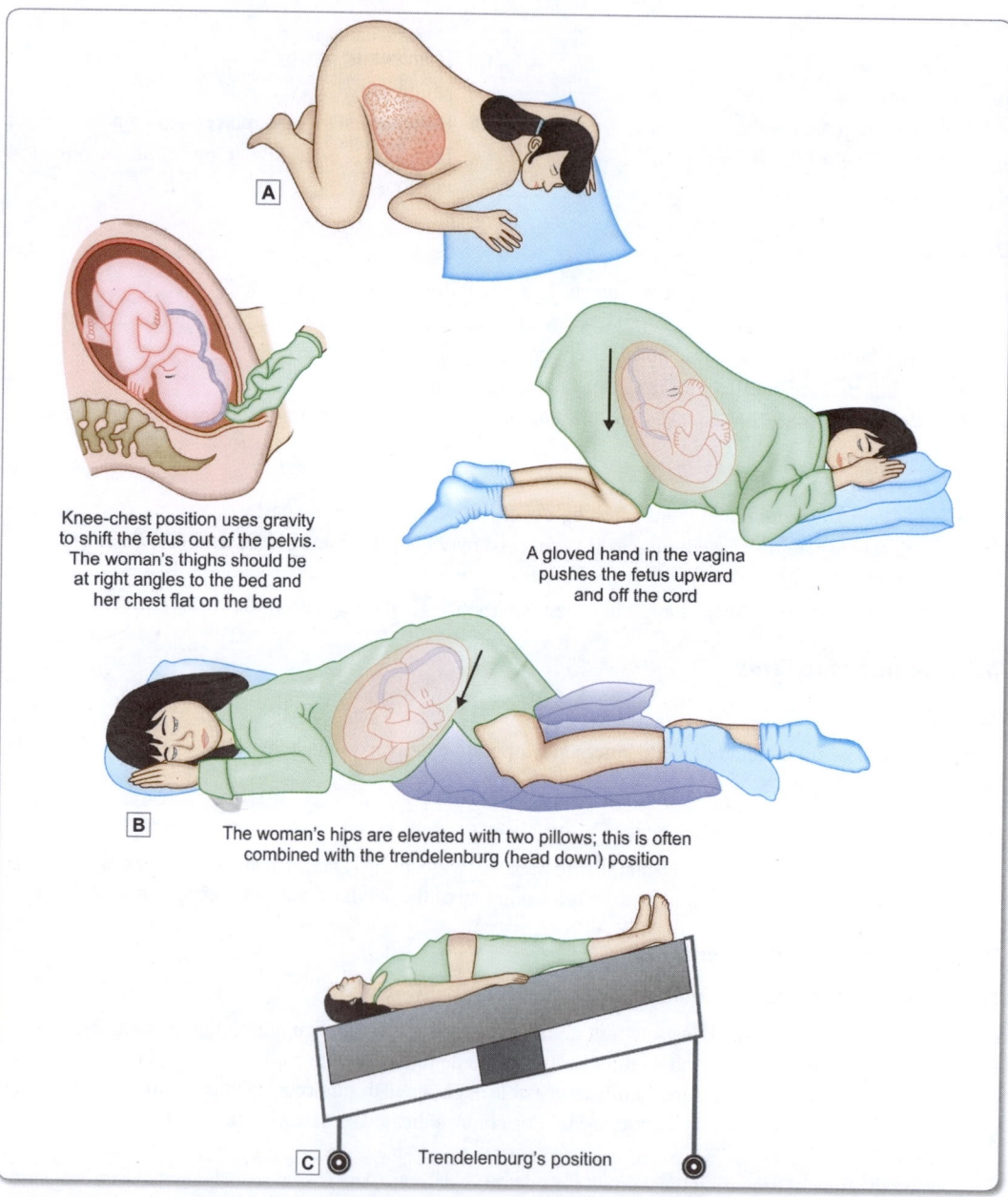

Knee-chest position uses gravity to shift the fetus out of the pelvis. The woman's thighs should be at right angles to the bed and her chest flat on the bed

A gloved hand in the vagina pushes the fetus upward and off the cord

The woman's hips are elevated with two pillows; this is often combined with the trendelenburg (head down) position

Trendelenburg's position

**Figs 36A to C:** Position of mother during cord prolapse. **A.** Knee chest position; **B.** Exaggerated Sims' position, **C.** Trendelenburg position

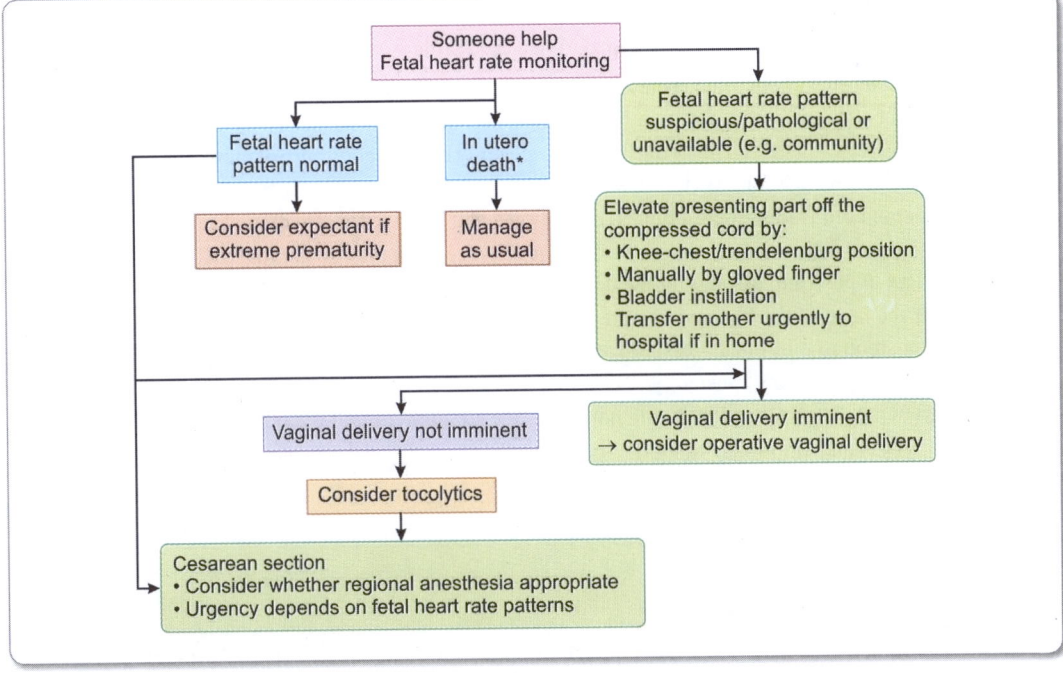

**Fig. 37:** Management of cord prolapse

## If Baby is Dead

- Confirm with ultrasound
- Wait for spontaneous expulsion or perform destructive operations.

## If Baby is Alive

- If immediate vaginal delivery not possible. Give first aid management to the mother which includes:
    - To lift the presenting part off the cord, by gloved fingers introduced into the vagina
    - Posture: Exaggerated and elevated Sims' position or Trendelenburg or knee-chest position
    - Transfer the patient to an equipped hospital
- If maternal and fetal health condition is favorable, perform vaginal delivery either by forceps/ventouse
- In case of breech presentation—Breech extraction in expert hands only
- Cesarean section is the treatment of choice
- Elevate presenting part off the compressed cord by:
    - Knee-chest/Trendelenburg's position
    - Manually by gloved finger
    - Bladder Instillation
- Transfer mother urgently to hospital if in home.

## Nursing Management of Cord Prolapse

- Identify prolapse cord and provide immediate intervention.
  - Assess a laboring client often if the fetus is preterm or small for gestational age, if the fetal presenting part is not engaged, and if the membranes are ruptured.
  - Periodically evaluate fetal heart rate (FHR), especially right after rupture of membranes (spontaneous or surgical), and again in 5–10 minutes.
  - If prolapse cord is identified, notify the physician and prepare for emergency cesarean birth.
  - If the client is fully dilated, the most emergent delivery route may be vaginal. In this case, encourage the client to push and assist with the delivery as follows.
  - Lower the head of the bed and elevate the client's hips on a pillow, or place the client in the knee-chest position to minimize pressure from the cord.
  - Assess cord pulsations constantly.
  - Gently wrap gauze soaked in sterile normal saline solution around the prolapsed cord.
- Provide physical and emotional support.
- Provide client and family education.

## Amniotic Fluid Embolism

### Definition

Amniotic fluid embolism occurs when amniotic fluid enters the maternal circulation through a tear in the membranes or placenta.

### Incidence

Overall incidence ranges from 1 in 80,000 pregnancies and 10% maternal death.

### Predisposing Factors

Amniotic fluid embolism can occur at any stage in gestation. It is mostly associated with labor, though cases in early pregnancy and postpartum have been reported. Factors are as follows:

- Transfer of amniotic fluid from the uterus to the maternal circulation can be insidiously associated with a tear in the membranes.
- Amniotic fluid under pressure may enter maternal circulation in the first phase of hypoxia during hypertonic uterine activity.
- Procedures such as insertion of an intrauterine catheter and artificial rupture of membranes are associated with the condition.
- In cases of placental abruption, the placental bed is disrupted and the barrier between the maternal circulation and amniotic sac may be breached.
- It can occur during a cesarean section, termination of pregnancy or in association with ruptured uterus.
- Trauma may occur during intrauterine manipulation such as internal podalic version.

## Pathophysiology of Amniotic Fluid Embolism

Figure 38 shows the pathophysiology of amniotic fluid embolism.

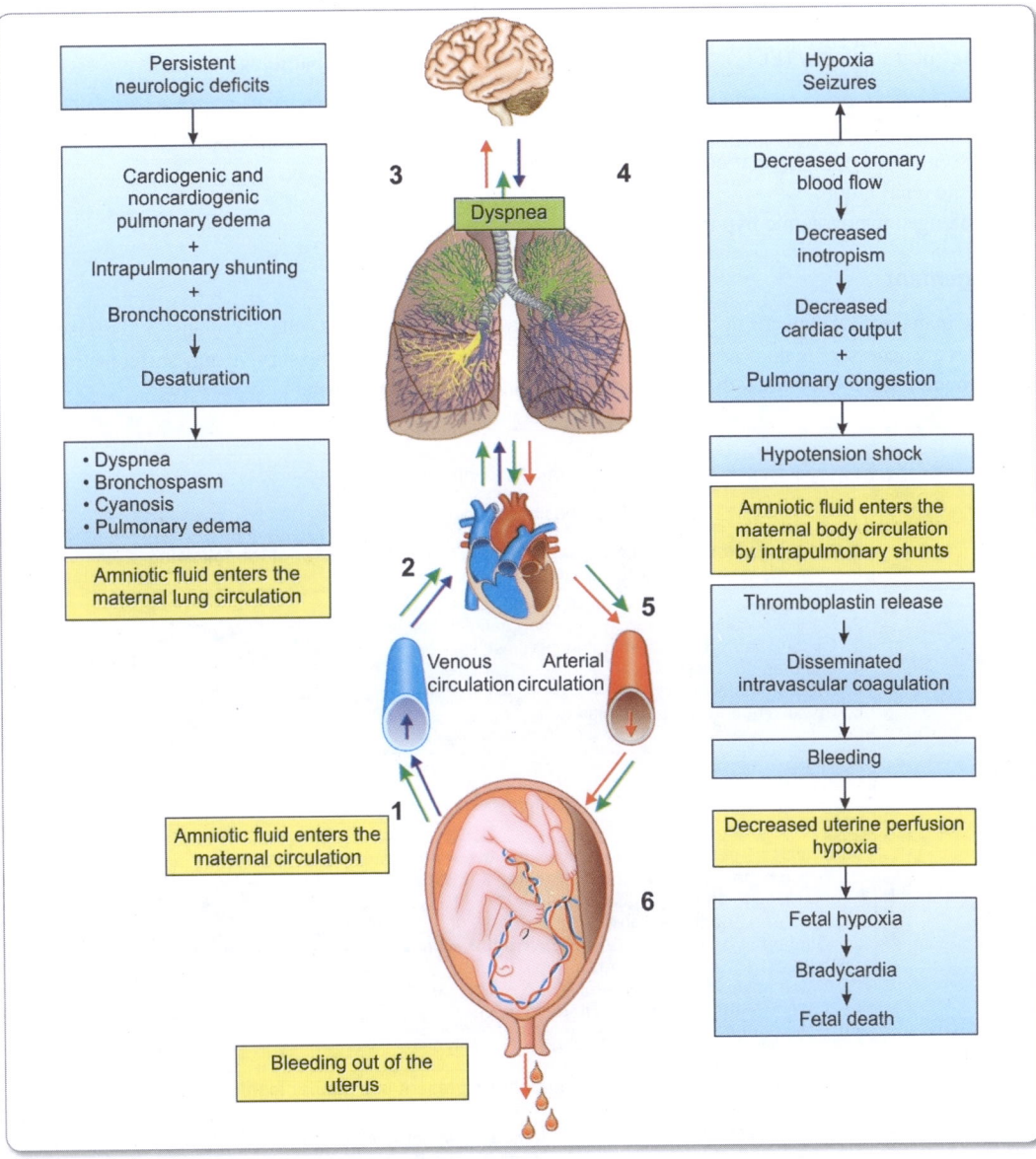

**Fig. 38:** Pathophysiology of amniotic fluid embolism

## Clinical Features

- Maternal respiratory distress
- Cyanosis
- Cardiovascular collapse
- Hemorrhage
- Convulsions, coma
- Fetal distress

## Laboratory Investigations

- Complete blood count
- Fibrinogen
- Arterial blood gases (ABG)
- Electrocardiography (ECG)
- Chest X-ray
- Echocardiogram
- Serum tryptase
- Cervical histopathology

## Complications

- Disseminated intravascular coagulation (DIC)
- Acute renal failure
- Prolonged hypovolemic hypotension

## Management

Specific management depends upon the symptoms. The mother may be in a state of collapse and resuscitative measures are necessary in that case. Administer oxygen therapy. Mothers who survive may suffer neurological impairment. Figure 39 exhibits the management of amniotic fluid embolism.

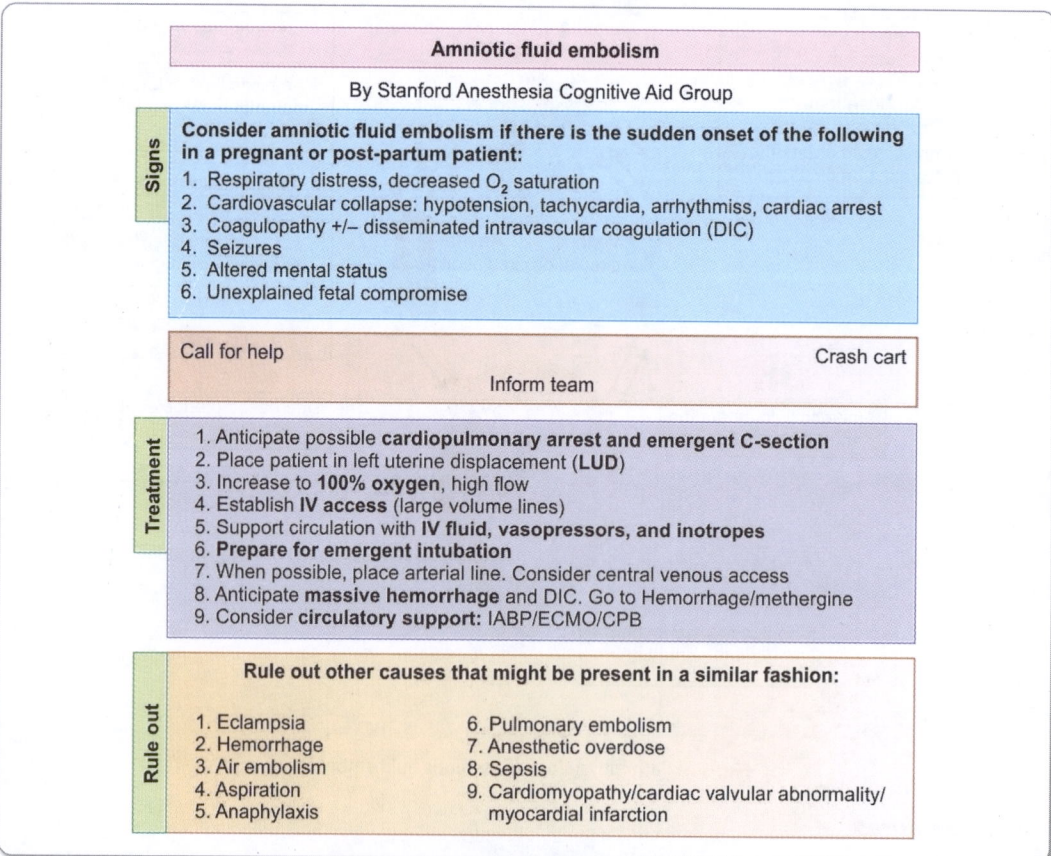

**Fig. 39:** Management of amniotic fluid embolism

*Abbreviations:* CPB, cardiopulmonary bypass; DIC, Disseminated intravascular coagulation; ECMO, extracorporeal membrane oxygenation; IABP, intra-aortic balloon pump

# Obstetric Shock

Shock is defined as a state of circulatory inadequacy with poor tissue perfusion resulting in generalized cellular hypoxia.

## Classification of Shock

### Hypovolemic Shock

It occurs due to inadequate circulating blood volume resulting from acute depletion. It may be:

### a. Hemorrhagic Shock

- Associated with postpartum or postabortal hemorrhage, ectopic pregnancy, placenta previa, abruptio placenta, rupture of the uterus and obstetric history
- Shock associated with DIC, intrauterine fetal death (IUFD) and amniotic fluid embolism.

### b. Nonhemorrhagic Shock

- **Fluid loss shock:** Associated with excessive vomiting, diarrhea, diuresis or too rapid removal of amniotic fluid.
- **Supine hypotensive syndrome:** Due to compression of inferior vena cava by the gravid uterus.

Table 7 exhibits the clinical presentation of different types of shock.

**TABLE 7:** Clinical presentation of different types of shock

| | | |
|---|---|---|
| **Hypovolemic** | Hypotension, tachycardia<br>Weak thready pulse<br>Cool, pale, moist skin urine output decreased | Decreased CO<br>**Increased SVR (systemic vascular resistance)** |
| **Cardiogenic** | Hypotension, tachycardia<br>Weak thready pulse<br>Cool, pale, moist skin<br>Urine output <30 mL/hr<br>Crackles, tachypnea | Decreased CO<br>**Increased SVR** |
| **Neurogenic** | Hypotension, bradycardia<br>Warm dry skin | Decreased CO<br>Venous and arterial vasodilation, loss sympathetic tone |
| **Anaphylactic** | Hypotension, tachycardia<br>Cough, dyspnea<br>Pruritus, Urticaria<br>Restlessness, decreased level of consciousness | Decreased CO<br>**Decreased SVR** |
| **Septic** | Hypotension, Tachycardia<br>Full bounding pulse, tachypnea<br>**Pink, warm, flushed skin**<br>Decreased urine output, fever | Decreased CO<br>**Decreased** SVR |

*Abbreviations:* CO, cardiac output; SVR, systemic vascular resistance

## Septic Shock (Endotoxic Shock)

Associated typically with septic abortion, chorioamnionitis, pyelonephritis and rarely postpartum endometritis. Hypotension is due to resulting in derangements in cellular and organ system dysfunction. Hypotension persists in spite of adequate fluid resuscitation.

## Cardiogenic Shock

It occurs due to impaired ability of the heart to pump blood. It is characterized by:

- ↓ systolic pressure (<80 mm Hg)
- ↓ cardiac index (<1.8 L/min/m²)
- ↑ left ventricular filling pressure (>18 mm Hg)

### Causes

Myocardial infarction, asystole/ventricular fibrillation, cardiac tamponade.

### Neurogenic Shock

- **Chemical injury:** Associated with aspiration of gastrointestinal contents during general anesthesia.
- **Drug-induced:** Associated with spinal anesthesia.

## Management

### Hemorrhagic Shock

Basic management of hemorrhagic shock is to stop the bleeding and replace the volume which has been lost. Urgent resuscitation is needed to prevent the mother's condition from deteriorating and causing irreversible damage.

**The priorities are to:**

- Maintain the airway:
  - Provide side lying position
  - Oxygen administration at rate of 6–8 L/min
  - Endotracheal intubation if unconscious
- **Replace fluids:** Plasma expander or fresh frozen plasma is given until whole blood is available.
- **Maintenance of cardiac efficiency:** Fluids and blood should be administered very carefully to avoid the risk of overloading the circulation and cardiac failure.
- **Avoid warmth:** Constriction of the peripheral blood supply occurs in response to the shock and keeping the mother warm may interfere with this response, causing further deterioration in her condition.
- **Control of hemorrhage:** Specific surgical and medical treatment for control of hemorrhage should start along with the general management of shock.
- **Monitor the mother:**
  - Level of consciousness
  - Sign of restlessness/confusion
  - Blood pressure every 30 minutes/continuously
  - Cardiac rhythm monitored continuously
  - Skin color and temperature hourly
  - Central venous pressure
  - Any bleeding

### Septic Shock

Principles of management are:

- To correct the hemodynamic instability due to sepsis
- Appropriate supportive care
- Remove the source of sepsis

*Management*

- **Antibiotics:** Broad spectrum antibiotics are given to start with and after confirming the sensitivity, specific antibiotics are given intravenously.
- **Intravenous fluids and electrolytes:** Septic shock associated with hemorrhagic hypotension is treated with liberal IV fluid infusion and blood transfusion. If there is renal dysfunction, avoid administering electrolytes.
- **Correction of acidosis:** Bicarbonate is administered to avoid acidosis.
- **Maintenance of blood pressure:** Inotropic agents are used to increase cardiac contractility. Vasodilators, nitroglycerin and diuretic are used to decrease after load and pulmonary edema.
- **Corticosteroids:** These are given to exert anti-endotoxin effect and to counteract anaerobic oxidative mechanism.
- As a prophylactic measure for DIC, heparin may be given. Fresh frozen plasma or whole blood may be used.
- In unresponsive septic shock following septic abortion or puerperal sepsis, hysterectomy may be done to eliminate the source of infection.

## Rupture of Uterus

**Definition:** A break in the continuity of the uterine wall any time beyond 28 weeks of pregnancy is called rupture of the uterus (Fig. 40).

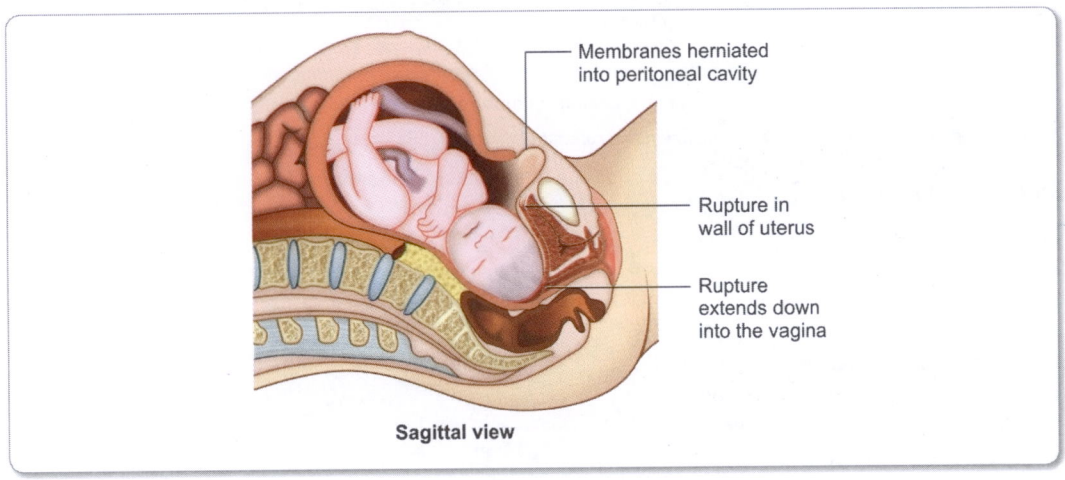

Membranes herniated into peritoneal cavity

Rupture in wall of uterus

Rupture extends down into the vagina

**Sagittal view**

**Fig. 40:** Rupture of uterus during labor

## Types

- **Complete rupture:** A tear in the wall of the uterus including the peritoneal coat and with or without expulsion of the fetus.
- **Incomplete rupture:** A tear of the uterine wall without involving the perimetrium.

## Incidence

Overall incidence varies from 1 in 2000 to 1 in 200 deliveries.

## Etiology of Rupture Uterus

Figure 41 shows the etiology of rupture uterus.

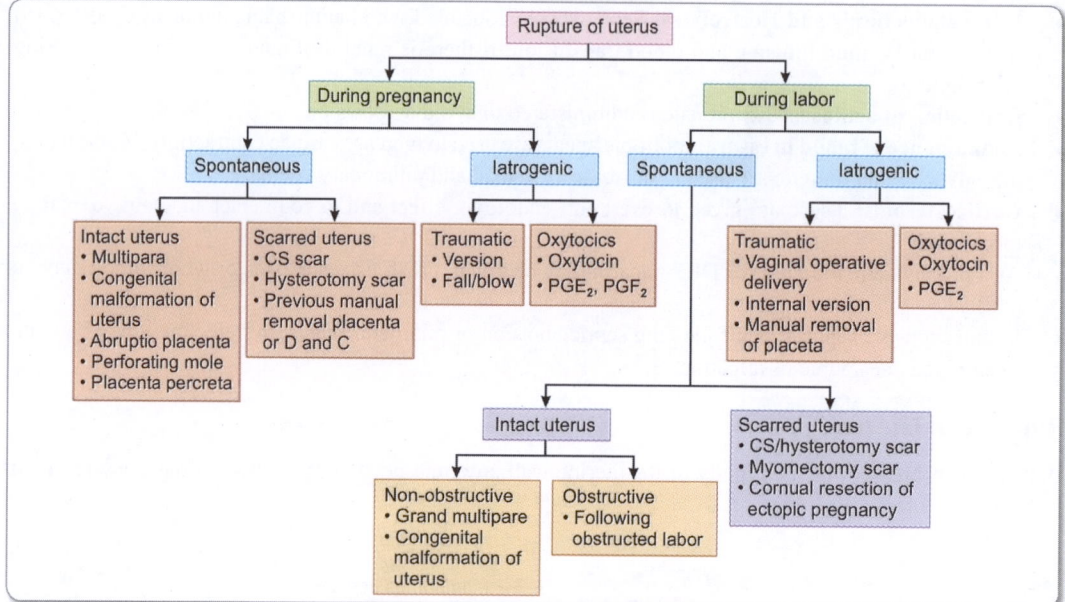

**Fig. 41:** Etiology of rupture of uterus

*Abbreviations:* CS, cesarean section, D & C, dilatation and curettage

## Signs and Symptoms

- Sudden collapse
- Severe abdominal pain
- Increased maternal pulse rate
- Alteration of fetal heart rate (FHR)
- Fresh vaginal bleeding
- Cessation of uterine contractions
- Change in contour of abdomen
- Sudden loss of FHR
- Palpable fetal parts as the presenting part regresses

Figure 42 shows the signs and symptoms of uterine rupture.

## Diagnosis of Rupture of Uterus

### During Pregnancy

- **Scar rupture (classical or hysterotomy):** The patient complaints of a dull abdominal pain over scar area with slight vaginal bleeding. Fetal heart sound (FHS) may be irregular or absent. The features may not be always dramatic in nature (silent phase). Sooner or later, the rupture becomes complete. There is a sense of something giving way accompanied by acute abdominal pain and collapse.
- **Spontaneous rupture in uninjured uterus:** It is usually confined to high parous women. The onset is usually acute but sometimes insidious. In acute types, the patient has acute pain in abdomen with

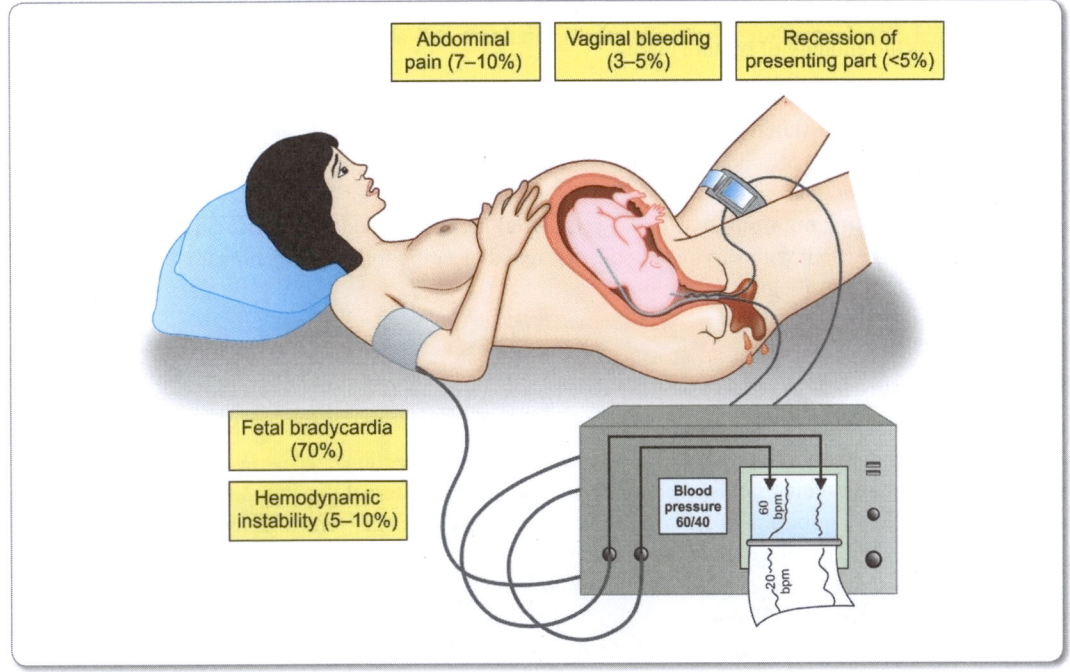

| Abdominal pain (7–10%) | Vaginal bleeding (3–5%) | Recession of presenting part (<5%) |

Fetal bradycardia (70%)

Hemodynamic instability (5–10%)

Blood pressure 60/40

60 bpm

20 bpm

**Fig. 42:** Signs and symptoms of uterine rupture

fainting attacks and she may collapse. However, with insidious onset, the diagnosis is often confused with concealed accidental hemorrhage or rectus sheath hematoma.

- **Rupture following fall, blow or external version or use of oxytocics:** Patient complains of acute pain in abdomen and slight vaginal bleeding. Rapid pulse and tender uterus raise the suspicion of rupture. Confirmation is done by laparotomy.

## During Labor

- **Scar rupture:**
  - **Lower segment scar rupture:** Onset is insidious. There is no classical feature of lower segment scar rupture. Confirmation is by laparotomy.
  - **Classical or hysterotomy scar rupture:** Features are same as those occur during pregnancy. Onset is acute.
- **Spontaneous obstructive rupture:** It has distinct premonitory phase prior to rupture.
  - **Premonitory phase:** Patient is multipara in labor with features of obstruction. Initially, the pains become severe in an attempt to overcome obstruction and come at quick intervals. Gradually, the pains become continuous and mainly confined to suprapubic region. On examination, patient is dehydrated and exhausted. Pulse rate and temperature rise.

## Phase of Rupture

- Sense of something giving way at the height of uterine contraction.
- Constant pain changed to dull aching pain with cessation of uterine contractions.

- General examination reveals feature of exhaustion and shock.
- Abdominal examination reveals (i) superficial fetal parts (ii) absence of FHS (iii) absence of uterine contour.
- **Vaginal examination reveals:** Varying degree of bleeding and recession of presenting part.
- **Spontaneous nonobstructive rupture:** Usually confined to parous women. The patient at the height of uterine contraction is suddenly seized with an agonizing bursting pain followed by a relief, with cessation of contractions.
- **Rupture following manipulative or instrumental delivery:** Sudden deterioration of the general condition of the patient with varying amount of vaginal bleeding following manipulative or instrumental delivery raises the suspicion.

## *Management*

### Preventive Measures

- High-risk mother should have mandatory hospital delivery.
- Avoid vaginal delivery if there is previous history of cesarean section.
- General anesthesia should not be used to give undue force in external version.
- Undue delay in the progress of labor in multipara with previous uneventful delivery should be viewed with concern and the cause should be sought for.
- Judicious selection of cases and careful watch are mandatory during oxytocin infusion either for induction/augmentation of labor.
- Internal podalic version should not be done in obstructed labor.
- Do not conduct forceps delivery or breech extraction through incompletely dilated cervix.
- Destructive operations should be performed by skilled personnel only.
- Exploration of the uterus should be done as a routine following delivery.
- In case of morbid adherent placenta, manual removal should be done by senior medical practitioner only.

### Definitive Management

Depending upon the state of the clinical condition, resuscitation needs to be done followed by laparotomy, or in acute conditions; resuscitation and laparotomy are to be done simultaneously. Following laparotomy, any of the following procedures may be adopted.

- Hysterectomy in spontaneous obstructive rupture, a quick subtotal hysterectomy is usually done.
- Repair is mostly applicable in the case of scar rupture where the margins are clean.
- Repair and sterilization (tubal ligation) are mostly done in patients with a clean cut scar rupture having desired number of children.

### Nursing Management

1. Monitor for the possibility of uterine rupture.
   - In the presence of predisposing factors, monitor maternal labor pattern closely for hypertonicity or signs of weakening uterine muscle.
   - Recognize signs of impending rupture, immediately notify the physician, and call for assistance.
2. Assist with rapid intervention.
   - If the client has signs of possible uterine rupture, vaginal delivery is generally not attempted.
   - If symptoms are not severe, an emergency cesarean delivery may be attempted and the uterine tear is repaired.

- If symptoms are severe, emergency laparotomy is performed to attempt immediate delivery of the fetus and then establish homeostasis.
3. Implement the following preparations for surgery.
   - Monitor maternal blood pressure, pulse, and respirations; also monitor fetal heart tones.
   - If the client has a central venous pressure catheter in place, monitor pressure to evaluate blood loss and effects of fluid and blood replacement.
   - Insert a urinary catheter for precise determinations of fluid balance.
   - Obtain blood to assess possible acidosis.
   - Administer oxygen, and maintain a patent airway.
4. Prevent and manage complications.
   Take these steps in order to prevent or limit hypovolemic shock:
   - Oxygenate by providing 8–10 L/min using a closed mask.
   - Restore circulating volume using one or more IV lines.
   - Evaluate the cause, response to therapy, and fetal condition.
   - Remedy the problem by preparing the client for surgery and administering antibiotics. Provide physical and emotional support.
   - Provide support for the client's partner and family members once surgery has begun.
   - Inform the partner and family how they will receive information about the mother and newborn and where to wait.

## Shoulder Dystocia

Shoulder dystocia (Fig. 43) means difficulty in the birth of the shoulders. Shoulder dystocia occurs when either the anterior or the posterior (rare) fetal shoulder impacts on the maternal symphysis or on the sacral promontory respectively.

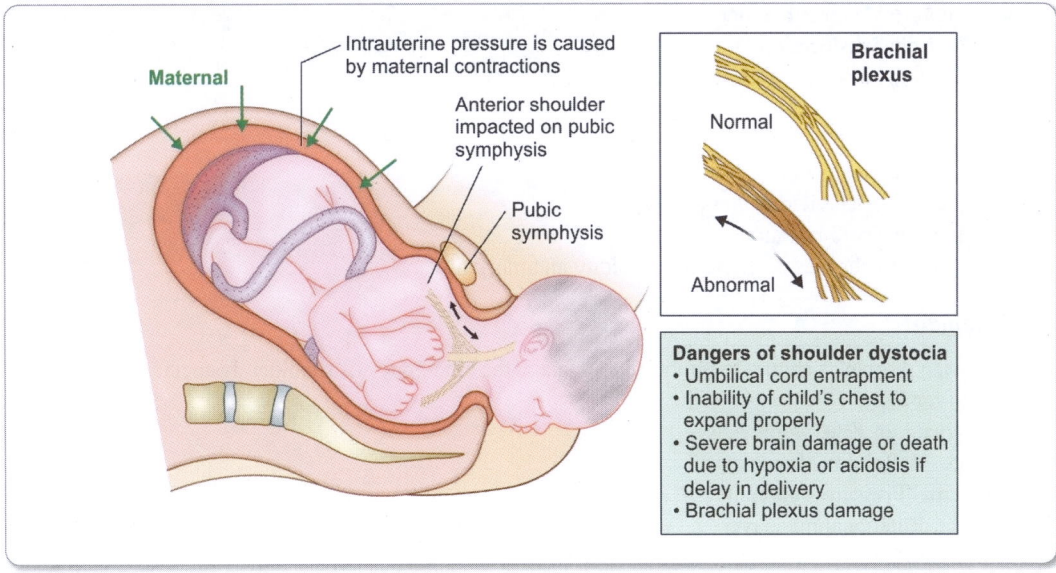

**Fig. 43:** Shoulder dystocia

## Incidence

Incidence varies between 0.2% and 1%

## Risk Factors

- Obstetric history of large babies
- Maternal diabetes
- Family history of large sibling
- Maternal obesity
- Fetal macrosomia
- Maternal age over 35 years
- High parity

- Induced labor
- Prolonged first and second stage of labor
- Secondary arrest of labor
- Post maturity
- Anencephaly
- Fetal ascites

## Diagnosis

- **Turtle neck sign:** Definite recoil of the head back against the perineum
- Inadequate spontaneous restitution
- Fetal face becomes plethoric
- Failure of shoulder to descend

## Complications

- **Maternal complications:**
  - Postpartum hemorrhage (PPH)
  - Cervical laceration
  - Vaginal tear
  - Perineal tear
  - Rupture of uterus/bladder
  - Sacroiliac dislocation
  - Increased chances of maternal morbidity
- **Fetal complications:**
  - Asphyxia
  - Brachial plexus injury
  - Fracture of clavicle, humerus
  - Sternomastoid hematoma
  - Increased chances of perinatal morbidity and mortality

## Management

The following principles should be followed to manage the emergency of shoulder dystocia:

- **H** Call for **H**elp
- **E** **E**valuate for **E**pisiotomy
- **L** **L**egs: McRoberts Maneuver
- **P** External **P**ressure–suprapubic
- **E** **E**nter: Rotational maneuver
- **R** **R**emove the posterior arm
- **R** **R**oll the patient to the hands and knees

**The obstetrician may try the following maneuvers to dislodge the shoulders and deliver the baby (Figs 44A to D):**

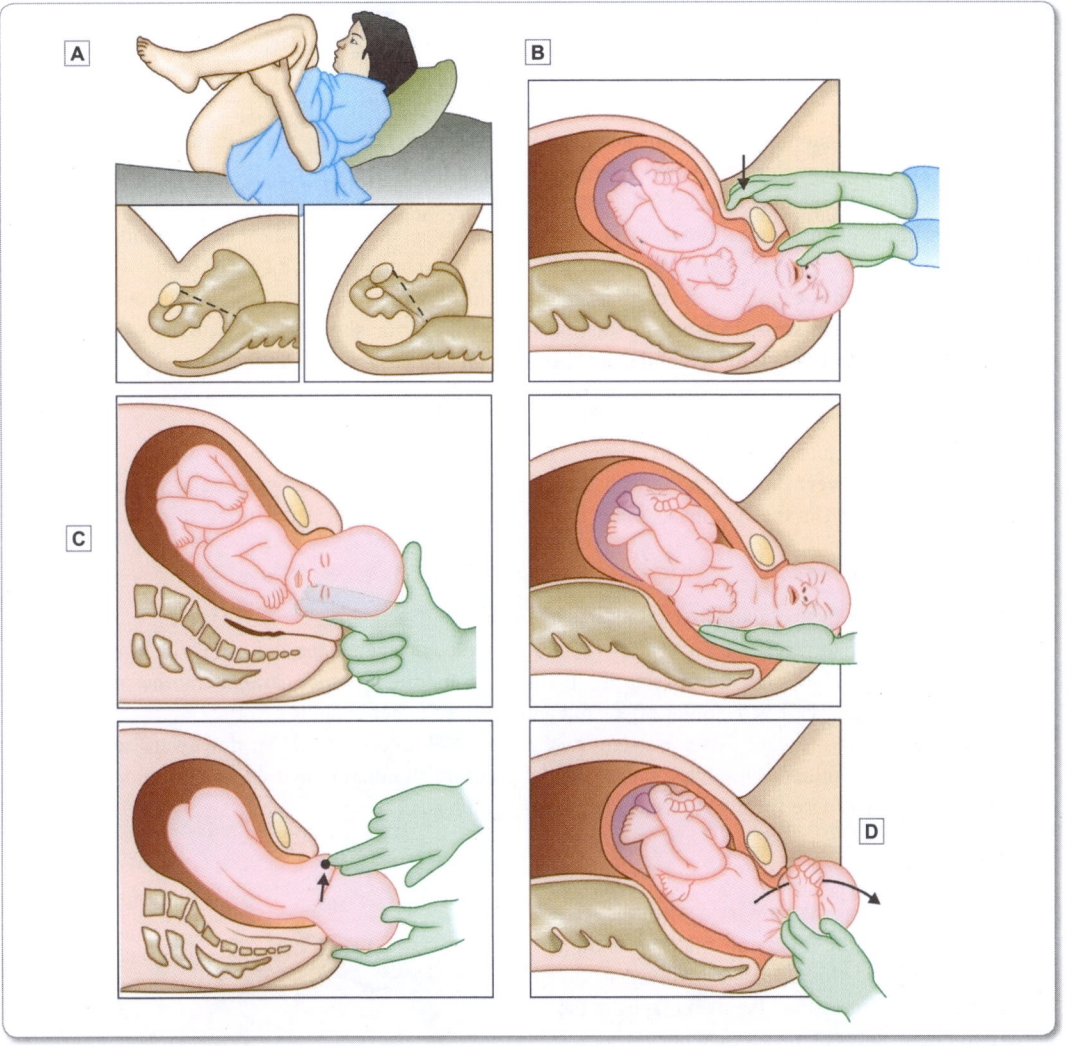

**Figs 44A to D:** **A.** The McRoberts maneuver is the least invasive maneuver to disimpact the shoulders in shoulder dystocia. Position the patient in the extreme lithotomy position with the hips completely fixed (knee-chest position); this may free the anterior fetal shoulder; **B.** Moderate suprapubic pressure will often disimpact the anterior shoulder. Desperate traction on the fetal head is not likely to facilitate delivery and might lead to trauma. Delivery of an infant with shoulder dystocia often results in fracture of the clavicle or humerus to accomplish delivery; **C.** Rubin or reverse Wood's screw maneuver: (1) Rotate the posterior shoulder (2) Deliver the rotated shoulder; **D.** Posterior shoulder delivery. Insert a hand and sweep the posterior arm across the chest and over the perineum. Take care to distribute the pressure evenly across the humerus to avoid unnecessary fracture

- **Suprapubic pressure:** Head and neck should be grasped and taken posteriorly while suprapubic pressure is applied by an assistant slightly towards the side of fetal chest. This will reduce the bisacromial diameter and rotate the anterior shoulder towards the oblique diameter.
- **Mc-Roberts maneuver:** Instruct the mother to lie flat and to bring her knees up to her chest as far as possible. This will rotate the angle of the symphysis pubis superiorly and use the weight of the mother's legs to create gentle pressure on her releasing the impaction of the anterior shoulder.

- **Rubin's maneuver:** On vaginal examination, identify the posterior shoulder in the direction of the fetal chest, thus rotating the anterior shoulder away from the symphysis pubis. By adduction of the shoulders, this maneuver reduces the 12 cm bisacromial diameter.
- **Wood's maneuver:** Through vaginal examination, identify the fetal chest. Then by exerting pressure on the posterior fetal shoulder, rotation is achieved. This maneuver abducts the shoulder, rotates them into a more favorable diameter and enables the completion of the delivery.
- **Extraction of the posterior arm:** The operator's hand is introduced into the vagina along the fetal posterior humerus in the sacral hallow. The arm is then swept across the chest and thereafter delivered by gentle traction. This procedure may cause either fracture clavicle or humerus or both.
- **"All four" position:** Changing the mother on to all four may increase the pelvic dimensions and allows the fetal position to shift. Downward traction on the posterior shoulder helps to free the impacted shoulder. It is mostly done for a mobile and slim woman in a community setting.

### Other Methods if Above Maneuvers have Failed

- **Cleidotomy:** Fracture of one or both clavicles to reduce shoulder girth.
- **Zavanelli maneuver:** Pushing the fetus back to the uterus and delivering by cesarean section.
- **Symphysiotomy:** Cut the symphysis pubis to increase the diameter of pelvic brim. It is rarely done.

### *Nursing Management*

- Identify shoulder dystocia and assist with management.
- Place the client in the McRobert's position (i.e. thighs pulled up against the abdomen with hips abducted).
    - The woman flexes her thighs sharply against her abdomen, which straightens the pelvic curve. A supported squat has a similar effect and adds gravity to her pushing efforts.
- Apply suprapubic pressure by an assistant pushes the fetal anterior shoulder downward to displace it from above the mother's symphysis pubis. Fundal pressure should not be used, because it will push the anterior shoulder more firmly against the mother's symphysis.

## Vasa Previa

Vasa previa (Fig. 45) is the term used when the fetal blood vessel lies over the OS in front of the presenting part. In vasa previa, blood vessels involved in the baby's circulation grow along the membranes in the lower part of the uterus at the cervical opening.

Normally in pregnancy, the blood vessels of the umbilical cord and the placenta are insulated inside amniotic sac. In case of vasa previa, the blood vessels are present at membranes without this protection such as incase of velamentous insertion or in multilobed placenta. Vasaprevia can occur as a complication of placenta previa or low-lying placenta. When the condition is not detected in advance, the blood vessels can rupture during labor.

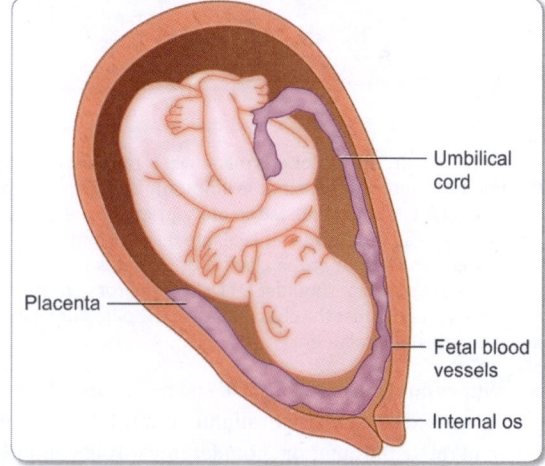

**Fig. 45:** Vasa previa

### *Risk Factors*

- Placenta previa
- Velamentous insertion of umbilical cord

- Multilobed placenta
- Multiple pregnancies

## Diagnosis

- Vasa previa may sometimes be palpated on vaginal examination, when the membranes are still intact. Pulsations felt may be synchronous with the fetal heart rate.
- Speculum examination may be done to visualize the blood vessel.
- It may also be visualized on ultrasound.
- Fresh vaginal bleeding, which commences at the time of rupture of membranes, may be due to ruptured vasa previa.

## Complications

Complications of vasa previa are displayed in Figure 46.

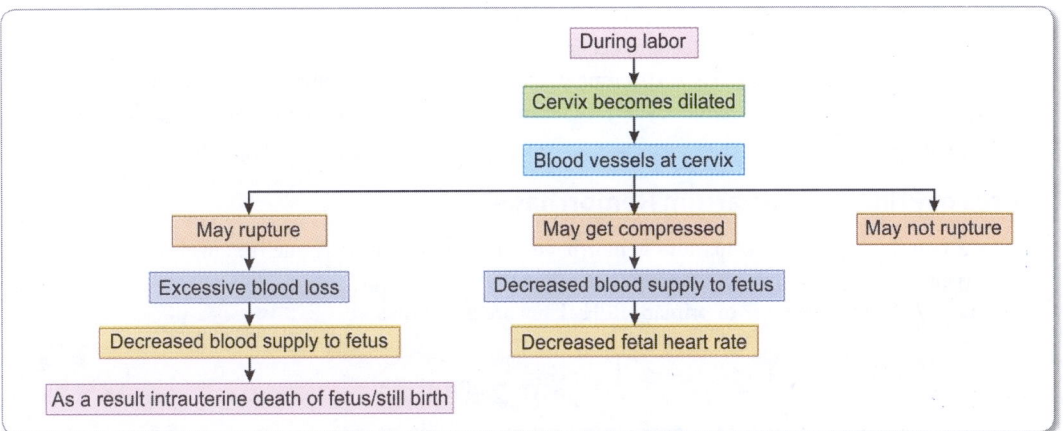

**Fig. 46:** Complications of vasa previa

## Treatment

- Hospitalize the mother in third trimester to ensure rapid access to medical care if blood vessels rupture.
- Assess the FHR at frequent interval.
- If in the first stage of labor and the fetus is alive, an emergency cesarean section is carried out.
- If the mother is in the second stage of labor, delivery should be expedited and a vaginal birth may be achieved. Mode of delivery depends on parity and fetal condition.
- The pediatrician should be present at delivery and if baby is alive, hemoglobin estimation is necessary after resuscitation. If required, start blood transfusion.

## Nursing Management

- Identify, and assist with treatment of the disorder.
  - Monitor fetal heart rate and status during labor.
  - Assist with diagnosis of the condition.
  - Anticipate and assist with emergency cesarean birth.
- Provide physical and emotional support.
- Provide client and family education. Explain emergency procedures to the client and family.

## POSTPARTUM HEMORRHAGE

Any amount of bleeding from or into the genital tract following birth of the baby to the end of the puerperium, which adversely affects the general condition of the mother, evidenced by rise in pulse rate and falling blood pressure is called postpartum hemorrhage.

### Incidence

Varies widely, approximately 1% among hospital deliveries.

### Types

- **Primary:** Hemorrhage occurs within 24 hours following the birth of the baby. In majority, hemorrhage occurs within two hours following delivery. It is of two types
  i. *Third stage hemorrhage:* Bleeding occurs before expulsion of placenta
  ii. *True postpartum hemorrhage:* Bleeding occurs subsequent to expulsion of placenta
- **Secondary:** Hemorrhage occurs beyond 24 hours and within puerperium, also called delayed or late puerperal hemorrhage.

### Causes of Primary Postpartum Hemorrhage

There are four Ts that cause postpartum hemorrhage—Tone (atonicity), Tissue (retained bits, blood clots), Trauma (genital tract injury) and Thrombin (coagulopathy).

Figure 47 shows the causes of primary PPH. They are as follows:

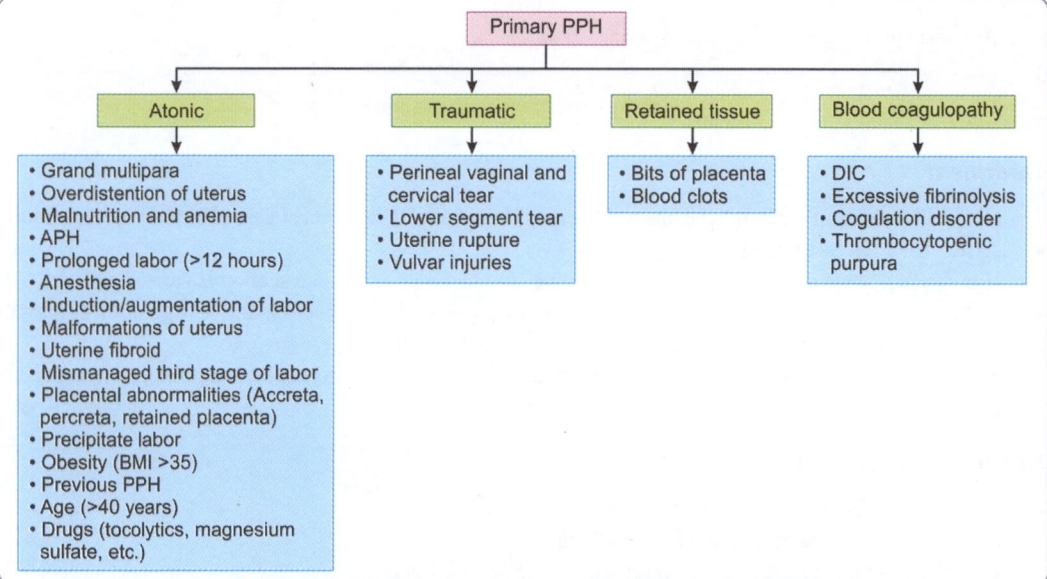

**Fig. 47:** Causes of primary PPH

*Abbreviations:* APH, antepartum hemorrhage; BMI, body mass index; DIC, disseminated intravascular coagulation; PPH, postpartum hemorrhage

## Atonic Uterus (80%)

Atonicity of the uterus is the most common cause of postpartum hemorrhage. With the separation of placenta, the uterine sinuses, which are torn, cannot be compressed effectively due to imperfect contraction, and retraction of uterine musculature and bleeding continue. The following conditions often interfere with retraction of uterus as a whole and of placental site in particular.

- **Grand multipara:** Inadequate retraction and frequent adherent placenta contribute to it.
- **Over distention of the uterus:** In case of hydramnios, multiple pregnancy and big baby (>4 kg).
- **Incomplete separation of placenta:** If the placenta remains fully adhered to uterine wall, it is unlikely to cause bleeding. If placental tissue remains partially embedded in spongy decidua, efficiency of contraction and retraction is interrupted.
- **Precipitate labor:** It may cause uterine muscles insufficient opportunity to retract.
- **Prolonged labor:** If active phase lasts >12 hours, uterine inertia may result due to muscle exhaustion.
- **Placental abruption:** Blood may have seeped between the muscle fibers, interfering with effective action.
- **Placenta previa:** The placental site is partly or wholly in the lower segment where the thinner muscle layer contains few oblique fibers, which result in poor control of bleeding.
- **General anesthesia:** Anesthetic agents may cause a uterine relaxation, particularly in inhalational agents, like halothane.
- **Mismanagement of third stage of labor:** 'Fundus fiddling' or manipulation of the uterus may precipitate arrhythmic contractions so that the only placenta separates partially, and retraction is lost.
- **Malformation of the uterus:** Implantation of placenta in the uterine septum of a septate uterus or in corneal region of a bicornuate uterus may cause excessive bleeding.
  Other causes are:
  - Obesity (BMI >35)
  - Previous postpartum hemorrhage
  - Age (>40 years)
  - Drugs: Use of tocolytic (ritodrine), $MgSO_4$, nifedipine

## Traumatic (20%)

Causes
- Perineal, vaginal and cervical tears
- Lower segment tears
- Uterine rupture
- Vulval injuries

## Retained Tissue

Bits of placenta and blood clots cause PPH due to imperfect uterine retraction.

## Blood Coagulation Disorders

- Blood coagulation disorders cause disseminated intravascular coagulation (DIC), excessive fibrinolysis, inherited coagulation disorders, idiopathic thrombocytopenic purpura.
- Postpartum hemorrhage may be the result of coagulation failure. The blood clotting failure possibly occurs due to diminished procoagulants or increased fibrinolytic activity. It can occur following severe preeclampsia, abruption placenta, amniotic fluid embolism, HELLP syndrome, IUD or sepsis.

## Signs and Symptoms

- Vaginal bleeding (common)
- Vulvovaginal/broad ligament hematoma (rarely)
- Pallor
- Rising pulse rate
- Falling blood pressure
- Altered level of consciousness
- Restless/drowsiness
- Enlarged uterus (concealed hemorrhage)
- Maternal collapse

## Diagnosis

- On speculum examination: Vaginal bleeding is visible outside, as a slow trickle. Rarely bleeding is totally concealed as either vulvovaginal/broad ligament hematoma.
- On abdominal examination:
  - *In case of traumatic hemorrhage:* Uterus is well contracted.
  - *In atonic hemorrhage:* Uterus is found flabby and become hard on massaging.

## Prophylaxis

- **Antenatal:**
  - Improvement of health status of women.
  - High-risk patients are to be screened and delivered in a well-equipped hospital.
  - Blood grouping and typing should be done for high-risk mothers, so that no time is lost during an emergency.
  - In case of previous history of cesarean section, prior to delivery ultrasound and MRI should be done for placental localization.
- **During labor:**
  - Active management of third stage of labor.
  - Continuous infusion of oxytocin for at least 1 hour after the delivery.
  - Baby should be pushed out by the retracted uterus and not be pulled out. Wait for 2–3 minutes to deliver the trunk after the head is born.
  - Avoid temptation of fiddling with or kneading the uterus, pulling the cord or creeds' expression of placenta.
  - In case of previous history of placenta previa, two units of cross match blood should be kept available.
  - Women delivered by cesarean section, oxytocin 5 international unit (IU) slow IV is to be given to reduce blood loss.
  - Exploration of uterovaginal canal for evidence of trauma following difficult labor or instrumental delivery.
  - Examination of placenta and membranes to make sure for its complete removal.
  - Observe the mother for two hours after delivery to make sure uterus is hard and contracted.

## Management of Third Stage Bleeding

- Control the bleeding by fundal massage and make it hard.
- Following delivery of anterior shoulder, injection Methergine 0.2 mg IV should be given.

- Start normal saline drip with oxytocin
- Arrange for blood transfusion
- Catheterize the bladder
- If placenta is separated, express the placenta out by controlled cord traction [CCT]
- If placenta doesn't separate, manual removal of placenta under general anesthesia
- In case of traumatic hemorrhage, it should be tackled by sutures

## Management of True Postpartum Hemorrhage

### Principles

- To find out the cause of bleeding
- Take prompt and effective measures to control bleeding
- To correct hypovolemia

The management of postpartum hemorrhage is shown in Figure 48.

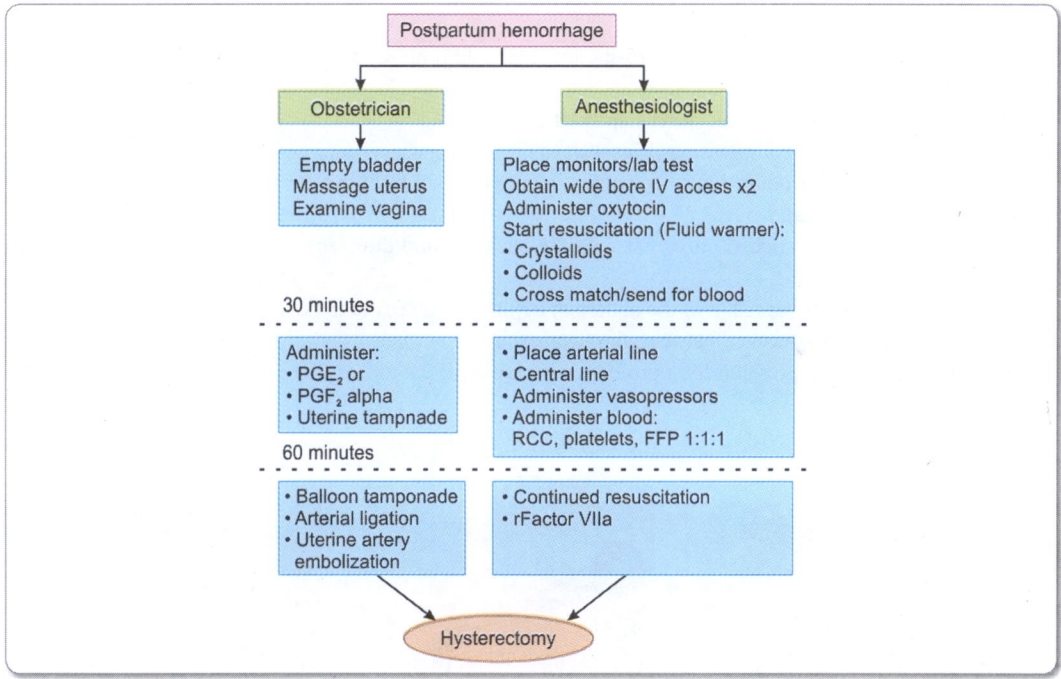

**Fig. 48:** Management of postpartum hemorrhage
*Abbreviations:* FFP, frozen fresh plasma; RCC, red cell concentrated

### Immediate Measures

If the blood loss is more than 1 L, the following measures are taken:

- Call for extra help
- Insert two large bore hole (14 gauge) intravenous cannulas
- Keep patient flat and warm
- Send blood for grouping and cross matching

- Start rapid infusion of 2 L of normal saline or plasma substitutes to re-expand the vascular bed
- Administer oxygen therapy
- Monitoring of pulse, blood pressure, fluids infused, urinary output, drugs given and central venous pressure (CVP)

### Actual Management

- **First step** is to feel the uterus for its consistency to determine the likely cause of bleeding. If the uterus is found atonic:
  - Massage the fundus to make it hard and express the blood clot
  - Methergine 0.2 mg is to be given intramuscularly
  - Empty the bladder
  - Examination of placenta and membranes for its completeness
- **Second step:** If the uterus fails to remain firm and relaxes again with more bleeding:
  - Explore the uterine cavity under general anesthesia
  - Inspect the cervix, vagina and periurethral region to exclude co-existent bleeding sites
  - I/M administration of methergine
  - In refractory cases, 0.25 mg of 15-methyl PGF$_2$ administered intramuscularly to bring back the uterine tone
  - If the uterus remains atonic, next step is taken.
- **Third step:** Bimanual compression (Figs 49A to C)
  - Whole hand is introduced into the vagina in cone-shaped fashion after separating the labia with the fingers of other hand
  - Vaginal hand is clenched into a fist with the back of hand directed posteriorly and the knuckles in the anterior fornix
  - The other hand is placed over the abdomen behind the uterus to make it anteverted
  - Uterus is firmly squeezed between the two hands
  - Continue the compression for a prolonged period until the tone of the uterus is regained

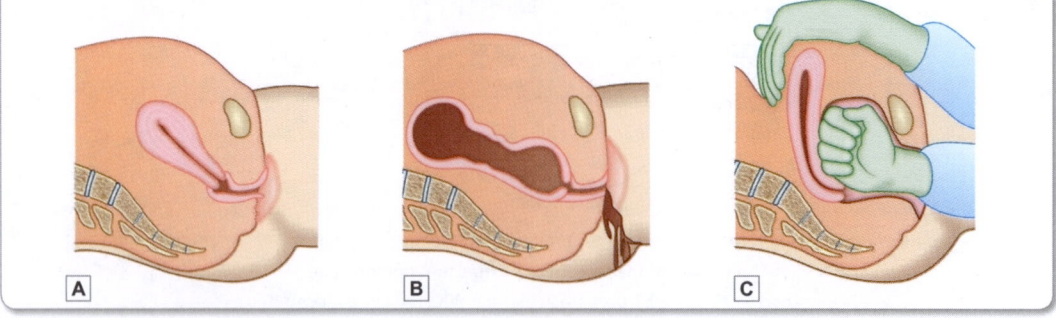

**Figs 49A to C:** Bimanual compression. **A.** Normal postpartum condition with contracted uterus preventing hemorrhage; **B.** Uterine atony allows hemorrhage to flow in the uterus; **C.** Manual fundal massage squeezing of the uterus in an attempt to stop the hemorrhage

- **Step 4: Hot intrauterine douche:** This method is an effective method to stimulate the uterus to regain its tone. The temperature of the fluid should be about 108°F and some antiseptic lotions are mixed in the douche. If this method fails, try next method.

- **Step 5: Tight intrauterine packing** (Fig. 50): This method is useful in case of uncontrolled PPH where other methods have failed and the patient is being prepared for transport to a tertiary care center. In this method, a long 5-meter gauge, 8 cm wide folded twice. The gauge should be soaked in antiseptic cream before introduction. Gauze is placed high up and packed into the fundal area first while the uterus is steadied by external hand. Gradually, the rest of the cavity is packed so that there is no free space inside the uterine cavity. A separate pack is used to insert inside the vagina. Placed abdominal binder. Antibiotic should be given and remove the plug after 24 hours. Action of intrauterine packing is to exert direct hemostatic pressure to the open uterine sinuses.

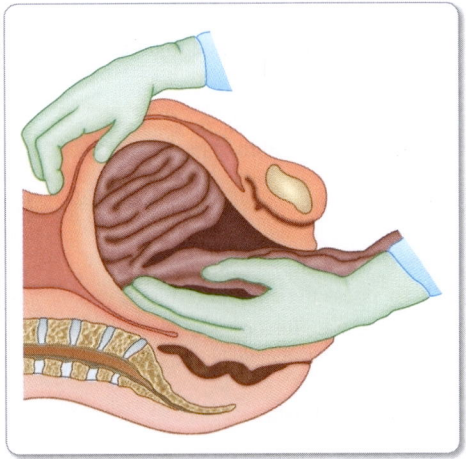

**Fig. 50:** Intrauterine packing

- **Step 6: Balloon tamponade** (Fig. 51): Sengstaken-Blakemore tube is inserted into the uterine cavity and balloon is inflated with normal saline (200–500 mL). It is kept for 4-6 hours. It is considered as the first line surgical management for most women with atonic PPH
- **Step 7: Hysterectomy:** If in spite of the above measures, the uterus fails to contract and blood coagulopathy is excluded, then hysterectomy may have to be performed.

## Secondary Postpartum Hemorrhage

Secondary PPH is bleeding from the genital tract more than 24 hours after delivery of the placenta and may occur up to 6 weeks after delivery. It is most likely to occur between 8 and 14 days after delivery.

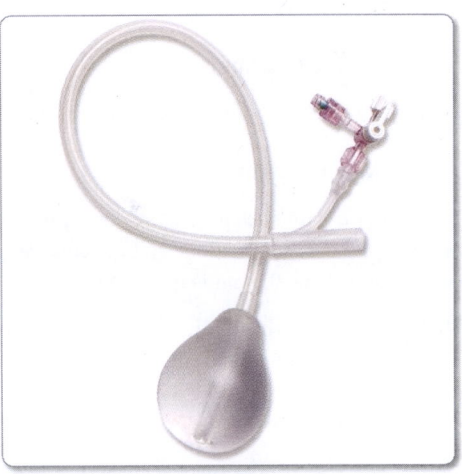

**Fig. 51:** Balloon tamponade

### Causes

- Retained placenta and membranes
- Infection of uterovaginal canal
- Separation of slough over a deep cervico-vaginal laceration
- Sub involution of placental site due to delayed healing process because of low-grade infection
- Secondary hemorrhage from cesarean section
- Withdrawal bleeding following estrogen therapy for suppression of lactation
- **Other causes:** Chorionic epithelioma, cancer of cervix, placental polyps, fibroid uterus

### Signs and Symptoms

- Heavy vaginal bleeding, offensive in nature
- Subinvolution of uterus and patulous os

- Pyrexia and tachycardia
- Anemia: Proportionate to blood loss

## Diagnosis

Ultrasound is useful to detect placenta and membranes inside the cavity.

## Management

### Principles

- To assess the amount of blood loss
- Blood transfusion
- To find out the cause and to take appropriate step to correct it

### Supportive Therapy

- Arrange resuscitative equipment
- If there is uterine bleeding, administer Ergometrine 0.5 mg IM
- Antibiotics as a routine

### Conservative Therapy

Bed rest and observation for 24 hours, if bleeding is mild.

### Active Management

- If there is retained product of conception in the uterine cavity, explore the cavity under general anesthesia
- Gentle curettage is done and the contents are sent for histopathological examination
- Ergometrine 0.5 mg is given IM

Secondary hemorrhage following cesarean section may at times require laparotomy for applying hemostatic sutures. Rarely, ligation of internal iliac artery or hysterectomy may become necessary.

## Nursing Care Plan for Postpartum Hemorrhage

### Subjective Data

- Pain in vaginal area (if due to hematoma)
- Dizziness

### Objective Data

- Uncontrolled bleeding
- Excessive saturation of perineal pads
- Hypotension
- Tachycardia
- Low hematocrit

**Nursing interventions have been tabulated as follows:**

| Nursing interventions | Rationale |
|---|---|
| • Check vital signs and also monitor signs of shock | • Decreased fluid volume will cause blood pressure to drop and patient will go into shock |
| • Assess the amount of blood loss | • Amount of blood loss and presence of blood clots can be helpful to decide treatment |
| • Check for vaginal hematoma | • If bleeding is due to vaginal hematoma, rest and application of an ice pack is very much effective |
| • Monitor intake and output; insert indwelling catheter for accurate measurement | • Decreased urine output (<30–50 mL/hr) may be a sign of hematomas that put pressure on the urethra, or may be a late sign of hypovolemic shock |
| • Note lab values to determine need for blood transfusions or signs of complications | • Watch hematocrit and clotting levels to know the necessity of blood transfusion and for signs and severity of DIC |
| • Administer IV fluids, medications and blood products as necessary | • Fluid replacement may be necessary and depending on the amount of blood lost. In case of decreased hematocrit level, a blood transfusion may be required. Oxytocin is sometimes given to initiate contractions that will help stop bleeding |
| • Perform uterine massage to stimulate contractions following delivery | • These contractions are helpful to stop uterine bleeding |
| • Observe and manage pain | • Continued, unrelieved pain may be due to hematomas or lacerations within the vagina |
| • Provide bedrest to the patient with legs elevated | • Rest and elevation of legs help venous return and minimize bleeding |
| • Assist the client and family to deal with physical and emotional stresses of postpartum complications | • To cope-up with the situation |
| • Prepare patient for surgery if indicated; remain on Nil per oral (NPO) status | • Patient remains NPO to prevent regurgitation |

## ATONIC UTERUS

Atonicity of the uterus is the most common cause (80%) of PPH. This is a failure of the myometrium at the placental site to contract and retract, and to compress torn blood vessels and control blood loss by a living ligature action. When the placenta is attached, the blood flow at the placental site is approximately 500–800 mL/min.

Nurse can take the help of the drug chart shown in Table 8 to be used in postpartum complications.

**TABLE 8: Drug chart used for postpartum complications**

| Classification | Used for | Selected interventions |
|---|---|---|
| Anticoagulants Heparin sodium injection (Hepalean) Lovenox | • Blocks the conversion of prothrombin to thrombin and fibrinogen to fibrin thus decreasing clotting ability<br>• Inhibits thrombus and clot formation | • Heparin IV should be administered as a "piggy back" infusion.<br>• Heparin SC is given deep into the site (abdomen), sites are rotated, do not aspirate, apply pressure (do not massage).<br>• Used to prevent and treat pulmonary embolism and thrombosis. |

*Contd…*

| Classification | Used for | Selected interventions |
|---|---|---|
| Warfarin sodium (Coumadin, Warfilone) | • Interferes with hepatic synthesis of vitamin K – dependent clotting factors (II, VII, IX, X) | • Women on anticoagulopathy therapy should not be given estrogen or aspirin.<br>• Obtain baseline coagulation studies.<br>• Obtain serial coagulation studies while the client is on therapy.<br>• Keep protamine sulfate readily available in case of heparin overdose.<br>• Assess client for bleeding from nose, gums, hematuria, and blood in stool.<br>• Observe color and amount of lochia. Institute pad count.<br>• Avoid IM injections to avoid formation of hematomas.<br>• Inform the client that this drug does not pass into breast milk.<br>• Monitor for the following side effects; hemorrhage, bruising urticaria, and thrombocytopenia.<br>• Women on anticoagulant therapy should not be given estrogen or aspirin.<br>• Obtain baseline coagulation studies while on therapy.<br>• Keep aquamephyton (vitamin K) on hand in case of Coumadin overdose.<br>• Assess client for bleeding from nose, gums, hematuria, and blood in stool.<br>• Observe color and amount of lochia. Institute a pad count.<br>• Avoid IM injections to avoid formation of hematomas.<br>• Inform the client that this drug passes into breast milk and its use is contraindicated during pregnancy. Monitor the side effects, such as hemorrhage, fever, nausea, and cramps. |

## Causes

(Causes of atonic uterus already discussed in the causes of primary PPH)

## Management

[Management of Atonic uterus (step 1 to 7) discussed in actual management of true PPH]

# PERINEAL INJURY/GENITAL TRACT INJURIES/BIRTH CANAL INJURIES

Injuries to the birth canal commonly occur during child birth and contribute significantly to maternal morbidity. The maternal genital tract injuries occur in both natural and instrumental deliveries. Avoidance, early detection and effective management can minimize the morbidity and prevent gynecological problems in future.

**Common sites of birth canal injuries are:**
- Vulva
- Perineum
- Vagina
- Cervix
- Uterus
- Visceral organs

## Vulva

During delivery, lacerations can occur on the vulval skin posteriorly. Even tear can occur on inner aspect of labia minora.

### Management

- Start IV line to maintain fluid deficit
- Insert urinary catheter into the bladder
- Repair the tear with interrupted catgut sutures
- Check vital sign to assess maternal condition

## Perineal Injuries

Perineal injuries commonly occur in primigravida and due to mismanaged second stage of labor. On the basis of extent of injury, it is classified as (Figs 52A to D):

- **First degree:** Involves lacerations of the fourchette (lower end of the posterior vagina) only.
- **Second degree:** Involves fourchette and superficial perineal muscles and in some cases the pubococcygeus muscles
- **Third degree (complete tear):** Involves in addition to the above structures and the anal sphincter.
- **Fourth degree (central tear):** Tear extends to the rectal mucosa.

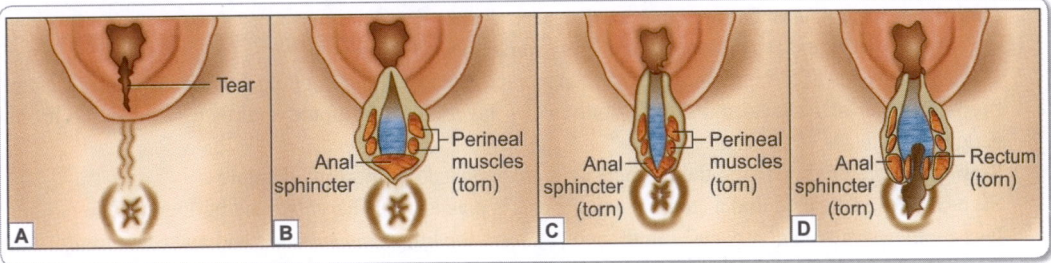

**Figs 52A to D:** Degree of perineal tear. **A.** First degree; **B.** Second degree; **C.** Third degree; **D.** Fourth degree

### Causes of Perineal Injury

Causes of perineal injury are shown in Figure 53.

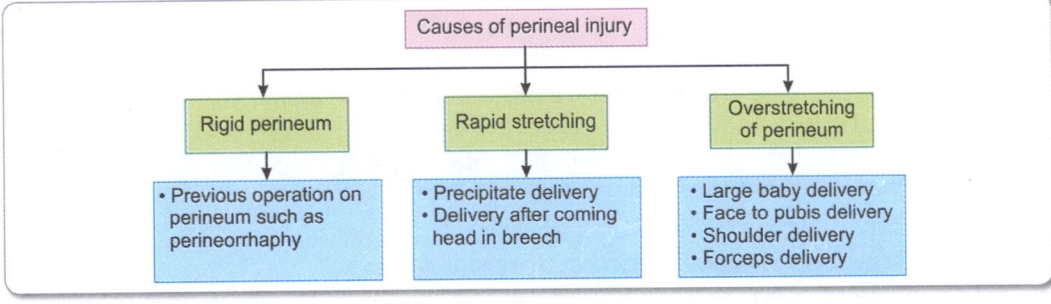

**Fig. 53:** Causes of perineal injury

Chapter 9 ● Management of High-risk Labor

## Prevention

- Maintain flexion of the head so that suboccipitofrontal diameter emerges out of the introitus.
- Avoid bearing down effort before complete cervical dilation to avoid forcible delivery of the head.
- Deliver the head in between contractions.
- Give timely episiotomy.
- Careful delivery of the shoulders.

## Management

- Tear must be repaired immediately following the delivery of placenta to minimize blood loss and infection.
- In case of delay beyond 24 hours, repair is to be withheld.
- Give antibiotics and also apply antiseptic dressing on the wound.
- Allow the wound to heal by granulation tissue or repaired only after the infection is controlled.
- Complete tear (3°) that are delayed beyond 24 hours are repaired after 3 months.

*The following steps are to be followed for repair of perineal tear:*

- **Step-1**
  - Provide lithotomy position
  - Perineal infiltration with 1% lignocaine hydrochloride (10–20 mL)
- **Step-2**
  - Rectal and anal mucosa sutured from above downward with chronic catgut no '0' by interrupted stitches using curved atraumatic needle
  - Muscle walls and facia then sutured using same material
  - The torn ends of the sphincter ani are then reconstituted with figure of eight using '0' chromic catgut.
- **Step-3:** Repair of perineal muscles is done in two layers by interrupted sutures using no. '0' chromic catgut.
- **Step-4:** The vaginal wall and the perineal skin are apposed by interrupted sutures
- **Step-5:** Area is cleaned and a sterile, sanitary pad is placed over the vulva and perineum. The mother's legs are then removed gently and simultaneously form the lithotomy supports and make her comfortable.

## After Care

- Instruct the woman regarding care of perineal wound.
- A low residual diet is given from 2nd day onward.
- Stool softener such as milk of magnesia is given twice daily.
- Intestinal antiseptics, such as metronidazole is given for 5–7 days.

# Vaginal Tears

Injury to the vagina occurs due to instrumental or manipulative delivery. The most common site is the lower third of the vagina. The lower end of the vagina may be torn transversely from its junction with the perineum, leaving a deep cavity behind an intact perineum. Injuries of the upper and lower third of vagina are rare. In such cases, the tears are extensive and often associated with active bleeding.

Rupture of the vault of vagina is called colporrhexis. It may be:

- **Primary:** In primary colporrhexis, only vault of vagina is involved.
- **Secondary:** When colporrhexis is associated with cervical tear. It is complete when peritoneum is opened up.

## Management

A vaginal tear is sutured by interrupted or continuous sutures using chromic catgut no. '0'. In case of extensive lacerations, in addition to sutures, homeostasis may be achieved by intravaginal plugging by roller gauze soaked with glycerin and acriflavine. The plug is removed after 24 hours. If the tear extends high up into the lower segment, laparotomy is to be done simultaneously with resuscitative measures.

## Cervical Tears

During first delivery, minor degree of cervical tear is invariable. The extensive injury is rare. This is the commonest cause of traumatic PPH. Causes of cervical tears are listed in Figure 54.

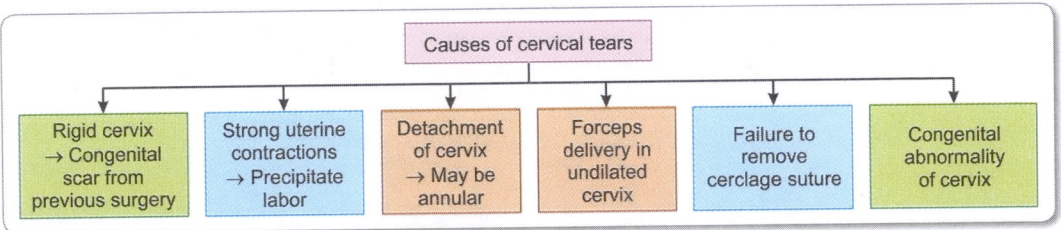

**Fig. 54:** Causes of cervical tears

## Signs

Excessive vaginal bleeding following delivery in the presence of a hard and contracted uterus is suggestive of cervical tear. Exploration of the uterovaginal canal under good light is essential to confirm the diagnosis and assess the tear.

## Complications

Complications of cervical tears are shown in Figure 55.

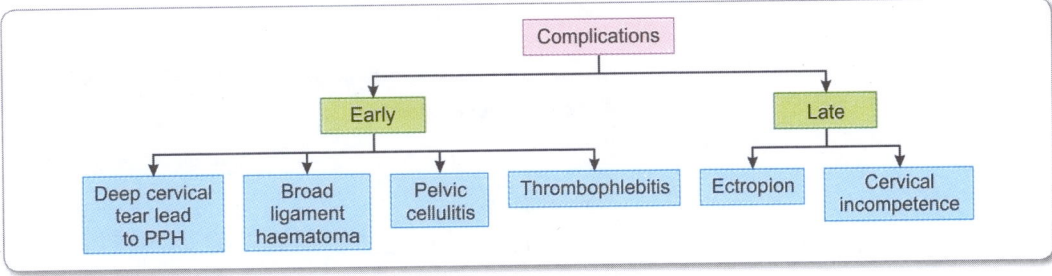

**Fig. 55:** Complications of cervical tears

*Abbreviation:* PPH, postpartum hemorrhage

## Management

Minor tears require no treatment. Deep cervical tears associated with bleeding should be repaired soon after delivery of the placenta. Repair should be done under general anesthesia in lithotomy position with a good light.

## Pelvic Hematoma

Collection of blood anywhere in the area between the pelvic peritoneum and the peritoneal skin are called pelvic hematoma (Figs 56A to C). Types of pelvic hematoma are shown in Figure 57.

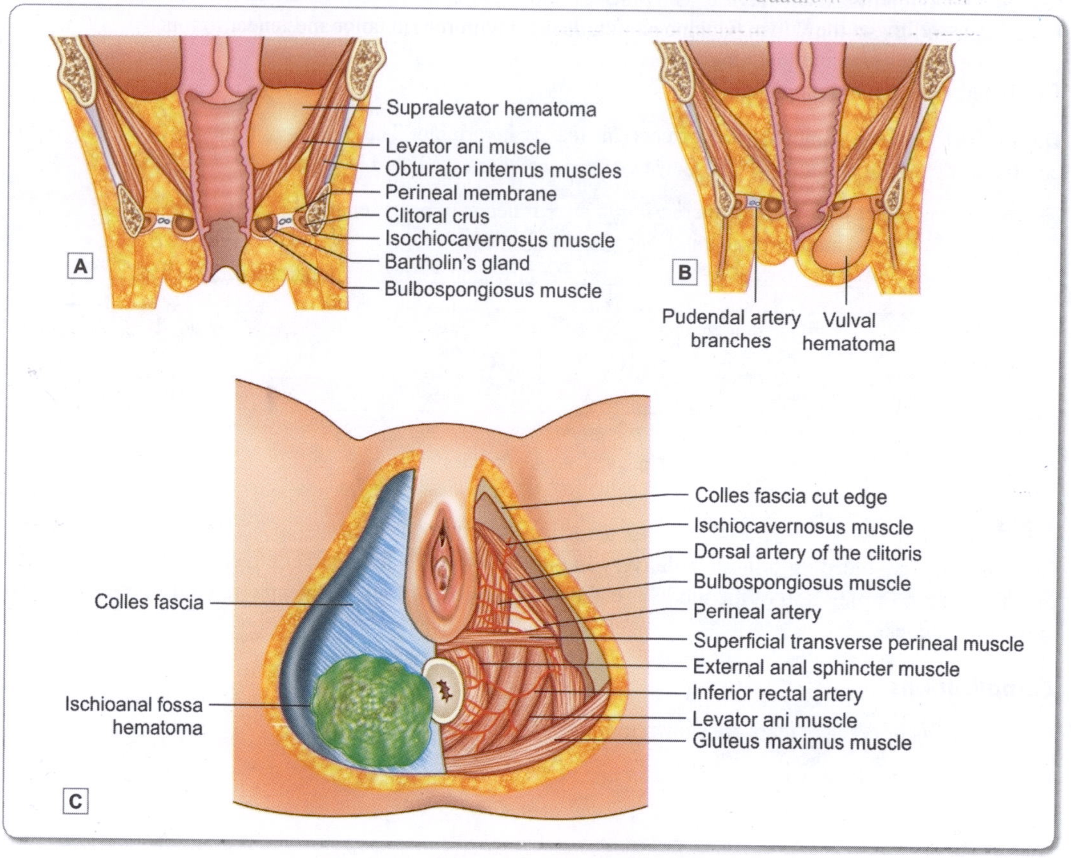

A
- Supralevator hematoma
- Levator ani muscle
- Obturator internus muscles
- Perineal membrane
- Clitoral crus
- Ischiocavernosus muscle
- Bartholin's gland
- Bulbospongiosus muscle

B
Pudendal artery branches    Vulval hematoma

C
- Colles fascia
- Ischioanal fossa hematoma
- Colles fascia cut edge
- Ischiocavernosus muscle
- Dorsal artery of the clitoris
- Bulbospongiosus muscle
- Perineal artery
- Superficial transverse perineal muscle
- External anal sphincter muscle
- Inferior rectal artery
- Levator ani muscle
- Gluteus maximus muscle

**Figs 56A to C:** Pelvic hematoma

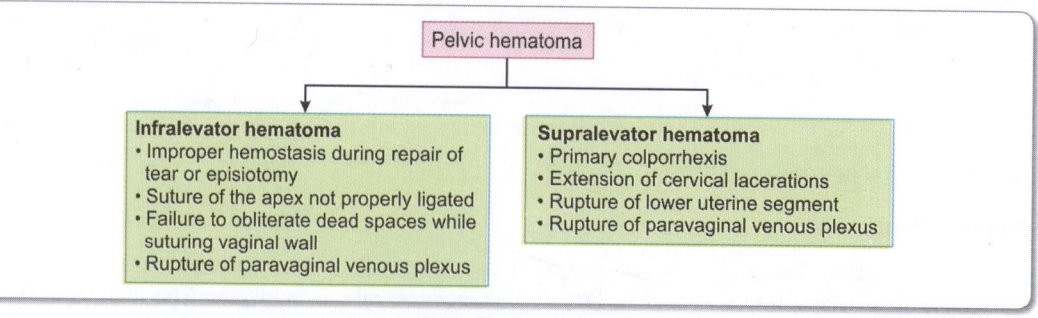

**Fig. 57:** Types of pelvic hematoma

Pelvic hematoma

**Infralevator hematoma**
- Improper hemostasis during repair of tear or episiotomy
- Suture of the apex not properly ligated
- Failure to obliterate dead spaces while suturing vaginal wall
- Rupture of paravaginal venous plexus

**Supralevator hematoma**
- Primary colporrhexis
- Extension of cervical lacerations
- Rupture of lower uterine segment
- Rupture of paravaginal venous plexus

## Manifestations

- Persistent, severe pain in the perineal region
- Rectal tenesmus or bearing down efforts
- Retention of urine
- Shock or collapse
- Tense swelling at the vulva, which becomes dusky and purple in color and tender to touch
- Pallor, rapid pulse and low blood pressure
- Tender pelvic lump on palpation

## Treatment

- Small hematoma (<5 cm) is treated conservatively with cold compresses
- When it is larger than 5 cm or increasing in size, it needs to be evacuated
- Administer blood and narcotic analgesics for pain relief
- Dead space is to be obliterated by deep mattress sutures and a close suction drain may be kept for 24 hours
- Prophylactic antibiotic is to be administered

## Rupture of Uterus

(Already discussed in obstetrical emergencies).

## Visceral Injuries

### Injury to Bladder and Urethra

Bladder injury mostly occurs due to long or difficult vaginal delivery. Delivery with forceps can result in injuries to the pelvic floor and anal sphincter muscles (Figs 58A and B). Prolonged pushing during a vaginal delivery also increases the likelihood of injury to the pelvic nerves and the bladder control problems that might follow. Urethral injury commonly occurs during instrumental delivery at the time of pubiotomy; due to ischemic sloughing, the mechanism is similar to that of bladder necrosis.

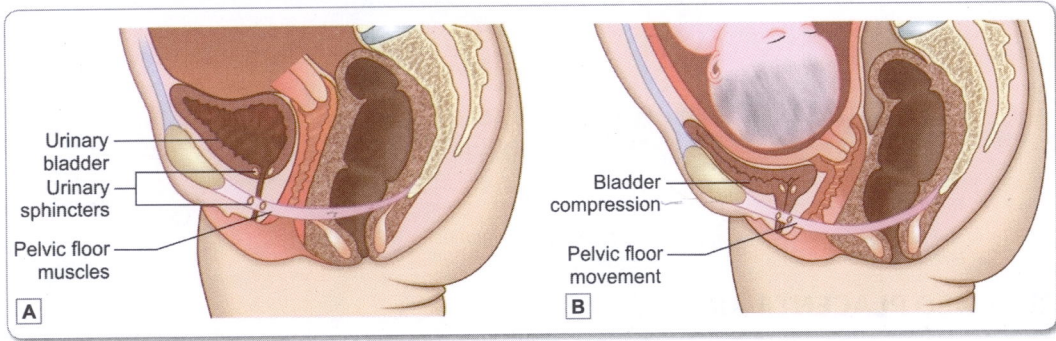

**Figs 58A and B:** Injury to the bladder

### Causes

Injury to bladder may be due to:

- **Trauma:**
  - During instrumental vaginal delivery such as forceps delivery or destructive operations.
  - Abdominal operation, such as hysterectomy for rupture of uterus or repeat cesarean section.

- **Sloughing fistula:** This results from prolonged compression of the bladder between the fetal head and symphysis pubis in obstructed labor.

### Clinical Manifestation

- **Traumatic:**
  - Urine dribbles out following the operative surgery
  - Blood-stained urine following cesarean section (CS) or hysterectomy sloughing fistula
- **Sloughing fistula:**
  - Dribbling of urine occurs after varying interval following prolonged labor (5–7 days)
  - Missing of a chuck of tissue seen on examination.

### Management

- If women's general condition permit and facilities are available, immediate repair is preferable.
- In unfavorable condition, self-retaining catheter is introduced and kept for 10–14 days.
- Urinary antiseptics are given and bladders wash is to be done daily.
- Spontaneous closure may occur and if not, repair is done after 3 months.

### *Injury to the Rectum*

The middle third of the rectum is protected by curved sacral hollow and upper third is protected by peritoneal lining hence rectal injury is rare (Fig. 59). In case of mid pelvic contraction, with flat sacrum, the head of the fetus compresses the rectum or a prolonged period that leads to necrosis of the anterior rectal wall and results in rectovaginal fistula (RVF). Repair of RVF should be postponed for at least 3 months.

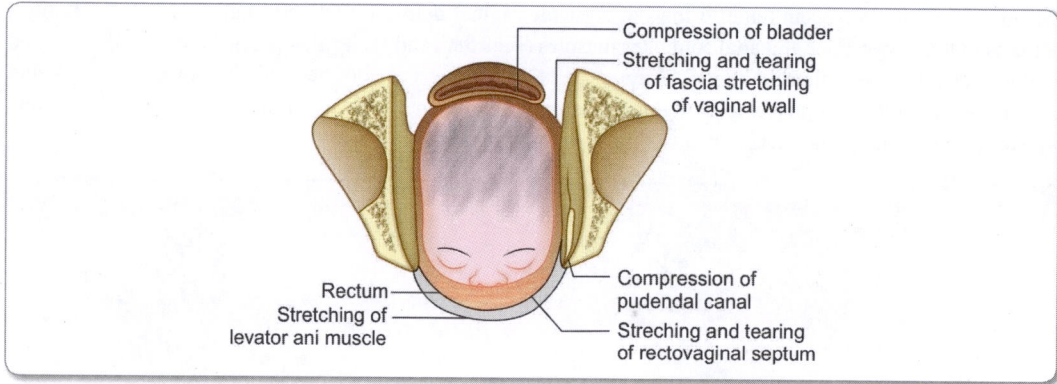

**Fig. 59:** Rectal injuries

# RETAINED PLACENTA AND MEMBRANES

Placenta is said to be retained when it is not expelled out even 30 minutes after the birth of the baby.

## Causes

There are three phases involved in the normal expulsion of placenta

1. Separation through the spongy layer of the decidua.
2. Descent into the lower segment and vagina.
3. Finally, its expulsion to outside.

Interference in any of these physiological processes, results in its retention:

- Placenta completely separated but is retained due to poor voluntary exclusive efforts.
- Simple adherent placenta is due to uterine atonicity in the case of grand multipara, over distension of uterus, prolonged labor and uterine malformation or due to bigger placental surface area.
- Morbid adherent placenta: Partial or rarely complete.
- Placenta incarcerated following partial or complete separation due to constriction ring, premature attempts to deliver placenta before it is separated.

## Diagnosis

Diagnosis of retained placenta is made by an arbitrary time (15 minutes) spent following delivery of the baby. Features of placental separation are assessed. The hour glass contraction or the nature of adherent placenta can only be diagnosed during manual removal.

## Dangers

- Hemorrhage
- Shock due to blood loss, frequent attempts of abdominal manipulation to express the placenta out
- Puerperal sepsis
- Risk of its recurrence in subsequent pregnancies

## Management

- Careful observation of the patient for arbitrary time limit of half an hour for evidence of any bleeding and to note the signs of separation of placenta.
- Empty the bladder by using rubber catheter.
- If the placenta is separated and retained, then extract the placenta by controlled cord traction (CCT) (Fig. 60).
- If unseparated retained placenta: Then manual removal is to be done under general anesthesia.
- In the case of retained placenta complicated by hemorrhagic shock or sepsis, follow the guidelines given here:

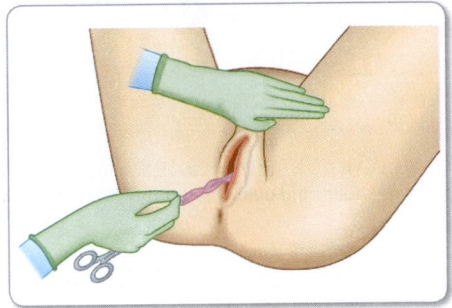

**Fig. 60:** Removal of placenta by cord controlled traction (CCT)

- **Retained placenta with shock but no hemorrhage:** To treat the shock and when condition improves, manual removal of the placenta is done.
- **Retained placenta with hemorrhage:** Same management as outlined for third stage hemorrhage.
- **Retained placenta with sepsis:** The woman is usually delivered outside and is admitted in the referral hospital after few hours or even days after delivery. Sepsis is a potential risk or may already be present. Intrauterine swabs are taken for culture and sensitivity test and broad-spectrum antibiotic is given. Blood transfusion is usually required. On examination, if the placenta is found separated, it is expelled out. If retained, manual removal is done, as soon as the patient's general condition permits.
- **Retained placenta with an episiotomy wound:** The bleeding point of episiotomy is to be secured by artery forceps. A manual removal is done without delay followed by repair of episiotomy wound.

Figures 61A to D give the various attempts done to clear retained placenta.

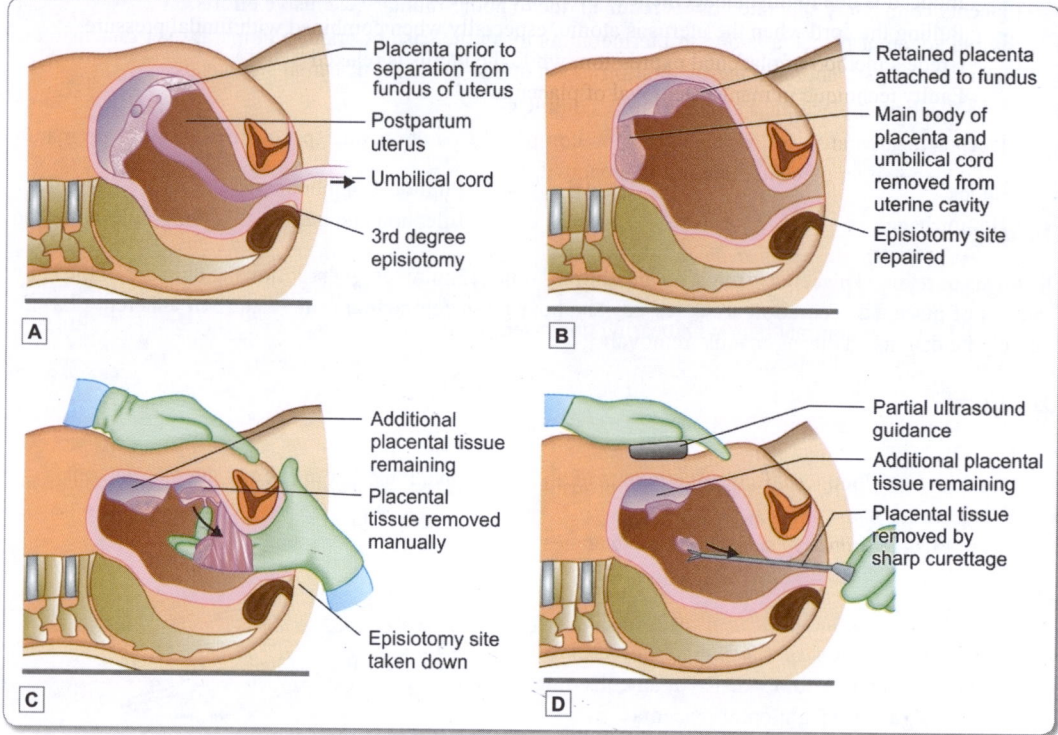

**Figs 61A to D:** Attempts to clear retained placenta following delivery. **A.** Initial postpartum condition; **B.** Condition following placental delivery; **C.** Attempted manual removal; **D.** Attempted removal by sharp curettage

## INVERSION OF THE UTERUS

When the uterus is turned inside out partially or completely, it is called inversion of uterus. It is the life-threating condition of third stage of labor. Incidence is 1:20,000 deliveries.

### Classification of Inversion

- **First degree:** There is dimpling of the fundus, which remains above the level of the internal os.
- **Second degree:** Uterus is inverted and fundus passes through the cervix, but lies inside the vagina.
- **Third degree:** Endometrium with or without the attached placenta is visible outside the vulva. The uterus, cervix and part of the vagina are inverted and visible.

### Causes

The inversion may be spontaneous or induced:

- **Spontaneous (40%):** Spontaneous is brought about by local atony of the placental site over the fundus associated with sharp rise of intra-abdominal pressure as in coughing, sneezing or bearing down effort. Fundal attachment of the placenta, short cord and placenta accreta are often associated.

- **Induced (60%):**
  - Induced is due to mismanagement of 3rd stage of labor
  - Pulling the cord when the uterus is atonic, especially when combined with fundal pressure
  - Crede's method of placental expression, while the uterus is relaxed
  - Faulty technique in manual removal of placenta.

## Complications

- Shock
- Hemorrhage
- Pulmonary embolism
- Infection and uterine sloughing, if left uncared

## Signs and Symptoms

- Acute lower abdominal pain with bearing down sensation
- Varying degree of shock
- On abdominal examination →
  - Dimpling or cupping of fundus
  - Fundus cannot be palpated
- Incomplete variety, a pear-shaped mass protrudes outside the vulva with broad end pointing downwards and looking reddish purple in color.

## Diagnosis

Based on signs and symptoms.

## Prevention

- Not to expel the placenta out when the uterus is in relaxed state
- Avoid pulling the cord simultaneous with fundal pressure
- Use appropriate steps for the manual removal of placenta

## Management

1. **Before shock develops:**
   - Call for extra help
   - Urgent manual replacement must be done
   - Put the patient under general anesthesia
   - Follow these steps for manual replacements of uterus (Figs 62A to C)
     - To push the fundus with the palm of the hand, along the direction of the vagina toward the posterior fornix.
     - To apply counter support by other hand placed on the abdomen.
     - After replacement, the hand should remain inside the uterus until the uterus becomes contracted by parenteral oxytocin or $PGF_{2\alpha}$
     - Remove the placenta manually after uterus becomes contracted; a partially separated placenta may be removed prior to replacement to reduce the bulk, which facilitates replacement
     - Arrange blood for transfusion if shock develops.

2. **After shock develops:**
   - Treatment of shock should be instituted vigorously. Morphine 15 mg I/M, dextrose saline drip and arrangement for blood transfusion is to be made.
   - Push the uterus inside the vagina if possible and to pack the vagina with antiseptic roller gauze.

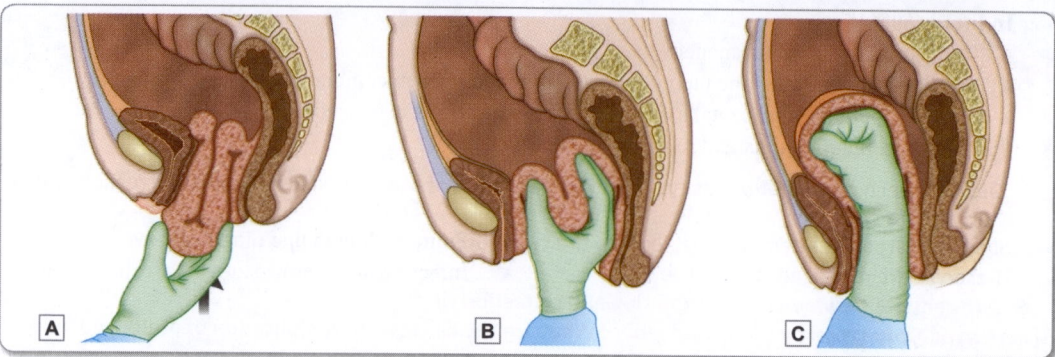

**Figs 62A to C:** Manual replacement of uterus

- Foot end of the bed to be raised
- Replacement of the uterus under general anesthesia to be done along with resuscitative measures.
3. **If manual replacement fails, then use the following measures:**
    - O'Sullivan hydrostatic method (Fig. 63): This involves instillation of warm saline through a douche nozzle. The pressure of the fluids builds up, as several liters are run into the vagina, and restores the uterus to the normal position, while the operator seals off the introitus by one hand inserted into the vagina.
    - If inversion fails due to development of constriction ring, drugs are used to relax constriction ring and facilitate the return of the uterus to its normal position.

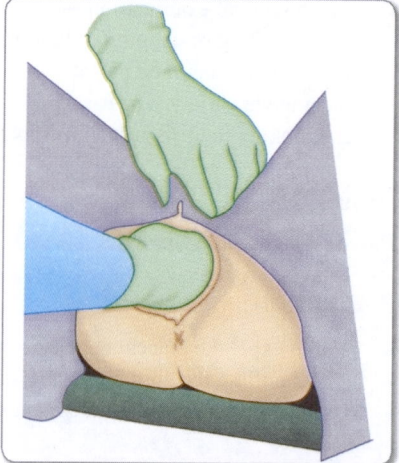

**Fig. 63:** O'Sullivan hydrostatic method

## Nursing Role in Inversion of Uterus

- Identify the signs of impending inversion, report the physician immediately, and call for assistance.
- Promptly assist with the resolution of uterine inversion.
- Immediate manual replacement of the uterus at the time of inversion will prevent cervical entrapment of the uterus; if reinversion is not performed on time, rapid and extreme blood loss may occur, resulting in hypovolemic shock.
- Take steps to prevent or limit hypovolemic shock:
    - Insert a large bore hole cannula for fluid replacement.
    - Check and record maternal vital signs every 5–15 minutes to establish a baseline and document change.
    - A fibrinogen level should be checked to determine the risk of blood clot formation.
    - Prepare the patient for anesthesia as needed.
    - Assist in cardiopulmonary resuscitation, if required.
- If manual reinversion is not successful, prepare the client and family for possible general anesthesia and surgery.

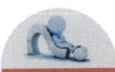

## Assess Yourself

### FREQUENTLY ASKED QUESTIONS IN EXAMS

1. Define breech presentation, its types and complication of breech. Explain the nursing responsibility during breech delivery.
2. Define postpartum hemorrhage. Explain the types of PPH, its causes and diagnostic evaluation.
3. Describe the management of true PPH.
4. Differentiate between contraction ring and retraction ring.
5. What do you mean by prolonged labor? What are the causes and complication of prolonged labor?
6. How can you manage a case of prolonged labor?
7. Write short notes on:
   1. Precipitate labor
   2. Contracted pelvis
   3. Cord prolapse
   4. Management of retained placenta
   5. Obstetrical shock

### MULTIPLE CHOICE QUESTIONS

1. **Contracted pelvis may be caused by the deficiency of which vitamin during early childhood:**
   a. Vitamin $B_{12}$
   b. Vitamin C
   c. Vitamin D
   d. Vitamin A

2. **When alae of both sides are absent and the sacrum directly fused with the innominate bones, the pelvis is known as:**
   a. Robert pelvis
   b. Naegele pelvis
   c. Android pelvis
   d. Anthropoid pelvis

3. **Pendulous abdomen in primigravidae is suspicious of:**
   a. Outlet contraction
   b. Inlet contraction
   c. Mid cavity contraction
   d. Whole pelvis contracted

4. **The cause of abnormal uterine contraction is:**
   a. Hydramnios
   b. Contracted pelvis
   c. Malpresentation
   d. All of the above

5. **To avoid supine hypotension in case of uterine inertia which position is favorable?**
   a. Right lateral
   b. Left lateral
   c. Semi fowler
   d. Squatting position

6. **A ring formed at the junction of upper and lower uterine segment around constricted part of the fetus is known as:**
   a. Retracting ring
   b. Spasmodic ring
   c. Constriction ring
   d. Shirodkar ring

7. **When the combined duration of 1st and 2nd stage of labor is less than 3 hours, it is called:**
   a. Prolonged labor
   b. Precipitate labor
   c. Normal labor
   d. Post-term labor

8. **When there is absence of progress in the absence of strong uterine contractions, the labor is known as:**
   a. Obstructed labor
   b. Prolonged labor
   c. Precipitate labor
   d. Normal labor

9. **The cause of prolonged labor is:**
   a. Fault in passage
   b. Fault in power
   c. Fault in passenger
   d. All of the above

10. **When cervical dilation and descent of presenting part is <1 cm/hr, the labor is:**
    a. Precipitate labor
    b. Prolonged labor
    c. Obstructed labor
    d. Normal labor

11. **When the membranes rupture between 37 and 40 weeks but before the onset of labor, it is known as:**
    a. Preterm PROM
    b. Term PROM
    c. Prolonged PROM
    d. Post term PROM

12. **Normal vaginal pH during pregnancy is:**
    a. 4.5–5.5
    b. 3.5–4.1
    c. 6.5–7.1
    d. 7.5–7.9

13. **When the cord is slipped down below the presenting part and lies in front of it in the intact bag of membranes is called:**
    a. Cord prolapse
    b. Cord presentation
    c. Occult prolapse
    d. True knots of cord

14. **When the fetal blood vessels lie over the os in front of the presenting part is called:**
    a. Cord prolapse
    b. Cord presentation
    c. Occult prolapse
    d. Vasa previa

15. **Definite recoil of the head back against the perineum is:**
    a. Turtle neck sign
    b. Chadwick sign
    c. Goodell's sign
    d. Dystocia

16. **A state of circulatory inadequacy with poor tissue perfusion resulting in generalized cellular hypoxia is called:**
    a. Vasa previa
    b. Card prolapse
    c. Obstetric shock
    d. Amniotic fluid embolism

17. **The shock that occurs due to intrauterine fetal death, amniotic fluid embolism, DIC is called:**
    a. Hypovolemic shock
    b. Septic shock
    c. Cardiogenic shock
    d. Neurogenic shock

18. **Uterine rupture occurs due to:**
    a. Previous cesarean section scar
    b. Hysterectomy scar
    c. Version
    d. All of the above

19. **Bleeding occurs subsequent to expulsion of placenta is called:**
    a. True PPH
    b. Third state hemorrhage
    c. Secondary hemorrhage
    d. Delayed puerperal hemorrhage

20. **When the uterus is inverted and fundus passes through the cervix, but lies inside the vagina is:**
    a. 1° inversion of uterus
    b. 2° Inversion of uterus
    c. 3° Inversion of uterus
    d. Complete Inversion of uterus

## Answer Key

| 1. c | 2. a | 3. b | 4. d | 5. b | 6. c | 7. b |
|------|------|------|------|------|------|------|
| 8. a | 9. d | 10. b | 11. b | 12. a | 13. b | 14. d |
| 15. a | 16. c | 17. a | 18. d | 19. a | 20. b | |

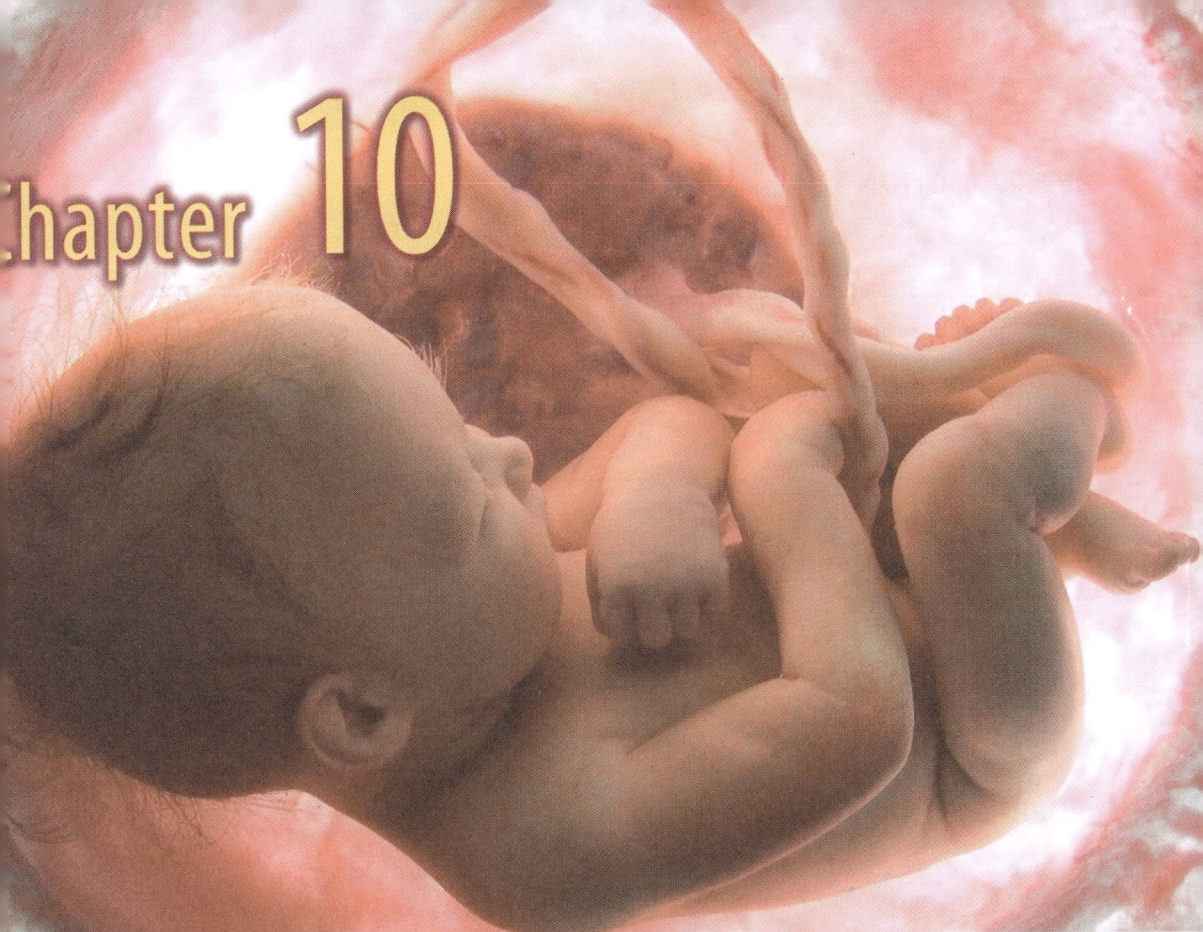

# Management of Complications of Puerperium

# INTRODUCTION

World Health Organization (WHO) describes the postnatal period as the most critical and yet the most neglected phase in the lives of the mothers and babies; most deaths occur during the postnatal period. Puerperal complications include many of those encountered during pregnancy, however some of them are most common at postpartum period.

The common postpartum complications are given in Figure 1.

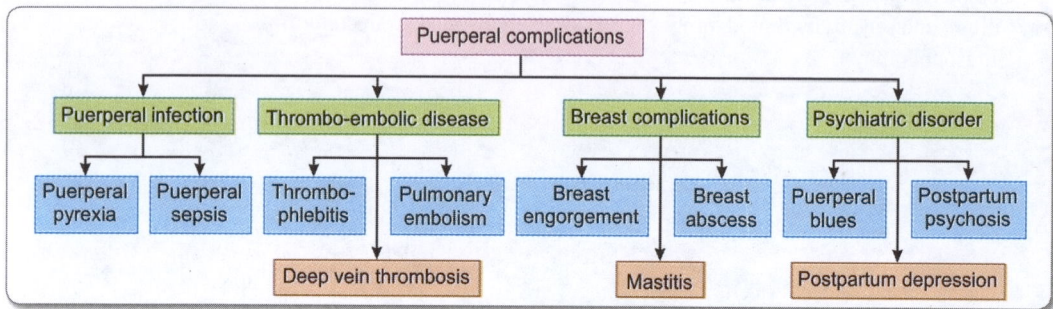

**Fig. 1:** Complications of puerperium

# PUERPERAL INFECTIONS

It is infection of the genital tract which has occurred as a complication of delivery.

Due to infection of the genital tract the woman may have:

- **Puerperal pyrexia:** A rise of temperature reaching 100°F (38°C) or more (measured orally) on two separate occasions at 24 hours apart, within first 10 days after delivery.
- **Puerperal sepsis:** An infection of the genital tract occurs as a complication of delivery.

## Causes

- Endometritis
- Atelectasis
- Wound infection
- Septic pelvic thrombophlebitis

## Signs and Symptoms

- Local infection
  - Rise of temperature
  - Malaise
  - Headache
  - Redness and swelling of the episiotomy or surgical wound
  - Pus formation in the episiotomy or lower segment cesarean section (LSCS) surgical wound
- Uterine infection
  - Rise in temperature with chills and rigor
  - Rapid pulse
  - Copious and offensive lochial discharge
  - Subinvolution of uterus
  - Breathlessness, abdominal pain and dysuria

- Spreading infection (sepsis)
  - Parametritis
  - Pelvic peritonitis
  - Pelvic abscess

## Investigations

- Complete blood count (CBC)
- Culture and sensitivity (blood, urine vaginal swab and wound swab culture)
- Ultrasonography

## Management

### Prophylactic Measures

A prophylactic measure includes:

- Antenatal prophylaxis:
  - Improvement of nutritional status
  - Removal of septic focus (skin, tonsils, etc.) from the body
- Intranatal prophylaxis:
  - Full surgical asepsis during delivery (clean surface, clean hands and clean instruments)
  - Screening of high risk patient (patient with chronic disease such as asthma, diabetes or history of any immune disorder)
  - Prophylactic use of antibiotic before cesarean section
- Postpartum prophylaxis:
  - Aseptic precautions for at least 1 week following delivery
  - Too many visitors are restricted
  - Use sterilized sanitary pads
  - Isolation of infected babies from mother.

### Treatment

General care includes:

- Isolation of the patient
- Provide adequate fluid and calories
- If mother is anemic, provide iron supplemental therapy or in severe case blood transfusion
- Indwelling catheter is to be used to empty the bladder due to pelvic abscess
- Antibiotic therapy:
  - **Gentamycin:** 2 mg/kg IV loading dose, followed 1.5 mg/kg IV every 8 hours (maintenance dose)
  - **Clindamycin:** 900 mg IV every 8 hourly
  - **Metronidazole:** 0.5 IV/8 hourly

Surgical treatment includes:

- **Perineal wound:**
  - Removal of stitches to facilitate drainage and relieve pain
  - Cleaning the wound with antiseptic solution and apply sterile dressing
  - After infection is controlled, resuturing should be done

- **Retained uterine product:** Dilatation and evacuation are to be done
- **Pelvic abscess:** Drained by colpotomy under ultrasonographic guidance
- **Wound dehiscence:**
  - Scrubbing of episiotomy and abdominal wound twice daily
  - Debridement of necrotic tissue
  - Resuturing done
  - Administer antimicrobial therapy
- **Laparotomy:** In the case of severe peritonitis, laparotomy is indicated. If no pathology is found, drainage of pus is effective
- **Hysterectomy:** In the case of rupture or perforation, multiple abscesses or gangrenous uterus

## THROMBOEMBOLIC DISORDERS

### Thrombophlebitis

It is a condition which originates in the thrombosed veins at the placental side by anaerobic streptococci or bacteroides. When localized in the pelvis, it is called pelvic thrombophlebitis.

There can be extra pelvic spread and can reach the lungs or kidney. In the case of retrograde extension of ileofemoral vein, the clinical pathological condition named phlegmasia alba dolens or white legs is produced.

#### Signs and Symptoms

- Mild fever
- Headache
- Tachycardia
- Pain in the affected leg
- Affected leg is swollen, white and cold
- Tenderness

#### Diagnosis

- Venous ultrasound
- Computed tomography (CT) scan
- Magnetic resonance imaging (MRI)
- Venography
- Phlebography

#### Management

- Anticoagulant therapy, i.e. heparin therapy is started and continued for 7–10 days or more. The dose depends upon the estimation of clotting time, which should be done daily. It is followed by warfarin (oral). The dose of warfarin is adjusted by estimating prothrombin time of blood.
- **Bed rest:** Restriction of movement until the clotting time has shown signs of improvement.
- Analgesics are given to relieve pain.
- After about a week, on subsiding pain, slight movement can be started but in case of suspected deep vein thrombosis (DVT), the patient is not allowed to walk about.

### Pulmonary Embolism

Whenever there is venous thrombosis in leg or pelvis, the thrombus (clot) breaks away from the vessel and enters the systemic circulation. When it reaches in pulmonary artery, it causes obstruction due to smaller lumen, the condition known as pulmonary embolism.

Pulmonary embolism is likely to occur in 80–90% cases due to DVT. The predisposing factors are:

- Cesarean section
- Obesity
- High parity (more than 5)
- Immobility (prolonged bed rest)
- Trauma to legs (fracture)
- Smoking

## Signs and Symptoms

- Tachycardia (>100 bpm)
- Dyspnea
- Pleuritic chest pain
- Cough
- Tachypnea (>20 breath/min)
- Hemoptysis (blood in sputum)
- Rise in temperature

## Diagnosis

- X-ray chest
- Arterial blood gas
- Electrocardiogram (ECG)
- Doppler ultrasound
- Lung scans
- Pulmonary angiography
- Magnetic resonance angiography

## Management

### Prophylaxis

- Use elastic compression stocking (Fig. 2) intermittent pneumatic compression devices during surgery
- Prevention of trauma, sepsis, anemia in pregnancy and labor
- Dehydration during delivery should be avoided

### Active Treatment

- Resuscitation:
  - Cardiac massage
  - Oxygen therapy
  - Intravenous heparin bolus dose of 5000 IU
  - Morphine 15 mg/IV
- Anticoagulant continued for 6 weeks to 6 months, until heparin level is maintained at 0.2–0.4 U/mL or activated partial thromboplastin time (APTT) is 1.5–2.5 times
- IV fluid support
- Maintain blood pressure either by dopamine/adrenaline
- Tachycardia is counteracted by digitalis

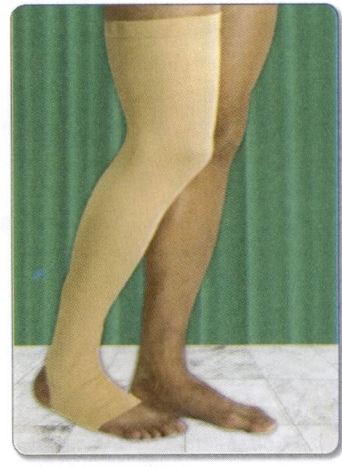

**Fig. 2:** Elastic compression stocking

- Surgical treatment includes:
  - Embolectomy
  - Placement of inferior vena caval filter (Fig. 3)
  - Ligation of inferior vena cava and ovarian veins.

## Deep Vein Thrombosis

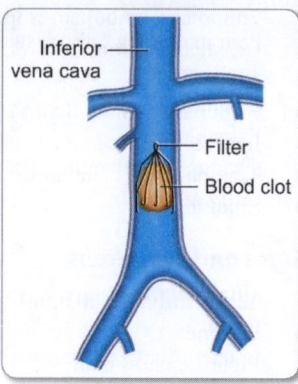

In deep vein thrombosis, a thrombus is formed in the deep vein of the legs. It is a rare complication during puerperium. However, it can be rapidly fatal if the clot breaks away from the vein in the leg and travels to heart, lungs or brain, blocking vital blood vessels.

### Causes

The blood clots of deep vein thrombosis can be caused by anything that prevents the blood from circulating or clotting normally, such as injury to a vein, surgery, certain medications and limited movement.

**Fig. 3:** Inferior caval filter

### Risk Factors

- **Inheriting a blood-clotting disorder.** Some people inherit a disorder that makes their blood clot more easily. This condition on its own might not cause blood clots unless combined with one or more other risk factors.
- **Prolonged bed rest, such as during a long hospital stay, or paralysis:** When the legs remain still for long periods, the calf muscles do not contract to help blood circulate, which can increase the risk of blood clots.
- **Injury or surgery:** Injury to veins or surgery can increase the risk of blood clots.
- **Pregnancy:** Pregnancy increases the pressure in the veins of pelvis and legs. Women with an inherited clotting disorder are especially at risk. The risk of blood clots from pregnancy can continue for up to 6 weeks after delivery.
- **Birth control pills (oral contraceptives) or hormone replacement therapy:** Both can increase the bloods, ability to clot.
- **Being overweight or obese:** Being overweight increases the pressure in the veins in the pelvis and legs.
- **Smoking.** Smoking affects blood clotting and circulation, which can increase the risk of DVT.
- **Cancer:** Some forms of cancer increase substances in the blood that cause the blood to clot. Some forms of cancer treatment also increase the risk of blood clots.
- **Heart failure:** This increases the risk of DVT and pulmonary embolism. Because people with heart failure have limited heart and lung function, the symptoms caused by even a small pulmonary embolism are more noticeable.
- **Inflammatory bowel disease:** Bowel diseases, such as Crohn's disease or ulcerative colitis, increase the risk of DVT.
- **A personal or family history of deep vein thrombosis or pulmonary embolism:** Increases the risk of developing a DVT.
- **Age.** Being older than 60 increases the risk of DVT, though it can occur at any age.
- **Sitting for long periods of time, such as when driving or flying:** When the legs remain still for hours, the calf muscles don't contract, which normally helps blood circulate. Blood clots can form in the calves of the legs if the calf muscles don't move for long periods.

## Clinical Features

- Pain in one leg only: Usually sudden onset
- Tenderness
- Swelling
- Palpable cord
- Change in limb color: The affected leg appears a bit red
- Calf pain

## Diagnosis

- **Ultrasound:** A transducer is placed over the part of the body where there's a clot sends sound waves into the area. As the sound waves travel through the tissue and reflect back, a computer transforms the waves into a moving image on a video screen. A clot might be visible in the image.

   Sometimes a series of ultrasound are conducted over several days to identify whether already formed blood clot is growing or any new clot forms.
- **Blood test:** Mostly the people who suffer from deep vein thrombosis have an elevated blood level of a substance called D dimer.
- **Venography:** In venography, a dye is injected into a large vein of the foot or ankle. An X-ray creates an image of the veins in the legs and feet, to look for clots.
- **CT or MRI scans:** Either can provide visual images of the veins and might show the presence of a clot.

## Treatment

- **Support stockings:** To treat deep vein thrombosis supportive stockings are used to prevent the clot from getting bigger and preventing it from breaking loose and causing a pulmonary embolism. It also reduces the chances of reoccurrence of deep vein thrombosis.
- **Blood thinners:** Anticoagulants, also called blood thinner and is commonly used to treat deep vein thrombosis. Anticoagulants can be injected or taken as pills, decrease the blood's ability to clot. They don't break up existing blood clots, but prevent the clots from getting bigger and reduce the risk of developing more clots.

   Heparin is typically given intravenously. Other similar anticoagulants, such as enoxaparin (lovenox), dalteparin (fragmin) or fondaparinux (arixtra), are injected under the skin.
- **Clot busters:** In case of severe deep vein thrombosis or pulmonary embolism, when the medications are not working, doctor might prescribe drugs that break up clots quickly, called clot busters or thrombolytics.

   Thrombolytics are given through an IV line to break up blood clots or through a catheter placed directly into the clot. It is reserved for severe cases of blood clots because it can cause serious bleeding.
- **Filters:** A vena cava filter prevents clots that break loose from lodging in the lungs.
- **Compression stockings:** These are worn in deep vein thrombosis, on the legs from the feet to about the level of the knees to prevent swelling.

# BREAST COMPLICATIONS

## Breast Engorgement

Breast engorgement (Fig. 4) is a condition which occurs due to:

- Excessive production of milk
- Obstruction in the outflow of milk
- Poor removal of milk by baby

### Onset

It usually manifests after the milk secretion starts (3rd or 4th postpartum day).

### Signs and Symptoms

- Both breasts feel tense, tender and firm
- Nipples become edematous and flushed
- The veins over the breasts become engorged and prominent
- Generalized malaise and rise in temperature
- Painful breastfeeding

### Prevention

- To initiate breastfeeding early and at frequent interval
- Exclusive breastfeeding on demand
- Feeding in sitting position.

### Management

- Support the breast with a binder or brassiere
- Manual expression of milk after each feeding and keeping the interval short between feeds
- Analgesics for pain
- Cause of poor sucking by the newborn should be corrected
- In severe cases, to remove milk from breast, breast pump may be helpful.

### Mastitis

Mastitis (Fig. 5) is an infection of milk ducts (lactiferous ducts) and tissues of the breast. It occurs frequently during the time of breastfeeding by cross infection from baby to mother. The causative organism is *Staphylococcus aureus*.

### Pathophysiology

The pathophysiology of cellulitis and mammary adenitis has been shown in Figure 6.

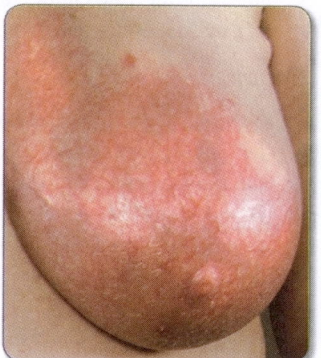

**Fig. 5:** Mastitis

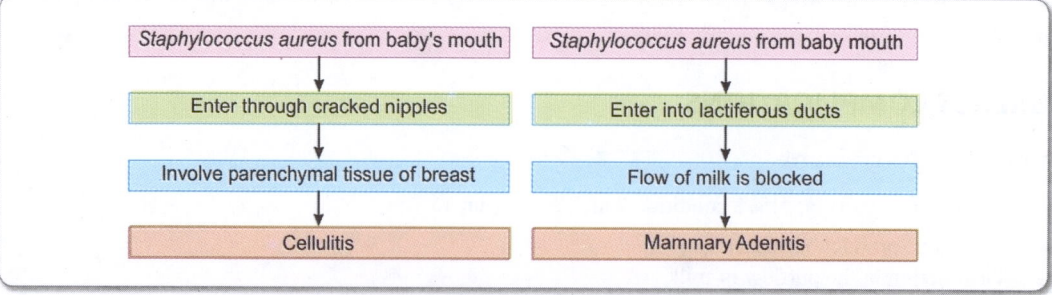

**Fig. 6:** Pathophysiology of cellulitis and mammary adenitis

## Signs and Symptoms

- Generalized malaise and headache
- Fever (102°F or over) with chills
- Severe pain and swelling in one quadrant of the breast with its apex at the nipple
- Overlying skin is hot and flushed, feels tense and tender

## Diagnosis

On microscopic examination, breast milk shows leucocytes more than $10^6$/mL and bacterial count more than $10^3$/mL indicates mastitis.

## Complications

Due to excessive destruction of breast tissue, breast abscess occurs.

## Management

- Prophylactic:
  - Thorough hand washing before each feed
  - Prevention of engorgement
  - Cleaning the nipples before and after each feed
  - Keep the nipple dry
  - Isolation of the infected baby
- Curative:
  - Isolation of mother and baby
  - Suspension of breastfeeding on the affected side until the infection is controlled
  - Manual expression of milk to relieve engorgement
  - Breast support
  - Plenty of oral fluids
  - Continue breastfeeding from uninfected side to establish let down
  - The infected side is emptied manually with each feed
  - Provide analgesics to relieve pain
  - Antibiotic therapy for at least 10 days

## Breast Abscess

Breast abscess (Fig. 7) is a condition in which there is acute inflammation and infection with a collection of pus within the breast tissue.

## Causes

- Bacterial infection: *Staphylococcus* or *streptococcus*
- Cracked nipples
- Tight bra put pressure on milk ducts
- Skipping breastfeeding sessions
- Stress and exhaustion in new mothers

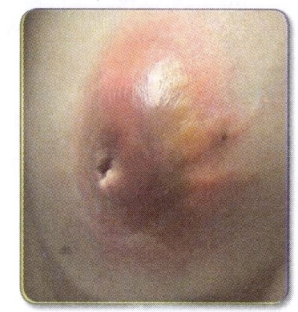

**Fig. 7:** Breast abscess

## Signs and Symptoms

- Flushed breast not responding to antibiotics promptly
- Brown-colored edema of the overlying skin

- Marked tenderness with fluctuation
- Swinging temperature
- Redness, hardness and colicky pain in breast

### Treatment

- Prevent irritation or cracking of the nipples
- Lose weight
- Clean the skin on the breast and nipple with extra care
- Supporting and bandaging the breast
- Manual expression of milk
- Not allowing the baby to feed from affected side
- Antibiotic such as penicillin to treat infection
- Surgery to open and drain the abscess

## URINARY COMPLICATIONS

### Urinary Tract Infection

A urinary tract infection (UTI) is an infection in any part of the urinary system—kidneys, ureters, bladder and urethra. Most infections involve the lower urinary tract—the bladder and the urethra. Women are at greater risk of developing a UTI compared to men.

### Causes

- Reoccurrence of previous cystitis/pyelitis
- Asymptomatic bacteriuria becomes overt
- Effect of frequent catheterization, either during labor or in early puerperium to relieve retention of urine
- Stasis of urine during early puerperium due to lack of bladder tone and less desire to pass urine

### Symptoms

- A strong, persistent urge to urinate
- A burning sensation when urinating
- Passing frequent, small amounts of urine
- Urine that appears cloudy
- Urine that appears red, bright pink or cola-colored—a sign of blood in the urine
- Strong-smelling urine
- Pelvic pain, in women—especially in the center of the pelvis and around the area of the pubic bone

### Types

Each type of UTI may result in more-specific signs and symptoms, depending on which part of urinary tract is infected (Table 1).

### Diagnosis

- History
- Physical examination
- Lab. parameters
  - Urinalysis with microscopy for WBC, bacteria
  - Urine culture for sensitivity

**TABLE 1:** UTI infection—signs and symptoms

| Part of urinary tract affected | Signs and symptoms |
|---|---|
| Kidneys (acute pyelonephritis) | • Upper back and side (flank) pain<br>• High fever<br>• Shaking and chills<br>• Nausea<br>• Vomiting |
| Bladder (cystitis) | • Pelvic pressure<br>• Lower abdomen discomfort<br>• Frequent, painful urination<br>• Blood in urine |
| Urethra (urethritis) | • Burning with urination<br>• Discharge |

## Complications

- Recurrent infections, especially in women who experience two or more UTIs in a six-month period or four or more within a year.
- Permanent kidney damage from an acute or chronic kidney infection (pyelonephritis) due to an untreated UTI.
- Increased risk in pregnant women of delivering low-birth-weight or premature infants.
- Sepsis, a potentially life-threatening complication of an infection, especially if the infection works its way up the urinary tract to the kidneys.

## Prevention

- **Drink plenty of liquids, especially water:** Drinking water helps dilute the urine and ensures that person urinate more frequently—allowing bacteria to be flushed out from the urinary tract before an infection can begin.
- **Drink cranberry juice:** Cranberry juice prevents UTIs, it might not be harmful.
- **Wipe from front to back:** Doing so after urinating and after a bowel movement helps prevent bacteria in the anal region from spreading to the vagina and urethra.
- **Avoid potentially irritating feminine products:** Using deodorant sprays or other feminine products, such as douches and powders, in the genital area can irritate the urethra.

## Treatment

Antibiotic treatment includes ciprofloxacin 100 mg twice daily, amoxicillin 250 mg three times daily of cephalexin 250 mg four times daily.

## Retention of Urine

Urinary retention is an inability to completely empty the bladder. This is a common complication in early puerperium.

## Symptoms

- Difficulty starting to urinate
- Frequent urination
- Difficulty in fully emptying the bladder

- Inability to feel when bladder is full
- Increased abdominal pressure
- Weak dribble or stream of urine
- Loss of small amounts of urine during the day
- Lack of urge to urinate
- Nocturia (waking up more than two times at night to urinate)
- Strained efforts to push urine out of the bladder

## Causes

Two types of urinary retention are: Obstructive and nonobstructive.

1. **Obstructive urinary retention:** In this, urine cannot flow freely through the urinary tract.
   Obstructive retention may result from:
   - Cancer
   - Kidney or bladder stones
2. **Nonobstructive urinary retention:** It is due to weak bladder muscle and nerve problems that interfere with signals between the brain and the bladder. If the nerves aren't working properly, the brain may not get the message that the bladder is full.
   The most common causes of nonobstructive urinary retention are:
   - Pelvic injury or trauma
   - Stroke
   - Impaired muscle or nerve function due to medication or anesthesia
   - Accidents that injure the brain or spinal cord
   - Vaginal childbirth

## Treatment

If simple measure fails to initiate micturition, an indwelling catheter is to be kept in place for about 48 hours. It is not only helpful in emptying the bladder but also helps in regaining the normal bladder tone and sensation of fullness. Following removal of catheter, the amount of residual urine is to be measured. If it is found to be more than 100 mL, continuous drainage is resumed. Appropriate urinary antiseptics should be administered for about 5–7 days.

## Incontinence of Urine

When the woman passes urine regularly it is called incontinence. The incontinence may be of the following types:

- Overflow incontinence is a form of urinary incontinence, characterized by the involuntary release of urine from an overfull urinary bladder, often in the absence of any urge to urinate.
- Stress incontinence occurs when physical movement or activity, such as coughing, sneezing, running or heavy lifting puts pressure (stress) on the bladder.
- True (continuous) incontinence in this case, urine escapes continuously by day and night. It is caused by: urinary fistula as vesicovaginal fistula, ectopia vesica.

Stress incontinence usually appears in late puerperium, whereas true incontinence in the form of genitourinary fistula usually appears soon following delivery or within first week of puerperium.

## Causes

### Temporary Urinary Incontinence

Certain drinks, foods and medications may act as diuretics—stimulating the bladder and increasing the volume of urine. They include:

- Alcohol
- Carbonated drinks and sparkling water
- Caffeine
- Artificial sweeteners
- Chocolate
- Chili peppers
- Heart and blood pressure medications, sedatives, and muscle relaxants
- Foods that are high in spice, sugar or acid, especially citrus fruits
- Large doses of vitamin C

  Urinary incontinence may also be caused by an easily treatable medical condition, such as:
  - **Urinary tract infection:** Infections can irritate bladder, causing the person to have strong urges to urinate.
  - **Constipation:** The rectum is located near the bladder and shares many of the same nerves. Hard, compacted stool in the rectum causes the nerves to be overactive and increases urinary frequency.

### Persistent Urinary Incontinence

Urinary incontinence can also be a persistent condition caused by underlying physical problems or changes, including:

- **Pregnancy:** Hormonal changes and the increased weight of the fetus can cause stress incontinence.
- **Childbirth:** Vaginal delivery can weaken the bladder muscles, damage bladder nerves and supportive tissue, leading to a dropped (prolapsed) pelvic floor. With prolapse, the bladder, uterus, rectum or small intestine can get pushed down from the usual position and protrude into the vagina. Such protrusions can cause urinary incontinence.
- **Changes with age:** Aging of the bladder muscle can decrease the bladder capacity to store urine. When the person gets older, involuntary bladder contractions become more frequent and result in urinary incontinence.
- **Menopause:** After menopause there is less production of estrogen hormone. This hormone keeps the lining of the bladder and urethra healthy. Deterioration of these tissues can aggravate incontinence.
- **Hysterectomy:** In women, the bladder and uterus are supported by many of the same muscles and ligaments. Any surgery that involves a woman's reproductive system, including removal of the uterus, may damage the supporting pelvic floor muscles, which can lead to incontinence.
- **Obstruction:** Any tumor or urinary stones anywhere along the urinary tract can block the normal flow of urine, leading to overflow incontinence.
- **Neurological disorders:** Brain tumor, multiple sclerosis, Parkinson's disease, stroke or a spinal injury can interfere with nerve signals involved in bladder control, causing urinary incontinence.

## Risk Factors

Factors that increase the risk of developing urinary incontinence include:

- **Gender:** Women are more likely to have stress incontinence. Normal female anatomy, pregnancy, childbirth and menopause account for this difference. On the other hand, men with prostate gland problems are at increased risk of urge and overflow incontinence.

- **Age:** As the person gets older, bladder and urethral muscles lose some of their strength and they increase the chances of involuntary urine release.
- **Being overweight:** Extra weight increases pressure on the bladder and surrounding muscles, which weakens them and allows urine to leak out when the person coughs or sneezes.
- **Smoking:** Use of tobacco use may increase the risk of urinary incontinence.
- **Family history:** If a close family member has urinary incontinence (urge incontinence), the risk of developing the condition is higher.
- **Other diseases:** Neurological disease or diabetes may increase the risk of incontinence.

### Diagnosis

- Stress incontinence is established by noting the escape of urine through the urethral opening during stress
- In true incontinence, fistula is established by noting the fistulas site by examining the patient in Sims' position, using Sims' speculum or by vaginal swab test, if fistula is tiny.

### Treatment

Treatment depends on the type of incontinence, its severity and underlying cause. A combination of treatment may be needed.

- **Behavioral techniques**
  - **Bladder training:** To delay urination after the person gets the urge to go.
  - **Double voiding:** Means urinating, then waiting for a few minutes and trying again.
  - **Scheduled toilet trips:** To urinate every 2–4 hours rather than waiting for the need to go.
  - **Fluid and diet management:** Example: Avoid alcohol, caffeine or acid foods. Reducing liquid consumption, losing weight or increasing physical activity, etc.
- **Pelvic floor muscle exercises:** Example: Kegel exercise to strengthen pelvic floor muscles that help to control urination.
- **Medication:** Example: Anticholinergics (ditropan, enablex), mirabegron, alphablockers (flomax, cardura) topical estrogen.
- **Medical devices:** Example: Urethral insert, pessary, etc.

## PSYCHIATRIC DISORDERS DURING PUERPERIUM

Postpartum period is demanding period characterized by overwhelming biological, social and emotional changes. It requires significant personal and interpersonal adaptation, especially in the case of primigravida. Childbearing from the standpoint of psychological medicine is the most complex event in human experience. Traditionally Inwood has classified postpartum psychiatric disorders (PPPD) as maternity blues, postpartum (postnatal) depression and puerperal psychosis (PP). However, the spectrum of postpartum phenomenology is widely characterized by range of emotions from transient mood liability, irritability and weepiness to marked agitation, delusions, confusion and delirium. Untreated postpartum depression can have adverse long-term effects. Therefore, a thorough knowledge of the same is important for all obstetrician and gynecologists.

### Etiology

The postpartum period is generally regarded as a period of maturation crisis similar to the adolescence and the menopause.

*The various stressors during the period include:*

## Biological Factors

- **Genetic factors:** Thuvel found that children of women treated with postpartum psychosis have a significantly higher prevalence of psychiatric disorders; a similarity was seen in grandchildren of these women but difference was not statistically significant.
- **Endocrinal factors:** Hypothalamic-pituitary gonadal axis: Progesterone and estrogen levels drop suddenly during the first 7–10 days postpartum, while prolactin levels rise by 3rd day and these changes are associated with affective disturbances. These relate only to postpartum blues. Bromocriptine, a drug which decreases prolactin levels and increases dopaminergic transmission is sometimes of benefit in treatment of bipolar depression.
- **Cortisol:** Like gonadal hormones, cortisol levels increase during pregnancy, peak at birth and decline suddenly after childbirth. Abnormal cortisol levels are often associated with postpartum blues.
- **Thyroid hormones:** Since the protein bound iodine levels during the first 9 months after childbirth are about 40% lower than those during the last trimester, a long-lasting depression of thyroxin production has been postulated for psychiatric symptoms.

## Biochemical Factors

- **Cyclic adenosine monophosphate:** These levels decrease during postpartum period and are associated with postpartum depression.
- **Amines:** Low levels of serotonin and tryptophan and high levels of norepinephrine metabolite have been found in postpartum blues.
- **Endorphins:** The endorphin levels vary with estrogens and decreased levels associated with mood swings.
- **Serum calcium:** An association between elevated serum calcium and puerperal psychosis has been noted.

## Psychosocial Factors

Pregnancy and the transition to motherhood give birth to a variety of psychosocial stressors. A woman has to adjust to changes in her body image, her relationships with her husband and family members, her responsibilities and the manner in which she is perceived in the society.

### Risk factors associated with postpartum disorders include

Primigravida, unmarried mother, cesarean section or other perinatal complications, past history of psychotic illness, family history especially mother and sister having postpartum disorder, stressful life events during pregnancy and delivery, history of sexual abuse, vulnerable personality traits and social isolation or unsupportive spouse.

## Clinical Features

There has been long controversy as to whether puerperal illnesses are separate, distinct illnesses or episode of a known psychiatric disorder such as affective disorders or schizophrenic psychoses occur coincidently in puerperium or are precipitated by it.

Postpartum disorders are classified as affective and others. Affective disorders are typically divided into three categories (Table 2).

### TABLE 2: Postpartum affective disorders

| Disorder | Prevalence | Onset | Duration | Treatment |
|---|---|---|---|---|
| Postpartum Blue | 30–75% | Day 3 or 4 | Hours to days | No treatment other than reassurance |
| Postpartum depression | 10–15% | 12 months | Week to months | Treatment usually required |
| Puerperal psychosis | 0.1–0.2% | 2 weeks | Week to months | Hospitalization usually required |

## Puerperal Blues

Postpartum blues are known as 'baby blues' or 'maternity blues' is a phase of emotional liability following childbirth, characterized by frequent crying episodes, irritability, confusion and anxiety. However, elation might also be observed during the first few days following childbirth. Postpartum blues is a very commonly observed puerperal mood disturbance, with estimates of prevalence ranging from 30% to 75%. The symptoms arise within the first 10 days and peak around 3–5 days. Generally, symptoms do not interfere with the social and occupational functioning of women, it is self-limiting with no requirement for active intervention except social support and reassurance from the family members. The symptoms include mood liability, irritability, tearfulness, and generalized anxiety and sleep and appetite disturbances. It can be attributed to changes in hormone levels compounded by stress following delivery. However, if it persists for 2 weeks, this may make a woman vulnerable to more severe forms of mood disorders.

## Postpartum Depression

- It is gradual in onset over first 4–6 months following delivery or abortion.
- Causes: Experiencing stress-inducing life events, low self-esteem, lack of support, demands of motherhood, severe maternal blues later on develop depression.
- Manifestations: Loss of energy and appetite, insomnia, social withdrawal irritability and suicidal behavior.
- Treatment
  - Administer selective serotonin reuptake inhibitors (SSRIs)
  - General supportive measures are essential as in blues.

## Postpartum Psychosis

**Postpartum psychosis** is a rare psychiatric emergency in which symptoms of high mood and racing thoughts, mania, depression, severe confusion, loss of inhibition, paranoia, hallucinations and delusions set in, beginning suddenly in the first two weeks after delivery. The symptoms vary and can change quickly. The most severe symptoms last from 2 to 12 weeks, and recovery takes 6 months to years.

### Causes

- Genetic component; while mutations in chromosome 16 and in specific genes involved in serotoninergic, hormonal, and inflammatory pathways have been identified.
- Family history of affective psychosis, prenatal depression and autoimmune thyroid dysfunction.

Many other potential factors are:

- Changing level of hormones in woman
- Lack of emotional support
- Low self-esteem
- Feeling of inadequacy
- Feeling isolated and alone
- Pregnancy and delivery complications
- Cesarean section
- Sex of the baby
- Length of pregnancy
- Changes in psychiatric medication
- Psychosocial factors

### Signs and Symptoms

There are many symptoms that occur in postpartum psychosis. These may include: ·
- Feeling 'high', 'maniac' or 'on top of the world'
- Low mood and tearfulness
- Anxiety or irritability
- Rapid changes in mood
- Severe confusion
- Being restless and agitated
- Racing thoughts
- Behavior that is out of character
- Being more talkative, active and sociable than usual
- Being very withdrawn and not talking to people
- Finding it hard to sleep, or not willing to sleep
- Loss of inhibitions
- Feeling paranoid, suspicious, fearful
- Feeling of being in a dream world
- Delusions: These are odd thoughts or beliefs that are unlikely to be true. For example, the patient might believe she has won the lottery. She may think her baby is possessed by the devil. She might think people are out to get her.
- Hallucinations: This means a person sees, hears, feels or smells things that are not really existing there.

### Management

- Mental health emergency: Requires immediate attention.
- A psychiatrist must be consulted urgently.
- Hospitalization is needed.
- Treat the problem with antipsychotic drugs, antidepressant/antianxiety.
- Because of suicidal thoughts, mother requires close observation.
- Electroconvulsive therapy (ECT) is considered if patient remains unresponsive or in depressive psychosis.
- Provide psychological counseling and support group therapy.

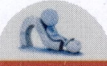

## ASSESS YOURSELF

### FREQUENTLY ASKED QUESTIONS IN EXAMS

1. Explain puerperal sepsis, its causes and management in detail.
2. Describe nursing management of postnatal mother with breast engorgement.
3. Describe the minor disorders of puerperium and its management.
4. Write short notes on:
   a. Mastitis
   b. Puerperal psychosis

### MULTIPLE CHOICE QUESTIONS

1. **Which is the first choice of drug in case of thrombophlebitis?**
   a. Warfarin
   b. Insulin
   c. Heparin
   d. Dopamine

2. **Which diagnostic test is of no value in case of thrombophlebitis?**
   a. X-ray
   b. Venous ultrasound
   c. CT scan
   d. MRI

3. **The dose of heparin in case of thrombophlebitis depends upon:**
   a. Prothrombin time
   b. Clotting time
   c. Activated partial thromboplastin time
   d. All of the above

4. **Which of the following is the clinical manifestation of pulmonary embolism?**
   a. Tachypnea
   b. Tachycardia
   c. Dyspnea
   d. All of the above

5. **Breast engorgement in puerperium usually occurs on:**
   a. 3–4th postpartum day
   b. Immediately after delivery
   c. On 2nd day
   d. After one week

6. **Surgical treatment of pulmonary embolism includes:**
   a. Embolectomy
   b. Placement of vena cava filters
   c. Ligation of inferior vena caval and ovarian vein
   d. All of the above

7. **Which postpartum psychiatric disorder is considered as mental health emergency that requires immediate attention:**
   a. Postpartum blues
   c. Postpartum depression
   b. Postpartum psychosis
   d. Postpartum anxiety

8. **Postpartum psychosis occurs:**
   a. Immediately following delivery
   c. At the end of first week
   b. 2–3 days following delivery
   d. Within 3 weeks of giving birth

9. **ECT is helpful to treat:**
   a. Postpartum blues
   c. Postpartum psychosis
   b. Postpartum depression
   d. Postpartum anxiety

10. **Mastitis is the infection and inflammation of:**
   a. Lactiferous ducts
   c. Bartholin's gland
   b. Sebaceous gland
   d. None of the above

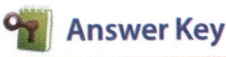 **Answer Key**

| 1. c | 2. a | 3. b | 4. d | 5. a | 6. d | 7. b |
|------|------|------|------|------|------|------|
| 8. d | 9. c | 10. a | | | | |

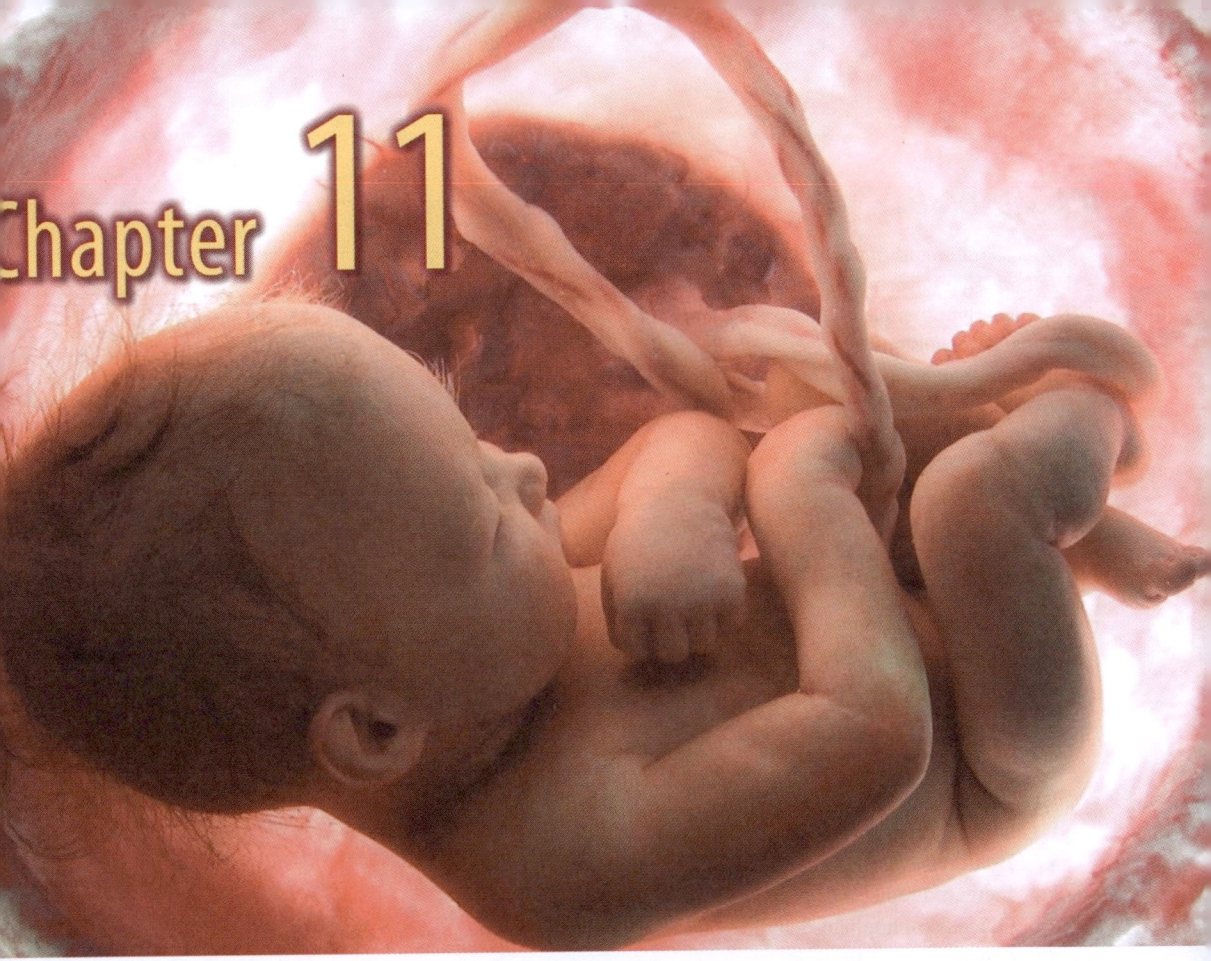

# Chapter 11

# High-risk and Sick Newborn

# HYPERBILIRUBINEMIA OF THE NEWBORN

When the bilirubin (unconjugated) level rises more than arbitrary cut-off point of 12 mg/dL, in a term infant, the condition is called "hyperbilirubinemia of the newborn".

The face and chest of the infant are usually stained yellow.

## Types

- **Unconjugated:**
  It can be caused by:
  - Hemolytic disease due to Rh and ABO incompatibility
  - Increased red cell fragility, prematurity
  - Glucose 6-phophate-dehydrogenase deficiency
  - Sepsis
  - Iatrogenic (drugs)
  - Breast milk jaundice
  - Cephalohematoma
  - Hemoglobinopathies
  - Infant of diabetic mother
  - Hypothyroidism
  - Idiopathic, etc.
- **Conjugated:**
  It can be caused by:
  - Neonatal hepatitis
  - Bacterial infection
  - Intrauterine toxoplasmosis, other infections, rubella, cytomegalovirus (CMV) and herpes infection (TORCH)
  - Trisomy 21
  - Galactosemia
  - Cystic fibrosis
  - Biliary atresia, etc.

## Diagnosis of Neonatal Hyperbilirubinemia

- **Clinical:** Evaluation of jaundice is done by blanching the skin with digital pressure. Clinical jaundice in a neonate indicates serum bilirubin of more than 5 mg/dL

- **Laboratory studies:**
  - Blood group (ABO, Rh) status: Mother and infants antibody screen of the mother
  - Direct Coombs test (Newborn): For alloimmunization disorder positive → Antibody study (Rh, ABO, Kell)
  - Total bilirubin, conjugated bilirubin and unconjugated bilirubin
  - Complete hemogram including reticulocyte count
  - Serum albumin: To detect total bilirubin binding sites and to assess the need of albumin infusion
  - Other laboratory tests
    - Urine for reducing substance (galactosemia) culture for infection
    - Hemoglobin electrophoresis
    - Osmotic fragility tests
    - Thyroid and liver function tests
    - G6 PD screening
    - Live function test (aspartate aminotransferase, alanine aminotransferase, prothrombin time)
- **Radiology and ultrasonography:** To detect intestinal obstruction, intraventricular hemorrhage and tumor.

## Complications

Most common complication of hyperbilirubinemia is kernicterus. It is a type of brain damage most often seen in babies. It is caused by an extreme buildup of bilirubin in the brain. Kernicterus has been reported to occur in near term infants with serum bilirubin level as low as 20.7 mg/dL and more recently, in preterm infants with peak total serum bilirubin as low as 13.1 mg/dL. Bilirubin is a waste product that's produced when liver breaks down old red blood cells, the body can remove them. Kernicterus is a medical emergency and babies with this condition need to be treated right away to bring down their bilirubin levels and prevent further brain damage. Complications of hyperbilirubinemia are given in Figure 1.

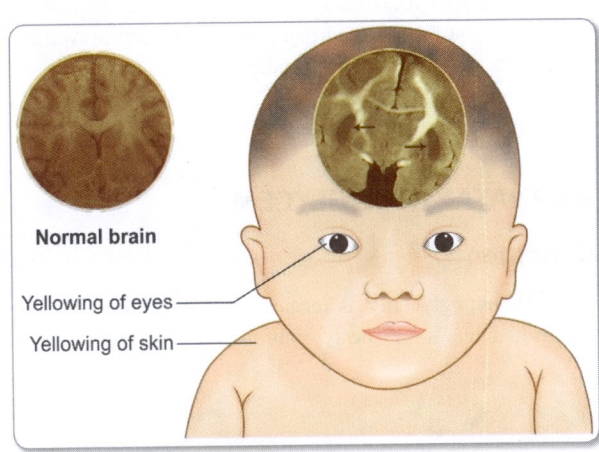

**Fig. 1:** Complication of hyperbilirubinemia

### Signs and Symptoms

- Poor feeding and sucking
- Excessive jaundice
- Hypotonia
- Fatigue and lethargy
- High-pitched crying
- Decreased appetite and less feeding than usual
- Inconsolable crying
- Missing reflexes
- Uncontrollable movements

- Vomiting
- Unusual eye movements
- Fever
- Seizures

## Causes of Kernicterus

Mostly, Kernicterus is caused by severe jaundice that isn't treated. Other risk factors include: Rh incompatibility, Polycythemia, Sulfonamide, Co-trimoxazole, Gilbert's syndrome, G6PDdeficiency.

## Treatment of Kernicterus

Same as Hyperbilirubinemia.

## Management

Three methods of treatment are used to reduce the level of unconjugated bilirubin.
- Phototherapy (light treatment) is the process of using light to eliminate bilirubin in the blood. Baby's skin and blood absorb these light waves and change bilirubin into products, which can pass from body through excretory waste.
  - **Side effects:** Redness and discomfort (sunburn), dry and itchy skin, folliculitis – inflammation of the hair roots may occur, sunlight-induced rash called polymorphic light eruption may develop whilst receiving ultraviolet light, bowel movements are sometimes loose and a greenish color and dehydration due to jaundice.
- Pharmacologic therapy (Ex: Phenobarbital therapy)
- Exchange transfusion

# NEONATAL HYPOGLYCEMIA

## Definition

Neonatal hypoglycemia is termed when the blood glucose level is <40 mg/dL, irrespective of period of gestational age. It may be symptomatic or asymptomatic (Fig. 2).

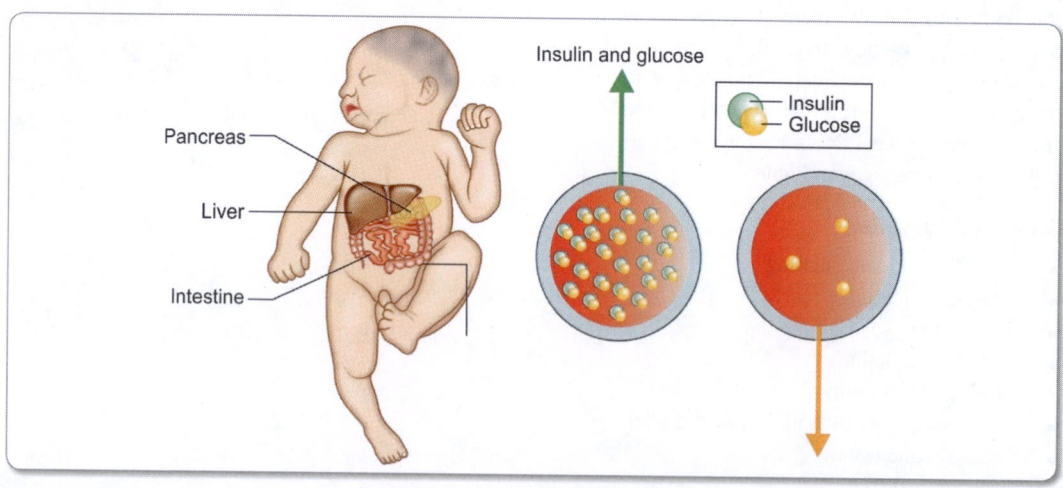

**Fig. 2:** Neonatal hypoglycemia

## Causes

- Low-birth-weight
- Newborn of diabetic mothers
- Secondary problem to perinatal stresses like:
  - Asphyxia
  - Hypothermia
  - Infection
  - Polycythemia
  - Respiratory distress
  - Neurological disturbances
- Intrauterine growth retardation (IUGR)
- Smaller twins
- Babies born to mother with pregnancy-induced hypertension (PIH)
- Rh incompatibility
- Maternal tocolytic agents
- Intractable hypoglycemia occurs due to metabolic/developmental disorders like:
  - Glycogen storage disease
  - Galactosemia
  - Fructosemia
  - Organic acidemia
  - Adrenal insufficiency

## Clinical Manifestations

- Refusal of feeds
- Sweating
- Tachycardia
- Limpness
- Jitteriness
- Tremors
- Twitching
- Pallor
- Hypothermia
- Lethargy
- Irritability
- Restlessness
- Convulsion
- Coma

### In Preterm Babies

- Apnea with cyanosis ⎤
- Tachypnea              ⎬ May occur
- Irregular breathing ⎦

## Management

### *In Asymptomatic Newborn*

- Early initiation of breastfeeding within first hour of birth
- Baby should be nursed in warm or thermoneutral environment with careful observation of "at risk" situation and prevention of hypoxia and hypothermia

Management of neonatal hypoglycemia has been shown in Figure 3.

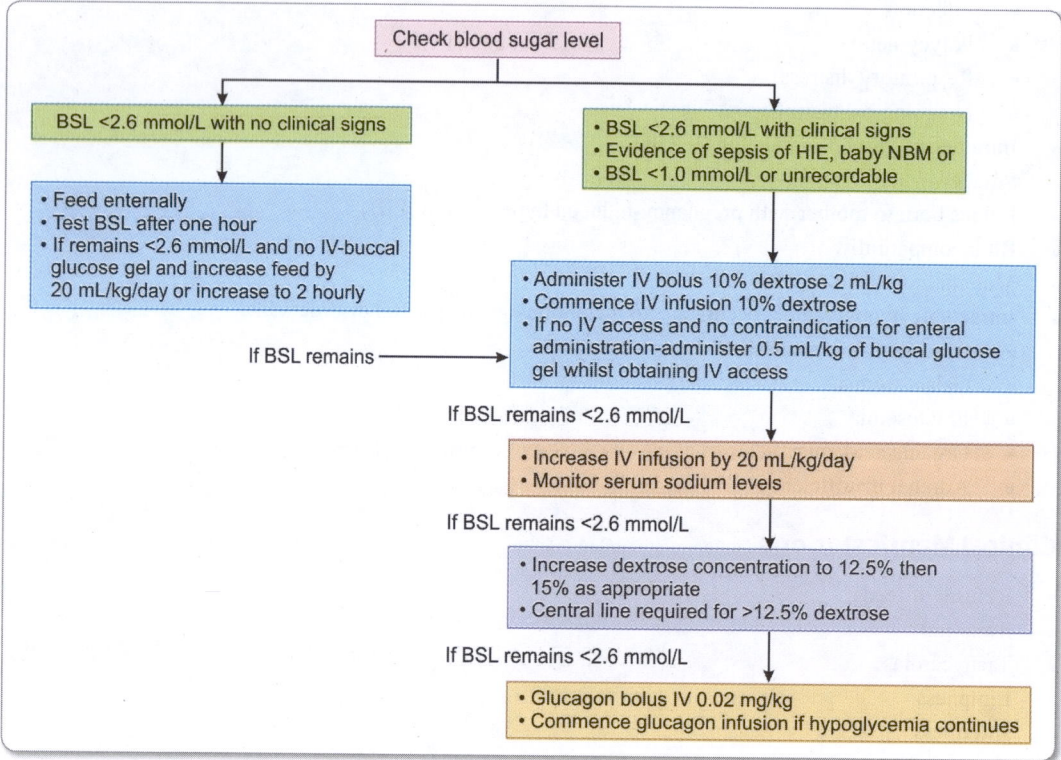

**Fig. 3:** Management of neonatal hypoglycemia

*Abbreviations:* BSL, blood sugar level; HIE, hypoxic ischemic encephalopathy; NBM, nil by mouth

### *In Symptomatic Newborn*

- In case of convulsion, 25% dextrose, 2 mL/kg I/V is given as a bolus.
- If there is no convulsion, 10% dextrose 2 mL/kg/IV bolus is given followed by continuous infusion of 10% glucose at a rate of 6–8 mg/kg/minute.
- Blood glucose level is checked every half hourly.
- Infusion rate to be reduced only if last two glucose estimation is more than 60 mg/dL, oral feeds are introduced gradually and glucose infusion is tapered off.
- If blood glucose is not corrected, then bolus administration of dextrose can be repeated and serum cortisol and insulin level to be checked.
- Hydrocortisone therapy is given 5 mg/kg/IV every 12 hours in intractable case.
- Glucagon and/or epinephrine, diazoxide may be given to the babies with maternal diabetes.

# NEONATAL HYPOTHERMIA

Hypothermia is a common alternation of thermoregulatory state of the neonates. Neonatal hypothermia occurs when the body temperature drops below 36.5° or 97.7°F in the newborn infant (World Health Organization [WHO]). Normal baby temperature is between 36.5°C and 37.5°C.

## Stages of Hypothermia

- 36–36.4°C (96.8–97.6°F)
  - Mild hypothermia (cold stress)
- 32–35.9°C (89.6–96.6°F)
  - Moderate hypothermia
- <32°C (89.6°F)
  - Severe hypothermia (neonatal cold injury)

## Factors Responsible for Neonatal Hypothermia

- Inadequate drying and wrapping
- Separation of baby from the mother
- Cold environment at the place of delivery and baby care areas
- Change of temperature from womb to cooler extrauterine environment
- Inadequate warming procedure before and during transport of the baby
- Excessive heat loss by evaporation, conduction, convection and radiation from wet baby to the cold linen, cold room and cold air
- **High risk neonates:** Low-birth-weight baby, birth asphyxia, congenital malformations and mother having anesthetic drugs.

## Signs and Symptoms

- **Early clinical signs**
  - Skin temperature of the neonate is below 36.5°C
  - Hands, feet, abdomen are cold to touch
  - Weak sucking ability, weak cry and lethargy
  - Blue hands and feet due to peripheral vasoconstriction
- **Late signs due to persistent hypothermia**
  - Gradual fall of baby temperature
  - Slow, shallow and irregular respiration
  - Slow heart rate
  - Lethargy and poor response
  - Pale body with face and extremities of bright red color
  - Central cyanosis may be present
  - Edema and sclerema may be present
  - Weight loss

## Prevention of Neonatal Hypothermia

### At the Time of Birth in Delivery Room

- Delivery room should be warm and free from draught air.
- Immediate drying and wrapping of the neonate in layers of soft clothes or prewarm towel should be done.

- Provision of extra warmth by radiant warmer or room heater or 200 W bulb, should be available.
- Baby should be kept by skin-to-skin contact or by the side of the mother so that mother's warmth will keep the baby warm.
- Fans to be kept off to prevent air movement, windows to be kept closed to prevent draught air.
- Baby bath should be postponed. Cleaning of blood and meconium should be done with lukewarm water.
- Allowing breastfeeding with half an hour of birth or as early as possible should be done to provide warmth, nutrition and protection.
- Continuous observation of thermal state and other vital signs should be done.
- Keep the baby in skin-to-skin contact with mother in kangaroo method to maintain temperature, facilitate bonding and breastfeeding.

### During Transportation

- Baby should be transferred after establishment of thermal stability.
- Assess the baby's condition and temperature.
- Baby can be transferred for skin-to-skin contact with mother in kangaroo method. Baby should be wrapped in prewarmed cloth. Baby's head, extremities should be covered properly. Avoid undressing the baby unnecessarily.
- Baby can be transferred within thermocol box with prewarmed linen, plastic bubble sheet or silver swaddler.
- Simple open transport trolley should be avoided.

### At Neonatal Care Unit

- Receive the neonate in prewarmed cloth.
- Cover the baby with adequate clothing.
- Keep the ambient atmospheric temperature warm for baby's weight and gestational age.
- Maintain humidity around 50%.
- Early feeding with breast milk should be done.
- Avoid dip bath until umbilical cord has fallen off. Sponge bath can be given with warm water in warm room quickly and gently and then wrapping promptly.
- Monitor baby's temperature every three hours, during initial postnatal days considering axillary temperature is as good as core temperature.
- Decrease the heat loss by convection, conduction and radiation.

### At Home

- Warmth should be maintained by warm room, skin-to-skin contact, adequate clothing, exclusive breastfeeding, bathing with warm water in warm room, oil massage and use of solar heat.
- Mother should be taught to assess the thermal state by touch.
- The warm and pink feet of the baby indicate baby is in thermal comfort.
- When feet are cold and abdomen is warm to touch, the baby is in cold stress.
- In hypothermia both feet and abdomen are cold to touch.

## Management of Neonatal Hypothermia

A hypothermic neonate should be rewarmed as quickly as possible. Rewarming procedure depends upon the severity of hypothermia and available facilities.

### In Moderate Hypothermia

- The neonate should be placed with mother in skin-to-skin contact in warm room and warm bed.
- Radiant warmer or incubator can be used if available.
- Rewarming should be continued till the temperature reaches normal range.
- Monitor temperature every 15–30 minutes.

### In Severe Hypothermia

- Rewarming should be done with air heated incubator or manually operated radiant warmer or thermostatically controlled heated mattress set at 37°–38°C.
- Room heater or 200 W bulb or infrared bulb can also be used.
- Monitor blood pressure, heart rate, temperature and blood glucose level.
- Preventive measures to reduce heat loss from the baby should be followed.
- Intravenous infusion with 10% dextrose, oxygen therapy and 'vitamin K' injection (1 mg for term baby and 0.5 mg for preterm baby) should be administered along with supportive care.

## NEONATAL CONVULSIONS

Neonatal convulsions are common life-threatening events in the newborn due to cerebral or biochemical abnormality. Newborn babies do not manifest febrile convulsions.

Common causes of neonatal convulsion are:
- Hypoxic ischemic encephalopathy (HIE)
- Hypocalcemia
- Hypoglycemia
- Septicemia

### Etiology of Neonatal Convulsions

- **Developmental neurological problems** like congenital hydrocephalus, microcephaly, polymicrogyria, agenesis of corpus callosum, etc.
- **Perinatal complications:** HIE, birth asphyxia, birth injury, intraventricular hemorrhage (IVH).
- Perinatal infections, like syphilis, toxoplasmosis, other infections, rubella, cytomegalovirus infection and herpes simplex (STORCH).
- Metabolic problems like hypocalcemia, hypoglycemia, hypomagnesemia, inborn errors of metabolism and pyridoxine deficiency.
- Drugs specifically in neonates born to narcotic addicted mothers, theophylline, phenothiazine, inadvertent injection of local anesthesia into fetal scalp.

### Types of Neonatal Convulsions

Five major types of neonatal convulsions are:

i. Subtle
ii. Generalized tonic
iii. Multifocal clonic
iv. Focal clonic
v. Myoclonic seizures

About 50% of all neonatal seizures are subtle type, which may manifest as eye movements (blinking, fluttering, deviation with jerking, eye opening sustained with ocular fixation) screaming, rowing and pedaling movements, apneic spells and bradycardia.

Pure tonic and clonic seizures are not seen in neonates as neonatal seizures are mainly subcortical in origin. Twitching, rolling of eyes, generalized tonic stiffness without clonic phase with apnea and respiratory irregularities or a change in baby's skin color and vacant look may indicate convulsive disorders and should be investigated.

## Investigations

- Blood examination for calcium, sugar, phosphorus and lumbar puncture for cerebrospinal fluid (CSF) study helps in diagnosis of the cause.
- Electroencephalogram (EEG), computed tomography (CT) scan, magnetic resonance imaging (MRI), Electrocardiography (ECG) and serology for STORCH infections help to exclude the exact cause
- Time of onset of convulsion, family history of convulsion, history of maternal drug addiction and infections are important aspects of investigation.

## Management

- Oxygen therapy
- IV infusion
- Thermal protection
- Prevention of aspiration and injury
- Respiratory support
- Anticonvulsant therapy (phenobarbitone, phenytoin, sodium valproate, etc.)

  Nelson's protocol for management of neonatal seizures is given in Figure 4.

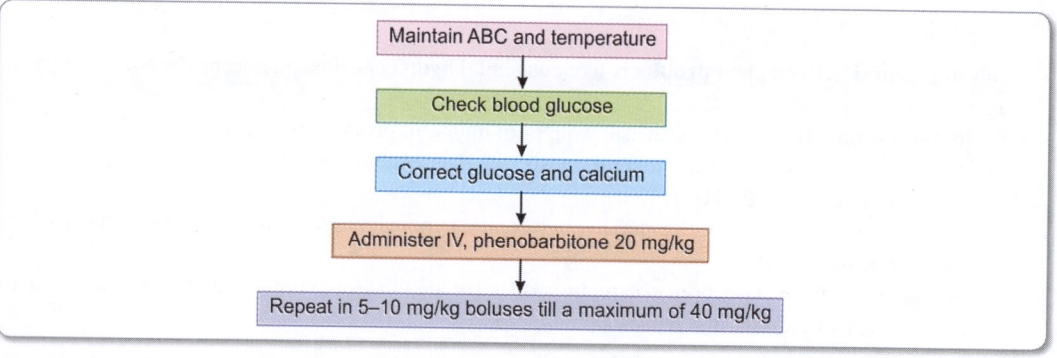

**Fig. 4:** Management of neonatal seizures

## Rh INCOMPATIBILITY

**Definition:** Rh incompatibility is a condition that occurs during pregnancy if a woman has Rh-negative blood and her baby has Rh-positive blood. Rh-negative and Rh-positive refer to whether the blood has Rh factor. Rh factor is a protein on red blood cells (Fig. 5).

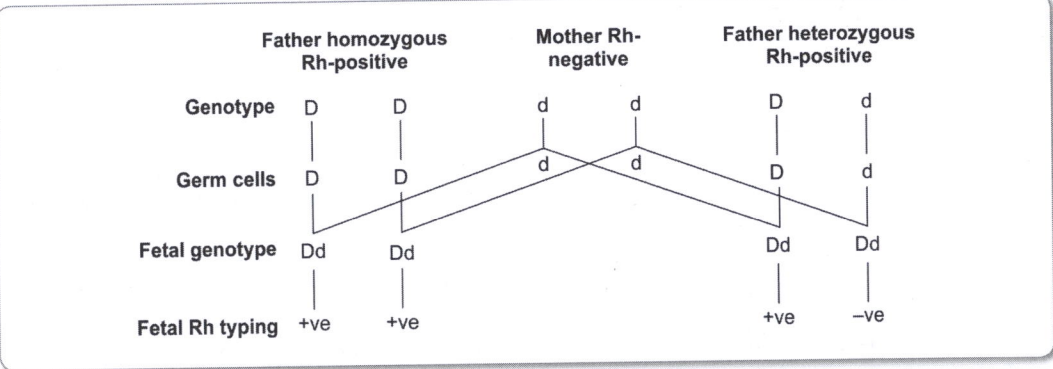

**Fig. 5:** Rh-positive husband mating with Rh-negative wife and resultant Rh-group of the baby

## Genetic Expression

The Father's genotype may be tested, when Rh-negative wife becomes pregnant, to find out whether he is homozygous or heterozygous. When the genotype of the father is heterozygous, half of his genes will be Rh-negative and compatible with Rh-negative mother; the other half being Rh-positive will be incompatible, and the children will be Rh-positive (Dd) and liable to be affected. When the father's genotype is homozygous, all his genes will be incompatible with Rh-negative mother and as such all the children will be Rh-positive (Dd) and may be affected by hemolytic disease.

## Clinical Manifestations

- **Hydrops fetalis:** This is the most serious form of Rh hemolytic disease. Excessive destruction of fetal blood cells leads to severe anemia, tissue anoxemia and metabolic acidosis. Hyperplasia of placental tissue occurs in an effort to increase the transfer of oxygen but the available fetal red blood cells are progressively diminished due to hemolysis. Because of fetal anoxemia, liver damage may occur that leads to hypoproteinemia, which causes generalized edema (hydrops fetalis), ascites and hydrothorax. Fetal death occurs sooner or later due to cardiac failure. The baby is either stillborn or macerated and even if born alive, dies soon after.
- **Icterus gravis neonatorum:** The baby is born alive without evidences of jaundice but soon develops it within 24 hours of birth when the fetus is *in utero*, there is destruction of fetal red cells with liberation of unconjugated bilirubin which is excreted through the placenta into the maternal system. Because of this, baby is not born with jaundice. However, as soon as umbilical cord is clamped, with continuing hemolysis, the bilirubin concentration is increased. If the bilirubin rises to the critical level of 20 mg per 100 mL, the bilirubin crosses the blood-brain barrier to damage the basal nuclei of brain permanently producing the clinical manifestation of kernicterus.
- **Congenital anemia of the newborn:** Although the anemia develops slowly within first few weeks of life, the jaundice is not usually evident. The destruction of the red cells continues up to 6 weeks after which the antibodies are not available for hemolysis. The liver and spleen are enlarged.

## Investigation for Rh Incompatibility

- **Blood test:** Blood testing for Rh and Abo grouping should be done at the first antenatal visit. If the woman is found Rh-negative, Rh grouping of the husband is to be done. If husband is found to be Rh-positive, further investigations are to be carried out.

- **Obstetric history:**
  - If woman is a primigravida with no previous history of blood transfusion, it is quite unlikely that the baby will be affected.
  - In a parous woman, a detailed obstetric history has to be taken. Example: history of stillbirth, neonatal death due to jaundice, etc. Also enquire about the administration of anti-D immunoglobulin following delivery or abortion.

- **Antibody detection:** In all the cases of Rh-negative woman irrespective of blood grouping and parity, IgG antibody is detected by indirect Coombs test. Quantitative estimation of IgG antibody should be done at weekly interval. If there is sudden rise in the titer from 1:8 to 1:256 is very much suggestive of fetal affection. Some centers consider the titer of 1:16 or antibody level more than 10 IU/mL as a critical one. Critical titer means anti-D antibody level that causes hydrops fetalis.

- **Doppler ultrasound:** Serial Doppler study of middle cerebral artery peak systolic velocity is the main predictor for fetal anemia. A value >1.5 multiples of the median (MOMs) for the corresponding gestational age, predicts moderate to severe fetal anemia.

- **Amniocentesis:** Amniocentesis and estimation of bilirubin in the amniotic fluid by spectrophotometer gives the prediction of severity of fetal hemolysis. The optical density of the liquor containing the bilirubin pigment is observed at 250–700 nm wavelength. The optical density difference at 450 nm wavelength gives the prediction of severity of fetal hemolysis. In the presence of bilirubin, there is 'deviation bulge' peaking at 450 nm wavelength. For any given period of gestation, the height of spectrophotometric 'deviation bulge' at $OD_{450}$ falls within one of the three zones when plotted in Liley's chart.

## Predictions

- **Liley's zone I (low zone):** The fetus is unlikely to be affected and the pregnancy can be continued to term.
- **Liley's zone II (mid zone):** Repeat amniocentesis by 2 weeks → Value upward → cordocentesis→ hematocrit < 30 % → Intrauterine transfusion to raise hematocrit 40–45%. Preterm delivery after 34 weeks.
- **Liley's zone III (high zone):** Fetus is severely affected and death is imminent. Pregnancy >34 weeks → delivery. Pregnancy <34 weeks → cordocentesis → hematocrit < 30% → Intrauterine transfusion to raise hematocrit 40–45%. Preterm delivery after 34 weeks.

## Prevention

- **To prevent active immunizations:** Rh anti-D immunoglobulin (IgG) 300 mg is administered IM to the mother during pregnancy or within 72 hours following delivery or abortion.
- **To prevent or minimize fetomaternal bleed:**
  - Use precautions during cesarean section to prevent blood spilling into peritoneal cavity and while removal of placenta.
  - Prophylactic ergometrine with delivery of the anterior shoulder preferably be withheld.
  - Amniocentesis should be done after sonographic localization of the placenta to prevent its injury.
  - Avoid external version in Rh-negative pregnancy.
  - Manual removal of placenta should be done gently.
  - Avoid abdominal palpation in case of abruption placenta.
- **To avoid mismatched transfusion**

## Management of Rh-negative Woman

Figure 6 shows the management of Rh-negative woman.

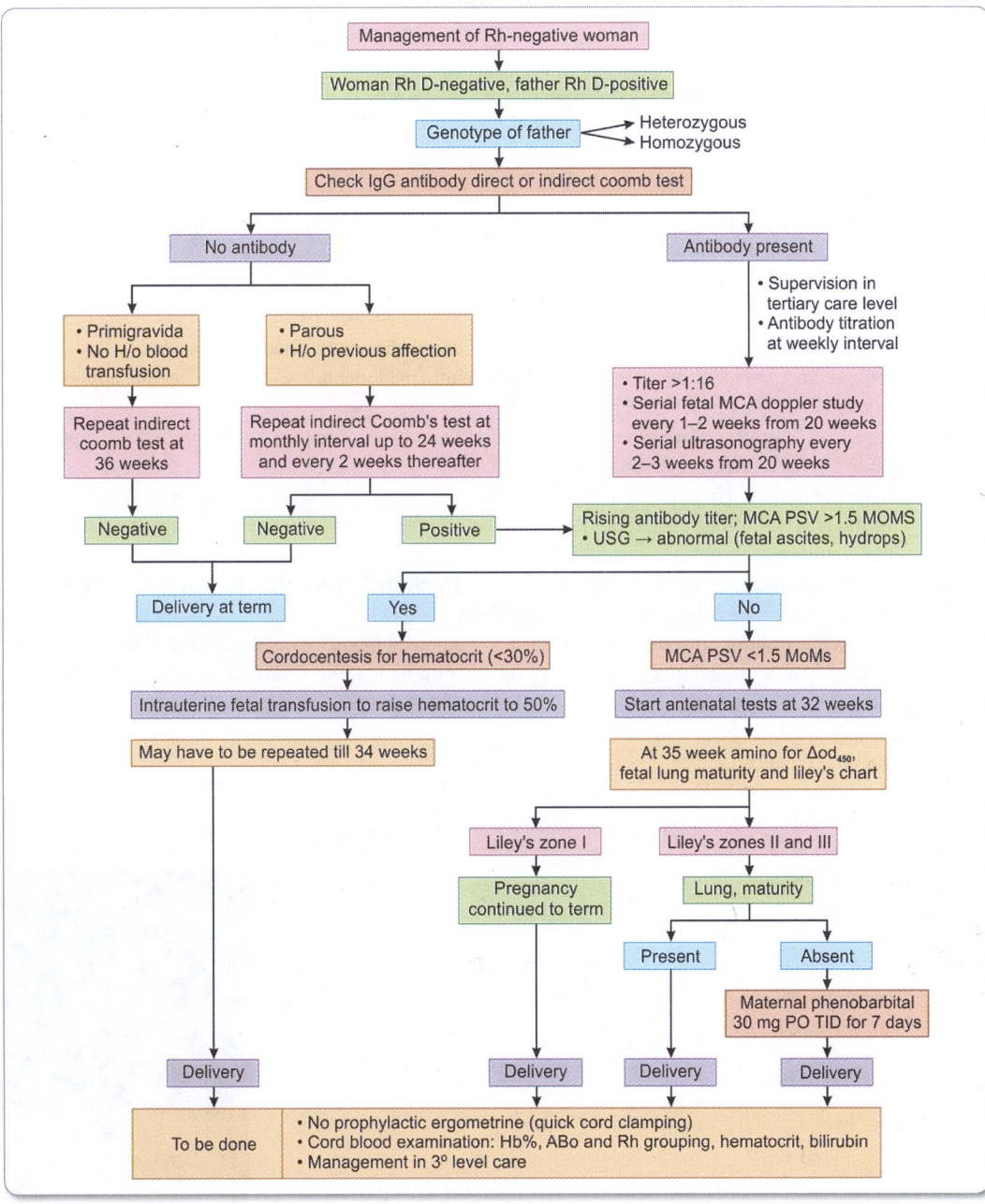

**Fig. 6:** Management of Rh-negative woman

*Abbreviations:* MCA PCV, Middle cerebral artery peak systolic velocity; MOMS, multiples of the median

# LOW-BIRTH-WEIGHT BABIES

A neonate with a birth weight of less than 2,500 g, irrespective of the gestational age are termed as low-birth-weight (LBW) babies. **They include both preterm and small for date (SDF) babies.**

## Preterm Baby

A baby born before 37 completed weeks of gestation calculating from the first day of last menstrual period is defined as preterm baby.

### Incidence

The incidence of preterm babies is about 20–25% and constitutes two third of LBW babies.

### Causes of Prematurity

- **Maternal causes**
  - **Uterine anomalies:** Cervical incompetence and congenital malformation of uterus
  - **Medical and surgical illness:** Acute fever, acute pyelonephritis, diarrhea, acute appendicitis, toxoplasmosis and abdominal operation
  - **Pregnancy complication:** Preeclampsia, antepartum hemorrhage (APH), premature rupture of membranes (PROM), polyhydramnios
  - **Chronic diseases:** Hypertension, nephritis, diabetes, heart diseases and severe anemia
  - **Genital tract infections:** Bacterial vaginosis, beta-hemolytic streptococcus, bacteroides, Chlamydia and mycoplasma
  - **Previous obstetric history:** There is an increased incidence in women who had previous history of induced spontaneous abortion or preterm delivery
  - **Low socioeconomic and nutritional status:** Women in low socioeconomic status appear to have shorter gestation period though there may be other compounding factors such as maternal illness.
- **Fetal causes**
  - Multiple pregnancy
  - Congenital malformations
  - Intrauterine death (IUD)
- **Placental causes**
  - Placenta previa
  - Abruptio placenta
  - Thrombosis
  - Infarction
- **Idiopathic**
  - Premature effacement of cervix due to irritable uterus
  - Early engagement of head

### Clinical Manifestations

- Weight of baby is 2500 g or less
- Length less than 44 cm
- Preterm baby has big head, small thoracic area and large abdomen
- Skull bones are soft, wide sutures and large fontanels
- Pinnae of ears are soft and flat (Fig. 7)

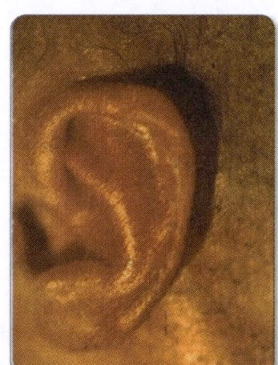

**Fig. 7:** Small amount of ear cartilage and/flattened Pinna

- Eyes are kept closed
- Skin is thin, red and shiny due to lack of subcutaneous fat
- Skin covered by plentiful lanugo and vernix caseosa
- Poor muscle tone
- Not well-defined plantar creases (Fig. 8)
- Undescended testis (Fig. 9)
- Exposed labia minora (Fig. 10)
- Nails not grown up to fingertips

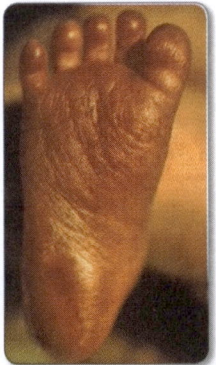 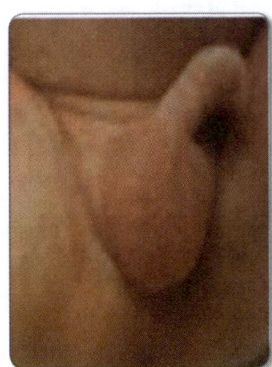 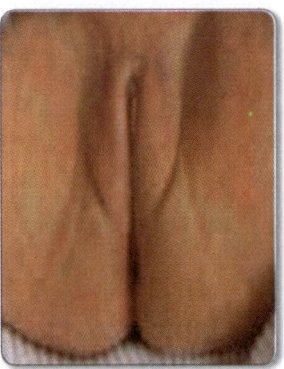

**Fig. 8:** Nondefined plantar creases and flat sole          **Fig. 9:** Undescended testis          **Fig. 10:** Exposed labia minora

## Complications

- Asphyxia due to anatomical and functional immaturity.
- Hypothermia due to reduced subcutaneous fat and brown fat.
- Pulmonary syndrome includes pulmonary edema, intra alveolar hemorrhage, respiratory distress syndrome (RDS), bronchopulmonary dysplasia.
- Cerebral hemorrhage due to soft skull bones, fragile subependymal capillaries and hypoprothrombinemia.
- Fetal shock due to improper resuscitative measures.
- Hypoglycemia due to lack of glycogen stores in the liver.
- Heart failure due to asphyxia or patent ductus arteriosus (PDA).
- Oliguria, anuria due to immature kidneys.
- Infection protective passive immunity is usually detained from the mother during the later months of pregnancy. As the transfer of protective immunoglobulins from the mother to a preterm baby is less, the incidence of infection is increased by 3–10 folds.
- Jaundice due to hepatic prematurity.
- Ductus persistent PDA inversely related to gestational age.
- Dehydration and acidemia due to immature kidneys.
- Anemia due to lack of iron store, hypofunction of bone marrow and excessive hemolysis.
- Apnea and sudden infant death syndrome due to immature autonomic nervous system.
- Retinopathy of prematurity.
- Increased length of hospital stay.

### *Management of Preterm Baby*

Figure 11 shows the various devices which are involved in the care of preterm baby.

#### Immediate Management following Birth

- Cord is to be clamped quickly to prevent hypovolemia.
- Cord length is kept long in case of exchange transfusion.
- Air passage should be cleared.
- Adequate oxygen supply should be provided.
- Baby should be wrapped including head in sterile warm towel.
- Administer vitamin K 1 g intramuscularly.
- Prevent from infections by aseptic techniques.

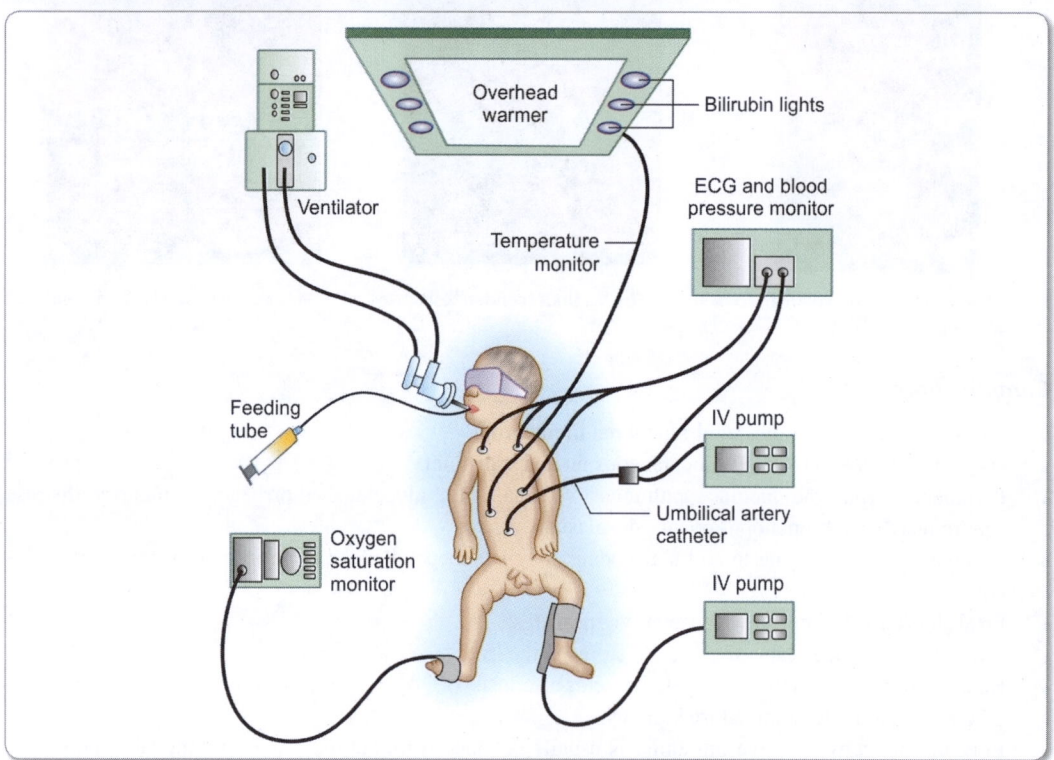

**Fig. 11:** Care of preterm baby
*Abbreviations: ECG, electrocardiogram; IV, intravenous*

#### Intensive Care Protocol

Preterm babies are functionally immature and special care is needed for their survival. Those requiring special care are judged by:

- Incapacity to regulate temperature
- Inability to control cardiopulmonary function
- Inability to suck the breast and to swallow

## Thermal Protection

As the preterm babies are extremely thermolabile, they can easily develop hyperpyrexia/hypothermia (Fig. 12).

*To prevent hypothermia, following guidelines are helpful:*

- Delay bathing
- Maternal contact
- Kangaroo mother care
- Warm room
- External heat source (incubator, radiant heat warmer)

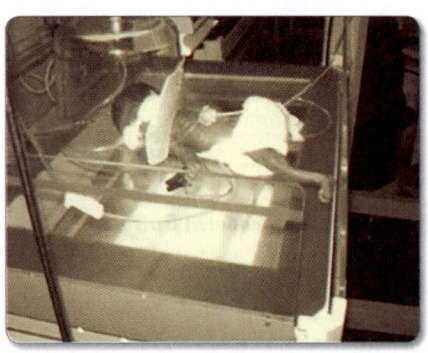

**Fig. 12:** Thermal protection

## Respiratory Support

- Clear the airway
- Administer oxygen (By using oxyhood)
- In severe conditions, endotracheal intubation and mechanical ventilation
- Arterial blood gases (ABG) sampling to monitor ventilator status
- Surfactant replacement therapy (Dexamethasone) 24–48 hours prior to delivery is helpful for fetal lung maturity in case of preterm delivery

## Infection

- Main sites of infection are respiratory tract, gastrointestinal tract, skin and umbilicus. Every precaution should be taken to prevent or minimize infection. The commonly used antibiotics are ampicillin 100 mg/kg/day or amikacin 10 mg/kg/day is to be given IM in two divided doses for 5–7 days.

## Nutrition (Fluids and Feeds)

- Preterm infants are often unable to suck and swallow. Therefore, the following guidelines are helpful to maintain nutritional pattern of the preterm baby:
  - Intravenous fluids for very small babies or who are sick
  - Expressed breast milk with gavage or katori and spoon
  - Direct breastfeeding

## Monitoring and Early Detection of Complications

- Weight and other clinical signs
- Electronic monitoring
- Biochemical monitoring
- Appropriate management of specific complications should be done

## Adequate Nursing Care

- The most single factor is high standard of nursing and one trained nurse can adequately take care of two or three newborn babies.
  - Check and record temperature twice daily
  - Baby should be weighed daily to know whether over- or under-hydrated
  - Constant supervision especially during the first 48 hours
  - Allow the mother to take care of the baby even in nursery
- Mother should be taught for the general care of the baby and manual expression of breast milk by pressing over the areola and the nipple.

## Favorable Signs of Progress in Preterm Baby

- Color of the skin remains pink all the time
- Smooth and regular breathing
- Increased vigor evidenced by movement of limbs and frequent crying
- Progressive weight gain

## Discharge of Preterm Baby

The premature babies are discharged:

- When they attain sufficient weight
- Attain good vigor
- Able to suck breast successfully

## Advices on Discharge

The following advices are given to the mother of preterm babies:

- Advice about feeding schedule
- Administer multivitamins and iron supplements as prescribed
- Frequent follow-up at well baby clinic for subsequent checkup, immunization and guidance

# Small for Dates

*(Syn: Intrauterine growth retardation (IUGR), chronic placental insufficiency)*
**Definition:** Intrauterine growth restriction (IUGR) is said to be present in those babies whose birth weight is below the tenth percentile of the average for gestational age.

## Types of IUGR

Based on clinical evaluation and ultrasonography (USG), the small fetuses are divided into two types:

- **Small and healthy fetus:** The birth weight is less than tenth percentile for their gestational age. They have normal subcutaneous fat and usually have uneventful neonatal course
- **Fetuses whose growth is restricted by pathological process (true IUGR):** Depending upon the relative size of the head, abdomen and femur, the fetuses are subdivided into:
  - Symmetrical or type I
  - Asymmetrical or type II

| Symmetrical IUGR | Asymmetrical IUGR |
|---|---|
| • Uniformly small | • Head larger than Abdomen |
| • Ponderal index → Normal | • Low |
| • Head circumference: Abdominal circumference ⎤ Normal<br>• Femur Length: Abdominal circumference ⎦ | • Elevated |
| • Causes: Genetic disease/Infection | • Chronic placental insufficiency |
| • Total cell number: Less | • Normal |
| • Cell size → Normal | • Smaller |
| • Neonatal course: Complicated with poor prognosis | • Usually uncomplicated having good prognosis |

Ponderal index is a way of characterizing the relationship of height to man for an individual.

$$PI = 100 \times \frac{Weight\ (g)}{Height\ (cm)^3}$$

Typical values are between 2.0 and 2.5. It is normal in symmetric IUGR and is low in asymmetric IUGR.

## Causes

The causes of intrauterine growth retardation have been shown in Figure 13.

- **Maternal history:** Ethnicity, racial and geographical areas, low social and economic status and short stature of mother (less than 150 cm), etc.
- **Maternal malnutrition:** Food deprivation, particularly during the last weeks of pregnancy, when mother is undernourished (weight under 40 kg) leads to the birth of malnourished baby.
- **Intrauterine infections** such as STORCH may lead to IUGR.
- **Placental factors:** Maternal problems such as toxemia of pregnancy and hypertension may be responsible for placental dysfunction, disorders of implantation of placenta, abruptio placenta, single umbilical artery, etc.

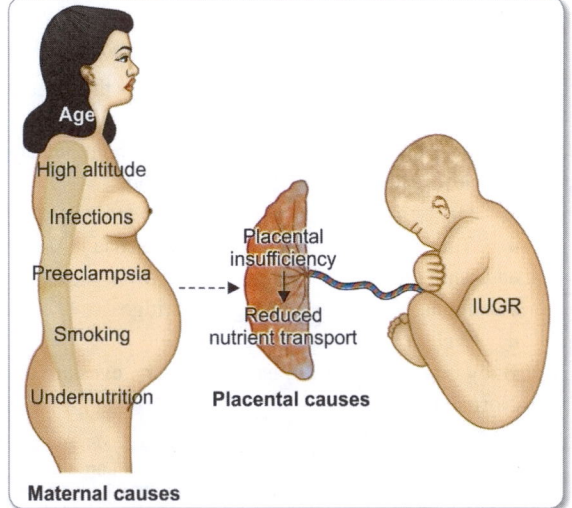

**Fig. 13:** Causes of intrauterine growth retardation

- **Multiple pregnancy:** After 35 weeks of gestation, mother is not capable of providing adequate nourishment to more than one fetus.
- **Maternal diseases:** Chronic diseases such as heart disease, tuberculosis, renal disease, bronchial asthma, etc. cause LBW babies.
- **Genetic/chromosomal disorders:** Some genetic disorders (Dwarfism) and chromosomal disorder (Turner's syndrome, Trisomies) present their adverse influences early during gestation, reducing both cell number and cell size, due to which resultant baby is small in all parameters.
- **Miscellaneous causes:** Teenage pregnancy, narcotic addiction, teratogenic agents, tobacco, smoking, high altitude, irradiation, etc.

## Diagnosis

It is made on the basis of clinical, biophysical methods and biochemical methods.

- **Clinical**
  - Clinical palpation of uterus for fundal height, liquor volume and fetal mass may be used to diagnose IUGR.
  - **Symphysis fundal height:** Measurement in centimeters closely correlates with gestational age after 24 weeks. A lag of 4 cm or more suggests IUGR.
  - **Maternal weight gain:** Remains stationary or at times falling during second half of pregnancy.
  - **Measurement of abdominal girth:** Stationary or falling values.
- **Biophysical**
  - Using head circumference/abdominal circumference ratio, 85% of IUGR fetuses are detected.
  - **Femur length:** Femur length (FL)/Abdominal circumference (AC) ratio greater than 23.5 suggests IUGR.

- **Amniotic fluid volume:** A vertical pocket of amniotic fluid <2 cm suggests IUGR.
- **Doppler velocimetry:** Elevated uterine artery systolic/diastolic ratio and presence of diastolic notch are associated with IUGR and IUD.
- **Ponderal Index (birth weight/Crown heel length):** PI below 10th percentile is taken as IUGR.
- **Biochemical:** Elevated level of erythropoietin in cord blood suggests IUGR.

### Clinical Manifestations

Clinical manifestations of IUGR have been shown in Figure 14.

- Weight deficit at birth about 600 g below the minimum percentile standard
- Length is unaffected
- Head circumference is relatively larger than the baby
- Physical features of IUGR babies include
  - Dry, wrinkled skin
  - Thin meconium-stained vernix caseosa
  - Thin umbilical cord
  - Pinna of ears has cartilaginous ridges
  - Well defined plantar creases
- Baby is alert, active and has normal cry, eyes are open
- Normal reflexes

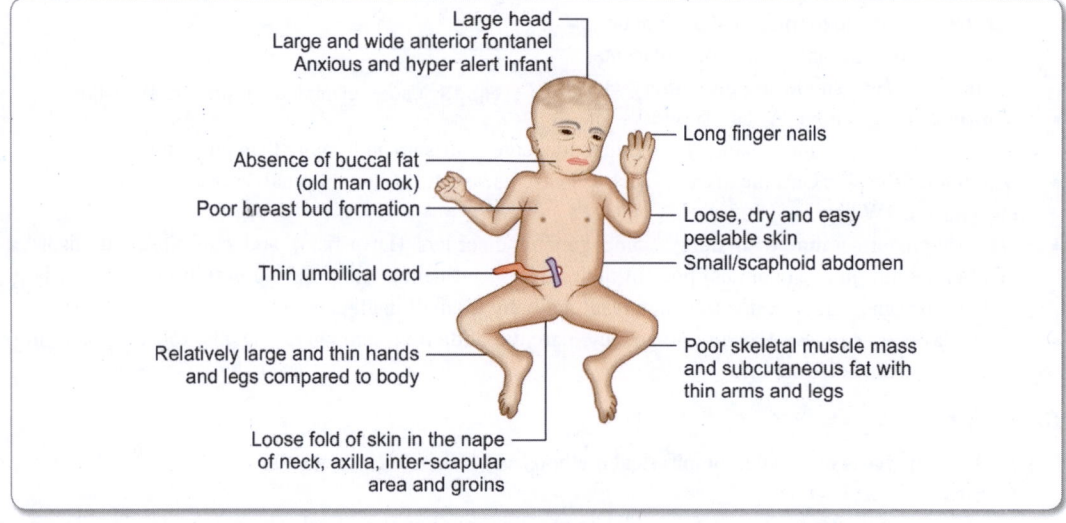

**Fig. 14:** Clinical manifestations of IUGR

### Complications

- Asphyxia (intranatal/neonatal)
- Hypoglycemia
- Meconium aspiration pneumonia
- Hyperthermia
- Pulmonary hemorrhage
- Polycythemia
- Necrotizing enterocolitis (NEC)
- Hyperviscosity syndrome
- Hyperbilirubinemia
- Intraventricular hemorrhage
- Difficulty in feeding and weight gain

## Management of IUGR

### Preventive Measures

- **Female literacy and formal education:** Mother should be educated before and during the pregnancy. Avoid harmful agents, education and training of the traditional birth attendants to provide the adequate care of the mothers during pregnancy and referral to a nearby health center in case of high-risk pregnancy is also helpful.
- **Maternal health status:** Adequate nutrition of the female throughout pregnancy. Good nutrition should be maintained continuously which keeps the mother free from medical ailments.
- **Antenatal care:** Antenatal checkups are essential. Early detection of high risk factors such as intrauterine infections, hypertension, toxemia of pregnancy and their early intervention can prevent the occurrence of IUGR.
- **Maternal infections:** Prevent the infections such as malaria, urinary tract infection, TORCH, etc. because these may lead to IUGR.

### Specific Management

- Objectives
  - To confirm IUGR and its type
  - To exclude congenital malformation and genetic disorders
  - To treat the specific cause if found
  - Fetal surveillance
    - Daily fetal movement count (DFMC)
    - Cardiotocography nonstress test
    - Biophysical profile
    - Umbilical artery Doppler flow velocimetry
- **If pregnancy ≥37 weeks (beyond 37 weeks):** Termination of pregnancy should be done
- **If pregnancy <37 weeks (before 37 weeks):** Assess mild IUGR or severe IUGR
  - **If mild IUGR:**
    - Adequate bed rest to mother (in left lateral position)
    - Administer folic acid tablets
    - Fetal monitoring till 37 weeks. Then at 37th weeks, termination of pregnancy should be done
  - **If severe IUGR:** Assess dual problems like prematurity or dysmaturity
    - Transfer the patient to equipped center or center with limited facilities
    - **In equipped center:** Assess fetal lung maturity by using lecithin sphingomyelin (L:S) ratio. If the fetal lungs are immature, give dexamethasone therapy 24–48 hours prior to delivery then termination of pregnancy should be done. If fetal lungs are mature, there is no need for surfactant and pregnancy can be terminated.
    - **In center with limited facilities:** In vitro transfer to a referral center. During hospitalization provide adequate hyperoxygenation and low dose aspirin. Continue the pregnancy up to 34 weeks, if possible, otherwise terminate it.

### Nursing Management

- Provide adequate fluid and electrolytes and nutrition.
  - Provide a high calorie formula for feeding (more than 20 calories per ounce) to promote steady weight gain (15–30 g/day growth plotted on curves shows a normal growth rate).
  - If the infant is breastfeeding, add human milk fortifier to expressed breast milk.

- Decrease metabolic demands when possible.
  - Provide small frequent feedings.
  - Provide gavage feedings if the infant does not have a steady weight gain.
  - Provide a neutral thermal environment.
- Decrease iatrogenic stimuli and prevent hypoglycemia
  - Monitor glucose screening.
  - Provide early feedings.
  - Provide frequent feedings (every 2–3 hours).
  - Administer IV glucose if blood sugar does not normalize with oral feedings.
- Maintain a neutral thermal environment.
- Monitor serum hematocrit (normal is 45–65%).
  - If an initial high hematocrit was obtained by heel stick capillary sample, a follow-up sample should be done by venipuncture
  - Observe for signs, symptoms, and complications of polycythemia
  - Ruddy appearance
  - Cyanosis
  - Lethargy, jitteriness, and seizures
  - Jaundice
  - Provide adequate hydration to prevent hyperviscosity.
- Assess the prenatal history for possible TORCH infections during pregnancy. Assess maternal and infant antibody titers. Use isolation precautions when congenital infections are suspected.
- Provide education and emotional support.
  - Explain the possible causes of IUGR.
  - Inform parents of the infant's goal weight for discharge.
  - Provide instructions on managing the infant at home.
  - Explain how to prepare a higher calorie formula or breastfeeding.
  - Explain the importance of follow-up with a developmental specialist who will screen for milestone achievements.

# ASPHYXIA

Birth asphyxia is defined as the nonestablishment of satisfactory pulmonary respiration at birth. Its literal meaning is "stopping of the pulse".

It is failure of initiation and maintenance of spontaneous respiration with hypoventilation, anaerobic glycolysis and lactic acidosis. It is characterized by progressive hypoxia, hypercapnia, hypoperfusion and metabolic acidosis.

## Causes of Asphyxia

- **Continuation of intrauterine hypoxia** (placental insufficiency)
  - The placenta, as a respiratory organ of the fetus, fails functionally either due to anatomical changes or due to inadequacy of uteroplacental circulation (e.g., abruptio placenta, hypertension in pregnancy, abnormal labor, placental abnormalities, cord compression, vascular anomalies in cord, etc.).
  - Maternal hypoxic states as in anemia, eclampsia, cyanotic cardiovascular disorders, status asthmaticus, dehydration and hypotension.

- **Prenatal and intranatal medication to the mother:** Morphine, pethidine and anesthetic agents depress the respiratory centers directly and the chance of development of asphyxia is increased.
- **Birth trauma to the neonate:** Malpresentation such as breech, oblique lie, occipitoposterior often requires manipulative and operative vaginal delivery (forceps or ventouse). Prolonged second stage of labor in contracted pelvis, often causes asphyxia.
- **Postnatal factors:** Postnatal asphyxia is secondary to pulmonary, cardiovascular and neurological abnormalities of the neonate.

## Phases of Asphyxia

Phases of asphyxia are shown in Figure 15.

- Primary apnea (30–60 seconds)
  - Short series of respiratory efforts
  - Convulsion or a series of clonic movements
  - Abrupt fall in heart rate
  - Then no muscle tone
  - Skin cyanotic and then blotchy
- Gasping (8 minutes)
  - 3–6 minutes
  - Heart rate and blood pressure continue to fall
- Secondary/terminal apnea

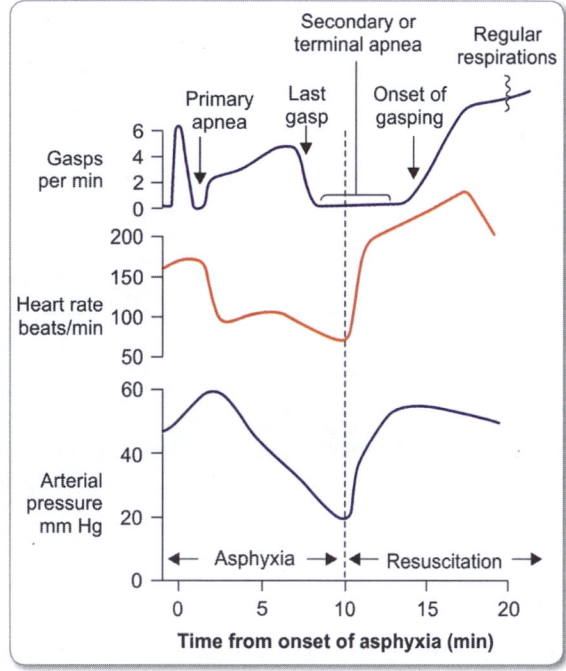

**Fig. 15:** Phases of asphyxia

## Signs and Symptoms

The signs and symptoms depend upon the etiology, intensity and duration of oxygen lack, plasma carbon dioxide excess and subsequent acidosis.

According to the intensity of signs and symptoms the condition has been classified as:

- **Asphyxia livida/stage of cyanosis:** It is due to respiratory failure with Apgar score 4–6.
- **Asphyxia pallida/state of shock:** Due to combined respiratory and vasomotor failure with Apgar score 0–3.

Depending upon Apgar scoring system, the score 0–3 indicates severe depression, the score 4–6 indicates moderate depression and score 7–10 indicates no depression. The evaluation to start resuscitation depends upon 3 important signs, i.e. respiration, heart rate and skin color. Based on these signs, prompt initiation of resuscitation can be done, not delaying one minute for Apgar scoring (Fig. 16). A delay could result in critical problem, especially in severely depressed baby.

| Component of acronym | Score of 0 | Score of 1 | Score of 2 (the best score, healthy) |
|---|---|---|---|
| 1. Skin color / Appearance | Overal blue/pale | Acrocyanosis (bluish discoloration of extremities), but trunk and head are pink | No blue cyanosis, the skin is pink all over |
| 2. Health rate beats per minute / Pulse | Absent | <100 bmp | >100 bmp |
| 3. Reflex irritability / Grimace | No response to stimulation | Grimace/ slight cry when stimulated | Vigorous cry in response to stimuli (like nasal suctioning); sneeze/cough/pulls away when stimulated |
| 4. Muscle tone / Activity | No movement, limpness | Some flexion | Vigorous, active movement of arms and legs |
| 5. Breathing / Respiration | Absent, apnoea | Slow, Weak or irregular | Strong, visible breathing and crying |

**Fig. 16:** Apgar score

## Complications

### Immediate

- **Cardiovascular:** Hypotension, cardiac failure
- **Renal:** Acute cortical necrosis, renal failure
- Liver function compromised
- **Gastrointestinal:** Ulcers and necrotizing enterocolitis
- **Lungs:** Persistent pulmonary hypertension
- **Brain:** Cerebral edema

### Delayed

- Retarded Mental and physical growth
- Epilepsy
- Minimal brain dysfunction

## Management

### Preventive Measures

- Early identification of high risk cases.
- Close fetal monitoring in high risk women to ensure early detection of fetal distress and timely termination of pregnancy and/or labor.

- Intrapartum use of electronic fetal monitoring and scalp blood PH assessment when indicated.
- Judicious administration of anesthetic agents and sedatives during labor.

## Definitive Management

Figure 17 shows guidelines for neonatal resuscitation.

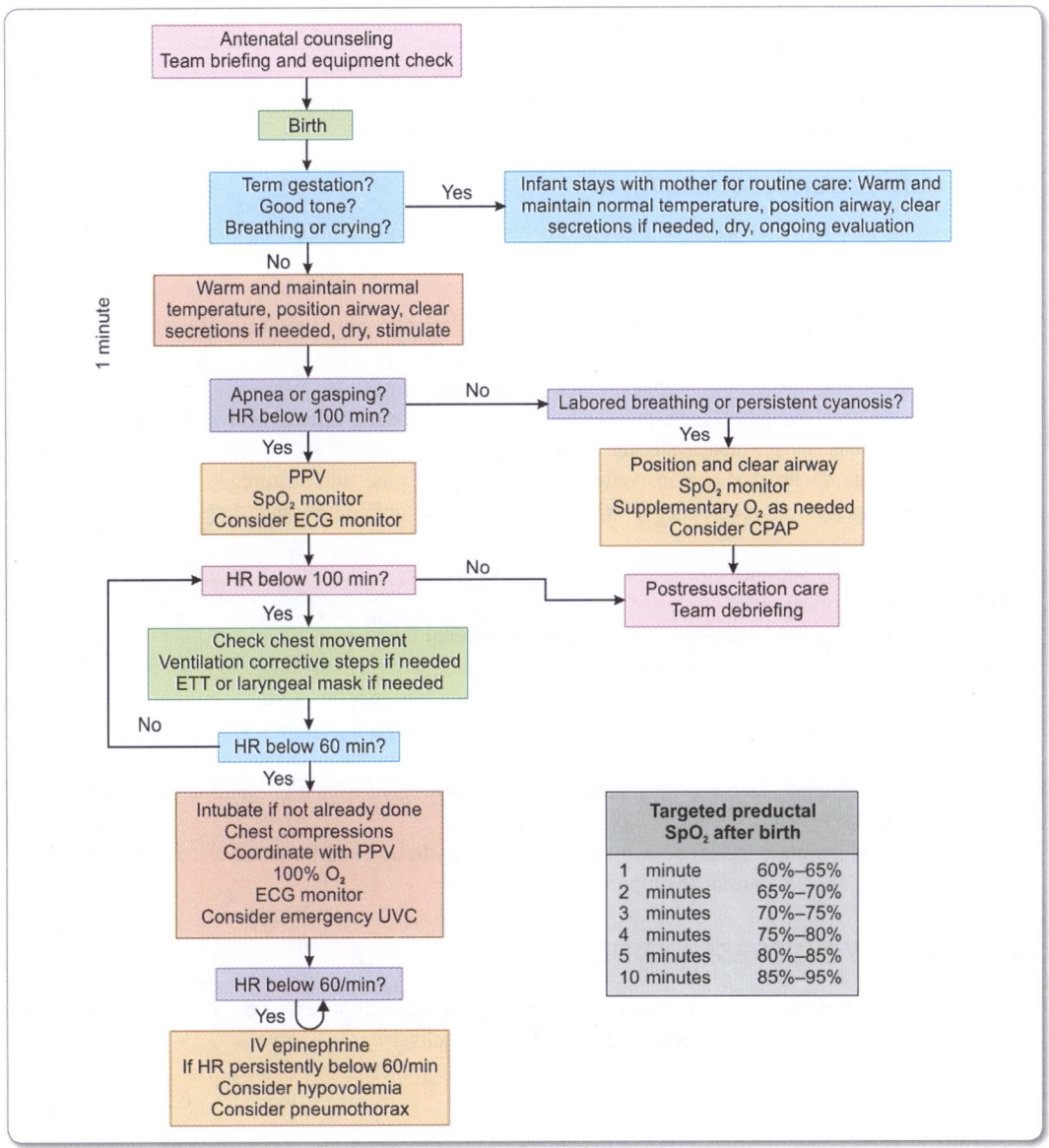

**Fig. 17:** 2015 guidelines for neonatal resuscitation

*Abbreviations:* CPAP, continuous positive airway pressure; ECG, electrocardiogram; ETT, endotracheal tube; HR, heart rate; PPV, positive pressure ventilation

### Medications

- **Epinephrine:** 0.1–0.3 mL/kg in 1:10,000 dilution is given IV when there is persistent bradycardia. Intratracheal administration can also be given. Repeated every 5 minutes.
- **Sodium bicarbonate:** To combat metabolic acidosis IV (4 mL/kg of 0.5 mEq/mL, 4.2% solution) is given.
- **Narcotic antagonist:** It is needed when mother has been given pethidine or morphine within 3 hours of delivery.
- **Naloxone** 100 ug/kg is given to the baby by IV, IM or endotracheal.
- **Volume expander:** It is needed when blood pressure is low and tissue perfusion is poor.
- **Dopamine infusion:** In case of hypotension.

### Nursing Management of Birth Asphyxia

- Observe the newborn that has been successfully resuscitated for the following constellation of signs.
  - Absence of spontaneous respirations
  - Seizure activity in the first 12 hours after birth
  - Decreased or increased urine output (which may indicate acute tubular necrosis or syndrome of inappropriate antidiuretic hormone)
  - Metabolic alterations (e.g., hypoglycemia and hypocalcemia)
  - Increased intracranial pressure marked by decreased or absent reflexes or hypertension
- Decrease noxious environmental stimuli.
- Monitor the infant's level of responsiveness, activity, muscle tone, and posture.
- Administer prescribed medications, which may include anticonvulsants (e.g., phenobarbital) as prescribed.
- Provide respiratory support.
- Monitor for complications:
  - Measure and record intake and output to evaluate renal function.
  - Check every voiding for blood, protein, and specific gravity, which suggests renal injury.
  - Check every stool for blood, suggesting necrotizing enterocolitis (NEC). NEC is a condition in which the bowel develops necrotic patches that interfere with digestion and possibly cause paralytic ileus, perforation, and peritonitis.
  - Take serial blood glucose determinations to detect hypoglycemia, and monitor serum electrolytes, as ordered.
- Administer and maintain intravenous fluids to maintain hydration and fluid and electrolyte balance.
- Provide education and emotional support.

## RESPIRATORY DISTRESS SYNDROME

**Definition:** Respiratory distress syndrome (RDS) occurs commonly in preterm neonates, babies of diabetic mother and infants delivered by cesarean section and breech delivery.

### Common Causes

- **A**spiration/**a**cute pancreatitis/**a**ir or **a**mniotic embolism
- **R**adiation
- **D**rug overdose/**d**isseminated intravascular coagulation/**d**rowning/**d**iffuse lung disease
- **S**hock/**s**epsis/**s**moke inhalation

## Pathogenesis

The pathologic finding is widespread atelectasis. A homogenous eosinophilic membrane (hyaline membrane) is found plastering the alveolar ducts and terminal bronchioles. Hyaline membrane is made up of proteins that are exuded into the alveoli and airways of a baby with RDS. It is caused by deficiency of surfactant in the baby's lungs. Surfactant production slowly increases from 20th week gestation with a surge at 30th–34th week and at term with the onset of labor.

A number of factors causing surfactant deficiency in the neonate include:
- Lower lecithin
- Hypoperfusion of pulmonary vascular bed
- Alternation in the fibrinolytic mechanism within the lungs

Due to less surfactant, as in premature baby, the pressure needed to open up and expand the alveoli is very high and much beyond the ability of the baby. Hence, there is collapse of lungs (atelectasis) and clinical manifestation of RDS appear.

## Signs and Symptoms

Baby presents the clinical manifestation abruptly 4–6 hours after birth as follows:
- Respiratory rate more than 60/minute
- Nasal flaring
- Rib retraction
- Expiratory grunting
- Cyanosis

## Diagnosis

X-rays show ground glass mottling due to extensive atelectasis process.

## Complications

- Intraventricular hemorrhage (IVH)
- Bronchopulmonary dysplasia
- Pulmonary hemorrhage
- Pneumothorax
- Retrolental fibroplasia (due to hyperoxygenation)
- Neurological abnormalities

About one-third babies with RDS die. Infant with mild affection may survive with prompt and effective management.

## Management

- **Preventive measures:**
  - Administration of betamethasone or dexamethasone before preterm delivery, especially to women who go into labor before 34th week of gestation.
  - Administration of prophylactic artificial surfactant into baby's lungs after delivery.
  - Assessment of lung maturity before premature induction of labor and to delay the induction as much as possible to avoid risk to the fetus.
  - Prevention of fetal hypoxia in diabetic mothers.

The management process of respiratory distress syndrome has been shown in Figure 18.

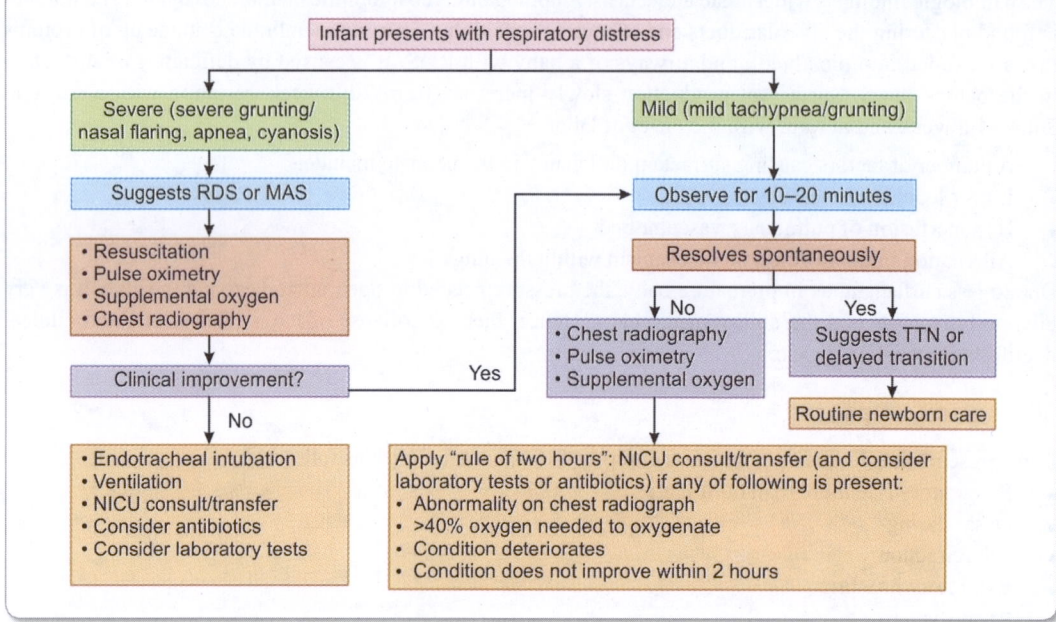

**Fig. 18:** Management of respiratory distress syndrome

*Abbreviations:* MAS, meconium aspiration syndrome; NICU, neonatal intensive care unit; RDS, respiratory distress syndrome; TTN, transient tachypnea of newborn

- **Definitive management**
  - Place the baby in neonatal intensive care unit (NICU) and nurse in a warm incubator with high humidity. Clear the airway by periodic endotracheal suctioning.
  - Provide warmed and humidified oxygen therapy.
  - Correction of hypovolemia with albumin or other colloid solution.
  - Correction of anemia, electrolyte imbalance, if any and prevention of infection.
  - Frequent monitoring of $pO_2$, $pCO_2$, pH and base excess to detect metabolic and respiratory acidosis and rectification accordingly.
  - Acidosis is corrected by I/V administration of sodium bicarbonate.
  - Direct tracheal instillation of surfactant therapy to reduce surface tension and stabilize alveolar air water interface.
  - **Feeding and nutrition:** Intragastric feeding is preferred. If there is chance for vomiting and aspiration, IV administration of 10% glucose may be given through a catheter inserted into umbilical/peripheral vein.

# NEONATAL SEPSIS

When pathogenic bacteria gain access in the blood stream, they may cause an over-whelming infection. The systemic bacterial infections of neonates are termed as neonatal sepsis, which incorporates septicemia, pneumonia, meningitis. It is caused by *Klebsiella pneumoniae, Staphylococcus aureus, Escherichia coli, Pseudomonas aeruginosa,* etc.

## Risk Factors

- Intrauterine infections
- Premature and prolonged rupture of membrane (PROM)
- Meconium stained liquor
- Repeated vaginal examination
- Maternal infections
- Lack of aseptic practices
- Birth asphyxia
- Resuscitation without aseptic precautions
- Low-birth-weight (LBW)
- Invasive procedures
- Superficial infections
- Aspiration of feed
- Lack of breastfeeding

## Sources of Infections

- Infusion sets
- Intravenous sites
- Face masks
- Feeding bottles
- Catheters
- Ventilators
- Resuscitators
- Incubators
- Baby care contaminated articles
- Infected care givers
- Unhygienic environment

## Types of Neonatal Sepsis

- **Early onset neonatal sepsis:** It develops before 72 hours of life due to intrauterine infections, maternal conditions and intranatal causes. It manifests frequently as pneumonia and less commonly as septicemia and meningitis.
- **Late onset neonatal sepsis:** It develops after 72 hours, may be at the end of first or in second week. It occurs due to nosocomial infection. The clinical presentations are those of septicemia, pneumonia or meningitis.

## Clinical Manifestations

- Early onset neonatal sepsis may be present as perinatal hypoxia, resuscitation difficulties and congenital pneumonia in the form of respiratory distress.
- Late onset neonatal sepsis in very small baby may be silent who may die suddenly without presenting any signs and symptoms.
  - Baby becomes lethargic, inactive, pale or unresponsive and refuses to suck
  - Hypothermia is common than fever
  - Poor cry, vacant look, comatose and not arousable baby with distention of abdomen, diarrhea, vomiting, less weight gain and poor neonatal reflexes

Chapter 11 ● High-risk and Sick Newborn

- Episodes of apnea or gasping
- In sick neonates, skin may become tight and gives a hide bound feel (sclerema) and poor perfusion
- In critical neonates circumoral cyanosis, shock, bleeding, excessive jaundice and renal failure occurs
- In case of pneumonia, child may have fast breathing, chest retraction, grunting, early cyanosis, apneic spells, inactive and poor feeding
- In case of meningitis, high pitched cry, fever, irritability, convulsions, twitching, blank look, neck retraction and bulging fontanelle can be seen
- Neonatal sepsis may be present with hypoglycemia, urinary tract infection (UTI), disseminated intravascular coagulation (DIC), necrotizing enterocolitis, etc.

## Investigations

- Blood culture
- Urine examination and culture
- Swab culture from septic umbilicus or from any other location of superficial infections
- Lumbar puncture for cerebrospinal fluid (CSF) study
- Chest X-ray
- Blood sugar
  - Serum bilirubin
  - Leukocyte count
  - Erythrocyte sedimentation ratio (ESR)
  - C-reactive protein (CRP)

## Management

Early recognition of problems and administration of effective and appropriate antibiotic therapy with optimal supportive care are mandatory management techniques to improve the survival of the neonates.

- Supportive care is provided to maintain normal body temperature, to stabilize the cardio- pulmonary status, to correct hypoglycemia and to prevent bleeding tendency. It includes:
  - Maintenance of warmth to ensure consistently normal temperature
  - Administration of intravenous fluids
  - Oxygen therapy should be provided if the neonate is having respiratory distress or cyanosis
  - Bag and mask ventilation with oxygen may be required if the infant is apneic or breathing is inadequate
  - Vitamin K, 1 mg IM should be given to control bleeding immediately after birth
  - Enteral feed is avoided if the neonate is very sick or had abdominal distension. Maintenance of fluid should be done by intravenous infusion.
  - Other supportive measures include gentle physical stimulation, nasogastric aspiration, close and constant monitoring of infant's condition and expert nursing care.
- Antibiotic therapy should be administered considering the common causative organism. A combination of ampicillin and gentamycin/amikacin is recommended for treatment of sepsis and pneumonia. In case of suspected meningitis, chloramphenicol should be added. Duration of antibiotic therapy should be individualized. In general, antibiotic should be given 0–14 days in septicemia and pneumonia, 14 days for UTI and 21 days for meningitis.
- **Other drug therapy:** Anticonvulsants in case of convulsions and corticosteroids in severely sick neonates with endotoxic shock, sclerema and adrenal insufficiency. Dopamine is used to treat shock and mannitol can be used in raised intracranial pressure (ICP).

- Phototherapy and exchange transfusion may be necessary in hyperbilirubinemia. Blood transfusion may be required in anemia and bleeding disorders.
- Administer immunoglobulin preparations containing type-specific antibodies to group-'b' streptococci.
- Treatment of superficial infections, like umbilical sepsis, pyoderma, oral thrush, conjunctivitis should be done appropriately.

# BIRTH INJURIES

## Definition

Birth injuries encompass any systemic damages incurred during delivery (hypoxic, toxic, biochemical, infection factors, etc.), but "birth trauma" focuses largely on mechanical damage. Birth trauma refers to damage of the tissues and organs of a newly delivered child, often as a result of physical pressure or trauma during childbirth.

## Etiology

- Primigravida
- Cephalopelvic disproportion (CPD), small maternal stature, maternal pelvic anomalies
- Prolonged or rapid labor
- Deep transverse arrest of descent of presenting part of the fetus
- Oligohydramnios
- Abnormal presentation (breech)
- Use of midcavity forceps or vacuum extraction
- Versions and extractions
- Very low-birth-weight infant or extreme prematurity
- Fetal macrosomia
- Large fetal head
- Fetal anomalies

## Common Birth Injuries

- **Soft tissue injuries** include:
  - Abrasions
  - Erythema petechiae
  - Ecchymosis
  - Lacerations
- **Skull injuries** include (Fig. 19):
  - Caput succedaneum
  - Cephalhematoma
  - Linear fractures
- **Facial injuries** include:
  - Subconjunctival hemorrhage
  - Retinal hemorrhage
- **Musculoskeletal injuries** include:
  - Clavicular fractures
  - Fractures of long bones
  - Sternocleidomastoid injury

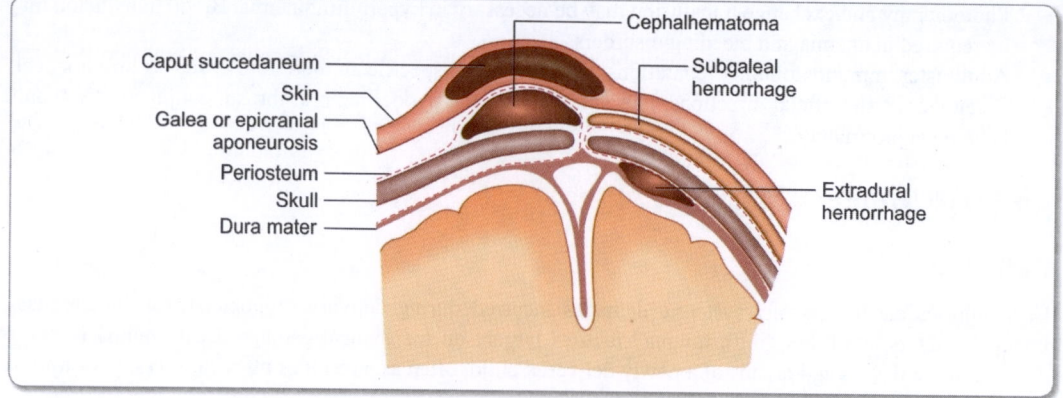

**Fig. 19:** Location of injury in soft tissue planes on the scalp and head

- Intra-abdominal injuries include:
  - Liver hematoma
  - Splenic hematoma
  - Adrenal hemorrhage
  - Renal hemorrhage
- Peripheral nerve injuries include:
  - Facial palsy
  - Unilateral vocal cord paralysis
  - Radial nerve palsy
  - Lumbosacral plexus injury
  - Erb's palsy

## Cephalhematoma

Cephalhematoma is a subperiosteal collection of blood secondary to rupture of blood vessels between the skull and the periosteum; suture lines delineate its extent. Most commonly parietal, cephalhematoma may occasionally be observed over the occipital bone.

The extent of hemorrhage may be severe enough to cause anemia and hypotension, although this is uncommon. The resolving hematoma predisposes to hyperbilirubinemia. Rarely, cephalhematoma may be a focus of infection that leads to meningitis or osteomyelitis. Linear skull fractures may underlie a cephalhematoma (5–20% of cephalhematomas). Resolution occurs over weeks, occasionally with residual calcification.

No laboratory studies are usually necessary. Skull radiography or computed tomography (CT) scanning is performed if neurologic symptoms are present. Usually, management solely consists of observation. Transfusion for anemia, hypovolemia, or both is necessary if blood accumulation is significant. Aspiration is not required for resolution and is likely to increase the risk of infection.

Hyperbilirubinemia occurs following the breakdown of the red blood cells (RBCs) within the hematoma. This type of hyperbilirubinemia occurs later than classic physiologic hyperbilirubinemia. The presence of a bleeding disorder should be considered. Skull radiography or CT scanning is also performed if a concomitant depressed skull fracture is a possibility.

## Caput Succedaneum

Caput succedaneum is a serosanguinous, subcutaneous and extraperiosteal fluid collection with poorly-defined margins; it is caused by the pressure of the presenting part against the dilating cervix. Caput succedaneum can also be caused by the use of vacuum extraction devices during a protracted delivery. Caput succedaneum extends across the midline and over suture lines and is associated with head molding. Caput succedaneum does not usually cause complications and is usually resolved over the first few days. Management consists of observation only.

## Erb's Palsy

Erb's palsy is caused by damage to the brachial plexus during delivery of the neonate (Fig. 20). This is mostly limited to the 5th and 6th cervical nerves.

### Risk Factors

| Risk factors in Erb's palsy | | |
|---|---|---|
| **Fetal factors** | **Maternal factors** | **Factors related to labor** |
| • Macrosomia | • Maternal propulsive forces | • Lateral traction exerted on head and neck during delivery in vertex presentation<br>• Arm extended overhead in breech presentation<br>• Excessive traction placed on shoulders during delivery |

### Presentation

The infant is unable to:
- Abduct the arm from the shoulder
- Rotate the arm externally from the shoulder
- Supinate the forearm

### Clinical Signs

- Characteristic position—adduction and internal rotation of the arm with the forearm pronated
- Forearm extension is normal
- Biceps reflex is absent
- Moro's reflex is absent on the affected side
- Sensory impairment on the outer aspect of the arm (unusual)
- Power of the forearm is normal (if impaired, it suggests injury to the lower part of the plexus)
- Hand grasp is normal unless the lower part of the plexus is also damaged

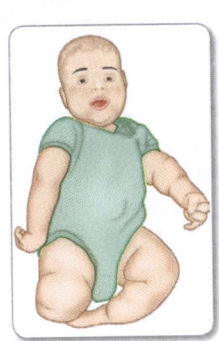

**Fig. 20:** Erb's palsy

### Investigations

- Magnetic resonance imaging (MRI) shows nerve root damage
- Electromyogram (EMG) and nerve root studies are not helpful in determining the extent of the damage severity.

### Management

- Intermittent immobilization and positioning to prevent contractures
- Positioning such that arm is abducted to 90°, externally rotated at the shoulder, supination of forearm and extension at wrist with the palm turned toward the face

- Gentle massage
- Physiotherapy with active and passive movement exercises by the end of the first week
- Electrical stimulation may prove to be beneficial
- Referral to a neurosurgeon if paralysis persists beyond three months or there is more proximal damage to the plexus
- Surgery can involve direct neurorrhaphy after neuroma resection, neurolysis to remove any scar tissue, nerve grafting with transplant of another nerve or nerve transfer from a local functioning nerve; however, results are mixed and pain, along with functional disability, persist in significant numbers.

### Facial Nerve Palsy

Facial nerve palsy (Fig. 21) due to birth trauma is the loss of controllable (voluntary) muscle movement in an infant's face due to pressure on the facial nerve in the face just before or at the time of birth.

#### Causes

Most of the time the cause is unknown. But a difficult delivery, with or without the use of an instrument called forceps, may lead to this condition.

Some factors that can cause birth trauma (injury) include:

- Large baby size (may be seen if the mother has diabetes)
- Long pregnancy or labor
- Use of epidural anesthesia
- Use of a medicine to cause labor and stronger contractions (oxytocin induction)

#### Symptoms

The most common form of facial nerve palsy due to birth trauma involves only the lower part of the facial nerve. This part controls the muscles around the lips. The muscle weakness is mainly noticeable when the infant cries.

The newborn infant may have the following symptoms:

- Eyelid may not close on affected side
- Lower face (below eyes) appears uneven during crying
- Mouth does not move down the same way on both sides while crying
- No movement (paralysis) on the affected side of the face (from the forehead to the chin in severe cases).

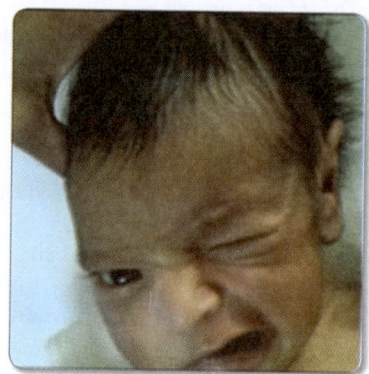

**Fig. 21:** Facial nerve palsy

#### Diagnostic Tests

A physical examination is usually all that is needed to diagnose this condition. In rare cases, a nerve conduction test is needed. This test can pinpoint the exact location of the nerve injury.

#### Management

- In most cases, the infant will be closely monitored to see if the paralysis goes away on its own.
- If the baby's eye does not close all the way, an eye pad and eye drops will be used to protect the eye.
- Surgery may be needed to relieve pressure on the nerve.
- Infants with permanent paralysis need special therapy.

## Torticollis

Torticollis also known as "wryneck", is a condition in which baby's head is tilted. The chin points to one shoulder, while the head tilts toward the opposite shoulder. It develops in newborns after a difficult childbirth or improper positioning in the womb, a condition known as congenital muscular torticollis or infant torticollis (Fig. 22).

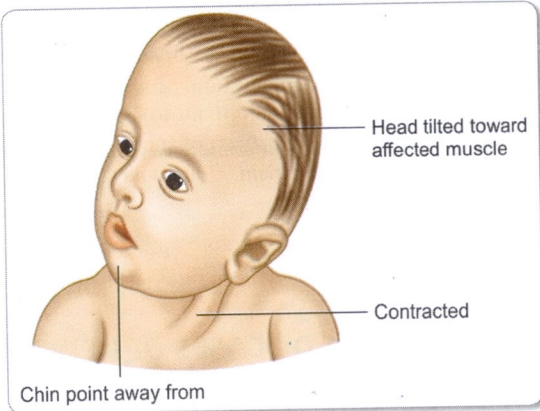

Fig. 22: Congenital muscular torticollis

*(Figure labels: Head tilted toward affected muscle; Contracted; Chin point away from)*

### Causes

- **Tightness in sternocleidomastoid muscles:** Congenital torticollis usually develops when the muscle connecting the breastbone and collarbone to the skull (sternocleidomastoid muscle) becomes tight. This tightness may be due to abnormal positioning in the womb (head tilted in one direction) or the muscle could have been damaged during childbirth. The condition is termed "congenital muscular torticollis".
- **Abnormalities in cervical vertebrae:** Less commonly, abnormalities in the formation of the cervical vertebrae may be the cause of congenital torticollis, a condition known as "Klippel-Feil syndrome". In such a case, the neck bones may be stuck together, abnormally formed, or a combination of both.
- **Inherited diseases:** Congenital torticollis in rare cases may occur as a result of serious medical conditions that cause damages to the nervous system or muscles such as brain and spinal cord tumor. The condition is also hereditary.

### Signs and Symptoms

Torticollis baby may show symptoms relating to turning of the head such as:

- Head tilted in one direction
- Looking over one shoulder instead of turning the head fully to follow movement
- Prefer breastfeeding on one breast as baby may have difficulty on the other side
- Have difficulty turning fully in a particular direction and gets frustrated when unable to do so

Other conditions that develop from torticollis include:

- Positional plagiocephaly (development of flat head) on one or both sides as a result of always lying in a particular direction
- Development of a tiny bump or lump in the neck, resembling a knot in a tense muscle.

### Treatment

- **Nonsurgical treatment:** There are many simple ways to stretch out and develop the weak muscles in a child with torticollis. For example, proper ways to hold him while feeding and specific ways to place him in his crib in order to encourage movement to his weaker direction will be recommended. If instructions are followed properly, recovery could be in two months or between 6 and 12 months in severe cases.
  - **Physical therapy:** Different bending and stretching exercises are helpful to strengthen neck muscles. Physiotherapist recommend a home exercise program that usually involves active and passive bending

and stretching motions during play and sleep to promote symmetrical movement. The success of the exercise program depends on how early treatment commences, the commitment of the parents and severity of muscle damage or presence of a tight muscle knot.

- ▪ **Tummy time:** This involves placing the baby on his stomach upon a blanket or soft surface and putting toys in front of him. Mother also plays with the toys and tries to catch his attention. The aim is to encourage him to lift his head up and see all the actions which help strengthen his neck muscles.
- **Surgical treatment:** In some cases, physical therapy alone for the treatment of torticollis may not be enough to provide full recovery. Pediatrician may refer the child to an orthopedic surgeon if by 18 months the baby still has weak neck muscles. It is always preferable to exhaust all efforts at recovery through physical therapy before opting for surgery. Surgical operations can help strengthen the muscles for full recovery to occur.

## HEMORRHAGIC DISEASES OF NEWBORN

Hemorrhagic diseases of the newborn are rare bleeding problem that can occur after birth. It is classified according to the timing of its first symptoms as early onset, classic onset or late onset. The disease is caused by vitamin K deficiency. As a result, it is often called vitamin K deficiency bleeding (VKDB). As a consequence of vitamin K deficiency, there is impaired production of coagulation factors II, VIII, IX and X, protein C and S by the liver, resulting in excessive bleeding. It commonly includes gastrointestinal hemorrhage, pericranial and intracranial hemorrhage and hemorrhagic diathesis.

### Gastrointestinal Hemorrhage

Bleeding from the gastrointestinal tract is a common and potentially, life-threatening condition in newborn, infants and children. A careful history taking and physical examination, as well as consideration of patient's age will suggest the most likely cause.

#### Causes of GI Hemorrhage

- Peptic esophagitis
- Swallowed maternal blood
- Mallory-Weiss tears
- Gastritis
- Gastric ulcer
- Duodenal ulcer
- Anal fissures
- Infectious colitis
- Intussusception
- Necrotizing enterocolitis (NEC)
- Meckel's diverticulum
- Hirschsprung's enterocolitis
- Colonic hemangiomas

#### Signs and Symptoms of GI Bleed

- Hematemesis
- Painless melena

- Melena with pain, obstruction, peritonitis, perforation
- Hematochezia with/without abdominal pain and diarrhea

## Diagnosis

- **History taking:** Careful history taking help to diagnose this condition. Sometimes food coloring agents can turn emesis and stool red, and bismuth and iron may make stools black
- **Blood test:** Confirmation of presence of heme protein is accomplished with a guaiac test
- **Gastric aspiration:**
  - A gastric aspirate positive for blood is highly specific for upper tract bleeding
  - A negative aspirate suggests lower tract bleeding
- **Endoscopy:** It includes:
  - Esophagogastroduodenoscopy in patients who have hematemesis or melena
  - Sigmoidoscopy in patients who have suspected colonic bleeding
  - Colonoscopy for the inspection of entire colon
  - Intraoperative endoscopy is done for those patients who continue to have significant bleeding when extensive endoscopic and radiologic test findings are negative and a small bowel source of bleeding is suspected.
- **Radiologic evaluation:**
  - A plain abdominal radiograph may exclude bowel obstruction and free intra-abdominal gas.
  - Barium studies is done in case of intussusception is suspected.
  - Bleeding scan is done in case of Meckel's diverticulum to detect ectopic gastric mucosa.
  - Angiography maybe used to detect bleeding sites in more difficult cases and requires a higher bleeding rate.
  - Enteroclysis involves intubation of the jejunum, the gradual instillation of barium, air or methylcellulose and evaluation of mucosal surface of the bowel through fluoroscopy. This technique may identify the site of small bowel bleeding in 5–10% patients.

## Management

- **Cardiovascular resuscitation** should be vigorous when orthostatic hypotension is present.
  - With massive bleeding, whole blood should be given to maintain intravascular volume. Once bleeding has stopped, packed cells alone may be given.
  - Vitamin K (1 mg per year of age, up to 10 mg); platelets and plasma should be given as needed to correct any coagulopathy.
- **Treatment of upper tract lesions:**
  - Mucosal lesion of the upper tract should be treated with antacids $H_2$ receptor antagonists or proton pump inhibitors
  - Esophageal varices may be treated with
    - Octreotide which is a synthetic analogue of somatostatin that will decrease splanchnic blood flow. A bolus of 1–2 mg/kg is administered followed by continuous infusion of 1–2 mg/kg/hr. Additional bolus may be administered in 2–4 hours, if bleeding persists.
    - Vasopressin infusion decreases portal preload pressure and therefore, decreases variceal blood flow. Bolus dose of 0.3 unit/kg followed by continuous infusion of 0.2–0.4 units/minute.
  - Sclerotherapy permits variceal obliteration by direct variceal injection of a sclerosant solution such as 5% morrhuate sodium.

- Transjugular intrahepatic portosystemic shunt is an angiographic technique in which stent is placed within the liver through hepatic parenchyma to connect intrahepatic branches of the portal and hepatic veins.
  - Surgery to decompress the portal system can be performed.
- **Treatment of lower tract lesions:** Depends on the cause (e.g., surgery is used for Meckel's diverticulum.

## Pericranial and Intracranial Hemorrhages

- **Subaponeurotic/subgaleal hemorrhage** is a collection of blood beneath the thin, tendinous sheet covering the skull and above the periosteum of the bones of the skull; this is large potential space that crosses cranial suture lines. Subaponeurotic hemorrhage generally follows head-trauma at birth. On examination, the scalp and head feel firm and boggy over a large area, and there may be scalp discoloration and a large amount of blood loss. Failure to recognize subaponeurotic hemorrhage may yield disastrous result because of shock
- **Cephalohematoma** is a subperiosteal collection of blood; hence, it does not cross cranial suture lines. It is seen after birth trauma and is self-limited, almost always disappearing without residual effects. Therapy to evacuate the collection of blood is contraindicated because it is associated with a significant risk of infection.
- **Subarachnoid hemorrhage** may occur after a normal or traumatic delivery. Bleeding is self-limited and symptoms (e.g., irritability, seizure activity) are resolved in few days
- **Subdural hemorrhage** is also seen with birth trauma. A significant amount of blood can accumulate and cause focal neurologic deficits due to pressure exerted on the brain. However, drainage is necessary only if symptoms are severe or do not get resolved.
- **Intraventricular hemorrhage** is seen almost exclusively in preterm infants and is the result of bleeding of the germinal matrix, frequently after an asphyxia insult
  - Small ventricular hemorrhage is confined to a germinal matrix (grade I) or associated with a small amount of blood in the ventricle (grade II) often resolve without sequelae
  - Large intraventricular hemorrhages that are associated with ventricular dilatation (grade III) or extension into the brain parenchyma (grade IV) is associated with permanent functional impairment and hydrocephalus.

## Hemorrhagic Diathesis

- Bleeding due to thrombocytopenia is common but usually superficial
- If there is associated DIC or extreme leukocytosis, occasionally there may be severe and life-threating bleeding (e.g., in the central nervous system)

### Clinical Features

- Petechiae, purpura or both
- Severe recurrent epistaxis
- Prolonged bleeding after dental extractions, surgical procedures or major trauma
- Recurrent hemarthrosis

### Diagnostic Tests

Laboratory tests to assess coagulation include:

- Platelet count
- Bleeding time

- Partial thromboplastin time (PTT)
- Prothrombin time (PT)

## Management

- Drugs that compromise platelet function (e.g., aspirin) must be avoided, as should deep venipunctures and intramuscular injections. The patients should be protected against trauma (especially to the head) prolonged immobilization should be avoided.
- When the nature of the defect is identified, specific replacement measures should be employed.
- If the bleeding is life threatening, fresh frozen plasma (10–20 mL/kg) can be used as a temporizing measure for defects in coagulation factors until a specific factor deficiency is identified.

# CONGENITAL ANOMALIES

Congenital anomalies can be defined as structural or functional anomalies (e.g., metabolic disorders) that occur during intrauterine life and can be identified prenatally at birth or sometimes may only be detected later in infancy, such as hearing defects. In simple terms, congenital refers to the existence at or before birth.

## Incidence

- Global incidence about 30–70/1000 (live birth)
- In India: 2.5–4%
- **Most common type of birth defect:** Central nervous system abnormalities (22%)

## Risk Factors

- Consanguinity (mental retardation)
- Advanced maternal age (Down's syndrome)
- Maternal malnutrition (iodine deficiency, folic acid deficiency)

## Etiology

- **Genetic factors**
  - Chromosomal abnormalities, e.g., Down's syndrome
  - Single gene disorders
    - Autosomal inheritance
    - X-linked or sex-linked inheritance
    - Dominant traits–one parent affected
    - Recessive traits–both parents
    - Recessive traits–son affected
    - Dominant traits–daughter affected
  - Polygenic or multifactorial inheritance
    - Combination of polygenic and environmental factors
- **Environmental factors**
  - **Drugs intake during pregnancy:** Steroids, anticonvulsants, cocaine, lithium, etc.
  - **X-ray exposure during** pregnancy.
  - **Maternal diseases:** Diabetes mellitus, endocrine abnormalities, iodine deficiency, folic acid deficiency and malnutrition.

- **Intrauterine infections:** Syphilis, toxoplasmosis, other infections, rubella, cytomegalovirus and herpes simplex infections (STORCH).
- **Abnormal intrauterine environment:** Bicornuate uterus, septate uterus and polyhydramnios, etc.
- **Environmental pollution:** Air.
- **Maternal addiction:** Alcohol, tobacco and smoking.

## Diagnostic Approaches

### Prenatal Diagnosis

- Antenatal screening
- Radiography
- Fetoscopy
- Ultrasonography (USG)
- Amniocentesis at 14–16 weeks
- Chorionic villus sampling (CVS)
- Maternal serum alpha fetoprotein testing (MSAFP)
- Amniography
- Protein assay, deoxyribonucleic acid (DNA) diagnosis

### Postnatal Diagnosis

- Maternal and family history
- Physical examination
- Radiography
- USG
- Blood test
- Biochemical assay
- Cytogenic study
- Hormonal assay

## Common Congenital Anomalies

### Abnormalities of Central Nervous System

- **Anencephaly:** It is the absence of a major portion of the brain, skull, and scalp that occurs during embryonic development. It is a cephalic disorder that results from a neural tube defect that occurs when the rostral (head) end of the neural tube fails to close, usually between the 23rd and 26th day following conception (Fig. 23A).
- **Meningoencephalocele:** It is a type of encephalocele, which is an abnormal sac of fluid, brain tissue, and meninges (membranes that cover the brain and spinal cord) that extend through a defect in the skull (Fig. 23B).
- **Meningocele:** A meningocele is a birth defect where there is a sac protruding from the spinal column. The sac includes spinal fluid, but does not contain neural tissue. It may be covered with skin or with meninges (Fig. 23C).
- **Meningomyelocele:** Meningomyelocele, also commonly known as myelomeningocele, is a type of spina bifida. Spina bifida is a birth defect in which the spinal canal and the backbone don't close before the baby is born. This type of birth defect is also called a neural tube defect (Fig. 23D).

- **Hydrocephalus:** It is usually due to blockage of cerebrospinal fluid (CSF) outflow in the ventricles or in the subarachnoid space over the brain (Fig. 23E).
- **Microcephaly:** It is a medical condition in which the brain does not develop properly resulting in a smaller than normal head. Microcephaly may be present at birth or it may develop in the first few years of life (Fig. 23F).
- **Syringomyelia:** It is the development of a fluid-filled cyst (syrinx) within the spinal cord. Over time, the cyst gets enlarged, damaging the spinal cord and causing pain, weakness and stiffness, among other symptoms.
  - **Others**
    - Agenesis of cranial nerves
    - Porencephaly

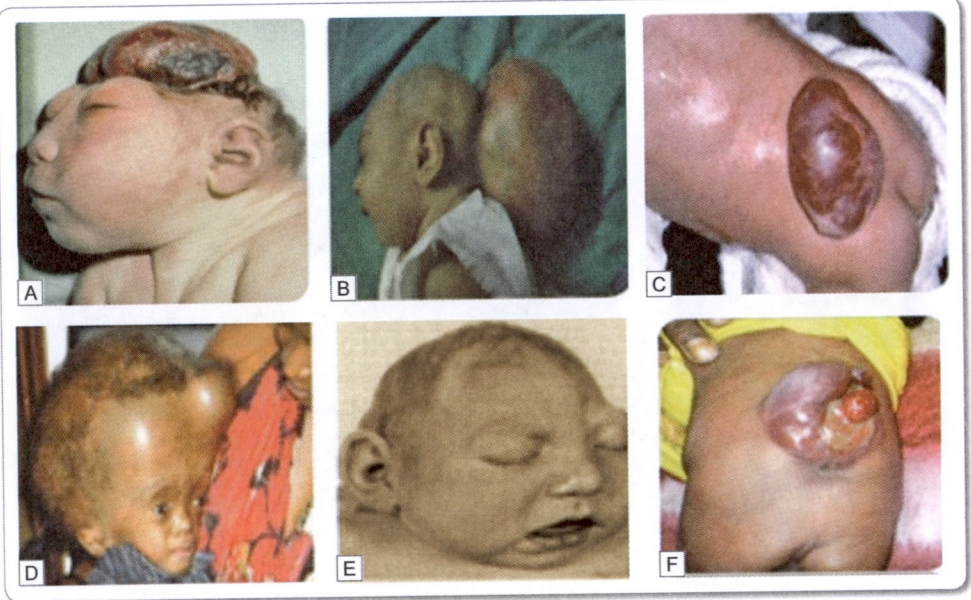

**Figs 23A to F:** Central nervous system abnormalities. **A.** Anencephaly; **B.** Meningoencephalocele; **C.** Meningocele; **D.** Meningomyelocele; **E.** Hydrocephalus; **F.** Microcephaly

## Congenital Heart Diseases

Figures 24A to D show different kinds of congenital heart diseases.

- **Ventricular septal defects (VSD):** It means a hole in the heart. It is a common heart defect which is present at birth. The oxygen-rich blood then gets pumped back to the lungs instead of out to the body, causing the heart to work harder.
- **Atrial septal defect (ASD):** An atrial septal defect (ASD) is an opening in the interatrial septum, causing a left-to-right shunt and volume overload of the right atrium and right ventricle. Children are rarely symptomatic, but long-term complications after 20 years of age include pulmonary hypertension, heart failure, and atrial arrhythmias.
- **Patent ductus arteriosus (PDA):** Before a baby is born, the fetus's blood does not need to go to the lungs to get oxygenated. The ductus arteriosus is a hole that allows the blood to skip the circulation to the lungs. However, when the baby is born, the blood must receive oxygen in the lungs and this hole is

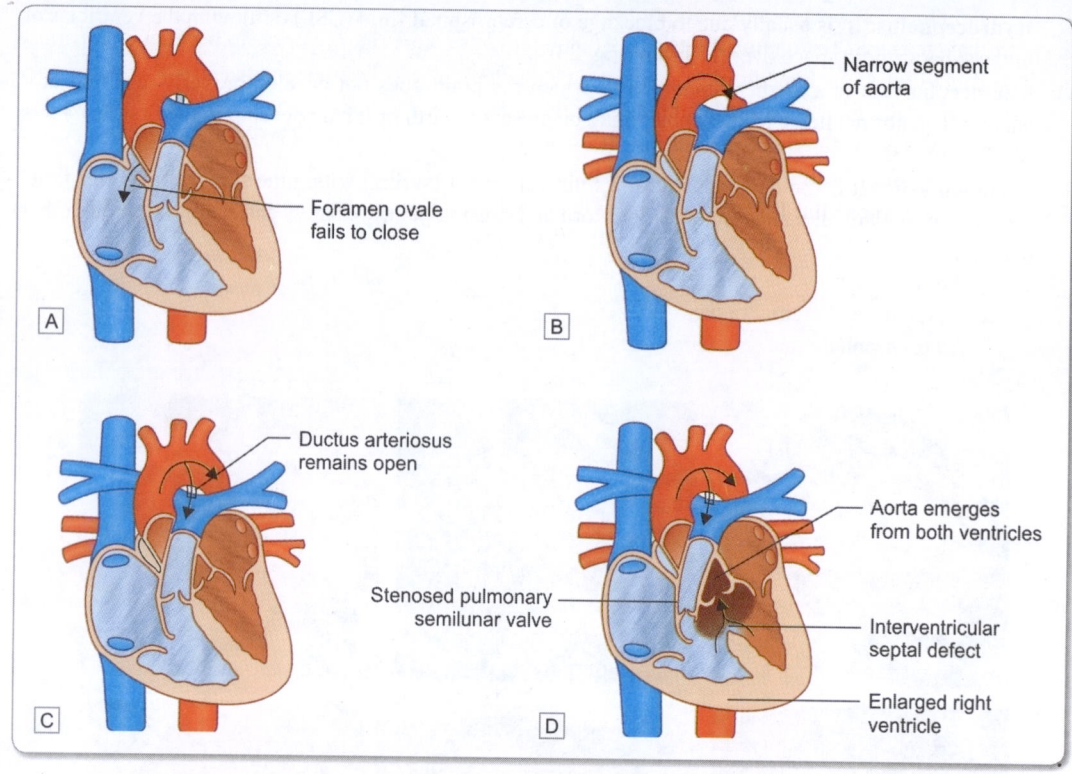

**Figs 24A to D:** Congenital heart diseases. **A.** Patent foramen ovale; **B.** Coarctation of the aorta; **C.** Patent ductus arteriosus; **D.** Tetralogy of Fallot

supposed to be closed. If the ductus arteriosus is still open (or patent) the blood may skip this necessary step of circulation. The open hole is called the patent ductus arteriosus.

- **Coarctation of aorta:** It is a congenital (present at birth) heart defect involving a narrowing of the aorta. The aorta is the large artery that carries oxygen-rich blood from the left ventricle to the body.
- **Transposition of great vessels:** In this condition, the two arteries that carry blood from the heart to the lungs and body are not connected as they should be.
- **Tricuspid atresia:** It is a heart defect present at birth in which a valve (tricuspid valve) between two of the hearts chambers is not formed. Instead, there is solid tissue between the chambers, which restricts blood flow and causes the right lower heart chamber (ventricle) to be underdeveloped.
- **Aortic stenosis:** It is the narrowing or blocking of the heart's aorta, which carries oxygen-rich (red) blood from the heart to the body.
- **Pulmonic stenosis:** It is a condition characterized by obstruction to blood flow from the right ventricle to the pulmonary artery.
- **Tetralogy of Fallot:** ToF is a cardiac anomaly that refers to a combination of four related heart defects that commonly occur together. The four defects are:
  1. Ventricular septal defect (VSD)
  2. Overriding aorta—the aortic valve is enlarged and appears to arise from both the left and right ventricles instead of the left ventricle as in normal hearts

3. Pulmonary stenosis—narrowing of the pulmonary valve and outflow tract or area below the valve that creates an obstruction (blockage) of blood flow from the right ventricle to the pulmonary artery

4. Right ventricular hypertrophy—thickening of the muscular walls of the right ventricle, which occurs because the right ventricle is pumping at high pressure:
   - **Mitral or aortic regurgitation:** It is also known as mitral valve insufficiency. It occurs when the mitral valve allows reversal of blood flow from the left ventricle (LV) to the left atrium.
   - **Dextrocardia:** It is a condition in which the heart is pointed toward the right side of the chest. Normally, the heart points toward the left.

## Gastrointestinal System Anomalies

Figures 25A to L show various anomalies related to gastrointestinal system.

- **Tracheoesophageal fistula:** It is a condition in which the esophagus and the trachea are abnormally connected, allowing fluids from the esophagus to get into the airways and interfere with breathing.

- **Esophogeal atresia:** It is a rare birth defect in which a baby is born without part of the esophagus (the tube that connects the mouth to the stomach). Babies with EA are also more prone to infections like pneumonia and conditions such as acid reflux.

- **Pyloric stenosis:** Pyloric stenosis is the narrowing of the lower portion of the stomach (pylorus) that leads into the small intestine. The muscles in this part of the stomach thicken, narrowing the opening of the pylorus and preventing food from moving from the stomach to the intestine.

- **Duodenal atresia:** It is the congenital absence or complete closure of a portion of the lumen of the duodenum. It causes increased levels of amniotic fluid during pregnancy (polyhydramnios) and intestinal obstruction in newborn babies.

- **Meconium ileus:** It is a condition where the content of the baby's bowel (meconium) is extremely sticky and creating a blockage in a part of the small intestine called the ileum.

- **Hirschsprung's disease:** It is a condition that affect the large intestine and causes problems with passing stool. It occurs as a result of missing nerve cells in the muscles of the colon.

- **Exomphalos:** It is weakness of the baby's abdominal wall where the umbilical cord joins it. This weakness allows the abdominal contents, mainly the bowel and the liver to protrude outside the abdominal cavity where they are contained in a loose sac that surrounds the umbilical cord.

- **Gastroschisis:** It is an opening in the abdominal wall through which the internal organs push outside of a baby's body. During fetal development, the abdominal wall fails to close properly, leaving an opening. The opening is usually to the right of the umbilical cord.

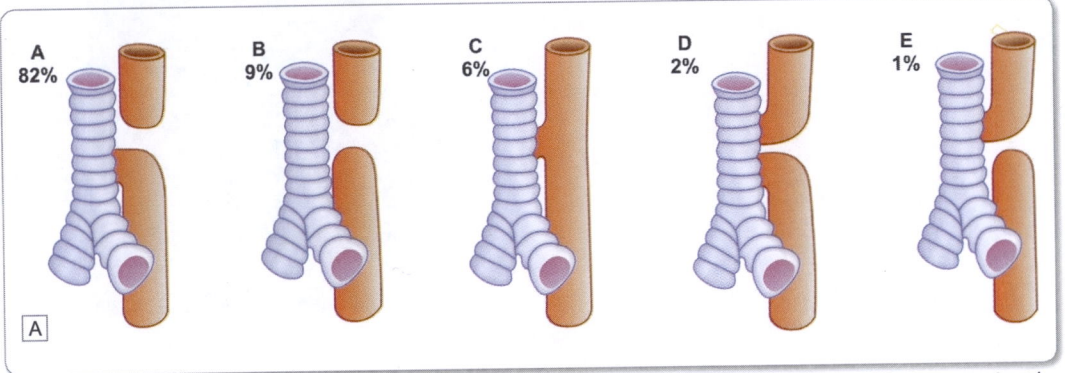

A — 82%    B — 9%    C — 6%    D — 2%    E — 1%

**Figs 25A:**

*Contd...*

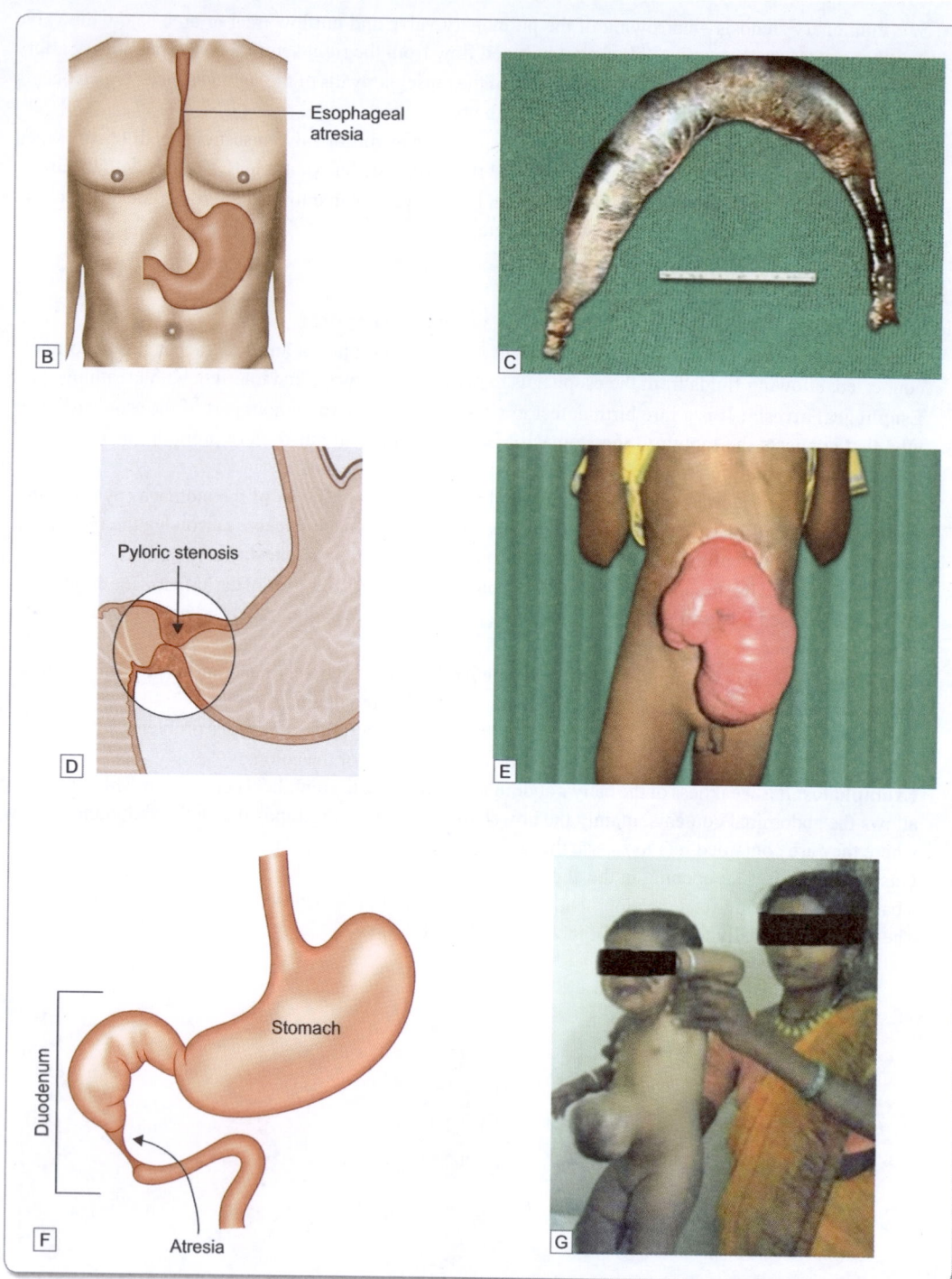

**Figs 25B to G:**

*Contd...*

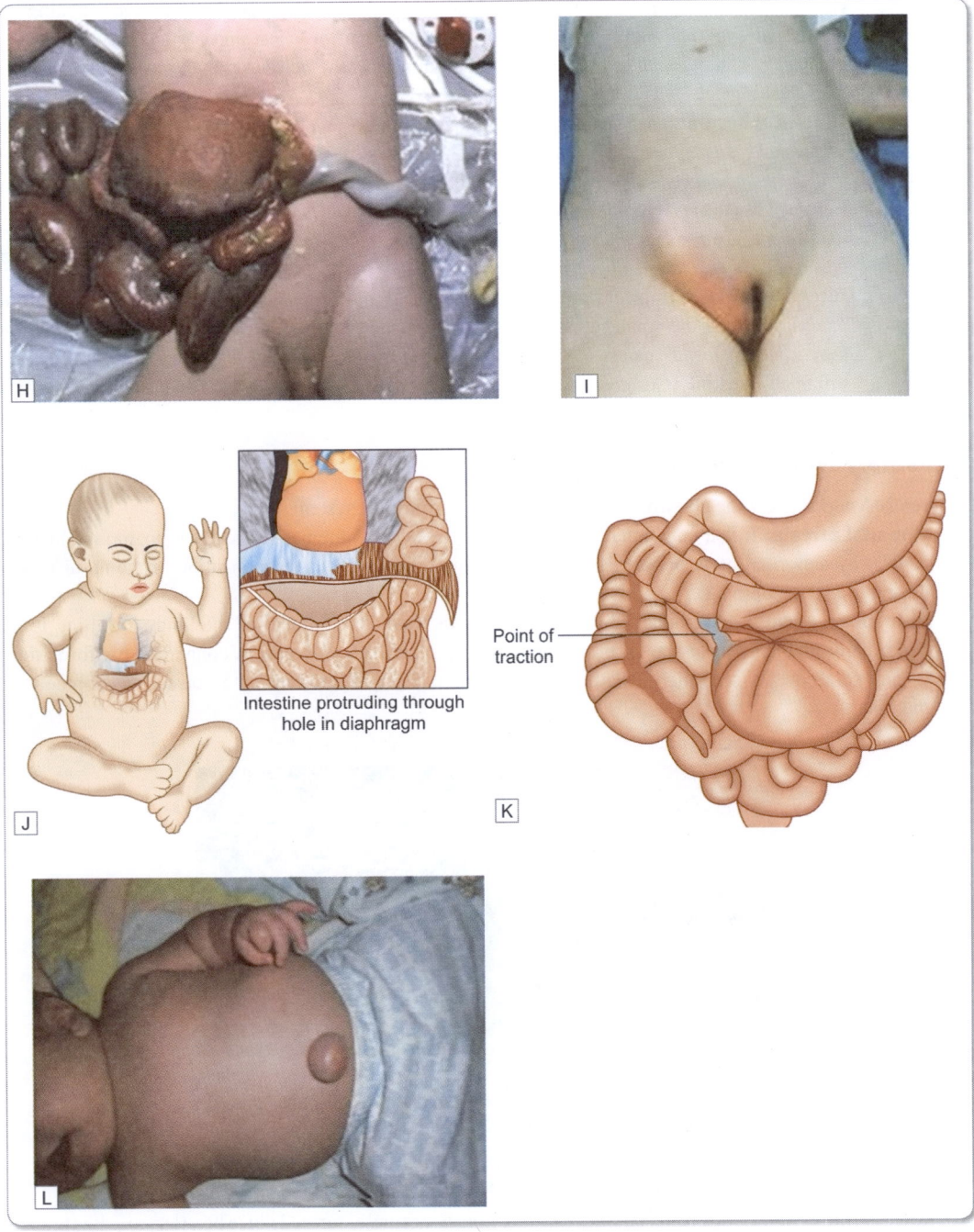

**Figs 25A to L:** Gastrointestinal abnormalities. **A.** Trachea-esophageal fistula; **B.** Esophageal atresia; **C.** Meconium ileus;
**D.** Pyloric stenosis; **E.** Hirschsprung disease (congenital megacolon); **F.** Duodenal atresia; **G.** Exomphalos; **H.** Gastroschisis;
**I.** Femoral hernia; **J.** Diaphragmatic hernia; **K.** Intestinal obstruction; **L.** Umbilical hernia

- o **Diaphragmatic hernia:** It is a birth defect in which there is an abnormal opening in the diaphragm. The diaphragm is the muscle between the chest and abdomen that helps in breathing. The opening allows part of the organs from the belly to move into the chest cavity near the lungs.
- o **Umbilical hernia:** It is a slight swelling or even a bulge near the belly button. The spot becomes larger and harder when the baby cries, coughs, or strains, due to the increase of pressure on the abdomen.
- o **Femoral hernia:** A femoral hernia occurs when tissue pushes through a weak spot in the muscle wall of the groin or inner thigh. Common causes include being overweight and overstraining while coughing, exercising, or passing stool.
- o **Intestinal obstruction:** Intestinal obstruction is a blockage that keeps food or liquid from passing through the small intestine or large intestine (colon). Causes of intestinal obstruction may include fibrous bands of tissue (adhesions) in the abdomen that form after surgery, an inflamed intestine (Crohn's disease), infected pouches in the intestine (diverticulitis), hernias and colon cancer.

## Respiratory System Abnormalities

Figures 26A and B show the abnormalities related to the respiratory system.

- **Choanal atresia:** It is a congenital disorder where the back of the nasal passage (choana) is blocked, usually by abnormal bony or soft tissue (membranous) due to failed recanalization of the nasal fossae during fetal development.
- **Pulmonary agenesis:** Pulmonary hypoplasia is incomplete development of the lungs, resulting in an abnormally low number or size of bronchopulmonary segments or alveoli. A congenital malformation, it most often occurs secondary to other fetal abnormalities that interfere with normal development of the lungs.

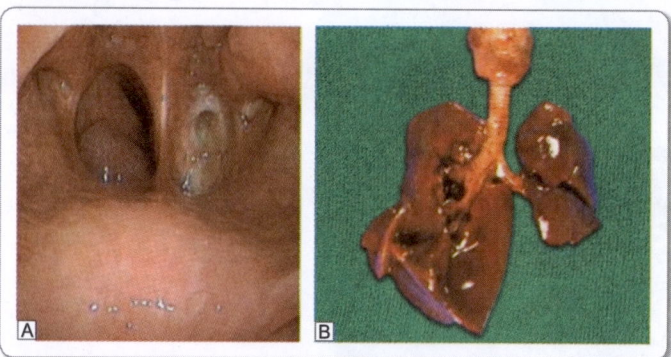

**Figs 26A and B:** Respiratory system abnormalities. **A.** Choanal atresia; **B.** Pulmonary agenesis

## Others

- **Congenital atelectasis:** It can result from a failure of the lungs to expand at birth.
- **Congenital stridor:** Congenital laryngeal stridor is an abnormally formed voice box (larynx). It is present at birth (congenital). During the baby's development, the larynx may not fully develop. The stridor is usually heard when the baby breathes in, but it can also be heard when the baby breathes out.
- **Congenital cyanosis:** Cyanosis is a bluish discoloration of the tissues that results when the absolute level of reduced hemoglobin in the capillary bed exceeds 3 g/dL. Neonatal cyanosis, particularly central

cyanosis, can be associated with significant and potentially life-threatening diseases due to cardiac, metabolic, neurologic, infectious, and parenchymal and nonparenchymal pulmonary disorders.

## Genitourinary System Abnormalities

Figures 27A to H show the abnormalities related to genitourinary system.

- **Renal agenesis:** It is a condition in which a newborn is missing one or both kidneys. Unilateral renal agenesis (URA) is the absence of one kidney. Bilateral renal agenesis (BRA) is the absence of both kidneys.
- **Hydronephrosis:** It occurs when a kidney has an excess of fluid due to a backup of urine, often caused by an obstruction in the upper part of the urinary tract.

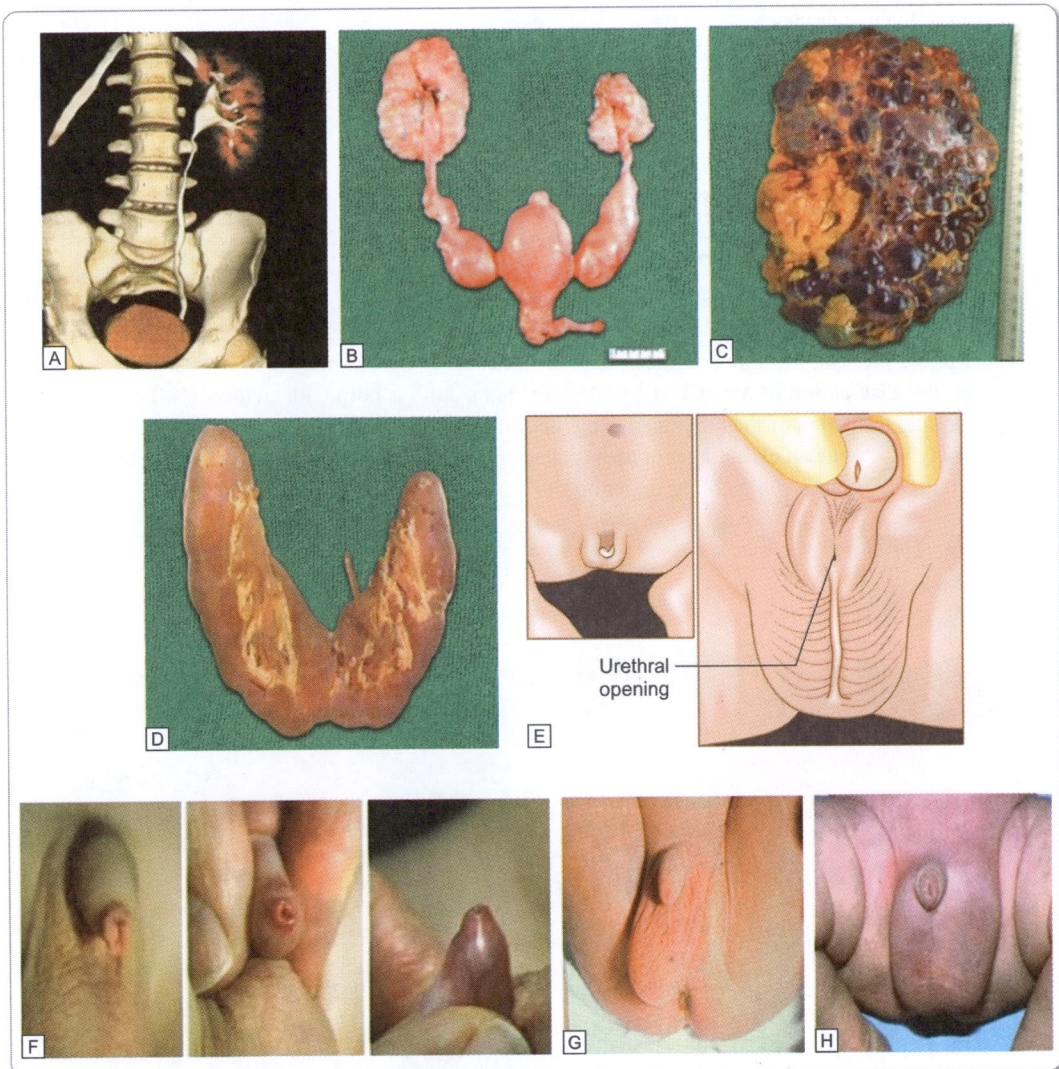

**Figs 27A to H:** Genitourinary system abnormalities. **A.** Renal agenesis; **B.** Hydronephrosis; **C.** Polycystic kidney; **D.** Horseshoe kidney; **E.** Hypospadias; **F.** Phimosis; **G.** Undescended testis; **H.** Hydrocele

- **Polycystic kidney:** Polycystic kidney disease (PKD) is an inherited disorder in which clusters of cysts develop primarily within the kidneys, causing the kidneys to enlarge and lose function over time. Cysts are noncancerous round sacs containing fluid.
- **Horseshoe kidney:** It is a congenital disorder in which the kidneys fuse together to form a horseshoe-shape during development in the womb.
- **Hypospadias:** It is a birth defect (congenital condition) in which the opening of the urethra is on the underside of the penis instead of at the tip.
- **Phimosis:** It is a condition in which the foreskin can't be retracted (pulled back) from around the tip of the penis. Phimosis can occur naturally or be the result of scarring.
- **Undescended testes:** Cryptorchidism (or undescended testes) is a condition seen in newborns when one or both of the male testes have not passed down into the scrotal sac.
- **Hydrocele:** It is a type of swelling in the scrotum that occurs when fluid collects in the thin sheath surrounding a testicle.

**Others**
- Posterior urethral valve (PUV)
- Congenital inguinal hernia
- Malformation of reproductive organs

## Musculoskeletal System Abnormalities

Figures 28A to I show the abnormalities related to musculoskeletal system.
- **Club foot (talipes):** Clubfoot is a birth defect where one or both feet are rotated inward and downward. The affected foot and leg may be smaller than the other.
- **Congenital dislocation of hip (CDH):** It occurs when a child is born with an unstable hip. It is caused by abnormal formation of the hip joint during the early stages of fetal development.
- **Polydactyly:** Having an extra finger or toe is called polydactyly. The extra digit may range from a small, raised bump to a complete, working finger or toe.

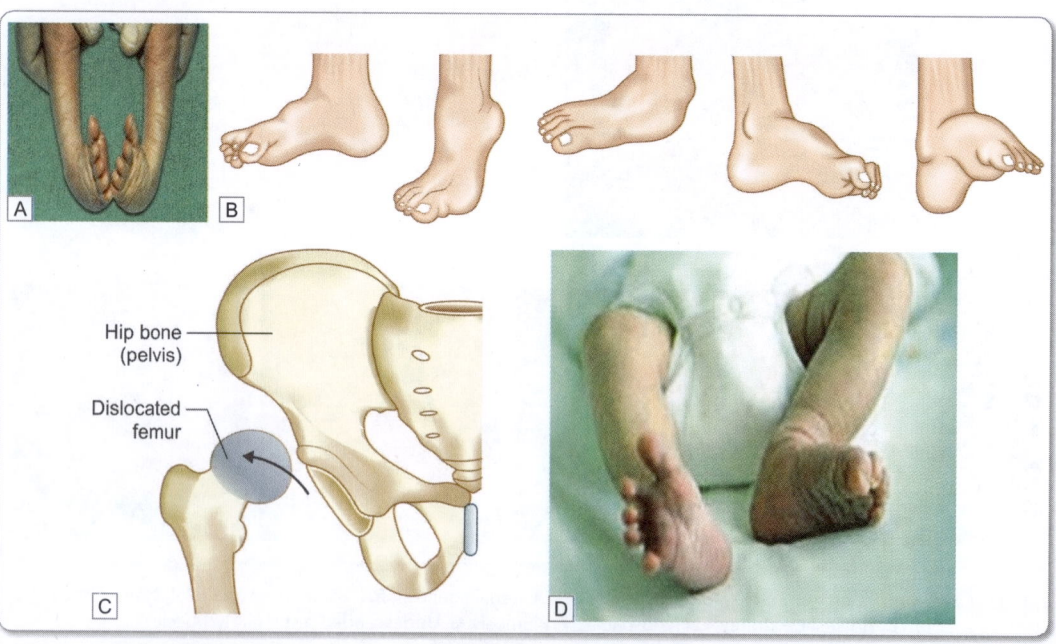

**Figs 28A to D:**

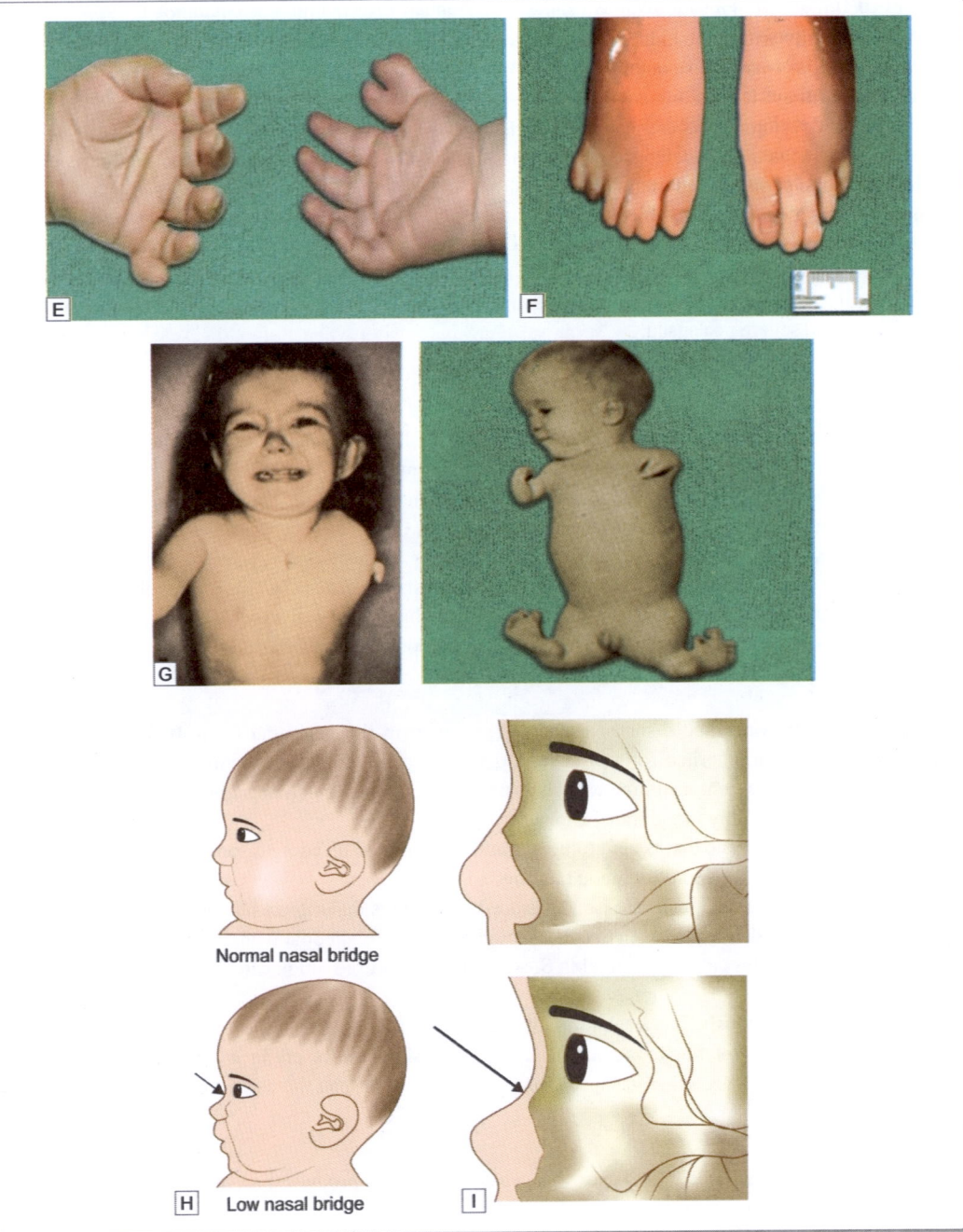

Normal nasal bridge

Low nasal bridge

**Figs 28A to I:** Musculoskeletal system abnormalities. **A.** Club foot (talipes); **B.** Club foot-types; **C.** Congenital dislocation of hip; **D.** Dislocated hip baby; **E.** Polydactyl; **F.** Webbed fingers; **G.** Amelia and phocomelia; **H.** Low nasal bridge; **I.** Hurler syndrome

- **Webbed fingers:** It is also known as syndactyly. Webbed fingers and toes occur when tissue connects two or more digits together.
- **Amelia and phocomelia:** It is the birth defect in which one or more limbs are missing.
- **Hurler's syndrome:** It is the most severe form of mucopolysaccharidosis type 1, a rare lysosomal storage disease, characterized by skeletal abnormalities, cognitive impairment, heart disease, respiratory problems, enlarged liver and spleen, characteristic faces and reduced life expectancy.
- **Marfan's syndrome:** It is an autosomal dominant genetic disorder with skeletal, cardiac and ocular involvement. Mutations in the fibrillin-1 gene (FBN1) on chromosome 15 are responsible for the development of MFS. Particularly pronounced features often include long extremities and fingers, joint laxity and contractures, a characteristic facial appearance with deeply set and downward slanting eyes and/or crumpled ears, loose and redundant skin, poor feeding, breathing difficulties, enlarged cornea or glaucoma, and severe prolapsed.

**Others**

- **Muscular dystrophy:** It is a disorder that weakens a person's muscles over time. Common signs are contractures (tightness) in the ankles, hips, knees and elbows. Some of these babies may also have respiratory problems because of weakness of breathing muscles.
- **Congenital scoliosis:** It is the presence of an abnormal curvature of the spine. The curvature causes the spinal column to bend left or right in the shape of an S or C.
- **Osteogenesis imperfecta:** Osteogenesis imperfecta is a rare heterozygous disorder of collagen production. It is characterized by osteopenia, Osteogenesis imperfecta (OI) is a rare inherited (genetic) bone disorder that is present at birth. It's also known as brittle bone disease. A child born with OI may have soft bones that break (fracture) easily, blue sclera, bone deformities, and progressive hearing loss.

## Blood Disorders

- **Thalassemia:** It is a blood disorder caused by a defect in the gene that controls the production of hemoglobin. It is an inherited form of anemia that most commonly affects children of Mediterranean, African and Asian descent. Children with thalassemia major may look pale and have shortness of breath and is treated by monthly blood transfusion.
- **Hemophilia:** It is not one disease but rather a group of inherited bleeding disorders that cause abnormal or exaggerated bleeding and poor blood clotting.
- **Sickle cell anemia:** Sickle cell disease is a group of disorders that affects hemoglobin, the molecule in red blood cells that delivers oxygen to cells throughout the body. People with this disorder have atypical hemoglobin molecules called hemoglobin S, which can distort red blood cells into a sickle, or crescent, shape.
- **Congenital spherocytosis:** It is an abnormality of red blood cells, or erythrocytes. The disorder is caused by mutations in genes relating to membrane proteins that allow for the erythrocytes to change shape. The abnormal erythrocytes are sphere-shaped (spherocytosis) rather than the normal biconcave disk shaped.

## Metabolic Disorders

- **Cystic fibrosis:** It is a hereditary disease that causes the body to produce thick and sticky mucus that can clog the lungs and obstruct the pancreas.
- **Glucose-6-phosphodiesterase (G6PD) deficiency:** It is a genetic disorder that occurs almost exclusively in males. It is an inborn error of metabolism that predisposes to red blood cell breakdown. Hemolytic anemia develops when red blood cells are destroyed faster than the body replaces them.

- **Phenylketonuria:** Phenylketonuria (fen-ul-key-toe-NU-ree-uh), also called PKU, is a rare inherited disorder that causes an amino acid called phenylalanine to build up in the body. PKU is caused by a defect in the gene that helps create the enzyme needed to break down phenylalanine. Without the enzyme necessary to process phenylalanine, a dangerous buildup can develop when a person with PKU eats foods that contain protein or eats aspartame, an artificial sweetener. Untreated, PKU can lead to intellectual disability, seizures, behavioral problems, and mental disorders.
- **Congenital lactose intolerance:** It is a condition that occurs due to the lack of enzyme lactase in the small intestines that break down lactose into glucose and galactose.
- **Wilson's disease:** Wilson disease is a genetic disorder that prevents the body from removing extra copper, causing copper to build up in the liver, brain, eyes, and other organs. Without treatment, high copper levels can cause life-threatening organ damage.
- Glycogen storage diseases.
- Inborn errors of metabolism.

## Endocrine Abnormalities

- **Congenital hypopituitarism (dwarfism):** It is a condition of short stature. There are two main categories of dwarfism. Disproportionate and proportionate. Disproportionate dwarfism is characterized by an average-size torso and shorter arms and legs or a shortened trunk with longer limbs. In proportionate dwarfism, the body parts are in proportion but shortened.
- **Congenital goiter:** It is a diffuse or nodular enlargement of the thyroid gland present at birth. Thyroid hormone secretion may be decreased, increased, or normal. Diagnosis is by confirming thyroid size with ultrasonography. Treatment is thyroid hormone replacement when hypothyroidism is the cause.

### Others

- **Congenital hypothyroidism (cretinism):** A condition characterized by physical deformity and learning difficulties that is caused by congenital thyroid deficiency.
- **Congenital adrenogenital hyperplasia:** Congenital adrenal hyperplasia (CAH) is a group of inherited genetic disorders that affect the adrenal glands, a pair of walnut-sized organs above the kidneys because of the lack of enzymes (proteins that cause chemical changes in the body), steroid 21-hydroxylase and as a result adrenal glands do not work properly. Figures 29A and B show Endocrinal abnormalitie.

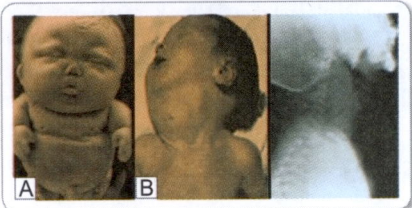

**Figs 29A and B:** Endocrinal abnormalities

## Chromosomal Abnormalities

- **Down's syndrome:** Down syndrome is a chromosomal condition that occurs when an error in cell division results in an extra chromosome 21. Down syndrome can affect a person's cognitive ability and physical growth and can also cause mild to moderate developmental issues, and present a higher risk of some health problems (Fig. 30).
- **Edward's syndrome:** Also known as trisomy 18, is a rare but serious genetic condition that causes a wide range of severe medical problems. Babies are often born small and have heart defects. Other features include a small head, small jaw, clenched fists with overlapping fingers, and severe intellectual disability.

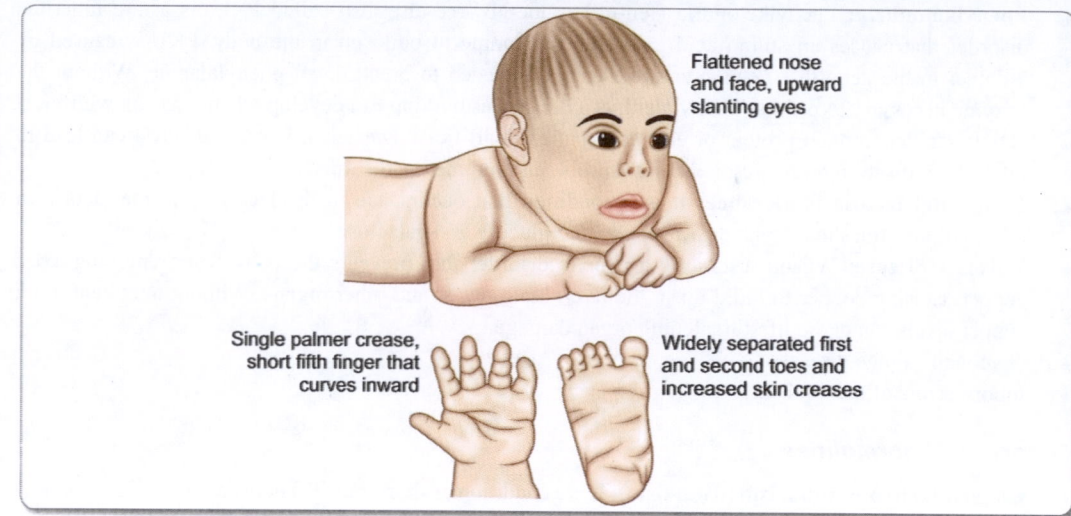

Flattened nose and face, upward slanting eyes

Single palmer crease, short fifth finger that curves inward

Widely separated first and second toes and increased skin creases

**Fig. 30:** Symptoms of Down's syndrome

## Others

- **Turner's syndrome:** Also known as 45, X or 45, X0, it is a condition in which a female is partly or completely missing an X chromosome. Signs and symptoms vary among those affected. Often, a short and webbed neck, low-set ears, low hairline at the back of the neck, short stature, and swollen hands and feet are seen at birth.
- **Klinefelter's syndrome:** It is a condition that occurs in men who have an extra X chromosome. The syndrome can affect different stages of physical, language, and social development. The most common symptom is infertility. Boys may be taller than other boys of their age, with more fat around the belly. After puberty, KS boys may have smaller testes and penis, breast growth, less facial and body hair, reduced muscle tone, narrower shoulders and wider hips, weaker bones, decreased sexual interest, lower energy, learning or language problems.

## Miscellaneous

- **Congenital cataract:** It can be dense, milky white opacities in the lens of an infant's eye(s) that prevent normal visual development. In some cases, contact lenses fitted on the eye's surface (cornea) may be used to help restore vision after the natural lens is removed during cataract surgery.
- **Congenital glaucoma:** A group of diseases in which high fluid pressure in the eye damages the optic nerve.
- **Color blindness:** Also known as color vision deficiency, is the decreased ability to see color or differences in color. Child with total color blindness (achromatopsia) may also have decreased visual acuity and be uncomfortable in bright environments.
- **Mental retardation:** Also known as general learning disability and intellectual disability (ID), is a generalized neurodevelopmental disorder characterized by significantly impaired intellectual and adaptive functioning.
- **Congenital biliary atresia:** Also known as extrahepatic ductopenia and progressive obliterative cholangiopathy, is a childhood disease of the liver in which one or more bile ducts are abnormally narrow, blocked, or absent.

- **Cleft lip:** It is an opening or split in the upper lip that occurs when developing facial structures in an unborn baby don't close completely. Cleft lip may be unilateral or bilateral.
- **Cleft palate:** It refers to a condition when the roof of the mouth contains an opening into the nose. These disorders can result in feeding problems, speech problems, hearing problems, and frequent ear infections (Figs 31A and B).

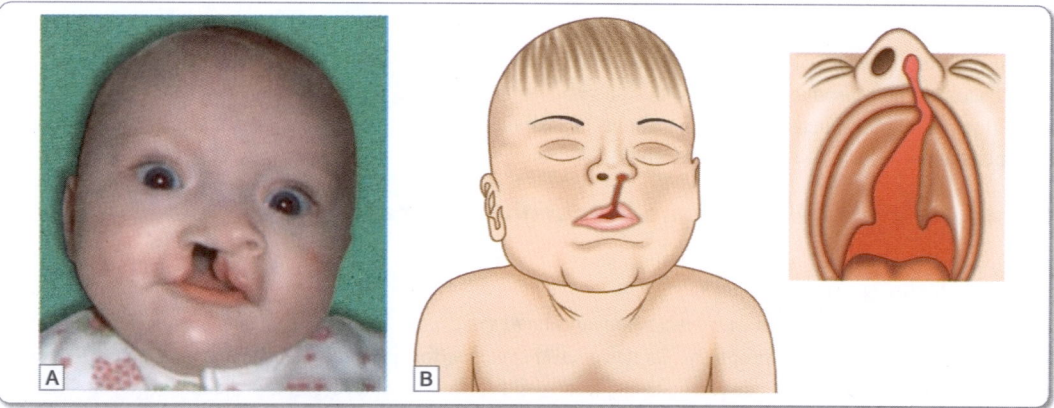

**Figs 31A and B:** Cleft lip and cleft palate. **A.** Cleft lip; **B.** Cleft palate

## Prevention

It is the process of advising individuals and families affected by or at risk of genetic disorders to help them understand and adapt to the medical, psychological and familial implications of genetic contributions to disease. The process integrates:

- Interpretation of family and medical histories to assess the chance of disease occurrence or recurrence
- Education about inheritance, testing, management, prevention, resources.
- Counseling to promote informed choices and adaptation to the risk or condition.
  It is of two types:
  1. Prospective genetic counseling:
     - It is for true prevention of disease
     - It aims at preventing or reducing heterozygous marriage by screening procedures and explaining the risk of affected children
  2. Retrospective genetic counseling:
     - It is conducted after the occurrence of hereditary disorders.

## Methods

- Contraception
- Medical termination of pregnancy (MTP)
- Sterilization
- Avoid consanguineous marriages
- Avoid late marriage and pregnancy >35 years
- Protection against mutagens such as X-rays, drugs and alcohol
- Promotion of health of girl child and prepregnant health status of the females by prevention of malnutrition, (anemia, folic acid deficiency, iodine deficiency, etc.)

Chapter 11 ☺ High-risk and Sick Newborn

- Encourage the immunization of all female child against Rubella
- Efficient antenatal care
- Immunization of anti-D immunoglobulin to Rh-negative mother within 72 hours of delivery, or even after abortion
- Prevention of intrauterine infection and promotion of sexual hygiene
- Promotion of therapeutic abortion after prenatal diagnosis
- Avoid smoking, tobacco chewing by mothers
- In the first trimester of pregnancy avoid intake of drug without consulting physician
- Discouraging reproduction after birth of a baby with congenital anomalies
- Educate the individual and families about the risk factors and etiological anomalies and their preventive measures

## Nursing Responsibilities towards Congenital Anomalies

- Collection of detail history especially history of prenatal, natal and postnatal period along with history of family illness
- Preparation of pedigree chart by interview and have visit
- Identification of present problems, its nature and severity, for necessary interventions
- Participation in diagnostic investigations, treatment, follow-up and research project
- Provide necessary information to the parents and family members
- Motivate the family members for genetic counseling and referring to the genetic clinic
- Provide emotional support and answer questions by the counselor
- Guide the family for rehabilitation of the child and for available social and economic support through social welfare agencies

# NEWBORN OF HIV-POSITIVE MOTHER

Children are innocent victims of human immunodeficiency virus (HIV)/acquired immunodeficiency syndrome (AIDS). HIV infection leads to AIDS. It is a fatal illness and a pandemic disease with a large number of infected children throughout the world.

## Mode of Transmission in Newborn/Children

- Vertical transmission (90%) from infected mother to fetus or from infected mother to child. Transmission may occur in uterus (30–35%) during delivery (60–65%) and through breastfeeding (1–3%)
- Blood and blood product transfusion
- Organ transplantation
- Contaminated needle prick
- Use of contaminated instruments during surgical procedure or any skin piercing instruments, during ear piercing, tattooing, acupuncture and circumcision

**Factors responsible to increase the rate of mother to child transmission includes (MTCT):**

- High level of viral load (viremia)
- Lack of matching antibody in the pregnant women
- Advanced maternal HIV disease
- Low maternal CD4 counts and high CD8 counts
- Maternal $P_{24}$ antigenemia

- Placental membrane inflammation
- Preterm infant
- First born twins
- Lack of antiviral therapy to infected pregnant women
- Breastfeeding

## Clinical Staging

The main symptoms of acute HIV infection are given in Figure 32. World Health Organization (WHO) clinical staging system of HIV infection and related disease in children is shown in this figure.

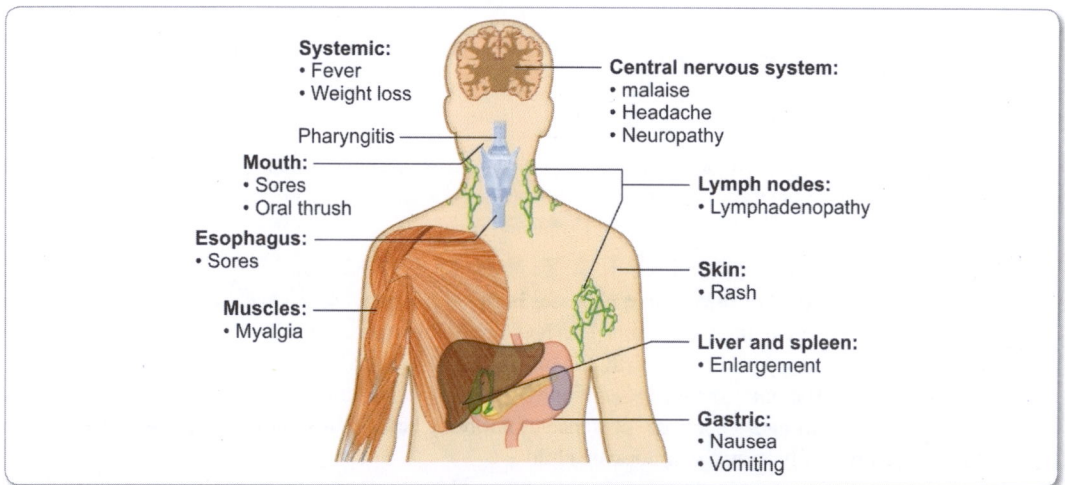

**Fig. 32:** Symptoms of HIV infections

### Stage I

- Asymptomatic
- Persistent generalized lymphadenopathy

### Stage II

- Unexplained chronic diarrhea
- Severe persistent or chronic candidiasis outside the neonatal period
- Weight loss or failure to thrive (FTT)
- Persistent fever
- Recurrent severe bacterial infections

### Stage III

- AIDS defining opportunistic infections (such as pneumonia, *Candida* infections)
- Severe failure to thrive
- Progressive encephalopathy
- Malignancy
- Recurrent septicemia/meningitis

## Diagnostic Criteria of Pediatric AIDS (According to WHO, 2015 Guidelines)

### Major Criteria

- Weight loss or abnormally slow growth
- Chronic diarrhea for over one month
- Prolonged/intermittent pyrexia from 1 month

### Minor Criteria

- Generalized lymphadenopathy
- Oropharyngeal candidiasis
- Recurrent common bacterial infections
- Persistent cough for over 1 month
- Generalized dermatitis
- Confirmed HIV infection in the mother

**Note:** *The existence of two major and two minor criteria in the absence of other known causes of immune deficiency is diagnostic of AIDS.*

## Diagnosis

The definitive diagnosis of HIV infection in neonates born to HIV infected mother is difficult due to various reasons. An HIV infected mother transmits her IgG antibodies to the newborn transplacentally. These neonates are usually antibody positive at birth, but only 15–30% is actually infected. Maternal antibodies are usually undetectable in 9 months, hence IgG antibody tests are not reliable indicators of infection status in a child before 18 months of age. Therefore, presence of antibody beyond this period is necessary to consider the child infected especially in an asymptomatic child.

The definite diagnostic test for HIV infection in the newborn includes:

- Detection of $P_{24}$ antigen
- Enzyme-linked immunosorbent assay (ELISA) (detection of IgA and IgM)
- Polymerase chain reaction (PCR) to detect viral nucleic acid in the peripheral blood

## Complications

- Recurrent infections
- Opportunistic infections
- Acute and chronic ear, nose and throat (ENT) infections
- Hearing loss
- Tooth and gums diseases
- Drug related toxicities
- Failure to thrive
- Developmental delay
- Malabsorption and wasting
- Chronic atopic dermatitis
- Cardiomyopathy
- Nephropathy
- Neuropathy
- Neutropenia

- Anemia
- Thrombocytopenia
- Psychological crisis

## Management

- Preventive measures are important aspects of management. If the child becomes infected, early diagnosis and prompt management should be initiated for the associated problems and opportunistic infections.
- Improvement of general health and promotion of living standard help in prolongation of life of the infected child.
- Specific supportive management should be provided for the clinical problems of HIV/AIDS.
- Nutritional support and management of diarrhea, cough, fever and pain, etc.
- Tuberculosis, pneumonia, candidiasis, Kaposi's sarcoma, Herpes zoster, etc. should be managed accordingly.
- Family counseling and social support are important aspects of supportive management.
- Specific therapy with antiretroviral drugs like zidovudine, didanosine, stavudine and lamivudine other drugs, like protease inhibitors (ritonavir, indinavir, saquinavir, nelfinavir) and nonnucleoside reverse transcriptase inhibitors (nevireapine, delavirdine) used as antiretroviral combinational therapy.

These drugs suppress HIV infection but do not cure the disease. It is helpful for prolongation of life in severely infected neonate.

## Nursing Care of Baby whose Mother is HIV Positive

| Step | Nursing intervention |
|------|----------------------|
| 1. | Use standard precautions. |
| 2. | Babies greater than 32 weeks gestation if in stable condition, after birth should be bathed as soon as possible using standard baby wash <br> • A nurse should wear a long sleeve gown and gloves whilst carrying out the bath <br> • Where possible include either parent in the bathing activity, however this should not delay the timing of the bath. |
| 3. | After baby is bathed vitamin K is given intramuscularly in right leg (Parent consent needed). |
| 4. | Baby is not given breast milk or breastfed (as there is increased risk of HIV transmission to baby). <br> • When gestationally appropriate, teach parents how to prepare and give a bottle feed to baby (see bottle feeding guideline). <br> • Ask parents to provide bottle and teat that they will use at home. <br> • Document feeding plan on observation chart. |
| 5. | Ensure baseline fasting blood sugar is taken. |
| 6. | Commence antiretroviral medication within 4 hours (follow Zidovudine guidelines) <br> • Liaise with ward pharmacists to arrange supply of discharge medication <br> • Educate parents how to administer the oral liquid; discuss the bottle label instructions with them. |
| 7. | **No bacille calmette guerin (BCG) vaccination or other live vaccines should be given until baby's status is clear.** |

## Prevention

Four basic approaches to control HIV/AIDS include:

- Prevention by health education to make life saving choices and avoiding blood HIV transmission.
- Antiretroviral treatment with combination therapy or postexposure prophylaxis.

- Specific prophylaxis for HIV manifestations for example, isoniazid for tuberculosis.
- Primary health approaches with integrated care in maternal and child health (MCH), family planning and health education.

# NEWBORN OF DIABETIC MOTHER

A fetus of a mother with diabetes may be exposed to high blood sugar (glucose) levels throughout the pregnancy.

## Diabetes in Pregnancy

There are two types of diabetes that occur in pregnancy:

1. **Gestational diabetes:** This term refers to a mother who does not have diabetes before becoming pregnant but develops a resistance to insulin because of the hormones of pregnancy.
2. **Pregestational diabetes:** This term describes a woman who already has insulin-dependent diabetes and becomes pregnant.

With both types of diabetes, there can be complications for the baby. It is very important to keep tight control of blood sugar during pregnancy.

## Causes of Diabetes in Pregnancy

The placenta supplies the growing fetus with nutrients and water. It also produces a variety of hormones to maintain the pregnancy. Some of these hormones (estrogen, cortisol and human placental lactogen) can block insulin. This usually begins about 20–24 weeks into the pregnancy.

As the placenta grows, more of these hormones are produced, and insulin resistance becomes greater. Normally, the pancreas is able to make additional insulin to overcome insulin resistance, but when the production of insulin is not enough to overcome the effect of the placental hormones, gestational diabetes results.

Pregnancy also may change the insulin needs of a woman with preexisting diabetes. Insulin-dependent mothers may require more insulin as pregnancy progresses.

## Signs and Symptoms

The newborn is often larger than most babies born after the same amount of time in the mother's womb (called gestational age).

Other symptoms, mostly caused by low blood sugar, may include:

- Blue or patchy (mottled) skin color, rapid heart rate, rapid breathing (signs of immature lungs or heart failure)
- Newborn jaundice (yellow skin)
- Poor feeding, lethargy, weak cry, seizures (signs of severe low blood sugar)
- Puffy face
- Reddish appearance
- Tremors or shaking shortly after birth

## Diagnosis

Before the baby is born:

- Ultrasound is performed on the mother in the last few months of pregnancy to monitor the baby's size.
- Lung maturity testing may be done on the amniotic fluid if the baby is going to be delivered more than a week before the due date.

After the baby is born:

- Tests may show that the infant has low blood sugar and low blood calcium.
- An echocardiogram may show an abnormally large heart, which can occur with heart failure.

## Complications (Actual or Potential)

The risk of stillbirth is higher in women with poorly managed type 1 diabetes. There is also an increased risk for a number of birth defects or problems:

- Congenital heart defects
- High bilirubin level (hyperbilirubinemia)
- Immature lungs
- Excessive birth weight
- Hypoglycemia
- Early or preterm birth
- Respiratory distress syndrome
- Type 2 diabetes later in life
- Neonatal polycythemia (more red blood cells than normal). This may cause a blockage in the blood vessels or hyperbilirubinemia
- Small left colon syndrome that causes symptoms of intestinal blockage

## Prevention

Prenatal care is essential to a healthy outcome when a mother has diabetes in pregnancy. Careful diet management, blood glucose monitoring, and insulin therapy can help keep a mother's blood glucose levels at normal levels and decrease many of the risks to her baby.

## Management

- **Monitoring of blood glucose level:** Blood may be drawn from a heel stick, with a needle in the baby's arm, or through an umbilical catheter (a tube placed in the baby's umbilical cord).
- **Maintain blood glucose level:** This may be as simple as giving a glucose and water mixture as an early feeding or the baby may need glucose given intravenously. The baby's blood glucose levels are closely monitored after treatment in case hypoglycemia occurs again.

  *Efforts are made to ensure the baby has enough blood glucose levels:*
  - Feeding soon after birth may prevent low blood sugar in mild cases. Even if the plan is to breastfeed, the health care provider may suggest some formula during the first 8–24 hours.
  - Low blood sugar that does not go away is treated with fluid containing sugar (glucose) and water given through a vein.
  - In severe cases, if the baby needs large amounts of sugar, the fluid and glucose must be given through an umbilical (belly button) vein for several days.

- Checking for hypocalcemia (low calcium levels)
- Giving oxygen or using a breathing machine (if respiratory distress occurs)
- Care for any problems arising from a birth injury
- Care for any problems that occur with a birth defect

Rarely, the infant may need breathing support or medicines to treat other effects of diabetes. High bilirubin levels are treated with light therapy (phototherapy). Rarely, the baby's blood will be replaced with blood from a donor (exchange transfusion) for this problem.

## LEVELS OF NEONATAL CARE

- **Level-I care:** About 80–90% of neonates require minimal care which can be provided by their mothers with support from family members and under supervision of basic health professionals. The neonates weighing above 2000 g or having gestational age of 37 weeks of more belongs to this category. This care can be given at home, sub-center and primary health centers. Essential perinatal care should be provided as basic care at birth, provision of warmth, maintenance of asepsis and promotion of breastfeeding.
- **Level-II care:** Neonates weighing between 1500 g and 2000 g or having gestational age of 32–36 weeks need specialized neonatal care supervised by trained nursing staff and pediatricians. This intermediate neonatal care should be provided by the equipped district hospitals, teaching institutions and nursing homes. There should be arrangement of resuscitation procedures, maintenance of thermoneutral environment, intravenous infusion, gavage feeding, phototherapy and exchange blood transfusions. Only 10–15% of all neonates require this care. It should be available at all hospitals where 1000–1500 deliveries take place per year.
- **Level-III care:** Neonates weighing less than 1500 g or born before 32 weeks of gestation require intensive care unit (ICU). Only 3–5% of all neonates need this care by skilled nurses and neonatologists, especially trained in neonatal intensive care. Apex institutions or regional perinatal centers equipped with centralized oxygen and suction facilities, incubators, ventilators, monitors and infusion pump, etc. are best suited to provide intensive neonatal care.

High risk pregnancies which are associated with birth of high risk neonates must be identified during pregnancy and referred to an appropriate center for skilled management and better outcome. At birth, detection of high risk neonates should be done at all levels of healthcare delivery system and appropriate referral is essential to different level of neonatal care for prevention and reduction of neonatal mortality and morbidity.

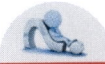

## ASSESS YOURSELF

### FREQUENTLY ASKED QUESTIONS IN EXAMS

1. Define the following:
   a. Hyperbilirubinemia
   b. Hypothermia
   c. Asphyxia
   d. Sepsis
   e. Neonatal convulsion

2. Define preterm baby. What are its causes, clinical manifestations and complications? As a nurse how you will manage a preterm baby?

3. Differentiate between symmetrical IUGR and asymmetrical IUGR.

4. Describe neonatal birth injuries and its management in detail.

5. Enlist the Congenital anomalies. Explain its preventive measures and describe the role of nurse in this case.

6. Define asphyxia neonatorum, its causes and complications. As a nurse how you will manage a neonate having Apgar score 3?

7. Write short notes on:
   a. Rh incompatibility
   b. Levels of care in NICU
   c. Newborn of HIV positive mother

### MULTIPLE CHOICE QUESTIONS

1. Low-birth-weight babies are:
   a. Less than 2500 g
   b. Less than 2000 g
   c. Less than 1500 g
   d. Less than 3000 g

2. A baby born before 37 completed weeks of gestation calculating from the 1st day of last menstrual period is called:
   a. Small for date baby
   b. Preterm baby
   c. Low-birth-weight baby
   d. None of the above

3. Urethral opening above the penis is called:
   a. Epispadiasis
   b. Hypospadiasis
   c. Hydrocele
   d. Phimosis

4. Small for dates is also called:
   a. IUGR
   b. Dysmaturity
   c. Chronic placental insufficiency
   d. All of the above

5. Ponderal index is calculated as:
   a. FL/AC ratio
   b. Weight/Crown heel length
   c. Amniotic fluid volume
   d. HC/AC ratio

6. Symphysis fundal height in centimeters closely correlates with gestational age after:
   a. 26 weeks
   b. 24 weeks
   c. 30 weeks
   d. 38 weeks

7. **Genetic counseling that is for true prevention of disease is:**
   a. Retrospective genetic counseling
   b. Integrated genetic counseling
   c. Prospective genetic counseling
   d. All of the above

8. **The main cause of hemorrhagic diseases in newborn is:**
   a. Vitamin K deficiency
   b. Vitamin C deficiency
   c. Vitamin A deficiency
   d. Vitamin D deficiency

9. **Which of the following coagulation factor impairment leads to hemorrhage in newborn?**
   a. Factor II
   b. Factor VII
   c. Factor IX and X
   d. All of the above

10. **Neonate born at 32 weeks weighing 2000 g, will receive which level of care:**
    a. Level I care
    b. Level II care
    c. Level III care
    d. None of the above

11. **Neonatal hypoglycemia is termed when the blood glucose level is:**
    a. Less than 60 mg/dL
    b. Less than 50 mg/dL
    c. Less than 40 mg/dL
    d. Less than 80 mg/dL

12. **Which type of seizures is not seen in neonates?**
    a. Subtle seizures
    b. Pure tonic and clonic seizures
    c. Myoclonic seizures
    d. Focal clonic seizures

13. **The systemic bacterial infections of neonates are termed as neonatal sepsis which incorporates:**
    a. Septicemia
    b. Pneumonia
    c. Meningitis
    d. All of the above

14. **The antibody that is transmitted by HIV positive mother to the fetus transplacentally is:**
    a. IgG
    b. IgM
    c. IgE
    d. IgF

15. **The exact diagnosis of HIV/AIDS in newborn is made after:**
    a. 7 months
    b. 9 months
    c. 12 months
    d. 18 months

16. **The most commonly used antiretroviral drugs in neonate are:**
    a. Zidovudine
    b. Stavudine
    c. Ritanavir
    d. Nelfinavir

17. **Neonatal hypothermia occurs when the body temperature drops below:**
    a. 38°C
    b. 40°C
    c. 37°C
    d. 36.5°C

18. **Stopping of the pulse means:**
    a. Hypoglycemia
    b. Hyperbilirubinemia
    c. Cyanotic heart diseases
    d. Asphyxia

19. **In case of asphyxia pallida, Apgar score is:**
    a. 7–10
    b. 4–6
    c. 0–3
    d. 3–6

20. **Apgar score 7–10 indicates:**
    a. Severe depression
    b. Moderate depression
    c. Mild depression
    d. No depression

21. **When an Rh-negative mother carries Rh-positive fetus and hemolysis occurs, the condition is known as:**
    a. Rh incompatibility
    b. ABO incompatibility
    c. Hemorrhagic disorders of the newborn
    d. Hydrops fetalis

22. **To diagnose Rh incompatibility, the most commonly used test is:**
    a. ELISA test
    b. PCR test
    c. Indirect Coomb test
    d. Western blot assay test 1

23. **To prevent active immunization, anti-D immunoglobulin is given within:**
    a. 72 hours following delivery or abortion
    b. Within 24 hours following delivery or abortion
    c. Within 48 hours following delivery or abortion
    d. Immediately after birth

24. **To prevent fetomaternal bleed, which injection is withheld during delivery:**
    a. Oxytocin
    b. Tocolytic
    c. Prostaglandins
    d. Ergometrine

25. **In hyperbilirubinemia, the bilirubin level rises more than arbitrary cut off point of:**
    a. 18 mg/dL
    b. 20 mg/dL
    c. 16 mg/dL
    d. 12 mg/dL

 **Answer Key**

| 1. a | 2. b | 3. a | 4. d | 5. b | 6. b | 7. c |
|------|------|------|------|------|------|------|
| 8. a | 9. d | 10. b | 11. c | 12. b | 13. d | 14. a |
| 15. d | 16. a | 17. d | 18. d | 19. c | 20. d | 21. a |
| 22. c | 23. a | 24. d | 25. d | | | |

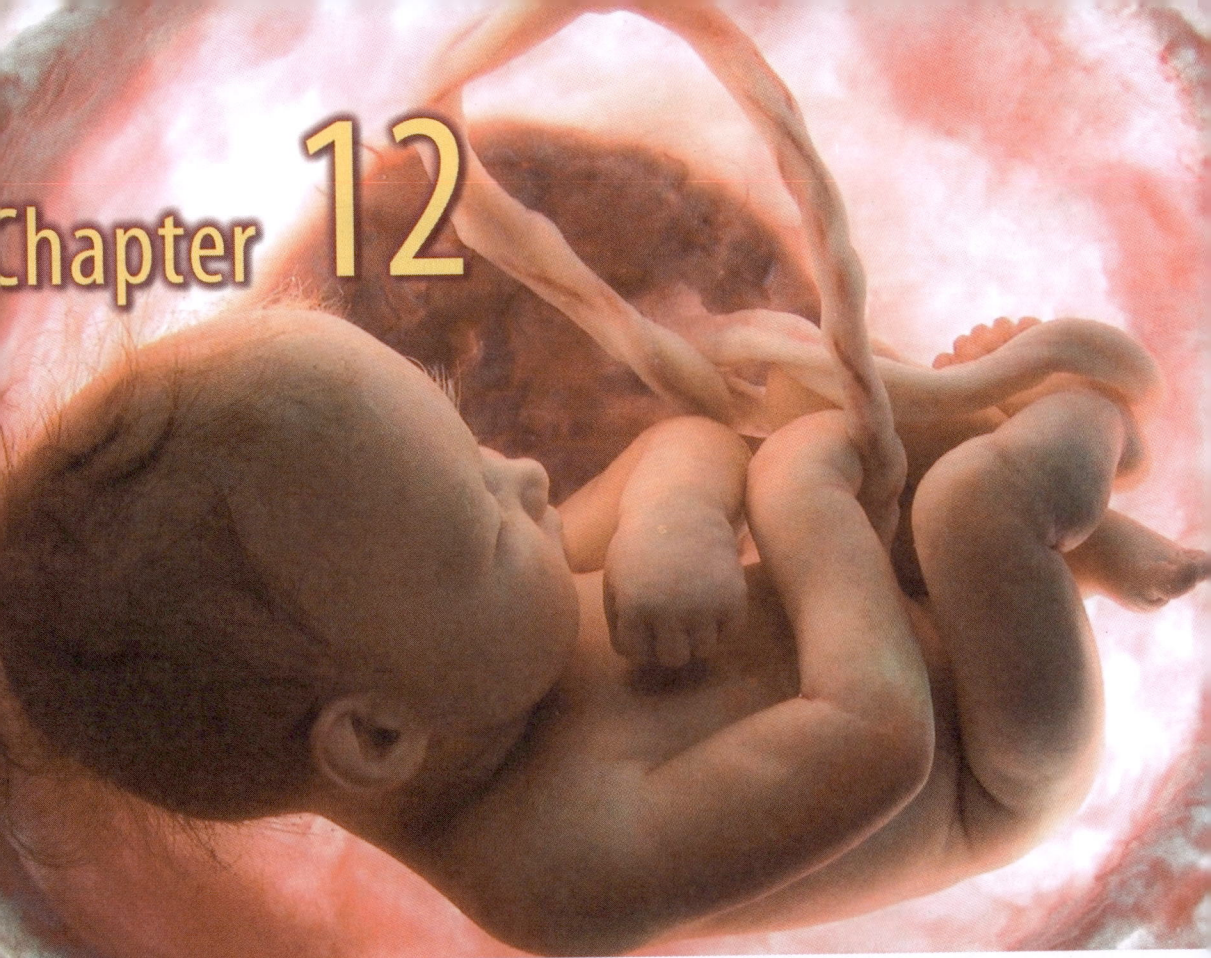

# Chapter 12

# Obstetric Operations

## INDUCTION OF LABOR

**Definition:** It is the deliberate initiation of labor by any method (medical, surgical or combined) before spontaneous onset after 28 weeks of pregnancy for the purpose of vaginal delivery.

It is indicated when there is risk to the life of mother or fetus if the pregnancy continues.

### Types of Induction

- **Elective induction:** It is the induction of labor for the convenience of woman, physician or hospital.
- **Indicated induction:** It is the induction of labor for the high risk pregnancies.

### Indications

- Post-term/prolonged pregnancy
- Previous history of intrauterine fetal death (IUFD)
- Preeclampsia/eclampsia
- Maternal medical complications, e.g., diabetes, renal problem, etc.
- Abruptio placenta
- Intrauterine growth retardation (IUGR)
- Premature rupture of membranes (PROM)
- Fetus with major congenital abnormality
- Oligohydramnios/polyhydramnios
- Unstable lie

### Contraindications

- Cephalopelvic disproportion, contracted pelvis
- Malpresentation
- Previous history of cesarean section/hysteria
- Placenta previa, vasa previa or unexplained vaginal bleeding
- Active genital herpes infection
- High risk pregnancies
- Pelvic tumors/cervical carcinoma
- Heart disease
- Cord prolapse
- Elderly primigravidae with medical or obstetrical problems

# Dangers of Induction

**Maternal complications:**
- Psychological upset when there is induction failure and cesarean section is done
- Prolonged labor
- Operative interference
- Increased need of analgesia during labor
- Increased morbidity

**Fetal complications:**
- Iatrogenic prematurity
- Hypoxia due to disordered uterine action, prolonged labor and operative interference

## Prerequisites for the Induction of Labor

### Maternal

- Confirm the indication of induction of labor
- Exclude the contraindication of induction of labor
- Assess Bishop's score (Table 1)

**TABLE 1: Bishop's preinduction cervical scoring system**

| Parameters | Score | | | |
|---|---|---|---|---|
| | **0** | **1** | **2** | **3** |
| **Cervix** | | | | |
| • Dilatation (m) | Closed | 1–2 | 3–4 | 5+ |
| • Effacement (%) | 0–30 | 40–50 | 60–70 | >80 |
| • Consistency | Firm | Medium | Soft | – |
| • Position | Posterior | Medium | Anterior | – |
| | –3 | –2 | –1, 0 | +1, +2 |
| **Head** | | | | |
| • Cervical tenth | >4 | 2–4 | 1–2 | <1 |

Total score = 13; favorable score = 6–13; unfavorable score = 0–5.

### Fetal

- Ensure fetal gestational age
- Estimate fetal weight
- Ensure fetal lung maturity
- Ensure fetal presentation and lie
- Confirm fetal wellbeing

## Methods of Induction of Labor

- **Medical:**
  - Oxytocin
  - Prostaglandins ($PGE_1$, $PGE_2$, $PGF_2\alpha$)
  - Mifepristone (progesterone receptor antagonist)
- **Surgical:**
  - Artificial rupture of membranes (ARM)
  - Stripping the membranes
- **Combined:**
  - Medical and surgical both

### Medical Method

Drug used for induction of labor are:

- **Prostaglandins:** Both $PGE_2$ and $PGF_{2\alpha}$ are used for induction of labor. $PGE_2$ is important for cervical ripening, whereas $PGF_{2\alpha}$ for myometrial contraction.
    - Dinoprostone ($PGE_2$ - 0.5 mg) gel is commonly used for cervical ripening. It is repeated after 6 hours and 3 or 4 doses are required. Advise the women for bed rest (30 minutes) after application of gel. Assess FHR and uterine activity.
    - Misoprostol ($PGE_1$): A dose of 25 µg vaginally every 4 hourly. Total 6–8 doses are used.
- **Oxytocin:** It stimulates uterine contractions. Oxytocin receptors present in the myometrium are more in the fundus than in the cervix. Receptor concentration increases during pregnancy and in labor.
- **Mifepristone:** Administer 200 mg mifepristone vaginally, daily for 2 days to ripen the cervix and induce labor pain. It blocks both progesterone and glucocorticoid receptors.

### Surgical Method

a.  **Artificial rupture of membranes:** It is commonly used method for induction with high success rate. The membranes below the presenting part overlying the internal OS are ruptured to drain amniotic fluid.

*Contraindication:* Not performed in case of polyhydramnios because sudden uterine decompression causes placental abruption.

### Procedure

- Assess FHR.
- Provide lithotomy position to the woman.
- Maintain surgical asepsis.
- Insert two fingers into the vagina after smearing with antiseptic solution. The membranes are swept free from lower segment as far as reached by the fingers.
- Insert long Kocher forceps with the blades closed or an amnion hook along the palmer aspect of the fingers up to the membranes.
- The blades are opened to seize the membranes and are torn by twisting movements. Amnion hook is used to scratch over the membranes.
- Escape of amniotic fluid occurs.
- Assess the following points after the rupture of membranes:
    - Color of liquor
    - State of cervix
    - Station of head
    - Detection of cord prolapse
    - Check FHR

### Complications

- Cord prolapse
- Sudden uterine decompression causes placental abruption
- Injury to cervix or presenting part
- Rupture of vasa previa leads to fetal blood loss
- Amnionitis

b.  **Stripping of membranes:** Digital separation of the chorioamniotic membranes from the wall of the cervix and lower uterine segment, is called stripping of the membranes. This procedure is done prior to artificial rupture of (fetal) membranes (ARM). The purpose is to release endogenous prostaglandins from the membranes and decidua. Manual exploration of the cervix causes Ferguson reflex which enhances oxytocin released from maternal pituitary, thus uterine contractions are enhanced.

## Combined Method

Both medical and surgical methods are used to increase the efficacy of induction by reducing the induction delivery interval. In this method, oxytocin infusion is started either prior to or following rupture of the membranes depending upon the state of cervix and head-brim relation. In case of nonengaged head, induce labor pain with prostaglandin or start oxytocin infusion followed by ARM.

## Nursing Role in Induction of Labor

- Obtain informed consent.
- Review patient history before Induction of labor (to ensure there are no contraindications or any caution).
- Perform abdominal palpation to confirm fetal presentation, position and degree of engagement of the presenting part.
- Maintain partograph to assess the progress of labor.
- Use aseptic technique during induction of labor.

### During prostaglandin administration:

- Instruct woman to pass urine before administering prostaglandin (because she will stay for long time in bed).
- The mother should remain in lateral or supine position with hip tilt for 30–60 minutes after administration of gel, for 2 hours after insertion of vaginal tablets so as to minimize leakage and improve effectiveness.
- Assess cervical dilatation after 6 hours of insertion. If no cervical response and no adverse effects, repeat the dose.
- Monitor the side effects of prostaglandins: Pyrexia, vomiting, diarrhea, back pain and warm feeling in vagina.
- Don't repeat the dose at least two hours after the administration of first dose of prostaglandins, and starting syntocinon infusion because prostaglandin increases the sensitivity of the uterus to syntocinon.
- If any adverse reactions occur, immediately inform the doctor to remove gel or suppository, if possible.

### During oxytocin infusion:

- Check respiration, BP, pulse, length, intensity, duration of contraction, FHR.
- Note the signs of water intoxication: Confusion, anuria, drowsiness, headache.
- Instruct the patient to report increase blood loss, abdominal cramp, fever, foul-smelling vaginal discharge.
- If uterine hyperstimulation or fetal distress occurs:
  - Stop oxytocin infusion immediately to prevent fetal anoxia and uterine rupture
  - Provide left lateral position to the woman to improve fetal-placental blood flow
  - Increase primary intravenous (IV) rate up to 200 mL/hr unless contraindicated to provide adequate intravascular volume, support maternal blood pressure (BP) and IV route for emergency medications.
  - Provide oxygen at the rate of 6–10 L/min by face mask to prevent fetal anoxia.
- Notify doctor if induction failed.
- If membranes are intact, discontinue induction and try again later.
- If membranes are ruptured, prefer cesarean section.

**After ARM:**

- The midwife should exclude the presence of cord prolapse.
- Note color, odor, consistency and quantity of amniotic fluid.
- Note presentation, position and station of fetal head.
- Check temperature every 2 hourly to detect developing infection.

## MANUAL REMOVAL OF PLACENTA

When the placenta is not expelled out spontaneously and retained inside the uterine cavity, manual removal of placenta is done.

### Steps of Manual Removal of Placenta

- **Step-I:** The operation is done under general anesthesia or sedation with 10 mg diazepam intravenously. Provide lithotomy position to patient and catheterize the bladder.
- **Step-II:** Separate the labia by fingers of one hand and other hand is introduced into uterine cavity after smearing with antiseptic solution in cone shape manner following the cord.
- **Step-III:** Counter pressure on the uterine fundus is applied by the other hand placed over the abdomen. The abdominal hand should steady the fundus inside the uterine cavity until the placenta is completely separated.
- **Step-IV:** As soon as placental margin is reached the fingers are insinuated between the placenta and the uterine wall with the back of hand in contact with the uterine wall. The placenta is gradually separated with a sideways slicing movement of the fingers, until whole of placenta is separated.
- **Step-V:** When the placenta is completely separated, apply traction on the cord by other hand and remove the placenta. The uterine hand is still inside the uterus for exploration of the cavity to be sure that nothing is left behind.
- **Step-VI:** Intramuscular methergine 0.2 mg is given and the uterine hand is gradually removed while massaging the uterus by the external hand to make it hard.
- **Step-VII:** After the completion of manual removal, inspection of cervicovaginal canal is to be made to exclude any injury.
- **Step-VIII:** The placenta and membranes are inspected for completeness and be sure that the uterus remains hard and contracted and the bleeding is arrested.

### Difficulties

- Hour glass contraction leading to difficulty in introducing the hand.
- Morbid adherent placenta may cause difficulty in getting to the plane of cleavage of separation.

### Complications

- Hemorrhage due to incomplete removal
- Injury to the uterus
- Infection
- Inversion
- Subinvolution
- Thrombophlebitis
- Embolism

# VERSION

It is a manipulative procedure designed to change the lie or to bring the comparatively favorable pole to the lower pole of the uterus.

## Types

- **Spontaneous:** When version process occurs spontaneously, more common in multipara
- **External:** Version is done solely by external manipulation
- **Internal:** Version is done by introducing one hand into the uterus and other hand on to abdomen
- **Bipolar:** The version is done introducing one or two fingers through the cervix and by other hand on the abdomen

## Indications

- **External version:** Done in case of:
  - Breech presentation
  - Transverse lie
- **Internal version:** Done in case of transverse lie in second baby of twins.

## Time of Version

Version can be performed from 36 weeks onwards. Version in early weeks is easy but chances of reversion are more. Late version is difficult to perform because of diminished liquor and increasing size of fetus.

## Prerequisites

- The cervix must be fully dilated.
- Liquor amnii must be adequate.

## Procedure of Version

### External Version (Cephalic)

#### Preliminaries

- Real time ultrasonography is done to confirm the diagnosis and adequacy of amniotic fluid volume.
- A reactive nonstress test (NST) should precede the maneuver.
- Empty the bladder.
- Ask the patient to lie on her back with the shoulders slightly raised and the thighs slightly flexed.
- Abdomen should be fully exposed.
- Presentation, and position of the back and limbs are checked.
- Check the fetal heart rate (FHR).
- Tocolytic drug (terbutaline 0.25 mg SC), if required can be administered.

The steps involved are:

**Step 1:** Mobilization of the buttocks using both hands to one iliac fossa toward which the back of the fetus lies.
**Step 2:** Rotation of the trunk holding the poles and maintaining flexion of the trunk.
**Step 3:** Change of hands to prevent crossing after the lie becomes transverse.
**Step 4:** The lie becomes longitudinal with the cephalic pole being brought to the lower pole of the uterus.

There may be bradycardia due to head compression which is expected to settle down by 10 minutes. If fetal bradycardia persists, the possibility of cord entanglement should be kept in mind and in such cases reversion has to be done. The patient is to be observed for thirty minutes.

**Instructions are:**

- Advise the patient for follow-up to check the corrected position.
- If there is vaginal bleeding or escape of liquor amnii or labor begins, report to physician.
- In case of Rh (Rhesus) negative nonimmunized women, give 100 ug anti-D-gamma globulin IM.

### Internal Version

Internal version is always a podalic version and is almost completed with the extraction of the fetus.

- The hand is to be introduced in a cone-shaped manner. If the podalic pole of the fetus is on the left side of the mother, the right hand is to be introduced and vice versa.
- The hand is to pass up to the breech and then along the thigh until a foot is grasped. The identification of the foot is done by palpation of the heel.
- While the leg is brought down by steady traction, the cephalic pole is pushed up using the external hand.
- After the delivery of one leg, deliver other leg and delivery is usually completed with breech extraction during uterine contractions.
- Explore the uterovaginal canal to exclude rupture of uterus or any other injury.

### Bipolar Version

It is a lifesaving procedure, especially in the rural areas where it is not possible to transport the patient with placenta previa to an equipped hospital. The indication of this procedure is lesser degree of placenta previa when the fetus is dead, deformed or previable. Cervix must be at least two fingers dilated to facilitate manipulation of head to one iliac fossa and to grasp one leg at the ankle. Simultaneous manipulation by external hand facilitates the procedure. Bringing down of one leg facilitates compression over the placenta and thereby stops the bleeding.

## Contraindications

- Antepartum hemorrhage
- Multiple pregnancy in external cephalic version
- Fetal causes: Congenital abnormalities, IUGR, IUFD, large fetus
- Premature rupture of membranes
- Congenital malformation of uterus
- Abnormal cardiotocography
- Contracted pelvis
- Previous cesarean section
- Rh incompatibility
- Obstetrical complications: Obesity, elderly primigravidae, oligohydramnios, preeclampsia.

## Complications of Version

- **Maternal**
  - Premature onset of labor
  - Premature rupture of membranes
  - Placental abruption and bleeding

- Increased chances of fetomaternal bleed
- Amniotic fluid embolism
- **Fetal**
  - Asphyxia
  - Cord prolapse
  - Intracranial hemorrhage
  - IUFD of fetus

## Nursing Responsibilities

- Advise the patient for follow-up to check the corrected position
- Report to the physician if there is vaginal bleeding or escape of liquor or labor starts
- Protect the Rh-negative nonimmunized women by intramuscular administration of 100 µg anti D-gamma globulin.
- Go for cardiotocography after the procedure to reassure about fetal heart rate (FHR).

## FORCEPS DELIVERY

**Definition:** Forceps delivery means using obstetric forceps (a pair of instruments designed to extract fetal head) for delivery when the mother is unable to deliver the baby by her own efforts.

### Types of Forceps

Figures 1A to D show various types of forceps.
- Long curved forceps with or without axis traction
- Short curved forceps
- Kielland's forceps

### Classification

According to level of fetal head at which the forceps are applied:

- **High forceps:** Refers to the application of forceps on fetal head where the biparietal diameter has not get passed the pelvic brim (In nonengaged head cesarean section is preferred to this type of forceps application).
- **Mid forceps:** Refers to the application of the forceps where the biparietal diameter has passed the brim of the pelvis, but not passed the level of ischial spines.
- **Low forceps:** Refers to the application of forceps where the biparietal diameter has passed the level of ischial spines.
- **Outlet forceps:** The forceps are applied on the fetal head lying on the perineum and is visible at the introitus in between contractions.

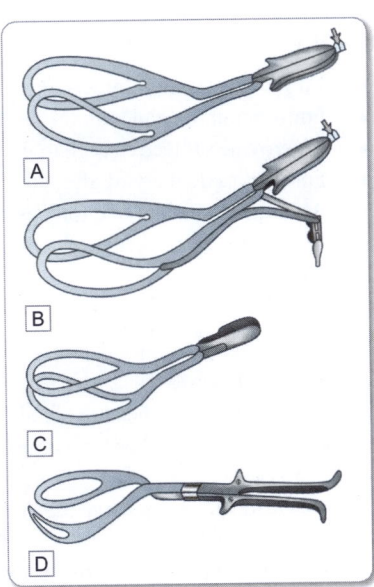

**Figs 1A to D:** Types of forceps; **A.** Long axis without axis traction; **B.** Long axis with axis traction; **C.** Wrigley's; **D.** Kielland

### Parts of Forceps

Figure 2 shows parts of forceps:

Each blade consists of following parts:

- Blade
- Shank

- Lock
- Handle with or without traction

There are two blades and are named right or left in relation to maternal pelvis in which they lie when applied. The blade has got two curves:

1. **Pelvic curve:** It is the outer curve that attaches towards the maternal pelvis.
2. **Cephalic curve:** It is the curve on the flat surface, which when articulated, grasps the fetal head without compression.

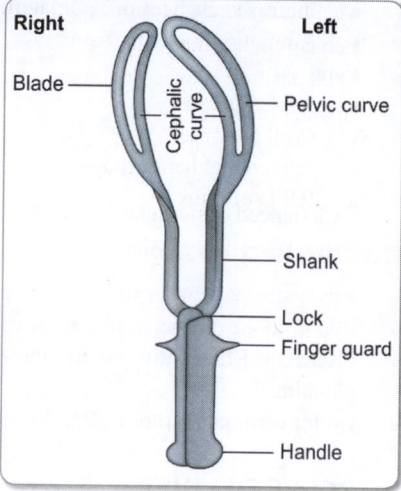

**Fig. 2:** Parts of forceps

## How to Identify the Blades

- **When articulated:** Place the instrument in front of the pelvis with the tip of the blades pointing upwards and the concave side of the pelvic curve forwards. The blade which corresponds to the left of maternal pelvis is the left blade and that to the right side is the right blade.
- **When isolated:**
  - The tip should point upwards.
  - The cephalic curve is to be directed inwards and the pelvic curve forwards.

## Functions of Forceps

- To provide traction force.
- For rotation of head with the help of Kielland's forceps.
- To provide protective cage to the head while head passes through the birth canal.
- For control delivery of after coming head in breech presentation.
- In cesarean section, one forceps blade can be used to deliver the head.
- When applied correctly, the compression effect of forceps should be minimal.

## Indications for Forceps Application

- **Fetal:**
  - Fetal distress
  - After coming head in breech delivery
  - In case of fetal compromise
- **Maternal**
  - Inadequate expulsive efforts
  - Maternal exhaustion
  - Avoidance of expulsive efforts as in case of cardiac disease, hypertensive crisis, spinal cord injury and cerebrovascular diseases
  - Prolonged second stage of labor
  - To cut short second stage of labor as in severe preeclampsia and post-cesarean pregnancy

## Prerequisites for Forceps Application

- Fetal head must be engaged
- Cervix must be fully dilated

- Membranes must be ruptured
- Pelvis is deemed adequate
- Fetal position is exactly known
- Bladder must be emptied
- Informed consent has been taken
- Adequate analgesia given to mother (Pudendal block)
- Experienced obstetrician/midwife
- Follow aseptic techniques.

## Steps of Forceps Application

### Step 1: Identification and Application of Blades

Firstly, identify the forceps as left or right by assembling them briefly. The left blade (lower blade) is to be introduced first. The four fingers of semi-supinated right hand are inserted along the left lateral vaginal wall, the palmer surface of the fingers rests against the side of the head. Hold the handle of left blade in a pen holding manner using three fingers of left hand—index, middle and thumb- and is held vertically almost parallel to the right inguinal ligament. The blade is introduced between the guiding internal fingers and the fetal head, manipulated by the thumb. As the blade is pushed up and up, the handle is carried downward and backward, transversing wide arc of a circle toward the left until the shank lies straight on the perineum. When correctly applied, the blade should be over the parietal eminence, the shank should be in contact with the perineum and the superior surface of the handle should be directed upward.

**Introduction of right blade:** Now introduce two fingers of left hand into the right lateral wall of the vagina alongside the baby's head. Hold the right blade in the right hand and introduce in same manner as with left one. (The blades are equidistant from the lambdoid suture indicating correct application.)

### Step 2: Locking of the Blades

The blades should be locked very easily when applied correctly. Minor difficulty in locking can be corrected by depressing the handles on the perineum. In case of major problem, remove the blades, find out the cause and then reinsert the blades.

### Step 3: Traction

The traction is given along the axis of birth canal in the following manner:
- Downward and backward
- Straight horizontal pull
- Upward and forward

### Step 4: Removal of Blades

Immediately after the delivery of head, the blades are removed one after the other (the right one first).

Following delivery of the head, usual procedures are to be taken as in normal delivery. Routine injection oxytocin 10 international unit (IU), intramuscular (IM) or intravenous (IV) methergine 0.2 mg is to be administered with the delivery of baby. Episiotomy is repaired in the usual method.

## Difficulties in Forceps Application

- The difficulties are mainly due to faulty assessment before the operative delivery is undertaken
- Difficulties in the application of blades are caused by incompletely dilated cervix and unrotated or nonengaged head.
- Difficulty in locking is caused by:
  - Application on unrotated head
  - Improper insertion of the blades
  - Failure to depress the handle against the perineum
  - Entanglement of the cord on fetal parts inside the blades

## Complications of Forceps Application

The complications of forceps at the time of application are shown in Table 2.

TABLE 2: Immediate and remote maternal and fetal complications

| Maternal | Fetal |
|---|---|
| **Immediate** | **Immediate** |
| • **Injury:** Vaginal laceration/tear, cervical tear, complete perineal tear<br>• **Nerve injury:** Femoral, lumbosacral with midforceps delivery<br>• **Postpartum hemorrhage:** Traumatic, atonic uterus or both may cause shock<br>• Anesthetic complications<br>• Puerperal sepsis<br>• Maternal morbidity | • Asphyxia<br>• Facial bruising<br>• Intracranial hemorrhage<br>• Cephalohematoma<br>• Hematoma<br>• Facial palsy<br>• Skull fracture<br>• Cervical spine injury |
| **Remote** | **Remote** |
| • Painful perineal scars, dyspareunia, low backache, genital prolapse, stress urinary incontinence and anal sphincter dysfunction | • Cerebral or spastic palsy |

## Nursing Interventions for Forceps Delivery

- Before forceps delivery is initiated, give clear explanation of the risks and benefits of forceps for the mother and fetus.
- Advise the patient that an attempt at instrumental delivery may not result in vaginal delivery, may avoid unrealistic expectations.
- Inform the patient that the forceps blades fit like two tablespoons around an egg. The blades come over the fetus ears.
- Check the prerequisites for forceps application.
- Obtain forceps designated by the physician.
- Check the reports and record the fetal heart rate before forceps are applied.
- Recheck the reports and record the fetal heart rate once again before traction is applied after application of the forceps. Compression of the cord between the fetal head and the forceps would cause a drop in fetal heart rate. The physician would then remove and reapply the forceps.
- After delivery, examine for any tears that might have been caused by the forceps. If there is any, repair it with catgut suture.
- Give support to the patient.
- Observe for signs and symptoms of complications.
- Assess the newborn for indications of injury.

- Following forceps delivery, documentation should include the indication for the procedure, a record of the discussion with the patient and a detailed description of the procedure itself.

# VENTOUSE

Ventouse is an instrumental device designed to assist delivery by creating a vacuum between suction cup and fetal scalp.

## Equipment

Ventouse consists of the following basic components.

- Suction cup (4 sizes—30, 40, 50 and 60)
- A vacuum pump
- Traction rod device

## Indications

- Deep transverse arrest with adequate pelvis
- Delay in descent of high head in case of second baby in twins
- Maternal exhaustion
- Inadequate expulsive efforts
- Prolonged second stage of labor
- Malposition—occipitolateral/occipitoposterior
- As an alternative to forceps operation except in:
  - Face presentation and after coming head in breech delivery
  - Fetal distress/prematurity

## Advantages of Ventouse

- Ventouse can be used in unrotated or malrotated occipitoposterior position of the head
- It can be applied even through incompletely dilated cervix
- Not a space occupying device like forceps blades
- Comfortable and has lower rates of maternal trauma and genital tract lacerations
- Analgesia need is less
- Lesser traction force is needed
- It can be safely used even when the head remains at a high level in second baby in twins.
- Requires less technical skill for the operator

## Contraindications for Ventouse

- Fetal distress
- Face presentation
- Prematurity, chance of scalp avulsion or subaponeurotic hemorrhage is more
- Fetal bleeding disorder

## Prerequisites

- No bony resistance below the head
- Head must be engaged
- Cervix at least 6 cm dilated

## Procedure

- Assemble all the articles related to ventouse and test prior to its use.
- Depending upon condition, give local anesthesia.
- Apply cup against fetal head near to occiput with knob of cup pointing towards the occiput.
- It will cause flexion of head and knob indicates the degree of rotation.
- Create a vacuum 0.2 kg/cm$^2$ by pump slowly taking at least 2 minutes.
- Have a check using the fingers around the cervix to ensure that no cervical or vaginal tissue is trapped inside the cup.
- Raise the pressure at the rate of 0.1 kg/cm$^2$ per minute until the effective vacuum of 0.8 kg/cm$^2$ is achieved in 10 minutes time.
- Apply traction at right angle to cup and in synchronous with uterine contractions.
- If there is no advancement during four successive tractions, then it should be stopped. The traction should not exceed for more than 30 minutes.

## Complications of Ventouse Delivery

### Fetal

- Sloughing of the scalp
- Cephalhematoma
- Cerebral trauma such as tentorial tear
- **Chignon:** Area of edema and bruising where the cup was applied.

### Maternal

Trauma to the mother is rare. Injuries may occur due to inclusion of the soft tissue such as cervix or vaginal wall inside the cup.

## Nursing Interventions for Ventouse Delivery

- Explain the procedure to the patient.
- Advising the patient that an attempt at instrumental delivery may not result in vaginal delivery; may avoid unrealistic expectations.
- Obtain the consent of the informed.
- Review patient history before applying ventouse (to ensure there are no contraindications or any caution).
- Do abdominal palpation to confirm fetal presentation, position and degree of engagement of the presenting part.
- Apply aseptic technique.
- Check the prerequisites for ventouse application.
- Select ventouse cup as per the size of fetal head.
- Checks reports and record the fetal heart rate before applying the cup and again after application of the ventouse.
- After delivery, examine for any tears that might have been caused by the forceps. If there is any, repair with catgut suture.
- Give support to the patient.
- Observe for signs and symptoms of complications.
- Assess the newborn for indications of injury.
- Record the whole procedure.

# CESAREAN SECTION

**Definition:** Cesarean section is an operative procedure whereby the fetuses after the end of $8^{th}$ week are delivered through an incision on the abdominal and uterine walls.

## Time of Operation

- **Elective cesarean:** When the operation is done at a prearranged time during pregnancy.
    - **Maturity is certain:** Operation is done about 1 week prior to the expected date of confinement.
    - **Maturity is uncertain:** Ultrasound assessment in first or second trimester, if available, is corroborated. Amniocentesis is used to assess fetal lung maturity. Otherwise wait for spontaneous onset of labor.
- **Emergency cesarean:** It is performed when adverse conditions develop during labor.

## Indications for Cesarean Section

### Elective Cesarean Section (Table 3)

Table 3 exhibits the indications for elective cesarean section.

**TABLE 3:** Indications for elective cesarean section

| Absolute indications | Relative indications |
|---|---|
| • Cephalopelvic disproportion (CPD)<br>• Major degree of placenta previa<br>• Multiple pregnancies<br>• Cancer of cervix<br>• Pelvic tumors<br>• Cervical fibroid | • Malpresentation<br>• Pregnancy induced hypertension (PIH)<br>• Medical/gynecological disorders such as:<br>  ▪ Chronic hypertension, chronic nephritis<br>  ▪ Diabetes mellitus<br>  ▪ Heart diseases<br>  ▪ Previous history of cesarean section or hysterectomy<br>  ▪ Antepartum hemorrhage (APH)<br>  ▪ Bad obstetric history of recurrent fetal loss |

### Emergency Cesarean Section

- Indications are:
    - Cord prolapse
    - Uterine rupture or scar dehiscence
    - Cephalopelvic disproportion diagnosed in labor
    - Fulminating PIH
    - Eclampsia
    - Failure to progress in the first or second stage of labor
    - Fetal distress
    - Abnormal uterine contractions

## Contraindications

- Dead fetus
- Premature baby, not able to survive inside the womb
- Presence of blood coagulation disorders

## Types of Operations

- **Lower segment cesarean section (LSCS):** In this operation, the extraction of the baby is done through an incision made in the lower segment through a transperitoneal approach. This method is commonly used in obstetric practice.

Figures 3A and B show the types of cesarean section.

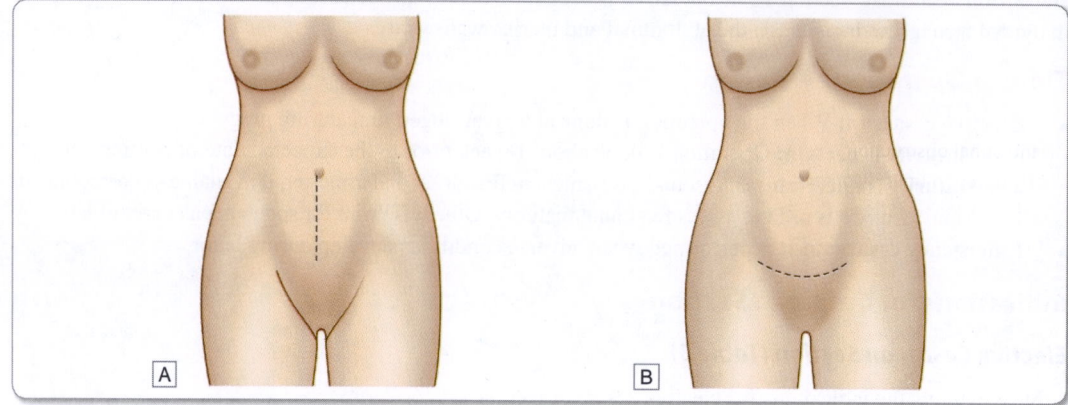

**Figs 3A and B:** Types of cesarean section

- **Classical cesarean section:** In this operation, the baby is extracted through an incision made in the upper segment of uterus. It is done only in following cases:
  - Gestation is less than 32 weeks before the lower segment has formed
  - Placenta previa
  - Hourglass constriction
  - Lower segment approach is difficult due to dense adhesions from previous operation or severely contracted pelvis with pendulous abdomen
  - Cancer of cervix or big fibroid in the lower uterine segment
- **Postmortem section:** Contemplating to have a live baby

## Complications of Cesarean Section

- **Intraoperative complications:**
  - Extension of uterine incision
  - Uterine lacerations
  - Bladder injury
  - Urethral injury
  - Gastrointestinal tract injury
  - Uterine atony
  - Postpartum hemorrhage (PPH)
- **Postoperative complications:**
  - Maternal (Immediate maternal and remote postoperative complications are shown in Table 4).
  - Fetal complication
    - Iatrogenic prematurity
    - Respiratory distress syndrome

**TABLE 4:** Immediate and remote postoperative complications

| Immediate maternal complications | Remote complications |
|---|---|
| • Postpartum hemorrhage (PPH)<br>• Shock<br>• Anesthetic hazards<br>• Infections<br>• Intestinal obstruction<br>• Thromboembolic disorders<br>• Wound complications<br>  ▪ Pus formation<br>  ▪ Hematoma<br>  ▪ Dehiscence<br>  ▪ Burst abdomen<br>• Secondary postpartum hemorrhage | • Gynecological<br>  ▪ Menstrual irregularities<br>  ▪ Chronic pelvic pain<br>  ▪ Backache<br>• General surgical<br>  ▪ Incisional hernia<br>  ▪ Intestinal obstruction<br>• Future pregnancy<br>  ▪ Scar rupture |

## Nursing Management

- **Psychological preparation:** Provide detailed explanations and reassurance. Women who have elective cesarean section, may be given the information in stages. If the possibility of cesarean section arises during labor, the midwife should begin to prepare the woman for this eventuality.
- **Preoperative preparation:**
    - Informed written permission for the procedure, anesthesia and blood transfusion is obtained.
    - Abdomen is scrubbed with soap and nonorganic iodide lotion. Hair may be clipped or shaved.
    - Nonparticulate antacid is given orally before transferring to theater to neutralize the existing gastric acid.
    - Ranitidine (H$_2$ blocker) 150 mg is given orally night before procedure and is repeated one hour before the surgery to raise the gastric pH.
    - Metoclopramide (10 mg IV) is given to increase the tone of lower esophageal sphincter as well as to reduce the stomach contents.
    - The stomach should be emptied by gastric suction, if necessary (emergency procedure).
    - Empty the bladder.
    - Check the fetal heart sound (FHS).
    - Neonatologist should be made available.
    - Arrange all the necessary equipment for surgery.
    - Provide dorsal position, a 15° tilt to her left side using a wedge till the delivery of baby.
- **Postoperative Care**
  *For First 24 Hours*
    - Close observation for first 6–8 hours is required.
    - Check pulse, blood pressure and amount of vaginal bleeding every hourly.
    - Administer fluid such as sodium chloride or ringer lactate drip until at least 2–2.5 L of the solution is infused.
    - Blood transfusion is required in anemic mother or if blood loss is more than average in cesarean section.

- Prophylactic antibiotics (cephalosporins, metronidazole) for all cesarean delivery is given for 2–4 doses.
- Analgesia such as pethidine hydrochloride 75–100 mg is administered.
- Ambulate the patient if condition permits, otherwise advise the client to move her legs and ankle and to breathe deeply to minimize deep vein thrombosis (DVT) and pulmonary embolism.
- Baby is put to breast for feeding after 3–4 hours when mother is stable and is relieved of pain.

*Day-1*
- Oral feeding in the form of plain/electrolyte solution/raw tea may be given.
- Active bowel sounds are observed by the end of the day.

*Day-2*
- Light solid diet of the patient's choice is given.
- If patient suffers from constipation, 3–4 teaspoon of lactulose is given at bedtime.

*Day 5–6*
- In transverse incision the abdominal (stitches are removed on Day 5th).
- In longitudinal, stitches are removed on day 6th.

## Discharge

- The patient is discharged on the day following removal of stitches.
- Advise the mother to take nutritious diet.
- Provide supplementary iron therapy.
- Advise mother regarding postnatal exercises.
- Instruct for breastfeeding and care of newborn.
- Gradual return to day-to-day activities.
- Avoidance of intercourse for a reasonable period of 4–6 weeks until cesarean scar is well healed.
- Family planning advice and guidance: Nonlactating women should practice some form of contraceptive measures after 3 weeks and lactating women should start 3-month after delivery.
- To have postnatal checkup after 6 weeks.

## STERILIZATION

**Sterilization:** Already discussed in Chapter 7: Management of Normal Puerperium.

## DILATATION AND EVACUATION (D AND E)

It is a procedure in which cervix is dilated and the products of conception are taken out from uterine cavity. It can be performed in two stages:

**One stage:** Dilatation of the cervix and evacuation of the uterus are done in the same sitting.

**Two stages**
- First phase includes slow dilatation of the cervix
- Second phase includes rapid dilatation of the cervix and evacuation

Indications for one-stage and two-stage operations are given in Figure 4.

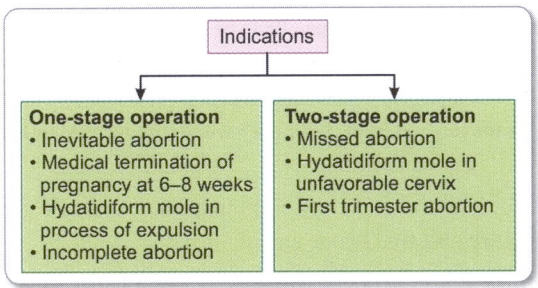

**Fig. 4:** Indications for one-stage and two-stage operations

## One-stage Operation

- Introduce posterior vaginal speculum and ask assistant to hold it.
- Grasp the anterior lip of cervix using Allis forceps.
- Measure the uterine length by introducing uterine sound. Also find out the position of uterus.
- Dilate the cervix by using metal dilators.
- Remove the products of conception using ovum forceps.
- Curette the uterine cavity gently by a flushing curette.
- Give IV methergine during procedure.
- Remove forceps and speculum and massage uterus bimanually.
- Make sure that uterus is firm and vaginal bleeding is minimal.
- Give perineal pad and shift to bed.

## Two-stage Operation

- **1st phase:** First dilate the cervix slowly by introducing laminaria tent into the cervical canal or insert misoprostol (PGE1) 400 mg, three hours before surgery.
- **2nd phase:** Further cervix is dilated by metal dilators and evacuation of uterus is done.

## Dangers of D and E Operation

The dangers involved in dilatation and evacuation operations are shown in Figure 5.

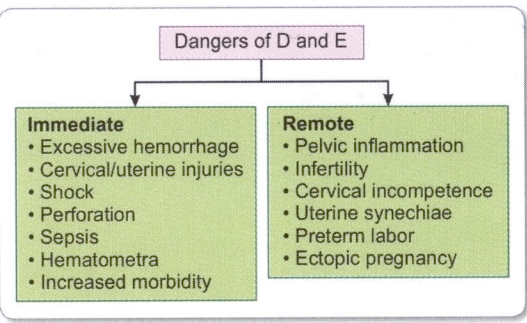

**Fig. 5:** Dangers of D and E

# SUCTION EVACUATION

Suction evacuation is a procedure in which the products of conception are sucked out from the uterus with the help of a cannula fitted to a suction apparatus.

## Indications

- Incomplete abortion
- Hydatidiform mole
- Medical termination of pregnancy (MTP)
- Inevitable abortion

## Procedure

- First vaginal examination is done to assess the size, position of uterus and to know the state of uterus.
- Cervix is dilated with metal dilators up to one size less than that of suction cannula.
- Administer methergine 0.2 mg IV.
- Appropriate size cannula is fitted to suction apparatus by a thick rubber or plastic tubing.
- Introduce the cannula into uterus, the tip is placed in middle of the uterine cavity.
- The pressure of suction is raised to 400–600 mm Hg.
- Move cannula up and down and rotate with uterine cavity with pressure on.
- Regulate the pressure by placing a finger over the hole at base of cannula.
- Check the suction bottle for products of conceptus and blood loss.
- Break the vacuum before withdrawing the cannula down through cervical canal to prevent injury to internal os.
- At the end of suction, curette uterine cavity by flushing curette.
- Introduce cannula again to suck out the remnants from uterine cavity.
- Assess for firmness of uterus and vaginal bleeding.
- Provide vulval pad and transfer the patient to bed from table.

## Complications

- **Immediate**
  - Excessive hemorrhage
  - Shock
  - Cervical/uterine injuries
  - Perforation of bowel, bladder, etc.
  - Sepsis
  - Hematometra
- **Remote**
  - Pelvic incompetence
  - Infertility
  - Cervical incompetence
  - Preterm labor
  - Ectopic pregnancy

## Post-abortal Care

- Emergency treatment of complications of any abortion (spontaneous or induced)
- Family planning counseling and referral services
- Linkages to other reproductive health services
- Male partner should be involved

# DESTRUCTIVE OPERATIONS

The destructive operations are designed to diminish the bulk of the fetus so as to facilitate the delivery of the fetus. The aim is to destroy the fetus in the womb to save the life of the woman.

Four types of operations are:
- Craniotomy
- Decapitation
- Evisceration
- Cleidotomy

## Craniotomy

It is an operation to make perforation on the fetal head, to evacuate the contents followed by extraction of fetus.

### Indications

- Cephalic presentation producing obstructed labor with dead fetus
- Hydrocephalus even in a living fetus
- Interlocking heads of twins

### Conditions to be Fulfilled

- Cervix must be fully dilated
- Baby must be dead except hydrocephalus

### Contraindications

- Severely contracted pelvis
- Rupture of the uterus

### Site of Perforation

- **Vertex:** On parietal bone, either side of sagittal suture
- **Face:** Through the orbit or hard palate
- **Brow:** Through the frontal bone

Suture is avoided to prevent collapse of the bone thereby preventing escape of brain matter.

### Preliminaries

- Give anesthesia (general, local or intravenous diazepam).
- Provide lithotomy position to the patient.
- Wash hand to maintain asepsis.

- Wear sterile cap, mask, gown and gloves.
- Vulva and vagina are to be swabbed with antiseptic solution.
- Drape the perineum and legs with sterile clothes.
- Empty the bladder.
- Perform vaginal examination.

## Procedure

- Introduce two fingers inside the vagina and place them on the proposed site of perforation.
- The Oldham perforator with the blades closed is introduced under the palmer aspect of the fingers until the tip reaches the proposed site of perforation.
- Ask the assistant to steady the head per abdomen in manner of first pelvic grip and perforate the skull by rotating movements.
- With the fingers, brain matter is evacuated so that skull is collapsed as much as possible.
- Extraction of fetus is done either by cranioclast or by two giant volsella by applying traction same as in forceps.
- After the delivery of placenta, explore the uterovaginal canal for any tear/laceration.

**Note:** Injection methergine 0.2 mg is to be given intravenously with the delivery of anterior shoulder. The rest of delivery is completed as in normal delivery.

# Decapitation

It is a destructive operation whereby fetal head is separated from trunk and delivery is completed with the extraction of trunk and that of decapitated head per vagina.

## Indications

- Dead fetus
- Interlocking head of twins

## Procedure

### Preliminaries

- Give anesthesia (general, local or intravenous diazepam).
- Provide lithotomy position to the patient.
- Wash hand to maintain asepsis.
- Wear sterile cap, mask, gown and gloves.
- Vulva and vagina are to be swabbed with antiseptic solution.
- Drape the perineum and legs with sterile clothes.
- Empty the bladder.
- Perform vaginal examination.

### Steps

- If the hand is not prolapsed, a hand is brought down. For this, roller gauze is tied on the wrist and ask the assistant to give traction toward the side away from fetal head to make the neck more accessible and fixed.
- Two fingers of right hand are introduced inside the vagina with the palmar surface downward and placed on the superior surface of the neck.

- The decapitation hook with knife is introduced into the vagina and knob pointing towards the fetal head.
- By upward and downward movements of the hook with knife, the vertebral column is severed. The decapitated head is pushed up and trunk is delivered by traction on the prolapsed arm.
- Delivery of the decapitated head by any method such as:
  - Using forceps
  - By hooking the index finger into the mouth
  - By holding the severed neck with giant vulsellum and delivery of head as that of aftercoming head in breech
- Routine exploration of the uterovaginal canal to exclude rupture of uterus or any other injury.

## Evisceration

The operation consists of removal of thoracic and abdominal contents through an opening on the thoracic or abdominal cavity at the most accessible site.

### Indications

- Gross fetal malformations such as fetal ascites or hugely distended bladder
- Neglected shoulder presentation with dead fetus

## Cleidotomy

It is the operation in which there is division of one or both clavicles so as to reduce the bulk of the fetus. The operation is done only on dead fetus with shoulder dystocia. The clavicles are divided by embryotomy scissors or long straight scissors introduced under the guidance of two fingers of left hand placed inside the vagina.

### Complications

- Injury to uterovaginal canal
- Postpartum hemorrhage-atonic/traumatic
- Shock due to blood loss/dehydration
- Puerperal sepsis
- Sub involution of uterus
- Vesicovaginal fistula/rectovaginal fistula

## Postoperative Care

- Bladder should be catheterized for 5–7 days in the cases where bladder distension was for prolonged time.
- Careful inspection of genital tract for signs of trauma including uterine exploration to rule out rupture
- Oxytocin infusion continued for 6–8 hours as the risk of atonic postpartum hemorrhage (PPH) following prolonged obstructed labor is high.
- Blood transfusion may be done, if required.
- Active management of third stage.
- Broad spectrum antibiotics.
- Thromboprophylaxis.
- As much possible the infant must be restored anatomically with suturing. This along with careful placement of blankets should help to reduce trauma to the parents when they realize that their newborn is dead.
- Psychological wellbeing of husband/wife and family members should be taken care of.
- Plans for subsequent pregnancy care.

## Nursing Care Plan for Destructive Operations

The following are the nursing care plan for destructive operations:

### Nursing Diagnosis

- Alteration in comfort due to pain related to delivery process:
    - Assess the duration, intensity and types of pain.
    - Provide comfortable left lateral position to the mother.
    - Provide psychological support to the mother.
- Potential for complication related to destructive operation:
    - Clean the perineal area with betadine.
    - Maintain aseptic technique.
    - Handle the case carefully.
    - Only experts should handle the case.
    - Assess for any types of laceration.
- Potential for infection related to destructive operation:
    - Maintain strict aseptic technique.
    - Avoid many visitors.
    - Clean the surrounding.
    - Assess for any scar.
- Fear and anxiety of parents related to delivery process:
    - Clarify the doubts of the mother.
    - Give information about progress of delivery frequently.
    - Provide proper explanation about baby's condition.
    - Provide psychological reassurance to the mother and family.

## MANUAL VACUUM ASPIRATION

It is done up to 12 weeks with minimal cervical dilatation. This is performed as an outpatient procedure using a plastic disposable cannula (up to 12 mm size) attached to a plastic syringe (double valve) of 60 mL. The cannula is inserted transcervically into the uterus and the vacuum is activated. A negative pressure of 660 mm Hg is created. Aspiration of the products of conception is done. This procedure takes less time (5–15 minutes) and is less traumatic.

### Complications

Similar to dilatation and evacuation (D&E).

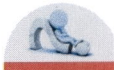

## ASSESS YOURSELF

### FREQUENTLY ASKED QUESTIONS IN EXAMS

1. Define induction of labor. Enlist its types, indications, methods of induction.
2. What do you mean by ventouse delivery? Enlist its indications, contraindications and complications.
3. Define cesarean section. Enlist its types and indications. Describe the nursing management of patient during cesarean section.

### MULTIPLE CHOICE QUESTIONS

1. Method of Induction of labor is/are:
   a. Oxytocin
   b. Prostaglandins
   c. Artificial rupture of membranes
   d. All of the above

2. When the version is done by introducing one hand into the uterus and other hand on the abdomen is:
   a. External version
   b. Internal version
   c. Spontaneous version
   d. Bipolar version

3. What are the conditions to be fulfilled before version?
   a. Cervix fully dilated
   b. Adequate amniotic fluid
   c. Live fetus
   d. All of the above

4. What is the ideal time to perform version by an obstetrician?
   a. Before 28 weeks
   b. At 30 weeks
   c. At 32 weeks
   d. 36 weeks onwards

5. Which of the following is the rotation forceps?
   a. Wrigley's forceps
   b. Kielland's forceps
   c. Das forceps
   d. Long curved forceps with traction

6. Which forceps is used when the biparietal diameter passed the pelvic brim but not pass the ischial spines?
   a. Midforceps
   b. High forceps
   c. Low forceps
   d. Outlet forceps

7. In which condition ventouse delivery is not possible?
   a. Inadequate expulsive efforts
   b. Maternal exhaustion
   c. Face presentation
   d. Prolonged second stage of labor

8. How much vacuum pressure is required to extract fetal head?
   a. $0.8 \text{ kg/cm}^2$
   b. $0.2 \text{ kg/cm}^2$
   c. $0.1 \text{ kg/cm}^2$
   d. $0.6 \text{ kg/cm}^2$

9. Which is the most common complication of ventouse delivery?
   a. Chignon formation
   b. Cerebral palsy
   c. Intracranial hemorrhage
   d. Perineal tear

10. When the cesarean section is done at prearranged time during pregnancy, it is called:
    a. Elective cesarean
    b. Classical cesarean
    c. Emergency cesarean
    d. None of the above

11. **What are the absolute indications of cesarean section?**
    a. Cephalopelvic disproportion
    b. Placenta previa
    c. Cancer of cervix
    d. All of the above

12. **In case of cesarean section with longitudinal incision the stitches are removed on:**
    a. Day 4th
    b. Day 5th
    c. Day 6th
    d. Day 7th

13. **Induction of labor is contraindicated in:**
    a. Elderly primigravida
    b. Previous cesarean
    c. Contracted pelvis
    d. All of the above

14. **During suction evacuation, required pressure is:**
    a. 100–200 mm Hg
    b. 200–300 mm Hg
    c. 400–600 mm Hg
    d. 700–900 mm Hg

15. **Cesarean section is must in which type of placenta previa?**
    a. Type II
    b. Type III
    c. Type IV
    d. All of the above

16. **Indication for classical cesarean section is:**
    a. Obstructed labor
    b. Cancer of cervix
    c. Placenta previa
    d. Both B and C

17. **Only common indication for internal version is:**
    a. Brow presentation
    b. Face presentation
    c. Delivery of 2nd twin
    d. Breech presentation

18. **Internal podalic version is done under:**
    a. Pudendal block
    b. IV calmpose
    c. Spinal anesthesia
    d. General anesthesia

19. **The most common contraindication for induction of labor is:**
    a. Diabetes
    b. Bad obstetrical history
    c. Poliomyelitis
    d. Heart disease

20. **On external cephalic version, fetal bradycardia occurs. The next course of action is:**
    a. Reversion to the original position immediately by external version
    b. Internal podalic version
    c. Cesarean section
    d. Rupture of membranes

## Answer Key

| 1. d | 2. b | 3. d | 4. d | 5. b | 6. a | 7. c |
|------|------|------|------|------|------|------|
| 8. a | 9. a | 10. a | 11. d | 12. c | 13. d | 14. c |
| 15. d | 16. d | 17. c | 18. d | 19. d | 20. a | |

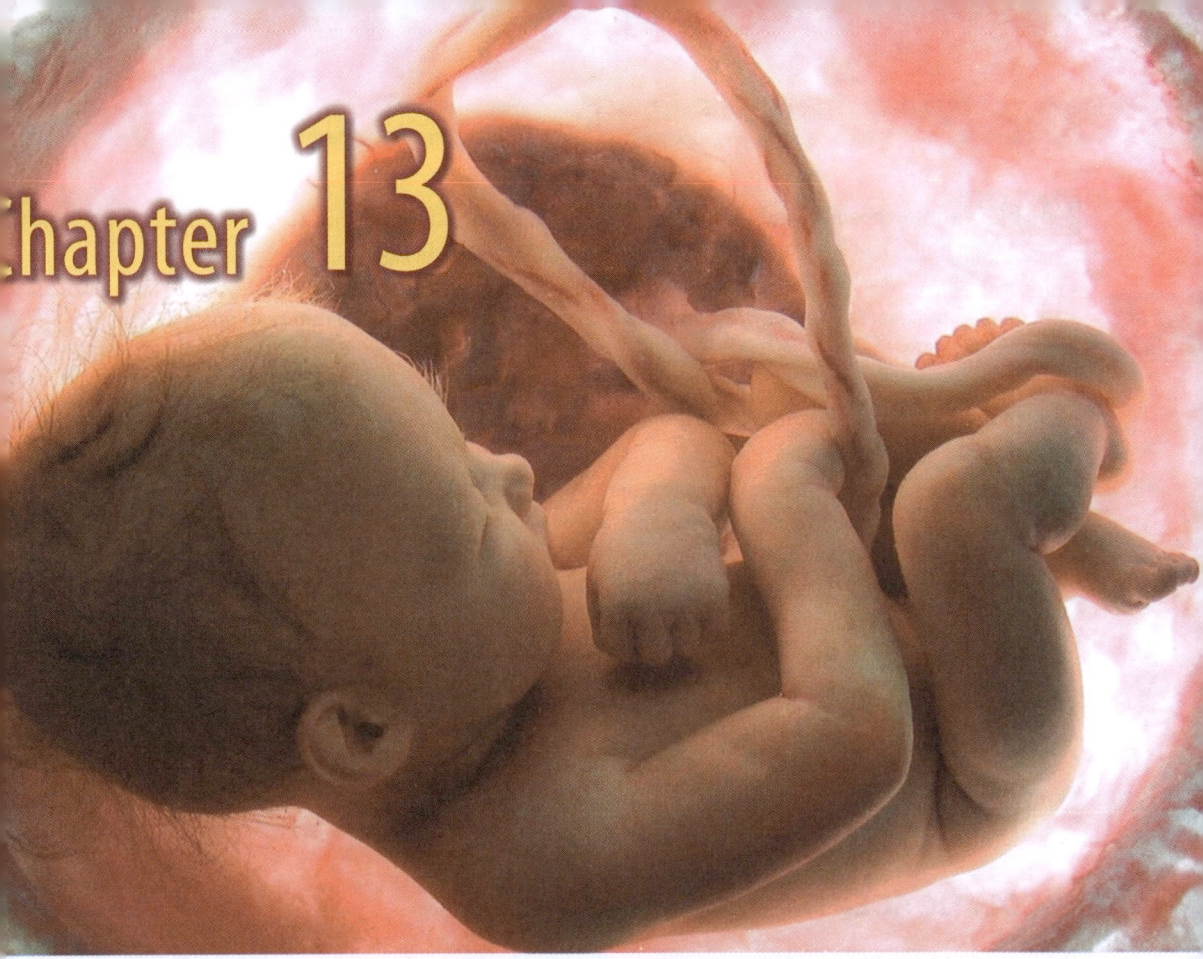

# Chapter 13

# Drugs used in Obstetrics

*Learning Objectives* .................................................................

**Upon completing this chapter, the learner will be able to:**

➡ Describe the use of oxytocic drugs and the nursing considerations related to each drug
➡ Explain the use of tocolytics for maternity clients
➡ Analyze anesthesia and analgesia in obstetrics
➡ Discuss the drugs used for newborn
➡ Understand the effects of teratogens on mother and baby

# UTEROTONICS

An uterotonic, also known as ecbolic, is an agent used to induce contraction or greater tonicity of the uterus. Uterotonics are used both to induce labor, and to reduce postpartum hemorrhage.

Some uterotonics act as analogues of oxytocin. An oxytocinergic, or oxytocic, means "having to do with oxytocin". The oxytocin receptors are the binding and activation site of oxytocin.

## Oxytocics

Oxytocics are the drugs that have power to excite contractions of uterine muscles (Table 1). Among a large number of drugs belonging to this group the important ones are:

• Oxytocin
• Ergot derivatives
• Prostaglandins.

# TOCOLYTIC AGENTS

Tocolytic drugs can inhibit uterine contractions and used to prolong the pregnancy in women who develop premature uterine contraction in addition to putting them to absolute bed rest and sedation, tocolytics are given to inhibit uterine contractions. Commonly used drugs are isoxsuprine (duvadilan) ritodrine hydrochloride (yutopar) and magnesium sulfate (Table 2).

# ANTIHYPERTENSIVES

Antihypertensive drugs are used when the blood pressure is 160/110 mm Hg to protect the mother from cerebral hemorrhage, cardiac failure and abruptio placentas. Aim is to reduce the blood pressure to a mean <125 mm Hg. First line drug is either methyldopa or labetalol. Second line drug is nifedipine (Table 3).

# ANTICONVULSANTS

Convulsions in pregnancy are largely due to eclampsia. Other causes are: epilepsy, cerebral malaria and cerebral tumors. The commonly used anticonvulsants are; diazepam, phenytoin and phenobarbitone. First choice of anticonvulsant drug is magnesium sulfate (Table 4).

# ANESTHESIA AND ANALGESIA

(*Note:* Already discussed in pain management during labor i.e. Chapter 5: Normal Labor and its Management)

**TABLE 1:** Oxytocics

| Drug | Mode of action | Indications | Contraindications | Dosage and route | Side effects | Nursing responsibilities |
|------|----------------|-------------|-------------------|------------------|--------------|--------------------------|
| Oxytocin (Pitocin/ Syntocinon) | Action on the physiological uterine contractile system and stimulate it law of polarity | • Therapeutic indication <br> • Diagnostic indication <br> **a. Therapeutic indications:** <br> **(i) Pregnancy** <br> **Early:** <br> • To accelerate abortion <br> • To stop bleeding after abortion <br> • As an adjunct to other abortifacient agents <br> **Late:** <br> • To induce labor <br> • To ripen the cervix before induction | • Heart diseases <br> • Abruptio placenta <br> • Contracted pelvis <br> • Grand multipara <br> • Malpresentation <br> • Fetal distress <br> • Obstructed labor <br> • Incoordinated uterine contractions <br> • History of cesarean section | • Route-IV <br> • For induction 2–5 units in 500 mL RL or NS with 15, 30 and 60 drops increasing at every 15-minute. <br> • For PPH 20 units in 500 mL NS and RL | **Maternal** <br> • Uterine hyper-stimulation <br> • Uterine rupture <br> • Water intoxication <br> • Hypertension <br> • Antidiuresis <br> **Fetal** <br> • Fetal distress | • Continuously monitor contractions, fetal and maternal heart rate, maternal blood pressure and ECG. Discontinue infusion if uterine hyperactivity occurs. <br> • Monitor patient closely during 1st and 2nd stages of labor because of risk of cervical lacerations, uterine rupture, maternal and fetal death. <br> • Assess fluid intake and output. Watch for signs and symptoms of water intoxication. <br> **Assessment and drug effects** <br> • Start flow charts to record maternal BP and other vital signs, input and output ratio, weight, strength, duration, and frequency of contractions, as well as fetal heart tone and rate, before instituting treatment. |
| | | **(ii) Labor** <br> • Augmentation of labor <br> • Uterine inertia <br> • Inactive management of 3rd stage of labor <br> • Following expulsion of placenta as an alternative to ergometrine | | | | • Monitor fetal heart rate and maternal BP, pulse after every 15-minute during infusion period; evaluate the intensity, frequency and duration of uterine contractions and record on partograph. If any change in rate and rhythm immediately inform to physician. Stop infusion to prevent fetal anoxia, turn patient on her side. Oxygen administration may be necessary. |

Contd...

| Drug | Mode of action | Indications | Contraindications | Dosage and route | Side effects | Nursing responsibilities |
|---|---|---|---|---|---|---|
| | | | | | | • If local or regional (caudal, spinal) anesthesia is being given to the patient receiving oxytocin, be alert to the possibility of hypertensive crisis (sudden intense occipital headache, palpitation, nausea, vomiting, sweating, bradycardia or tachycardia, constricting chest pain fever, marked hypertension, stiff neck, photophobia, dilated pupils). |
| | | (iii) **Puerperium**<br>• To control PPH<br>• To prevent breast engorgement<br><br>**b. Diagnostic indications**<br>• Contraction stress test<br>• Oxytocin sensitivity test | | | | • Monitor input and output during labor. If patient is receiving drug by prolonged IV infusion, watch for symptoms of water intoxication (drowsiness, listlessness, headache, confusion, anuria, weight gain). Report changes in alertness and orientation and changes in input and output ratio (i.e., marked decrease in output with excessive intake).<br>• Check fundus frequently during the first few postpartum hours and several times daily thereafter.<br>• Incidence of hypersensitivity or allergic reactions is higher when oxytocin is given by IM or IV injection rather than by IV infusion (diluted solution).<br>• Patient and family education. |

*Contd...*

| Drug | Mode of action | Indications | Contraindications | Dosage and route | Side effects | Nursing responsibilities |
|---|---|---|---|---|---|---|
| **Ergot derivative (methergine)** | Acts directly on myometrium producing tetanic contraction of the uterus with complete loss of polarity. | • To stop the atonic uterine bleeding after<br>   ◦ Labor<br>   ◦ Abortion<br>• To cut short 3$^{rd}$ stage of labor. (administered after expulsion of anterior shoulder of fetus) | • High blood pressure<br>• Rh-ve factor<br>• Abruptio placenta<br>• Multiple pregnancy before the delivery of last fetus E.g., 2$^{nd}$ fetus for twin pregnancy<br>• Heart disease<br>• Preeclampsia/eclampsia | • 0.25 mg IV<br>• 0.5 mg IM<br>• 1 mg orally | • Nausea<br>• Vomiting<br>• Rise of blood pressure<br>• Gangrene of toe (rare)<br>• Interfere with lactation. | • Assess vital sign of mother immediately after administration.<br>• Administer antiemetics for uncontrollable vomiting.<br>• Assess for lactation process. |
| **Prostaglandins preparations**<br>• Vaginal suppository<br>• Vaginal pessary<br>• Gel form<br>• Parenteral | PGF$_{2\alpha}$ acts on myometrium to excite uterine contractions and PGE$_2$ acts mainly on the cervix cervical ripening | • Induction of abortion<br>• Induction of labor<br>• Cervical ripening<br>• Acceleration of labor<br>• PPH management | • Hypersensitivity<br>• Uterine scar | • Vaginal suppository 20 mg PGE$_2$ or 50 mg PGE$_{2a}$<br>• Cervical gel (cerviprime) 0.5 mg (per vaginal)<br>  PGE2 1 mg/mL (parenteral<br>• PGF$_{2a}$ 2.5 mg /10 mL via IV | • Tachysystole<br>• Meconium passage by fetus<br>• Rupture of uterus | Same as oxytocins and ergot derivatives |

*Abbreviations:* FHS, fetal heart sound; NS, normal saline; PPH, postpartum hemorrhage; RL, Ringer's lactate

**TABLE 2:** Tocolytic agents

| Drug | Indications | Action | Dosage and route | Side effects | Contraindi-cations | Nursing considerations |
|---|---|---|---|---|---|---|
| • Isoxsuprine (duvadilan) | • Treatment of premature labor pain<br>• Threatened abortion<br>• Night cramps<br>• Cerebral and peripheral vascular disease | Acts directly on vascular smooth muscle causes cardiac stimulation and uterine relaxation | **Initial**<br>IV 100 mg in 5% dextrose. **Rate:** 0.2 ug/min<br>**Maintenance:**<br>IM 10 mg 6 hourly for 24 hours, tablet 10 mg 6–8 hourly | • Hypotension<br>• Tachycardia<br>• Nausea<br>• Vomiting<br>• Pulmonary edema<br>• Respiratory distress syndrome<br>• Hyperglycemia | • Hypersen-sitivity | **Assess:**<br>• Pulse and BP during treatment<br>• Intensity and length of uterine contractions<br>• Fetal heart tones<br>**Administer** with meals to reduce gastrointestinal upset<br>**Evaluate:**<br>• Therapeutic response<br>• Reduced uterine contractions<br>• Absence of preterm labor<br>• Increase pulse volume<br>**Teach patient:**<br>• To avoid hazardous activities until stabilized on medications, dizziness may occur<br>• Slowly change the position or fainting may occur<br>• To notify physician if rash, palpitations or severe flushing develops |
| • Ritodrine hydrochloride (yutopar) | Treatment of preterm labor in patients with a pregnancy of 20 or more weeks' gestation | **Uterine relaxant:**<br>Acts directly on vascular smooth muscle causes cardiac stimulation and uterine relaxation | **Initial:** IV drip 100 mg in 5% dextrose<br>**Maintenance:**<br>Tablet 10 mg 6–8 hourly | • Hyperglycemia<br>• Headache<br>• Restlessness<br>• Sweating<br>• Chills<br>• Drowsiness<br>• Nausea<br>• Vomiting<br>• Anorexia<br>• Malaise | • Hypersen-sitivity<br>• Eclampsia<br>• Hyperten-sion<br>• Dysrhyth-mias | **Assess:**<br>• Maternal and fetal heart rate<br>• Intensity and length of uterine contractions<br>• Fluid intake to prevent fluid overload, discontinue if this occurs<br>**Administer:**<br>• Only clear liquids<br>• Using infusion pump/monitor carefully<br>• Provide left lateral recumbent position to decrease hypotension and increase renal blood flow<br>**Evaluate:**<br>• Therapeutic response<br>• Decreased intensity<br>• Length of contraction<br>• Absence of preterm labor<br>• Decrease blood pressure<br>**Teach patient:** To remain in bed during infusion |

**TABLE 3:** Antihypertensives

| Drug | Indication | Mechanism of action | Dosage and route | Side effects | Contraindications | Nursing responsibilities |
|------|-----------|--------------------|-----------------|-------------|-------------------|-------------------------|
| Methyl-dopa | • Hypertension<br>• Hypertensive crisis<br>• Renal impairment<br>• Preeclampsia<br>• Eclampsia<br>• Treat preterm labor | Stimulates central α-adrenergic receptors or acts as false transmitter resulting in reduction of arterial pressure. | • Orally 250 mg b.i.d.- may be increased to t.i.d. depending upon the response<br>• IV infusion 250–500 mg | **Maternal-**Postural hypotension, hemolytic anemia, sodium retention, sedation<br>**Fetal:** Intestinal ileus | • Hepatic disorder<br>• Psychic patient<br>• Congestive cardiac failure | **Assess:**<br>• Intake output and weight daily<br>• Blood pressure and pulse × 4 hourly<br>• Liver function test<br>**Administer:** 1 hour before food<br>**Evaluate:**<br>• Therapeutic response: decreased BP after 1–2 weeks<br>• Edema in feet, legs daily<br>• Skin turgor and dryness of mucus membranes for hydration status<br>• Teach client<br>• Not to discontinue drug abruptly<br>• Not to use the counter medications<br>• To report bradycardia, dizziness, confusion and depression.<br>• Avoid alcohol, smoking and excess sodium intake<br>• Wear support hose to minimize orthostatic hypotension. |
| Labetalol | • Hypertension<br>• Preeclampsia<br>• Eclampsia | Nonselective beta-blocker | Orally -100 mg t.i.d may be increased up to 800 mg daily.<br>IV infusion (hypertensive crisis) 1–2 mg/min<br>Until desired effect | • Orthostatic hypertension<br>• Bradycardia<br>• Hepatic disorder<br>• Sinus bradycardia<br>• Bronchial asthma<br>• Chest pain<br>• Drowsiness<br>• Headache<br>• Nightmares<br>• Lethargy<br>• Thombocyto-penia<br>• Sore throat<br>• Dry burning eyes | • Hepatic disorder<br>• Sinus bradycardia<br>• Bronchial asthma | **Assess:**<br>• Intake output and weight daily<br>• Blood pressure and pulse check × 4 hourly<br>• Apical or radial pulse before administration.<br>**Administered:**<br>• Before meal or at bed time<br>**Evaluate:**<br>• Therapeutic response used BP after 1–2 weeks<br>• Evaluate skin turgor, edema, dryness of mucous membrane for dehydration<br>**Teach client**<br>• Not to discontinue drug abruptly<br>• Do not use over the counter medications.<br>• To report bradycardia, dizziness confusion or depression<br>• Avoid alcohol, smoking and excess sodium intake<br>• Wear support hose to minimize effects of orthostatic hypotension |

Contd...

| Drug | Indication | Mechanism of action | Dosage and route | Side effects | Contrain dications | Nursing responsibilities |
|------|-----------|---------------------|------------------|--------------|--------------------|--------------------------|
| Hydrala-zine | Severe hypertension | Vasodilates arteriolar smooth muscles by direct relaxation, reduction in BP with reflex increase in cardiac function. | • Orally 100 mg/day in four divided doses. <br>• IV 5–10 mg every 20 minutes maximum 20 mg | **Maternal** hypotension, tachycardia, arrhythmia, palpitation, fluid retention <br>**Neonatal** thormbo-cytopenia | • Because of variable sodium retention, diuretics should be used. <br>• To control arrhythmias, propranolol may be administered intravenously. | **Assess** <br>• Vital signs of patient, i.e. blood pressure and pulse at frequent interval <br>• Check intake output and weight daily <br>• Provide recumbent position to the patient during administration of drug and keep the patient in same position for at least 1 hour <br>**Evaluate** <br>• Edema in feet and legs daily <br>• Check skin and mucous membrane for hydration <br>• Check patient for rales, dyspnea, tachycardia, headache and nausea <br>**Teach client** <br>• To take this drug with meal <br>• Notify the physician if chest pain severe fatigue muscle or joint pain occur |
| Nifedipine | • Hypertension (high blood pressure) <br>• Angina (chest pain) <br>• Treat pre-term labor <br>• Dysmenor-rhea | • Calcium channel blockers <br>• Direct arte-riolar vaso-dilation by inhibition of slow inward calcium channels in vascular smooth muscles | Orally 5–10 mg tid, maximum dose 60–120 mg/day | Flushing Hypotension Headache Tachycardia Inhibition of labor | Simultaneous use of magnesium sulfate could be hazardous due to synergistic effect | **Assess** <br>• Therapeutic level of drug (0.025–0.1 mg/mL) <br>**Administer** <br>• Before meals and at night <br>• Evaluate therapeutic response, cardiac status, blood pressure, pulse, respiration and ECG <br>**Teach client** <br>• To limit caffeine consumption <br>• To avoid over the counter drugs unless directed by the physician |

Contd...

| Drug | Indication | Mechanism of action | Dosage and route | Side effects | Contraindications | Nursing responsibilities |
|------|-----------|---------------------|------------------|--------------|-------------------|--------------------------|
| Sodium nitroprusside | To produce controlled hypotension to reduce surgical bleeding. | Direct vasodilator (arterial and venous) | IV infusion 0.25- 8 μg/kg/min | **Maternal:** Nausea Vomiting Severe hypotension **Fetal:** Toxicity due to accumulation | • Drug should be used in critical care unit for short time. • Compensatory hypertension is possible | **Assess:** • Serum electrolytes blood urea nitrogen (BUN) and creatinine • Hepatic function (AST, ALP, ALT) • Blood pressure and ECG • Weight, intake and output **Administer:** • Using an infusion pump only • Wrap bottle with aluminum foil to protect from light **Evaluate:** • Therapeutic response decreased blood pressure absence of bleeding • Edema: Feet and legs • Hydration status |

*Abbreviations:* ALP, alkaline phosphatase; ALT, alanine aminotransferase; AST, aspartate aminotransferase; ECG, electrocardiogram

**TABLE 4: Anticonvulsants**

| Drug | Indications | Mode of action | Dosage & Route | Side effects | Nursing consideration |
|---|---|---|---|---|---|
| Magnesium sulfate | It is a valuable drug lowering seizure threshold in women with pregnancy induced hypertension. The drug is used in preterm labor to decrease uterine activity. | • Decrease the acetylcholine release from the nerve ending and reduces the motor end plates sensitivity to Acetylcholine.<br>• It blocks the calcium channel blockers<br>• It causes vasodilation ↑sed cerebral, renal and uterine blood flow<br>• Decreased intracranial edema | **Loading dose:** 4 gm, IV over 3–5 minutes followed by 10 g deep IM (5 g in each buttock)<br>**Maintenance dose:** 5 gm IM 4 hourly in alternate buttock. | **Maternal:** Severe CNS depression, evidence of muscular paresis.<br>**Fetal:** Tachycardia, hypoglycemia. | **Assess:**<br>• Vital signs × 15 minutes<br>• Magnesium level in the blood. (Normal level 4–7 mEq/L)<br>• During labor, assess uterine contraction and its intensity<br>• Urine output, if >30 mL, notify physician<br>• Reflex: Knee jerk, patellar reflex.<br>**Administer:**<br>• Using infusion pump or monitor carefully circulatory collapse may occur.<br>• If antidote (calcium gluconate) is available to manage toxicity.<br>**Perform/provide:**<br>• Seizure precautions: Place client in stimulus free environment, padded side rails.<br>• Left lateral position to decrease hypotension and increase renal blood flow. |
| Diazepam (Valium) | Used to relieve anxiety, muscle spasms, and seizures | Depresses subcortical level of CNS, anticonvulsant and antianxiety. | Initially 20–40 mg IV. To be followed by an infusion containing 500 mL of dextrose with 40 mg of diazepam, the drip rate being 30 drop/min or adjusted as per need. | **Mother:** Hypotension<br>**Fetus:** Respiratory depressant effect which may last for even three weeks after delivery. Hypotonia, thermoregulatory problems in newborn. | **Assess:**<br>• Blood pressure if systolic pressure falls 20 mm Hg, hold drug and inform to physician<br>• Blood studies: CBC<br>• Hepatic studies<br>**Administer:**<br>• Through large vein to decrease chances of extravasation<br>• With milk or food to avoid gastrointestinal Symptoms'<br>**Provide:**<br>• Safety measures during ambulation and at bed rest<br>**Teach patient:**<br>• Avoid alcohol consumption.<br>• Not to discontinue medication abruptly<br>• To rise slowly because fainting may occur |

*Contd...*

| Drug | Indications | Mode of action | Dosage & Route | Side effects | Nursing consideration |
|---|---|---|---|---|---|
| Phenytoin sodium | Seizures, status epilepticus (tonic-clonic). | Inhibits spread of seizure activity in motor Cortex | **Eclampsia:** 10 mg/kg IV. at the rate not more than 50 mg/min followed 2 hours later by 5 mg/kg. **Epilepsy:** 300–400 mg daily orally in divided doses | **Maternal:** Hypotension, Cardiac arrhythmias and Phlebitis at injection site. **Fetal:** Fetal hydantoin syndrome | **Assess:**<br>• CBC, platelets every 2 weeks until stabilized<br>• If Neutrophils count is less than 1, 600/mm$^2$ discontinue medication<br>■ **Administer:** After dilution with normal saline<br>■ **Evaluate:**<br>  ○ Mental status, sensorium, affect memory.<br>  ○ Respiratory depression<br>  ○ **Blood dyscrasias:** Sore throat, bruising.<br>■ **Teach patient and family members:** To notify physician if undue symptoms arise |

*Abbreviations:* CBC, complete blood count; CNS, central nervous system

# DIURETICS

Diuretics, also called water pills, are medications designed to increase the amount of water and salt expelled from the body as urine. Diuretics work by removing sodium and chloride from the body through the urine, and the sodium and chloride in turn draw excess water from the body. The amount of sodium chloride (NaCl) in the body, as previously discussed, has a marked effect on the amount of water retained by the body; hence most diuretics have their effects by reducing total body (NaCl) content. Diuretics decreases blood pressure broadly by two actions:

1. By decreasing plasma volume.
2. By depleting sodium in the body.

## Uses of Diuretics

The diuretics are used in the following conditions during pregnancy:

- Pregnancy induced hypertension with pathological edema.
- Severe anemia in pregnancy with heart failure.
- As an adjunct to antihypertensive drugs such as diazoxide or hydralazine.
- Eclampsia with pulmonary edema.
- Prior to blood transfusion in severe anemia.

## Types of Diuretics

The three types of diuretic medications commonly used in pregnancy are: (1) thiazide, (2) loop, and (3) potassium-sparing diuretics. All of them make the body excrete more fluids in the form of urine.

### Thiazide Diuretics

Thiazide diuretics act on distal convoluted tubule which inhibits NaCl reabsorption. They are most often used to treat high blood pressure. These drugs not only decrease fluids in the body, but they also cause blood vessels to relax. Thiazides are sometimes taken with other medications to lower blood pressure. Examples of thiazides include:

- Chlorothiazide
- Chlorthalidone
- Hydrochlorothiazidet
- Metolazone
- Indapamide

### Loop Diuretics

**Loop diuretics** act on loop of Henle (thick ascending limb) which selectively inhibits NaCl reabsorption. Loop diuretics are the most powerful diuretics and used in severe hypertension. Often, Furosemide used in hypertension emergencies to prevent the volume expansion during the administration of powerful vasodilators. Examples of these drugs include:

- Torsemide
- Furosemide
- Bumetanide
- Ethacrynic acid

### Potassium-sparing Diuretics

**Potassium-sparing diuretics** act on late distal convoluted tubule (LDCT) and collecting tubule. Potassium-sparing diuretics are useful both in avoiding excessive potassium depletion and in enhancing the natriuretic effects of other diuretics. Examples of potassium-sparing diuretics include:

- Amiloride
- Spironolactone
- Triamterene
- Eplerenone

## Side Effects

- Nausea
- Thirst and dry mouth
- Dizziness
- Constipation
- Muscle cramps (loss of calcium)
- Hyperuricemia (Increased levels or uric acid cause gout arthritis)
- Hypercalcemia (related to thiazide diuretics only)
- Metabolic acidosis [carbonic anhydrase inhibitor (CAI), K-sparing diuretics)]
- Metabolic alkalosis (thiazide diuretics, loop diuretics)
- Hypokalemia (related to loop diuretics, thiazide diuretics)
- Hyperkalemia (related to potassium-sparing diuretics)

## Nursing Interventions

- Collect complete health history, especially electrolyte balance and renal function.
- Check the vital signs and compare it with the baseline values specially blood pressure.
- Observe for any change in consciousness, dizziness, fatigue, postural hypotension.
- Find out patient's medication history including alcohol and nicotine consumption to avoid drug interaction.
- Monitor hearing and vision because some loop diuretics are ototoxic and thiazide diuretic produce visual change by increasing digoxin level.
- Collect blood and urine specimen for laboratory analysis.
- Monitor for fluid intake by measuring intake, output and daily weight.
- Monitor laboratory values specially potassium and sodium levels, BUN, serum uric acid.
- Identify possible drug allergies of patient.

## Patient Education

- Explain the right use of diuretics with dosage.
- Advise the patient to take medicine with meal only.
- Report any visible signs and symptoms of proximal edema, potential sign of heart failure or pulmonary edema.
- Immediate contact to physician if feeling dizzy or change in level of consciousness.
- To avoid postural hypotension, advise the patient to change position slowly.
- Check BP as specified by the health professionals.
- When going outside, wear dark glasses or light color cloth because some diuretics cause photosensitivity.
- Mention possible side effects of diuretics such as dry mouth, increase in urination.
- Advise the patient to take potassium-containing diet if using loop or thiazide diuretics.
- Avoid potassium-containing diet if using potassium-sparing diuretics.
- Take health care advice before taking any vitamin/minerals or other supplements.

# DRUGS USED FOR NEWBORN

Shortly after the baby is born, he/she receives the first shots and medications for some very serious health issues, including a rare bleeding disorder and a few sexually transmitted diseases.

Vitamin K, antibiotic ointment in the eyes, and a Hepatitis B vaccination are given to the child. There might be other medications too, depending on the pediatrician and hospital adhere to and any other medications that baby needs. **Vitamin K, Hepatitis B vaccine and bacille Calmette Guerin (BCG) vaccines are strongly encouraged.** These medications might be given immediately after birth.

## Vitamin K

Most states mandate that all babies receive vitamin K as soon as possible after birth. Intramuscular injection is given in the vastus lateralis thigh muscle. A onetime only prophylactic dose of 0.5–1 mg is given intramuscularly in the birthing area within 1 hour of birth.

If mother receives anticoagulant during pregnancy, an additional dose may be ordered by the physician and is given 6–8 hours after the first injection, IM/subcutaneous concentration: 1 mg/0.5 mL (neonatal strength) can use 10 mg/mL concentration to minimize volume injected.

### Neonatal Side Effects

Pain and edema may occur at injection site. Allergic reaction such as rash and urticaria, may also occur.

### Nursing Implications

- Document the administration of the medication to newborn to prevent an accidental doubling of the dose.
- Observe for bleeding (usually occurs on second or third day). Bleeding may be seen as generalized ecchymosis or bleeding from umbilical cord, circumcision site, nose or gastrointestinal tract.
- Observe for jaundice and kernicterus, especially in preterm infants.
- Observe for signs of local inflammation.
- Apply pressure to the injection site to prevent further bleeding.
- Protect drug from light.
- Give vitamin K before circumcision procedure.

## Antibiotic Ointment in the Eyes

Bacteria that normally live in a woman's vagina may be passed to the baby during childbirth. More serious eye damage may be caused by:

- **Gonorrhea and chlamydia:** These are infections spread from sexual contact.
- The viruses that cause genital and oral herpes: These may lead to severe eye damage. Herpes eye infections are less common than those caused by gonorrhea and chlamydia.
  Because of this, newborn commonly suffer from the following complications:
- **Ophthalmic neonatorum (Conjunctivitis):** It is defined as inflammation of conjunctiva during first month of life. The clinical picture varies and the discharge may be watery, mucopurulent to frank purulent in one or both eyes. The eyelids maybe sticky or markedly swollen. Cornea maybe involved in some cases. Treatment includes: 1% silver nitrate solution (1–2 drops to each eye), 0.5% erythromycin ophthalmic ointment, 2.5% Povidone iodine solution (1 drop) each eye is administered with in 1 hour of birth and continued for few days. Complications may include: blindness, inflammation of the iris and scar or hole in the cornea.

- **Sticky eyes:** Mucus also may be present; especially collecting on the eyelid margin and causing the eyelashes stick together. It is common during first two–three days after birth. Symptoms include swollen eyelids and redness of eyes. To help relieve symptoms, keep the area clean by regularly wiping baby's eyes with a clean, moist cloth. Gently massaging the corners of the eyes may help to open or unblock the tear duct.

## Hepatitis B Vaccine

**Hepatitis** B causes serious liver inflammation due to infection with the hepatitis B virus. It is spread through having contact with the blood, semen, vaginal fluids, and other body fluids of someone who already has a hepatitis B infection. A series of three vaccinations prevents people from getting hepatitis B, which can cause liver failure.

The World Health Organization (WHO) recommended schedule for hepatitis B immunization of children consists of a dose within 24 hours of birth followed by a second and third dose of hepatitis B containing vaccines at intervals of at least 4 weeks.

Dose and route: Hepatitis B vaccine (0.5 mL, IM). The vastus lateralis muscle in the anterolateral thigh is the recommended site for IM vaccination in infants <12 months of age, due to its larger muscle size.

## BCG Vaccine

Bacille Calmette-Guérin (BCG) is a vaccine given to babies to protect them from serious forms of tuberculosis (TB) such as TB Meningitis (an infection of the brain) and Miliary TB (widespread infection).

### Indications

Infants under two years of age who are at risk for TB such as:

- Those from northern communities where there are high rates of TB
- Infants from families or communities with a history or risk of exposure to TB

BCG vaccine is not required for those who already have a positive skin test.

### Side Effects

Normally, once the BCG is given (upper right arm), a small pimple appears in 1–3 weeks and lasts up to 6–8 weeks. A small scar will remain when the vaccination heals.

However, some possible side effects that may occur include:

- Drainage or a small scab over the site. If the injection site is draining, put dry gauze dressing on the area and allow it to dry and prevent the baby from scratching the area. There is no need to put a band-aid, cream or ointment on the site. It will normally resolve itself, usually within one to three months.
- On rare occasions, an abscess (painful swelling that contains pus), forms at the injection site and/or lymph glands in the armpit or neck can get larger.

## Commonly used Antibiotics for Newborn

- **First line antibiotics:** Penicillin, ampicillin, cefotaxime and gentamicin
- **Second line antibiotics:** Cloxacillin and amikacin
- **Third line antibiotics:** Piperacillin-tazobactam, ciprofloxacin and vancomycin

## Choice of Antibiotics

Empirical antibiotic therapy should be unit-specific and determined by the prevalent spectrum of etiological agents and their antibiotic sensitivity pattern. Antibiotics once started should be modified according to the sensitivity reports.

## Emergency Medications and Therapy for Neonates

Table 5 exhibits emergency medications and therapy for neonates.

**TABLE 5:** Emergency medications and therapy for neonates

| Medication | Indications | Dosage and route | Special consideration |
|---|---|---|---|
| Furosemide | Volume overload, pulmonary edema | 1 mg/kg/dose, IM, IV | |
| Lorazepam | Anticonvulsant | 0.05 mg/kg/dose IV, infuse over 3–5 minutes | May cause respiratory depression and hypotension, may repeat in 10–15 minutes |
| Naloxone | Narcotic reversal | 0.1 mg/kg IM/IV (IV preferred; IM acceptable but delayed onset of action). | Not recommended as part of initial resuscitation of newborns with respiratory depression in delivery room. If respiratory depression continues, naloxone may be given if mother had narcotics within 4 hours of delivery. |
| Phenobarbital | Anticonvulsant | 15–20 mg/kg IV load over 15–30 minutes | Respiratory depression possible if Diazepam used first. Follow with maintenance dose. |
| Phenytoin | Anticonvulsant | 15–20 mg/kg IV load | IV rate 0.5 mg/kg/min maximum; mix only with NS. |
| Sodium bicarbonate | Documented metabolic acidosis with adequate ventilation, hyperkalemia | 1–2 mEq/kg IV over at least 30 minutes or more | Use 0.5 mEq/mL; infuse over 30 minutes or more. |
| Volume expansion | | | |
| Normal saline (preferred) or lactated Ringer's solution | Volume expansion | 10 mL/kg IV over 5–10 minutes; may repeat | Check hematocrit and serum glucose before and after dose. |
| Rh-negative packed RBCs | Volume expansion (severe anemia/blood loss) | 10 mL/kg IV over 5–10 minutes; may repeat | If time permits, blood should be cross-matched to the mother. |
| Atropine | Bradycardia | 0.01–0.03 mg/kg/dose IV, IM, ETT; repeat every 10–15 minutes | For ETT use, dilute with NS. |
| Calcium gluconate (10%) (100 mg/mL) | Hyperkalemia Hypocalcemia | Ca gluconate 100–200 mg/kg slow IV over 10–30 minutes (1.0–2.0 mL/kg) | Infuse slowly; caution with digitalized patient; tissue necrosis if extravasation. Can also use calcium chloride 20–30 mg/kg. |
| Dextrose | Hypoglycemia Hyperkalemia (used with insulin) | 100–500 mg/kg/dose IV (1–5 mL/kg/ dose D10W) | D10 = 100 mg/mL; D12.5 = 125 mg/mL; D25 = 250 mg/mL (D25 only in central line). |

*Contd...*

| Medication | Indications | Dosage and route | Special consideration |
|---|---|---|---|
| Dubatamine | Cardiogenic shock, hypotension due to refractory CHF | 2–15 mcg/kg/min, increase every 10 minutes to maximum 40 mcg/kg/min | Mix in D5W, NS, RL. |
| Dopamine | Hypotension, agonal heart | 5 mcg/kg/min, increase to a maximum of 40 mcg/kg/min | Mix in D5W, NS, RL. |
| Cardioversion/defibrillation | VT, VF, SVT, atrial fib/flutter | 1–4 joules/kg, increase 50–100% each time | Synch switch off for ventricular fibrillation. |
| Epinephrine (1:10,000) | Asystole, bradycardia, hypotension (acute) | 0.1–0.3 mL/kg/dose of 1:10,000 IV; ETT only 0.5–1 mL/kg/dose of 1:10,000 (dilute with NS) | Do not use 1:1000; for ETT use, dilute in 1–2 mL NS; NRP, AHA, AAP suggests higher dose if by ETT. |

*Abbreviations:* AAP, American Academy of Pediatrics; AHA, American Heart Association; CHF, coronary heart failure; ETT, endotracheal tube; NRP, neonatal resuscitation program; NS, normal saline; RL, Ringer's lactate; SVT, supraventricular tachycardia; VF, ventricular fibrillation; VT, ventricular tachycardia

## TERATOGENS: EFFECTS OF DRUGS ON MOTHER AND BABY

The teratogens may be chemical agents (drugs) or physical agents (radiations, heat). They cause permanent alteration in the structure and/or function of an organ, acting during embryonic or fetal life. The dose (amount) and duration of teratogen exposure may cause variable response from no effect level to lethal level. Final results of abnormal development are:

- Death
- Malformation
- Growth restriction
- Functional disorder

Table 6 enlists the teratogenic effects of various drugs.

**TABLE 6:** Drugs with established teratogenic effects

| Drug | Teratogenic effects |
|---|---|
| Cytotoxic drugs | Multiple fetal malformations and abortion |
| Androgenic steroids, hydroxyprogesterone | Masculinization of female offspring |
| Lithium | Cardiovascular anomalies, neonate goiter, hypotonia and cyanosis |
| Diethylstilbestrol | Vaginal adenosis, cervical hoods, uterine hypoplasia of female offspring |
| Antithyroid drugs | Goiter, mental retardation |
| Oral antidiabetic drugs | Abnormalities in eye, central nervous system, skeletal system and neonatal hypoglycemia |
| Vitamin D | Cardiopathies, mental retardation, hypercalcemia |
| Lysergic acid diethylamide (LSD) | Chromosomal abnormality and stunted growth |
| Anticonvulsant phenytoin valproate | Mental retardation, cardiac abnormalities, limb defects, neonatal bleeding, epilepsy |

Table 7 gives the effects of various drugs on fetus.

**TABLE 7: Fetotoxic drugs**

| Drugs | Effect on fetus |
|---|---|
| Aspirin | Premature closure of ductus arteriosus, persistent pulmonary hypertension, kernicterus |
| Corticosteroids | Fetal and neonatal adrenal suppression |
| Aminoglycosides | Auditory or vestibular damage |
| Chloramphenicol | Peripheral vascular collapse |
| Tetracycline | Dental discoloration (yellow) and deformity, inhibition of bony growth |
| Long-acting sulfonamides | Neonatal hemolysis, jaundice, kernicterus |
| Nitrofurantoin | Hemolysis in newborn with glucose 6-phosphate dehydrogenase deficiency |
| Vitamin K | Hyperbilirubinemia and kernicterus |
| Alcohol and smoking | IUGR, preterm labor, mental retardation |
| Narcotics | Depression of CNS, apnea, bradycardia, and hypothermia |
| Anesthetic agents | Convulsion, bradycardia, acidosis hypoxia, hypertonia |
| Antihistamines | Tachycardia, vomiting, diarrhea |
| Anticoagulants | Optic atrophy, microcephaly, chondrodysplasia punctata |
| Diuretics | Fetal compromise due to placental insufficiency |
| Beta blockers | IUGR, fetal bradycardia, hypoxia |

*Abbreviations:* CNS, central nervous system; IUGR, intrauterine growth restriction

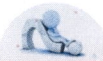

## Assess Yourself

### FREQUENTLY ASKED QUESTIONS IN EXAMS

1. What are the indications, side effects, dose/route and contraindications of oxytocin?
2. Write down the nursing management of patient with oxytocin infusion.
3. Write short note on prostaglandins.
4. Discuss MgSO$_4$ in detail.
5. Explain about Ergot derivatives (Methergine).
6. What are the commonly used drugs for newborns?

### MULTIPLE CHOICE QUESTIONS

1. Water intoxication is the common side effect of which drug?
   - a. Oxytocin
   - b. Methergine
   - c. MgSO$_4$
   - d. Prostaglandin

2. Which drug may cause gangrene of toe?
   - a. Oxytocin
   - b. Methergine
   - c. Prostaglandins
   - d. Diuretics

3. The action of PGE$_2$ is:
   - a. Cervical dilation
   - b. Myometrial contractions
   - c. Stimulation of uterus
   - d. None of the above

4. Which drug may be used to relieve breast engorgement in postpartum period?
   - a. Methergine
   - b. Bromocriptine
   - c. Oxytocin
   - d. Prostaglandins

5. How much dose of oxytocin is helpful to control PPH?
   - a. 5–8 units
   - b. 2–5 units
   - c. 10–12 units
   - d. 10–20 units

6. First line antihypertensive is:
   - a. Methyldopa
   - b. Nifedipine
   - c. Hydralazine
   - d. Sodium nitroprusside

7. Tocolytic drugs are used to:
   - a. Induce contractions
   - b. Inhibit uterine contractions
   - c. Cervical dilation
   - d. All of the above.

8. Which is the most commonly used tocolytic drug used nowadays?
   - a. Duvadilan
   - b. Yutopar
   - c. MgSO$_4$
   - d. Nifedipine

9. The therapeutic level of nifedipine is:
   - a. 0.025–0.1 ug/mL
   - b. 0.5–1 ug/mL
   - c. 2 ug/mL
   - d. 0.01–0.1 ug/mL

10. Which drug is wrapped in aluminum foil to protect from light?
    - a. Nifedipine
    - b. Sodium nitroprusside
    - c. MgSO$_4$
    - d. Methyldopa

11. **The aim of antihypertensive to reduce blood pressure to a mean:**
    a. <100 mm Hg
    b. <125 mm Hg
    c. <150 mm Hg
    d. <120 mm Hg

12. **The most common side effect of methyldopa on fetus is:**
    a. Intestinal ileus
    b. Thrombocytopenia
    c. Cardiac failure
    d. Palpitation

13. **What happens in neonates because of maternal intake of lithium?**
    a. Cardiovascular anomalies
    b. Abortion
    c. Vaginal adenosis
    d. Epilepsy

14. **The side effect of aminoglycosides on fetus is:**
    a. Auditory damage
    b. Neonatal hemolysis
    c. Jaundice
    d. Kernicterus

15. **The phenytoin is:**
    a. Antihypertensive
    b. Tocolytic
    c. Anticonvulsant
    d. Diuretics

 **Answer Key**

| 1. a | 2. b | 3. a | 4. b | 5. d | 6. a | 7. b |
|------|------|------|------|------|------|------|
| 8. a | 9. a | 10. b | 11. b | 12. a | 13. a | 14. a |
| 15. c | | | | | | |

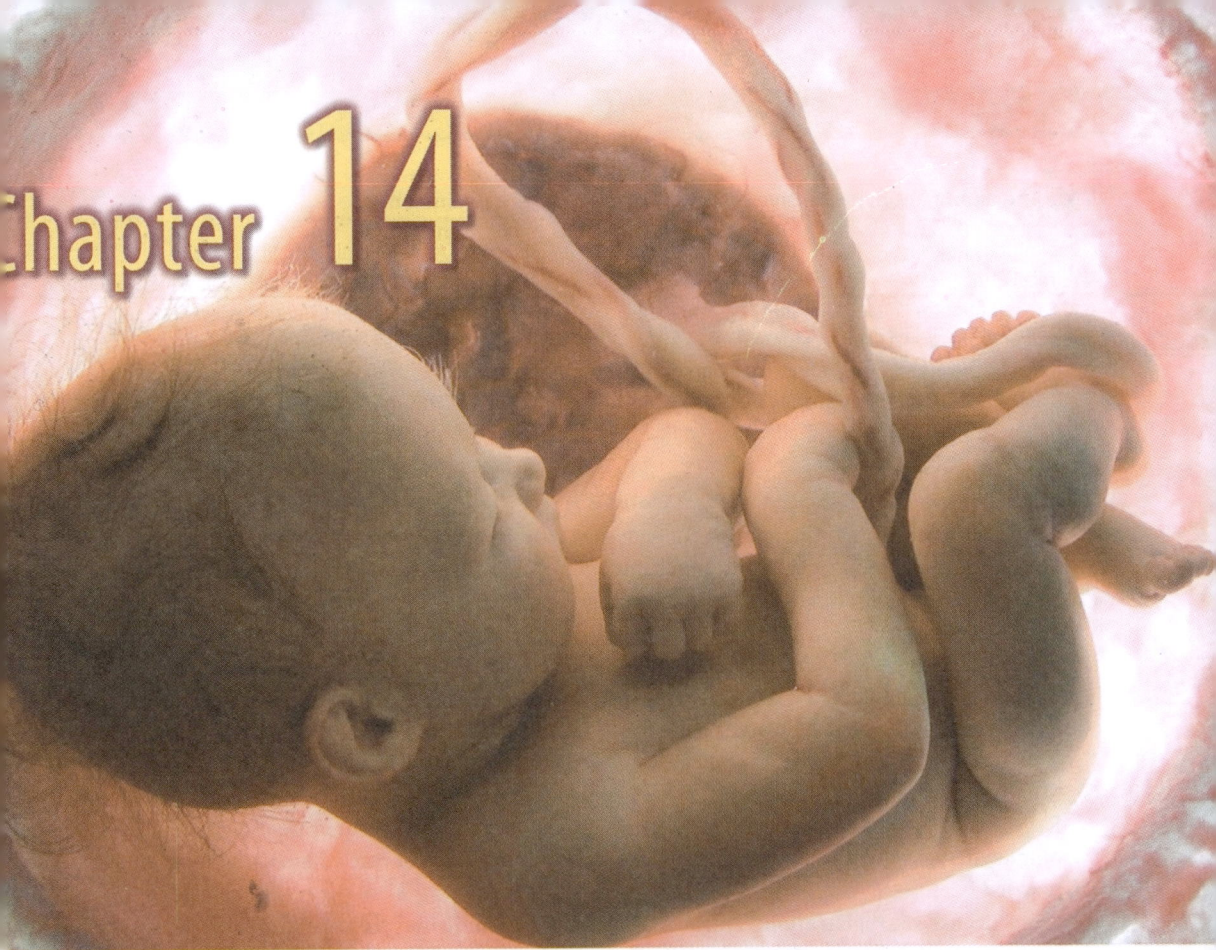

# Chapter 14

# Ethical and Legal Aspects Related to Midwifery

*Learning Objectives* .......................................................

**Upon completing this chapter, the learner will be able to:**

➡ Describe the legal and ethical issues related to midwifery practice

➡ Explain the mother and child tracking system

➡ Discuss maternal and newborn death review

## DEFINITIONS

- **Ethics:** Ethics are the principles of conduct governing one's relationship with others. They are basic beliefs about values of right and wrong that provide a framework for decisions and actions.

- **Laws:** Laws are rules of conduct or action recognized as binding or enforced by a controlling authority, such as the local, state or national government. They are designed to prevent the actions of one party from infringing on the rights of another party.

  Laws and ethics are often seen as complementary to each other, but at same time they are also seen as opposite sides of a coin. Midwives must follow standards and regulations that range from the national level to the individual area of practice, such as hospital, labor and delivery unit.

- **Standards of practice:** National standards provide an expectation of the delivery of care to clients. Regulations and policies at institutional levels provide for delivery of safe care. Educational programs of midwifery ensure that all new nurses/midwives can safely deliver care within the scope of midwifery practice.

- **State license or registration:** Practice of nursing and midwifery is regulated by state registration councils through license to practice. If a nurse/midwife moves to a different state, she must obtain registration in that state in order to practice there. The state license is meant to protect the consumers by ensuring that the midwife has appropriate education and can provide safe care.

- **Institutional policies:** Policies and regulations of an institution govern the nursing and midwifery care to clients seeking health care in that place.

- **Community standards:** A midwife's performance will be evaluated according to the availability of medical and nursing knowledge that would be used in the management of similar patients under similar circumstances by competent midwives, given the facilities, resources and option available.

## ETHICAL PRINCIPLES

- **Beneficence:** It means to act in the best interests of the patient and to balance benefits against risks. The benefits that medicine is competent to seek for patients are the prevention and management of disease, injury, handicap and unnecessary pain and suffering, and the premature or unnecessary death.

- **Respect for autonomy:** It means to respect the rights of individual. Respect for autonomy enters the clinical practice by the informed consent. This process is usually understood to have three elements, disclosure by the physician to the patient's condition and its management, understanding of that information by the patient and a voluntary decision by the patient to authorize or refuse treatment.

- **Nonmaleficence:** It means that the health personnel should prevent causing harm and is best understood as expressing the limits of beneficence. This is commonly known as "Primum non nocere" or first to do no harm.

- **Justice:** Justice signifies, to treat patients fairly and without unfair discrimination, there should be fairness in the distribution of benefits and risks. Medical needs, and medical benefits should be properly weighted
- **Confidentiality:** It is the basis of trust between health professionals and patient. By acting against this principle, one destroys the patient trust.
- **Informed consent:** The process of obtaining permission after explaining the expected risk and benefit is called informed consent. Patient or individual who requires health care services has got the right to make his/her own decision about the opinions for treatment or other related issues.
- **Truthfulness:** The fact of being realistic or true to life is called realism. It is the basic principle of the natural moral law, and people everywhere recognize that honesty in dealing with others is a prerequisite for societal order and well-being.

## CODE OF ETHICS FOR NURSES IN INDIA

- **The nurse respects the uniqueness of individual in provision of care:**
  A nurse:
  - Provides care of individuals without consideration of caste, creed, religion, culture, ethnicity, gender, socioeconomic and political status, personal attributes, or any other grounds.
  - Individualizes the care considering the beliefs, values and cultural sensitivities.
  - Appreciates the place of individual in the family and community and facilitates participation of significant others in the care.
  - Develops and promotes trustful relationship with individual(s).
  - Recognizes uniqueness of response of individuals to interventions and adapts accordingly.
- **The nurse respects the rights of individuals as partner in care and help in making informed choices:**
  A nurse:
  - Appreciates individual's right to make decisions about his/her care and therefore gives adequate and accurate information for enabling the person to make informed choices.
  - Respects the decisions made by individual(s) regarding their care.
  - Protects public from misinformation and misinterpretations.
  - Advocates special provision to protect vulnerable individuals/groups.
- **The nurse respects individual's right to privacy, maintains confidentiality, and shares information judiciously:**
  A nurse:
  - Respects the individual's right to privacy of his/her personal information.
  - Maintains confidentiality of privileged information except in life-threatening situations and uses discretion in sharing information.
  - Takes informed consent and maintains anonymity when information is required for quality assurance/academic/legal reasons.
  - Limits the access to all personal records written and computerized to authorized persons only.
- **Nurse maintains competence in order to render quality nursing care:**
  - Nursing care must be provided only by registered nurse.
  - A nurse strives to maintain quality nursing care and upholds the standards of care.
  - A nurse values continuing education, initiates and utilizes all opportunities for self-development.
  - A nurse values research as a means of development of nursing profession and participates in nursing research adhering to ethical principles.

- **The nurse if obliged to practice within the framework of ethical, professional and legal boundaries:**
  A nurse:
  - Adheres to code of ethics and code of professional conduct for nurses in India developed by Indian Nursing Council.
  - Familiarizes with relevant laws and practices in accordance with the law of the state.
- **Nurse is obliged to work harmoniously with members of the health team:**
  A nurse:
  - Appreciates the team efforts in rendering care
  - Cooperates, coordinates and collaborates with members of the health team to meet the needs of people.
- **Nurse commits to reciprocate the trust invested in nursing profession by society:**
  A nurse:
  - Demonstrates personal etiquettes in all dealings.
  - Demonstrates professional attributes in all dealings.

## CODE OF PROFESSIONAL CONDUCT FOR NURSES IN INDIA

- **Professional responsibility and accountability:**
  A nurse:
  - Appreciates sense of self-worth and nurtures it.
  - Maintains standards of personal conduct reflecting credit upon the profession.
  - Carries out responsibilities within the framework of the professional boundaries.
  - Is accountable for maintaining practice standards set by Indian Nursing Council.
  - Is accountable for own decisions and actions.
  - Is compassionate.
  - Is responsible for continuous improvement of current practices.
  - Provides adequate information to individuals that allows them informed choices.
  - Practices healthful behavior.
- **Nursing practice:**
  A nurse:
  - Provides care in accordance with set standards of practice.
  - Treats all individuals and families with human dignity in providing physical, psychological, emotional, social and spiritual aspects of care.
  - Respects individuals and families in the context of traditional and cultural practices, promoting healthy practices and discouraging harmful practices.
  - Presents realistic picture truthfully in all situations for facilitating autonomous decision-making by individuals and families.
  - Promotes participation of individuals and significant others in the care.
  - Ensures safe practice.
  - Consults, coordinates, collaborates and follows up appropriately when individuals' care needs exceed the nurse's competence.
- **Communication and interpersonal relationships:**
  A nurse:
  - Establishes and maintains effective interpersonal relationships with individuals, families and communities.
  - Upholds the dignity of team members and maintains effective interpersonal relationship with them.

- Appreciates and nurtures professional role of team members.
- Cooperates with other health professional to meet the needs of the individuals, families and communities.

- **Valuing human being:**

  A nurse:
  - Takes appropriate action to protect individuals from harmful unethical practice.
  - Considers relevant facts while taking conscience decisions in the best interest of individuals.
  - Encourages and supports individuals in their right to speak for themselves on issues affecting their health and welfare.
  - Respects and supports choices made by individuals.

- **Management:**

  A nurse:
  - Ensures appropriate allocation and utilization of available resources.
  - Participates in supervision and education of students and other formal care providers.
  - Uses judgment in relation to individual competence while accepting and delegating responsibility.
  - Facilitates conductive work culture in order to achieve institutional objectives.
  - Communicates effectively following appropriate channels of communication.
  - Participates in performance appraisal.
  - Participates in evaluation of nursing services.
  - Participates in policy decisions, following the principle of equity and accessibility of services.
  - Works with individuals to identify their needs and sensitizes policy makers and funding agencies for resource allocation.

- **Professional advancement:**

  A nurse:
  - Ensures the protection of the human rights while pursuing the advancement of knowledge.
  - Contributes to the development of nursing practice.
  - Participates in determining and implementing quality care.
  - Takes responsibility for updating own knowledge and competencies.
  - Contributes to core of professional knowledge by conducting and participating in research.

# ETHICAL DECISIONS AND REPRODUCTIVE HEALTH OF WOMEN

- **Ethics in gynecologic practice:** Beneficence-based and autonomy-based clinical judgments in gynecologic practice are usually in harmony, like management of ruptured ectopic pregnancy. Sometimes, they may come into conflicts. In such situation, one should not override the other. Their differences must be negotiated in clinical judgment and practice to determine which management strategies protect and promote the patient interest.
- **Ethics in obstetric practice:** There are obvious beneficence-based and autonomy-based obligations to the pregnant woman. While the health professional perspective on the pregnant women's interest provides the basis of beneficence based obligations, her own perspective on those interests provides the basis for autonomy-based obligations. Because of insufficiently developed central nervous system, the fetus cannot meaningfully be said to possess values and on its interest. Therefore, there is no autonomy based obligation to the fetus.
- **Ethics and assisted reproduction:** It involves many issues like donor insemination. *In vitro* fertilization (IVF), egg sharing freezing and storing of embryos, embryo research and surrogacy. Still there are many issues involved in IVF. First there is big question whether *in vitro* embryo is a patient or not. It is

appropriate to think that it is a previable fetus and only the women can give it the status of patient. Hence, preimplantation diagnostic counseling about how many embryos to be transferred should be evidence-based. Donor insemination raises the issues whether the child should be told about his genetic father or not. Egg sharing is also surrounded by many ethical issues. Ethics change from time to time keeping pace with changing social values, the sonologist issue being example. It was considered unethical few years back, now in recent issue of India Today, a lengthy article has appeared supporting surrogacy with the name of the center, the photos of the physician and number of happy surrogate mothers.

- **Ultrasonography:** There are many issues involved, like competence and referral, disclosure, confidentiality and routine screening. The foremost issue is that the sonologist must be competent enough to give a definitive option. Now routine screening is adopted at 18–20 weeks, but prior to screening the prenatal informed consent for sonogram must be taken. Strict confidentiality should be maintained.
- **Genetics and ethics:** The process of genetic research raises difficult challenges, particularly in the area of consent, community involvement and commercialization.
  Result of genetic research should be provided to subjects only if the tests have sufficient clinical validity. Results should never be disclosed to relatives, except in case of pedigree research.
- **Conception and the young girl:** Sometime teenaged girls request for oral contraception. They are already in an active sexual relationship. They do not want that their parents should know about them taking contraceptives. Lord Fraser's ethical recommendations include:
  - Assess whether the patient understands advice
  - Encourage the parent involvement
  - Take into account whether the patient is likely to have sexual intercourse without contraceptive treatment
  - Assess whether the physical, mental health would likely to suffer, if contraceptive advice is not given.
- **Embryonic stem cell research and ethics:** This involves many ethical issues and first and foremost is destroying a life by destroying the fertilized embryo. This raises the fundamental question of when life starts. Does human life begin at gastrulation (next step after blastula), at neurulation (formation of primitive streak, first sings of movement) or at the moment of sentience (consciousness)? When can embryo first feel pain or first suffer? The goal should be to minimize the exploitation of human embryos at any stage of development.

## POTENTIAL AREAS OF LITIGATION IN OBSTETRICS

### Antepartum Care

- **History collection:** Recently, preconceptual care is stressed more than antenatal care, especially when viewed in the context of its effect on pregnancy. Proper history taking can be a clue for further diagnosis and management of many cases. Avoidance of any relevant factors can cause maternal and fetal hazards.
- **Investigations:** One must not forget to do routine check-up, like hemoglobin, ABO, Rh grouping, blood sugar, hepatitis B virus surface antigen (HbsAg), venereal disease research laboratory (VDRL) and human immunodeficiency virus (HIV). The HIV testing must be done only after informed consent; otherwise the patient may sue the doctor. High-risk pregnancies are only picked up by thorough history taking, routine examinations and investigations. High risk patients and failure of timely referral create medicolegal issues.
- **Subsequent visits:**
  - **Antenatal screening for congenital abnormalities:** In patients having history of congenital abnormal babies at least basic screening is very necessary to avoid litigations. Other examinations,

like chorionic villus sampling, amniocentesis or some biochemical investigations may be necessary depending on the individual case. Patient's counseling is very necessary regarding false positive and negative test thereby avoiding legal problems.

- **Intrauterine growth retardation (IUGR):** Failure of timely detection of IUGR may cause intrauterine death of fetus and the doctor may have to face the court proceedings for this reason.
- **Multiple pregnancy:** It is a high-risk pregnancy involving two fetal lives. Management problem in such a case may cause fetal complication which will invite legal problems.
- **Intrauterine fetal death:** The cause of intrauterine death of fetus must be explored. As routine autopsy in India is not performed and unexplained fetal death may impose problems of medical litigation.
- **Sex selection and PNDT Act:** In view of falling sex ratio the Indian Government promulgated Diagnostic technique Act in 1994. The Act was evolved to identify genetic and congenital abnormalities related to sex. Unfortunately, this test was misused. Prenatal sex determination and selective female feticide become widespread all over in India in spite of amendment of PNDT Act in 2002. The amended Act prohibits unnecessary sex determination without any disease problem and aims at preventing selective abortions of female fetuses. However, still unethical practice of selective abortions is going on all over India.

- **Abortion:** A nurse assists in performing abortions under the Medical Termination of Pregnancy (MTP) Act and takes care of the patients following the procedure. A nurse has the right to refuse to assist in the procedure if the abortion is illegal.

## Intrapartum Care

- Proper intrapartum management during labor is essential for a healthy mother and a healthy child. Newer methods, like use of partograph during labor, pulse oximeter or fetal electrocardiogram (ECG) analysis can prevent birth asphyxia and appropriate therapy minimizes litigations.
- **Cesarean section:** Delayed decision of cesarean must be avoided as this leads to undesirable situations, like obstructed labor causing maternal and fetal morbidity and mortality.
- **Difficult vaginal delivery (shoulder dystocia):** Various clinical risk factors, like diabetes leading to big baby, etc. must be identified to predict and prevent this condition and associated injuries, like Erb's palsy. In this situation, emergency obstetrics care must be provided by experienced obstetrician, otherwise litigation problems might arise.
- **Breech presentation:** Timely decision to be taken whether to deliver the baby with breech presentation by vaginal route or cesarean delivery so as to avoid legal problems.
- **Multiple pregnancy:** Involves enormous risk and modern concept is to be delivered by cesarean section.
- **Instrumental delivery (forceps/vacuum):** High forceps must be avoided; only low forceps can be indicated in special circumstances to expedite the labor process. Ventouse must be avoided in premature baby and fetal distress. Concerned personnel may be sued due to untoward effects, like facial palsy or visceral injury to mother and baby.
- **Analgesia and anesthesia:** Expert anesthetist is required to prevent medical litigations.
- **Emergency obstetric care:** Every year more than, 5,00,000 women die during child birth in the world; out of which 1/5th, i.e. 1,00,000 women die in India alone, with present situation when there is no improvement of infrastructure, yet doctors have the risk of facing medicolegal problems regarding emergency obstetric care.

### Postpartum Care

- **Postnatal complete perineal tear (obstetric and sphincter injuries):** Significant perineal pain, dyspareunia, maternal morbidity and mortality and anal incontinence are problem areas. Forceps delivery is associated with increased perineal injury. Patients must be counseled about the risk of anal sphincter injury when operative delivery is contemplated, thus avoiding litigations.
- **Perinatal morbidity**
  - **Brain damage:** Any neurological and psychological deficiencies can be the major litigation issues where compensations are claimed. A health professional will be sued if it is proved in the court.
  - **Damage to bones and viscera:** This may occur specially during breech delivery. Health professional must be very conscious during face, legs and arm delivery in breech.
- **Nursing care of newborn:** Newborn requires professional and specialized care. Failure of the neonatal nurse to meet her obligations can result in liability in employment or even a civil suit.
- **Failure in assessing:** Failure in assessing and reporting changes in client's condition for timely action can be considered a malpractice that brain damage has occurred during intrapartum period due to negligence of health professional.
- **Drugs:** Food and drug administration (FDA) recommendations of drugs should be followed. The health professional must not use off license drugs. If damage occurs; he/she will be blamed of negligence when a licensed alternative drug is used.

## WAYS TO MINIMIZE MEDICOLEGAL PROBLEMS IN MIDWIFERY

- **Awareness of medicolegal problems:** Health practitioner should be aware about the changes in laws that may influence the practice.
- **Code of ethics:** The code of ethics for the midwife should be followed.
- **Good interpersonal relationship and clear communication:** The patient must not be given false hopes/ and needs to understand what to expect from the treatment. The health professionals must be polite and courteous showing sympathy towards patient.
- **Proper counseling:** Good counseling instills enormous confidence and faith. It helps to remove fear and misconceptions that may exist in the mind of the patient.
- **Informed consent:** After proper counseling, informed consent must be taken.
- **Standard health services:**
  - **Improving infrastructure:** Facilities available in the institution should be displayed. Health authorities should set norms for the health sector as a whole.
  - **Quality of care:** A good consultant is needed. Also, active pre and postoperative care needed.
- **Adequate training**
  - **Nursing education:** Improve the standard of nursing education as they came in direct contact with patients.
  - **Continuing education:** Regular continuing medical education and workshops should be attended.
  - **Audits:** Morbidity and mortality audits should be regularly done. Regular meeting of the staffs.
  - **Second opinion/referral:** Timely referral should be kept in mind.
- **Documentation and record keeping:** History, physical examination, drug allergies, chronic medications, plan of management, date and time of investigations done, operative and investigative notes, record of discussions with patient and relative, note to be kept of patients not following instruction, etc. should be documented.
- **Risk management:** Risk management involves limiting health risk to the patient and also reduce legal risks to the care provider. It should not primarily be about avoiding or mitigating claims but rather a tool for improving the quality of care.

- **Public awareness program and health education:** Public awareness includes health awareness by professional bodies and media.

## MATERNAL AND NEWBORN DEATH REVIEW

Mortality audit (also known as "death review") is a process to document the medical causes of each death and the contributing systemic failures across many cases to identify solutions and to take action.

It is a systematic way of improving quality of care by collecting and analyzing data, linking solutions to identified problems, and ensuring accountability for changes to improve care.

To foster an environment of collaboration rather than blame, it might be helpful if a written code of practice is established by the mortality audit (also known as "death review") steering team, and agreed through discussion with facility staff and management. For the written code of practice, use of wording specific to each team is encouraged, which can be signed by each individual before each review meeting. An attendance sheet could also be signed at the end of the meeting, so that those who were there to sign in at both the beginning and end of the meeting can be credited for staying and participating throughout the meeting.

Steering committee should include a diverse group of members, as appropriate. Members may include representatives from the district health office, the facility administration, the departments of neonatology/pediatrics, obstetrics, midwifery/nursing, anesthesia, pathology, pharmacy and statistics, as well as a community liaison.

**The key roles of the steering committee are to:**

- Help initiate the case review and mortality audit process and decide on the approach and its scope
- Oversee data collection, analysis and case selection for review meetings, including assigning responsibility for this task if not included in existing job descriptions.
- Develop a schedule for the audit meetings, invite participants and ensure adequate facilitation.
- Assist with dissemination of recommendations and advocate for their implementation.

### Perinatal Mortality Audit Cycle

Perinatal mortality audit cycle has been shown in Figure 1.

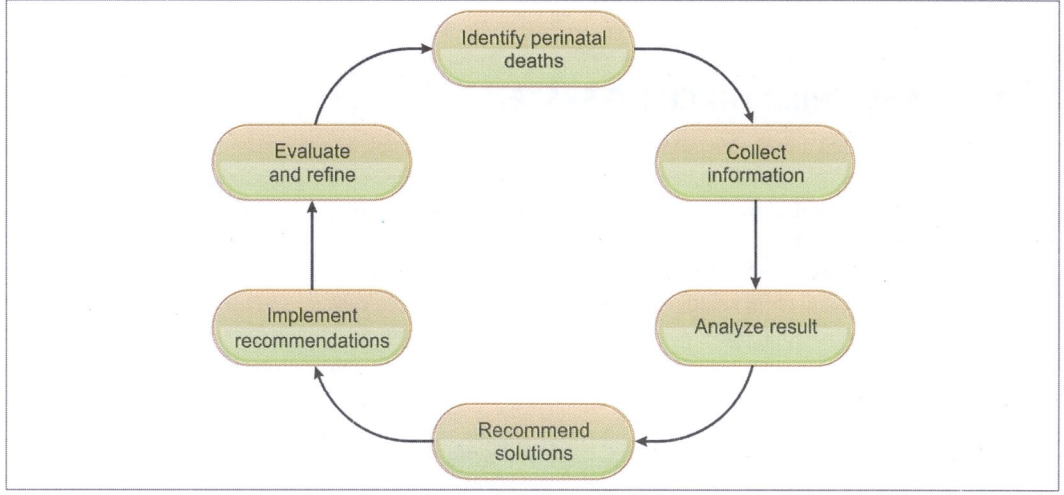

**Fig. 1:** Perinatal mortality audit cycle

### Steps

- Understand the steps of the perinatal mortality audit cycle and underlying principles.
- Establish or strengthen any local, regional or national stillbirth and neonatal mortality audit steering committee to oversee the process.
- Ensure confidentiality and a legal and ethical framework.
- Identify data and map all existing data and services.
- Plan data collection:
  - Obtain permission and engage the local community in the review process.
  - Set up the mortality audit steering committee.
  - Plan how you will identify cases.
  - Decide how to select a subset of identified cases for detailed review.
  - Decide which data to collect on each case.
  - Pilot-test and refine data collection instruments.
  - Plan review of cases—who will do it and how.
  - Plan data analysis.
  - Educate and sensitize health-care team members.
  - Set ground rules for review meetings.
- Implement the system:
  - Identify cases.
  - Collect the data.
  - Supervise data collectors.
  - Prepare data for review.
  - Hold mortality audit meeting to review data.
  - Analyze the results.
  - Use findings to create a list of possible actions (during the review meeting).
  - Develop, prioritize and disseminate recommendations.
  - Forward data, case notes and recommendations to the next review level.
  - Publish the results.
  - Evaluate and improve the system.
- Assess the achievements of the perinatal mortality audit cycle, and expand and improve linkages.

## MOTHER AND CHILD TRACKING SYSTEM

Mother and child tracking system (MCTS) is a technology-enabled application which will facilitate monitoring of universal access to maternal and child health services by all pregnant women and children. The system is developed jointly by the Ministry of Health and Family Welfare and National Informatics Center and it was launched by the Government of India in December 2009 in collaboration with states/union territories. It is an innovative application of the information technology directed towards improving the efficiency of maternal and child health services. MCTS is designed to capture and track all pregnant women right from conception up to 42 days postpartum and all newborn up to five years of age to ensure that the pregnant woman and children receive 'full' set of medical services thereby contributing to the reduction of maternal, infant and child mortality and achieving the goals laid down in the National Rural Health Mission as well as Millennium Development Goals.

**The broad objectives of the program through the software are:**

- To reduce infant mortality rate (IMR)
- To improve the nutritional level of the child

- To ensure completion of immunization in children by tracking the proper growth of the individual child
- To reduce mother mortality rate (MMR) and reduce total fertility rate (TFR)

MCTS serves two purposes. It facilitates the service provider at the grass roots level in delivering services to women and children according to their specific needs. At the same time, MCTS supports health and family welfare managers and policy makers in measuring and monitoring the efficiency of the maternal and child health services in terms of needs, effectiveness and capacity, efficiency and evaluating up to what extent the increase in efficiency in the delivery of maternal and child health services have contributed to the decrease in maternal, infant and child mortality. In this way, MCTS facilitates justification of investments in the public health and family welfare services delivery system.

## Services Offered

- **Registration of pregnant women:** When a pregnant woman comes to any health facility/sub-center and gets herself registered and receives first antenatal care (ANC) service then she is registered for getting the full health services.
- **ANC, delivery and postnatal care (PNC) services:** During the pregnancy period, MCTS records four ANC services given to a pregnant woman and then captures delivery details, like date of delivery, place of delivery and its outcome and then PNC Service. Workplan for the auxiliary nursing and midwifery (ANM)/accredited social health activists (ASHA) is generated so that no woman is left without services.
- **Registration of children for immunization:** In order to give 30 immunizations to every child, he/she is registered in MCTS application.
- **Immunization services to children:** Immunization is given to every child as per the schedule and work plan is generated to be consumed by ANM/ASHA from the MCTS application so that no child is left.
- **Integration with other applications, like public financial management system (PFMS), mobile device reporting (MDR), mother and child tracking facilitation center (MCTFC), Mobile Academy, Kilkari, etc.** Integrated with: 1. PFMS to make the DBT based JSY payments to the beneficiary. 2. MCTFC to access the quality of service being delivered in the field. 3. Kilkari Services, a dedicated IVRS platform to educate beneficiary about the pregnancy and child care.
- **Unstructured supplementary service data (USSD) technology to update the service live on the MCTS portal:** Data is updated through USSD by the ANMs on real time basis on the MCTS portal from the remotest part of the country.

## Initiatives taken by Government of India for their Effective Operationalization

- Call center established in ministry of health and family welfare (MoHFW) for verification of data is entered in MCTS. Another call center is being established at national institute of health and family welfare (NIFHW), New Delhi.
- Facility of communicating monthly Work Plan to ANMs/ASHAs through SMS in English and Hindi has been operationalized.
- SMS alerts to beneficiaries about services due have also been started. SMS related to mother and child registration status and telephonic verification status are sent daily to senior officials, like State Health Secretary, managing director of national rural health mission (NRHM) Regional Director, State Coordinators, District Collector, District Program Manager, etc.
- States/union territories have been asked to constitute State and District *e* -Mission Teams to regularly monitor the progress of implementation.
- States/union territories have been asked to nominate the District and Block Program Manager (NRHM) as the Nodal Officer for MCTS at district and block levels.

Chapter 14 ◗ Ethical and Legal Aspects Related to Midwifery

- Working groups on Technology Options and Business Processes Reengineering constituted to assess field difficulties along with the proposed solutions.

## Outcomes and Expectations

MCTS is expected to contribute significantly towards universal access of all pregnant women and children to maternal and child health services thereby facilitating and accelerating reduction in maternal, infant and child mortality. MCTS is being implemented all over the country. Once fully scaled up, MCTS will be accessible throughout the country. It will be accessible to the entire population of the country, irrespective of the region, caste, living status, etc.

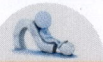

## ASSESS YOURSELF

### FREQUENTLY ASKED QUESTIONS IN EXAMS

1. Explain in detail about mother and child tracking system (MCTS).
2. Describe the legal and ethical issues in midwifery practice.

### MULTIPLE CHOICE QUESTIONS

1. Agreeing to others proposal, to give assent is called:
   a. Justice
   b. Consent
   c. Dilemmas
   d. Beneficence

2. Failure to satisfy ethical or moral obligations is called:
   a. Dilemmas
   b. Breach of duty
   c. Negligence
   d. Malpractice

3. Established rules or test model by authority are called:
   a. Norms
   b. Standards
   c. Ethics
   d. None of the above

4. Key elements of informed content are:
   a. Use of language that is understood
   b. Biased information
   c. Risk and benefits of each proposed action
   d. Verification that information given was understood

5. Basic beliefs about values of right and wrong that provide a framework for decisions and action are called:
   a. Ethics
   b. Norms
   c. Laws
   d. None of the above

6. Death review is also known as:
   a. Mortality audit
   b. Morbidity audit
   c. Neonatal mortality
   d. Fertility Calculation

7. Mother and child tracking system was launched by Government of India in:
   a. January 2010
   b. December 2009
   c. October 2009
   d. January 2014

8. **Mother and child tracking system (MCTS) has been developed jointly by the efforts of:**
   a. Ministry of Health and Family Welfare and National Information Center
   b. NRHM and National Informatics Center
   c. MCH programs and IT companies
   d. Directorate of Health services and National Informatics Center

9. **The broad objectives of MCTS are:**
   a. To reduce infant mortality rate
   b. To improve nutritional level of child
   c. To reduce mother mortality rate
   d. All of the above

10. **Service offered by MCTS are:**
    a. Registration of pregnant women
    b. Antenatal, delivery, postnatal services
    c. Registration of children for immunization
    d. All of the above

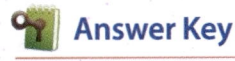 **Answer Key**

| 1. c | 2. b | 3. b | 4. c | 5. a | 6. a | 7. b |
|------|------|------|------|------|------|------|
| 8. a | 9. d | 10. d | | | | |

# Section II

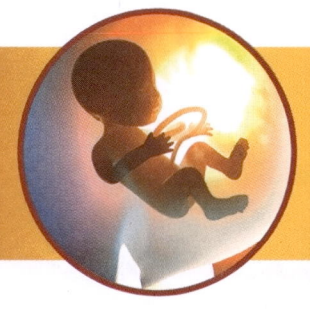

# Gynecological Nursing

## Section Outline

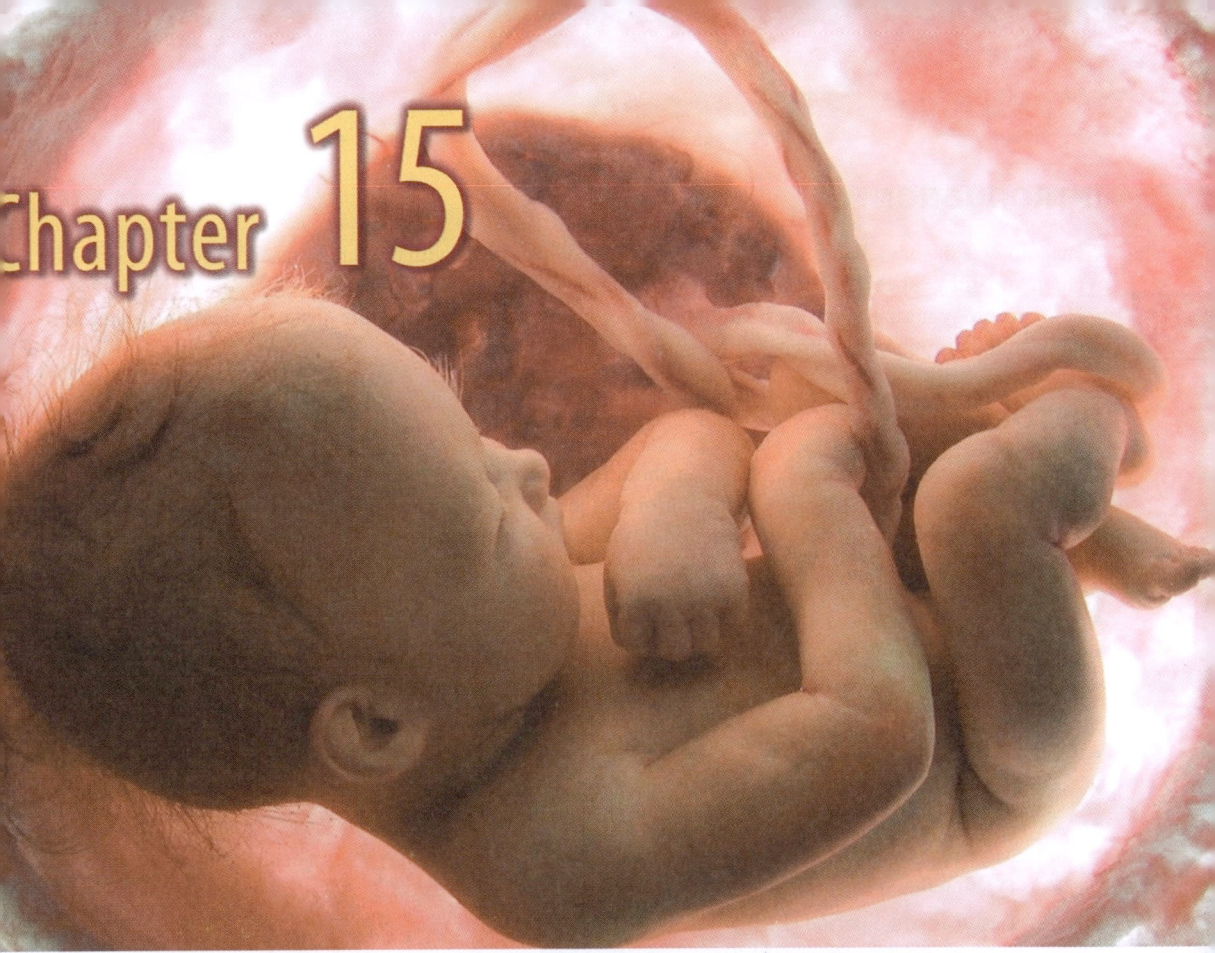

# Chapter 15

# Introduction

# INTRODUCTION

Gynecology is the branch of physiology and medicine which deals with the functions and diseases specific to women and girls, especially those affecting the reproductive system.

Gynecology normally means treating women who are not pregnant, while obstetrics deals with pregnant women and their unborn children, but both are interrelated to each other.

# HISTORY TAKING

The history taking and clinical examination should be thorough and meticulous keeping in mind the patient as a whole. To obtain a good, relevant and informative history, it is important to establish good rapport with the patient. A careful history taking is started in the following manner:

- Name _____
- Age _____
- Address _____
- Marital status _____
- Parity _____
- Social status _____
- **Chief complaints:** With regard to their onset, duration, severity, use of medications and progress
- **Menstrual history:**
  - Menarche/cycle/duration/amount of blood flow_____/____/_____/
  - Dysfunctional uterine bleeding (DUB) if any____
  - Last menstrual period (LMP)
  - Premenstrual syndrome (PMS)/menstrual irregularities/mid cycle abdominal pain
  - Age of menopause in mother/elder sister_____/_____
- **Obstetric history**

| Year and date | Pregnancy events | Labor | Type of delivery | Puerperium | Baby status |
|---|---|---|---|---|---|
| | • Full term | • Normal | • Normal vaginal delivery (NVD) | • Postpartum hemorrhage | • Sex and weight |
| | • Post-term | • Obstructed labor | • NVD with episiotomy | • Postpartum infection | • Condition at birth |
| | • Preterm | • Others | • Cesarean section/forceps/ventouse | • Contraception | • Duration of breastfeeding |
| | | | • Medical termination of pregnancy<br>• Self-abortion | | • Immunization |

- **Marital history:**
  - Age of marriage _____
  - Married for _____
  - Consanguineous marriage: Yes/No
- **Gynecological history:**
  - Reproductive tract infection/salpingitis/endometriosis/tubo-ovarian abscess _____/____/_____/

- Ectopic pregnancy/infertility_____/_____
- Human immunodeficiency virus (HIV)/Hepatitis/Syphilis toxoplasmosis, other infections, rubella, cytomegalovirus and herpes simplex (STORCH)_____/_____
- **Past medical history**
  **Chronic illness:** Hypertension ----------Diabetes _____
  **Genetic disorders:** _____ Psychiatric disorders: _____ Others: _____
- **Past surgical history:**
  - General surgery _____ Obstetrical surgery _____ Gynecological surgery _____ Nature of operation _____ Anesthetic procedure _____ Bleeding or clotting complication (if any) _____
- **Family history:** It is of occasional value. Malignancy of the breast, colon, endometrium, genital tract is also related. Similarly, history of tuberculosis in any of the family members can give clue to the diagnosis of genital tuberculosis.
- **Personal history:** Occupation, Marital status—married, widow, divorced or separated should be enquired. If married, details of sexual history should be taken, especially in case of infertility. Sexual history includes any sexual dysfunction or dyspareunia. Contraceptive practice, if any should be enquired especially relevant in pill users or cases having intrauterine contraceptive device (IUCD), as these methods often produce some adverse symptoms. History of taking drugs for a long time or allergy to certain drugs is to be noted.

## PHYSICAL EXAMINATION

The physical examination includes:

- General and systemic examination
- Gynecological examination
  - Breast examination
  - Abdominal examination
  - Pelvic examination

## General and Systemic Examination

- The general and systemic examination should be thorough and meticulous.
- Height _____ Weight _____
- Temperature _____ Pulse_____/min, respiration_____/min, BP_____mm Hg.

### Tick (P) for Information

- **Build:** Obese/average/thin
- **Nutrition:** Good/average/poor
- **Pallor:** Lower palpebral conjunctiva/dorsum of the tongue/nail buds
- **Tongue, teeth, gums and tonsils:** Glossitis stomatitis
- Heart/lungs/liver/spleen
- **Neck:**
  - Neck veins _____ Distended/normal
  - Thyroid gland _____ Palpable/normal
  - Lymph nodes _____ Palpable/normal

- Edema of legs:
  - Physiological edema
  - Pitting edema

## Breast Examination

- Inspect and palpate the breast to assess (Fig. 1):
  - Development of secondary sexual characteristics
  - Any abnormality or disparity in the breasts
  - Presence of nipple abnormalities like retracted/cracked/protruded nipples
  - For any breast infection
  - Tumor/lump in breast
  - Fibroadenoma/fibroadenosis
  - Focal venous engorgement
  - Edema, induration, Peau d'orange skin
  - Nipple discharge (clear-galactorrhea/blood stained)

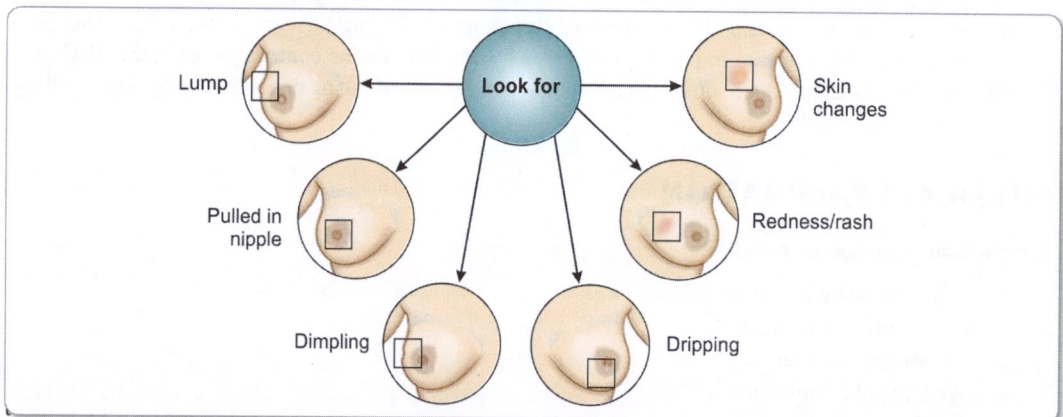

**Fig. 1:** Breast examination

## Abdominal Examination

### Prerequisites

- Empty the bladder.
- Provide dorsal supine position to the patient with legs slightly flexed to relax the abdominal muscles.
- Stand on the right side of the patient.
- Provide privacy.
- Establish good rapport with the patient and explain the whole procedure to win the confidence.

### Actual Steps

Figures 2A to C shows striae gravidarum; everted umbilicus and peritonitis respectively.
- **Inspection:** Inspect the skin condition of the abdomen for:
  - Presence of old scar, prominent veins
  - Striae gravidarum
  - Incisional hernia/divarication of rectus abdominis muscles

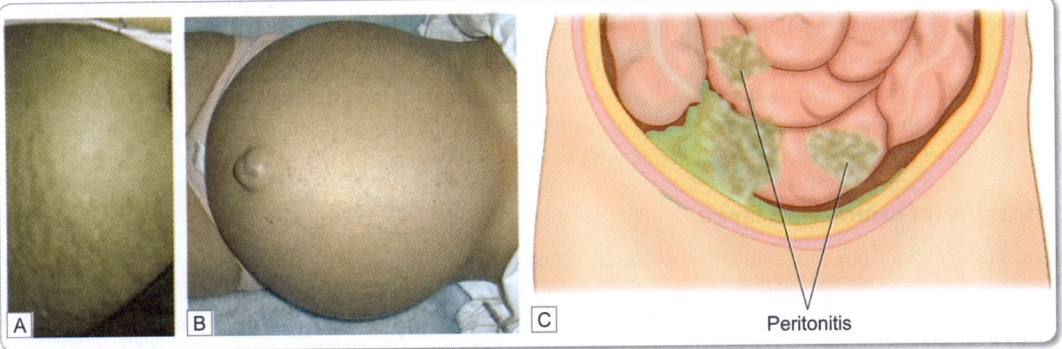

**Figs 2A to C:** **A.** Striae gravidarum; **B.** Everted umbilicus and **C.** Peritonitis

- ■ **If intestinal obstruction:** Abdomen is distended and respiration is thoracic type
- ■ **If pelvic peritonitis:** Lower abdomen distended with decreased inspiratory movements
- ■ In ascites–fullness of flanks
- ■ Any tumor
- • **Palpation:** Palpate the abdomen to assess:
  - ■ Rigidity of abdominal muscles, voluntary guarding and tenderness
  - ■ Mass/tumor in lower abdomen, its location, size, consistency, feel, surface mobility
  - ■ Routine palpation of the viscera (for any organomegaly) include liver, spleen, cecum, appendix, pelvic colon, gallbladder and kidneys
- • **Percussion** of the abdomen should be performed to identify:
  - ■ Organ enlargement
  - ■ Tumor
  - ■ Ascites
    - o **If pelvic tumor:** Dullness on percussion with resonance on the flanks
    - o **If retroperitoneal tumor/intestinal adhesions:** It will be resonant
    - o **If ascites:** Fluid thrill also present
- • **Auscultation:** Not required in gynecological examination
  - ■ **In paralytic ileus:** Hypoactive bowel sounds
  - ■ **In intestinal obstruction:** Hyperactive bowel sounds
  - ■ **If patient is pregnant:** Auscultation of fetal heart sound (FHS)

## Pelvic Examination

It includes:
- • Inspection of the external genitalia
- • Vaginal examination
- • Rectal examination
- • Rectovaginal examination

### Prerequisites

- • Ask the patient to empty the bowel and bladder.
- • Allow the patient/relative/friend to stay with her.
- • If minor/unmarried patient, take written consent.

- A good source of light should be available.
- Collect all the articles required for the procedure.
- Use aseptic/barrier techniques during procedure.
- Provide dorsal position with knees flexed and thighs abducted (lateral/Sims' position/lithotomy may be provided in gynecological procedures according to physician choice).
- Establish good rapport with the patient and explain whole procedure to win their confidence.

### Inspection of External Genitalia

Inspect the vulva from above downwards for any congenital abnormality:

- Abnormal hair growth (pattern of pubic hair), lice and boils
- Skin lesions, leukoplakia
- Itching marks, dermatitis
- Uterovaginal prolapse/condylomata
- Clitoral growth
- Swelling over labia (Bartholin's gland)
- Varicose veins of vulva
- Carcinoma of vulva, vagina and perineum
- Urethra—for redness, discharge, prolapsed mucosa
- Hymen—Intact/perforate
- Ask the patient to cough to see—urine leakage, prolapse of tissue like cystocele, rectocele, cervical competence.
- Check for hemorrhoids and fissure, fistula and perineal tear.

Figure 3 shows the inspection technique of external genitalia.

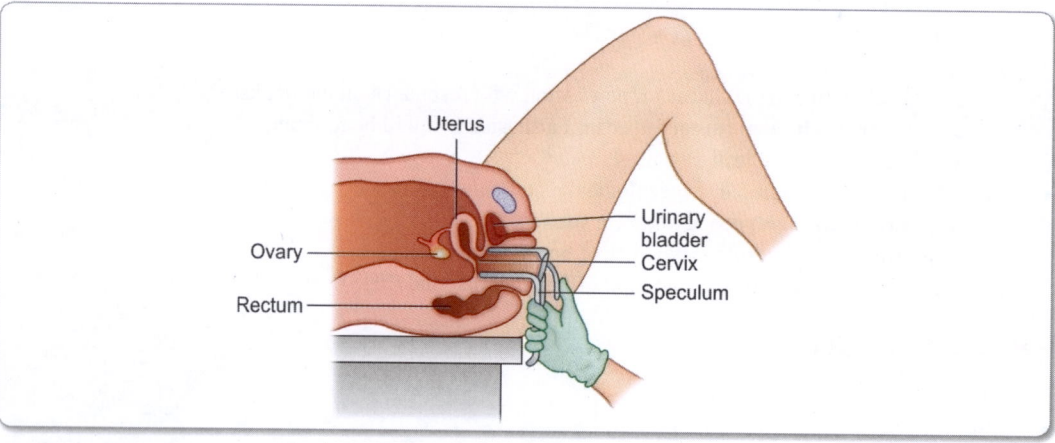

**Fig. 3:** Inspection of external genitalia

### Vaginal Examination

It is done either by speculum examination (Cusco's speculum/Sims' speculum) or bimanual examination (digital examination).

- **Speculum examination** is used to detect the vaginal wall and cervix for masses, ulceration or unhealthy discharge. Pap smear, cervical and scrape cytology and endocervical sampling for cytological examination is also obtained through speculum examination.

- *Bimanual examination* is done using a gloved index and middle fingers of the right hand lubricated with sterile lubricant. Note the following areas as shown in Figure 4:
    - **Urethra:** Pressed from above downwards to see any discharge
    - **Labia majora:** For any swelling of Bartholin's gland
    - **Cervix:** Consistency, firmness, length, position, movement and shape
    - **Uterus:** Note the position, size, shape, consistency and mobility (normally, uterus is anteverted, pear-shaped, firm and freely mobile in all directions).
    - **Uterine tubes/ovaries:** Normal fallopian tubes and ovaries are not felt as it is mobile and sensitive to manual pressure.
    - **Pouch of Douglas:** Examined through posterior fornix. Feel for any nodularity, mass, tenderness or any fullness.
    - To assess strength of levator ani muscles, ask the patient to contract the muscles of the pelvis.

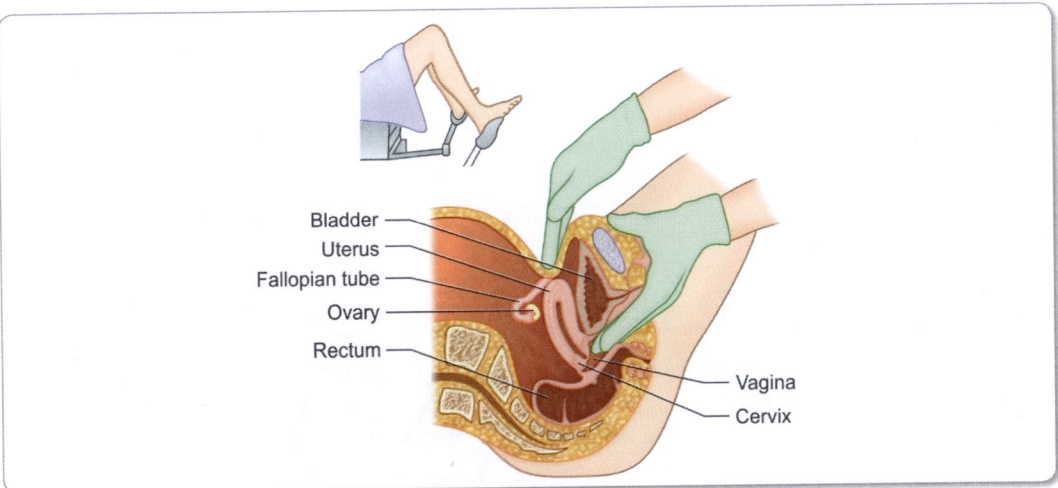

Bladder
Uterus
Fallopian tube
Ovary
Rectum
Vagina
Cervix

**Fig. 4:** Bimanual examination

## Rectal Examination

Rectal examination can be done in isolation or as an adjunct to vaginal examination (Fig. 5). The lower bowel should preferably be empty. The rectoabdominal procedure is almost same as that of vaginal examination except that only gloved index finger smeared with Vaseline is to be introduced into the rectum.

### Indications

- Imperforate hymen
- Severe vaginitis
- Unmarried patient
- Carcinoma of cervix
- Atresia of vagina
- To identify rectocele and differentiate it from enterocele

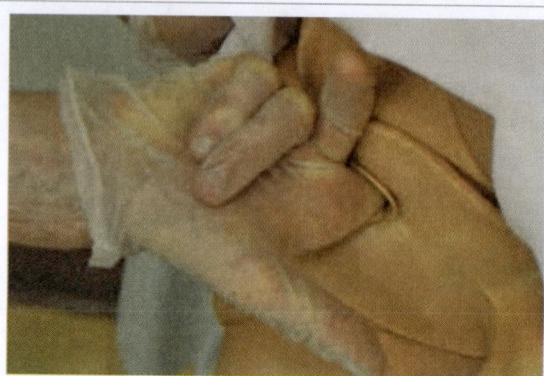

Rotate the
finger 360°
to assess the
anal canal

**Fig. 5:** Rectal examination

### *Rectovaginal Examination*

In this, the index finger is put in vagina and middle finger in the rectum. It is required to differentiate rectal growth and their extension into the vagina and vice-versa (Fig. 6).

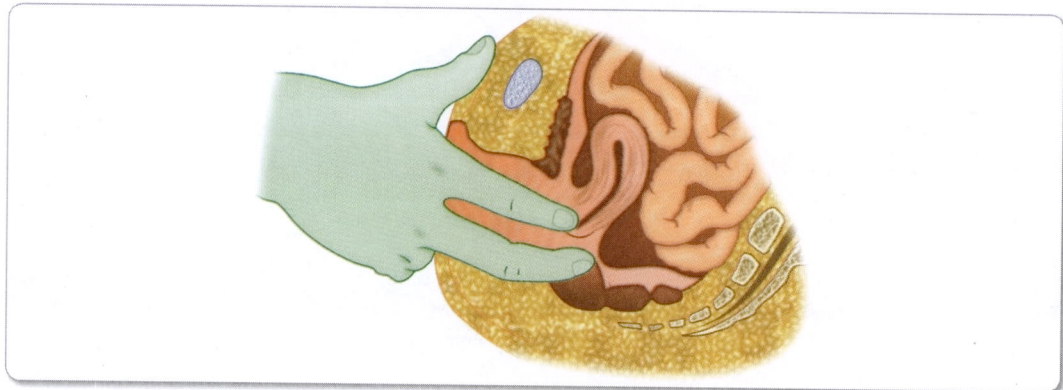

**Fig. 6:** Rectovaginal examination

## INVESTIGATIONS IN GYNECOLOGY

### Ultrasonography

Transabdominal ultrasound, transvaginal ultrasound are shown in Figure 7. It has become a common diagnostic modality in gynecology. It is widely used in:

- Infertility work up (sonohysterosalpingography), folliculometry, detection of ovulation and oocyte retrieval *in vitro* fertilization (IVF)
- Evaluation of pelvic mass
- Ectopic pregnancy
- Endometrial disease
- To locate missing intrauterine device

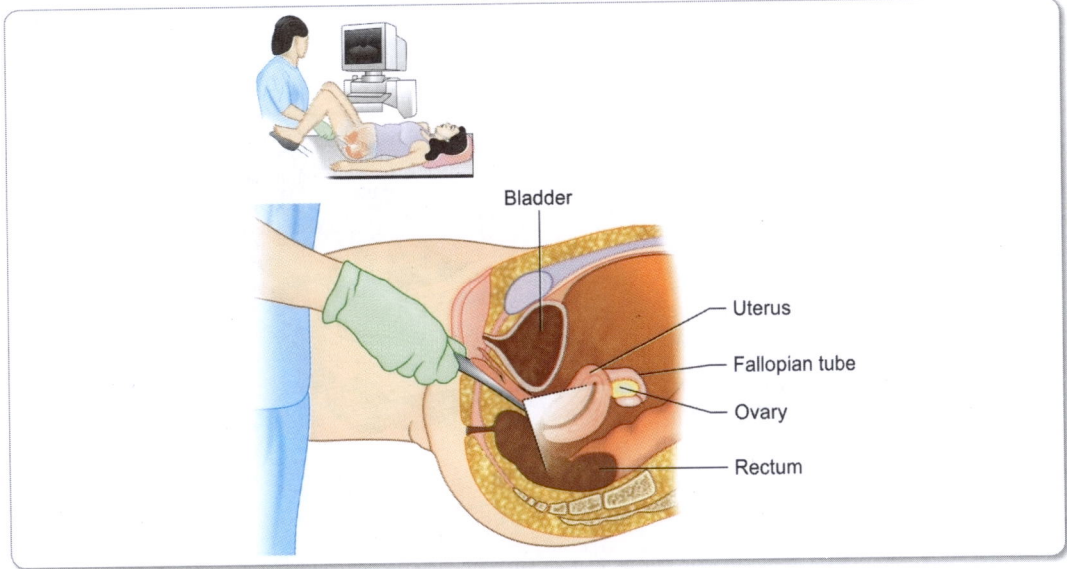

**Bladder**

**Uterus**

**Fallopian tube**

**Ovary**

**Rectum**

**Fig. 7:** Transvaginal sonography

## Computed Tomography (CT)

It is useful in the diagnosis of lymph node metastasis and depth of myometrial invasion in endometrial cancer. It may be employed in selected cases to detect microadenoma of pituitary or metastatic lesions in the brain or liver.

## Magnetic Resonance Imaging (MRI)

MRI uses radio waves (nonionizing) and magnetic fields. It accurately shows parametrial invasion of cervical cancer but cannot reliably identify the lymph node metastasis. It can measure the depth of myometrial penetration in endometrial carcinoma preoperatively. Tumor volume can be measured with 3D imaging system. It is safe in women with pregnancy or intrauterine device (IUD) as shown in Figure 8.

## Endometrial Sampling

Endometrial sampling (Fig. 9) can be performed in the outpatient department (OPD) using a narrow plastic cannula (pipette). It is helpful to:

- Diagnose infertility
- Abnormal perimenopausal bleeding
- Dysfunctional uterine bleeding

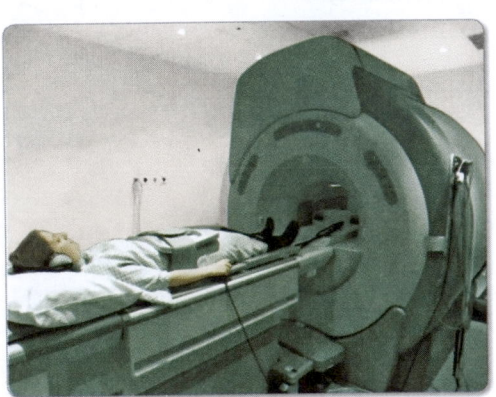

**Fig. 8:** MRI machine

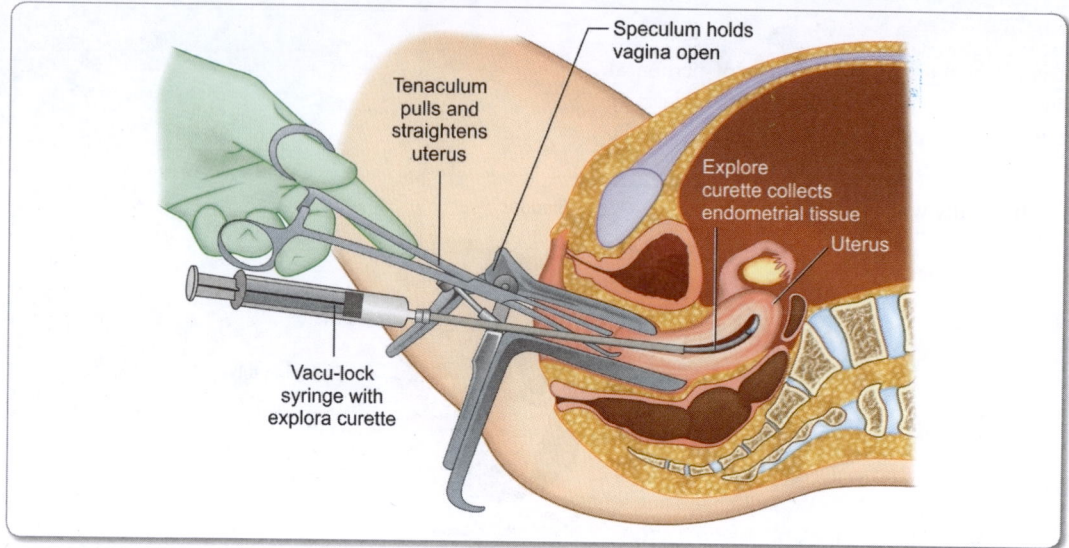

**Fig. 9:** Endometrial sampling

## Culdocentesis

Culdocentesis is the transvaginal aspiration of peritoneal fluid from the pouch of Douglas (Fig. 10). Indications are:

- Ectopic pregnancy
- Hemoperitoneum
- Pelvic abscess

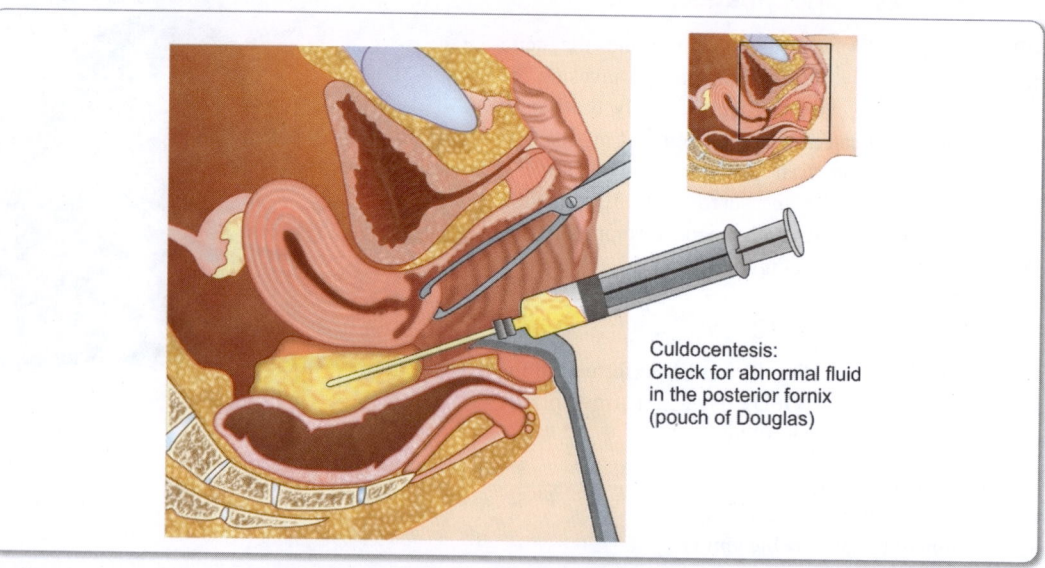

**Fig. 10:** Culdocentesis

## Laparoscopy

It is a technique of visualization of peritoneal cavity by means of a fiber optic endoscope introduced through the abdominal wall (Fig. 11).

Indications are:

- Infertility work-up
- Chronic pelvic pain
- To exclude pelvic lesions
- To identify uterine fibroid, ovarian cyst
- Following pelvic surgery (tuboplasty after endometriosis treatment, etc.)

## Hysteroscopy

It is an operative procedure where by the endometrial cavity can be visualized with the help of fiber optic telescope (Fig. 12).

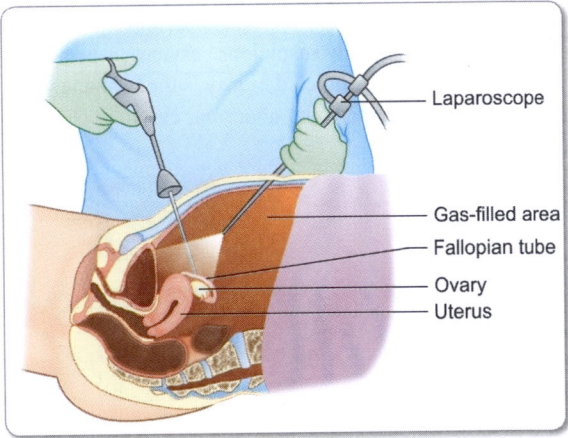

**Fig. 11:** Laparoscopy

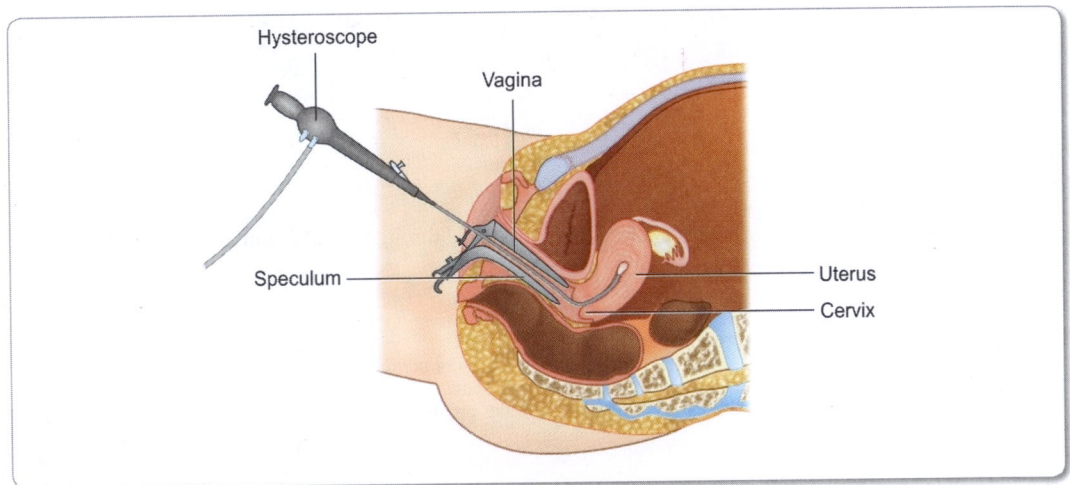

**Fig. 12:** Hysteroscopy

Diagnostic indications:

- To exclude uterine polyp, submucosal fibroid or products of conception
- Missing IUD
- Intrauterine adhesions
- Congenital uterine septum in recurrent abortion

Operative indications:

- Polypectomy and myomectomy
- Endometrial ablation
- Endometrial resection
- Metroplasty

- Tubal cannulation
- Sterilization
- Laser coagulation
- Endometrial biopsy

## Colposcopy

Colposcopy is a lower power binocular microscope. It is employed in the cases with abnormal cervical smear and with clinically suspicious cervices, especially with history of contact bleeding even if the smear is negative. Colposcopy directed biopsy is the best one when the lesion is not clinically detected. Colposcope is used to evaluate women with abnormal cytology (Fig. 13).

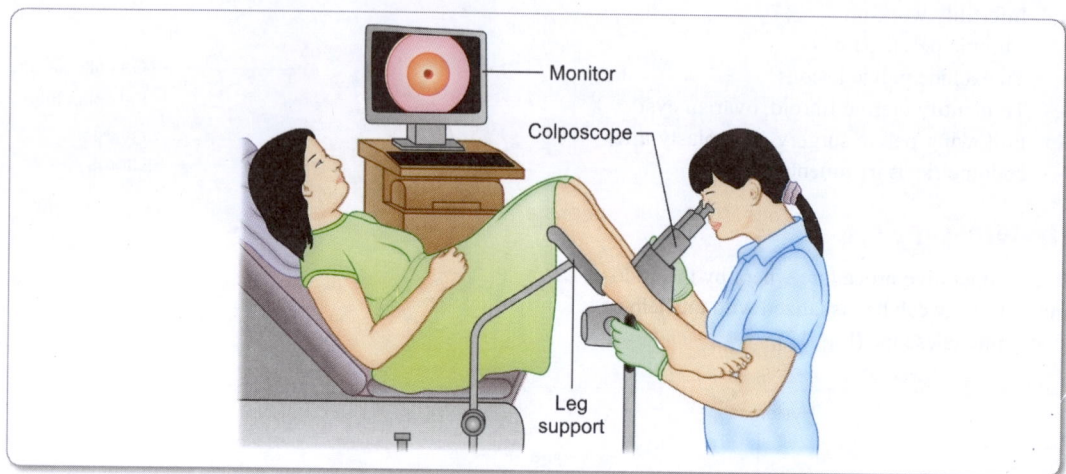

**Fig. 13:** Colposcopy

## Salpingoscopy

It is the evaluation of tubal mucosa with a telescope, introduced through the abdominal ostium of the tube.

## Pap Smear (Cervical Smear Test)

It is the most effective cancer screening procedure. It reduces the incidence of cancer cervix by 80% when used regularly (Fig. 14).

## Laser in Gynecology

It is used in gynecology for tissue cutting, coagulation or vaporization. Laser effect depends as power (Watts), spot size, power density and lower tissue contact time. Commonly used laser systems in gynecology are $CO_2$, ND:YAG, KTP 532 and Argon.

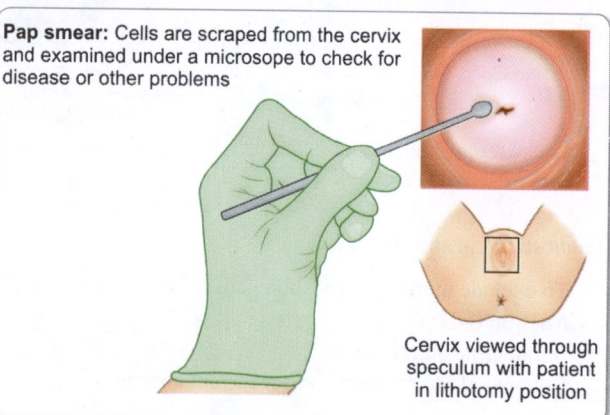

**Fig. 14:** Pap smear

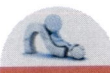

## ASSESS YOURSELF

### FREQUENTLY ASKED QUESTIONS IN EXAMS

1. **Define the following:**
   a. Gynecology
   b. Laparoscopy
   c. Pap smear
   d. Culdoscopy

2. **Discuss the steps of history taking in gynecological procedures.**

3. **Describe the diagnostic tests that are commonly used to diagnose gynecological problems.**

### MULTIPLE CHOICE QUESTIONS

1. **Visualization of peritoneal cavity by means of fiber optic endoscope introduced through the abdominal wall is called:**
   a. Hysteroscopy
   b. Laparoscopy
   c. Laser therapy
   d. Colposcopy

2. **Visualization of endometrial cavity with the help of fiber optic telescope is called:**
   a. Hysteroscopy
   b. Coloscopy
   c. Hysterosalpingography
   d. Salpingoscopy

3. **The common diagnostic test used to diagnose cervical cancer:**
   a. Pap smear
   b. Urine test
   c. MRI
   d. Vaginal ultrasonography

4. **Evaluation of tubal mucosa with a telescope is known as:**
   a. Laparoscopy
   b. Salpingoscopy
   c. Hysterosalpingoscopy
   d. Culdocentesis

5. **Endometrial sampling is performed to diagnose:**
   a. Dysfunctional uterine bleeding
   b. Abnormal perimenopausal bleeding
   c. Infertility
   d. All of the above

6. **Commonly used laser system in gynecology is:**
   a. $CO_2$
   b. ND:YAG
   c. Argon
   d. All of the above

7. **Uses of laser in gynecology are all except:**
   a. Tissue cutting
   b. Coagulation
   c. Vaporization
   d. Cannulation

8. **Which one of the following step in case of abdominal examination is least effective?**
   a. Inspection
   b. Palpation
   c. Percussion
   d. Auscultation

 **Answer Key**

| 1. b | 2. a | 3. a | 4. b | 5. d | 6. d | 7. d |
|------|------|------|------|------|------|------|
| 8. d |

Chapter 15 ➲ Introduction

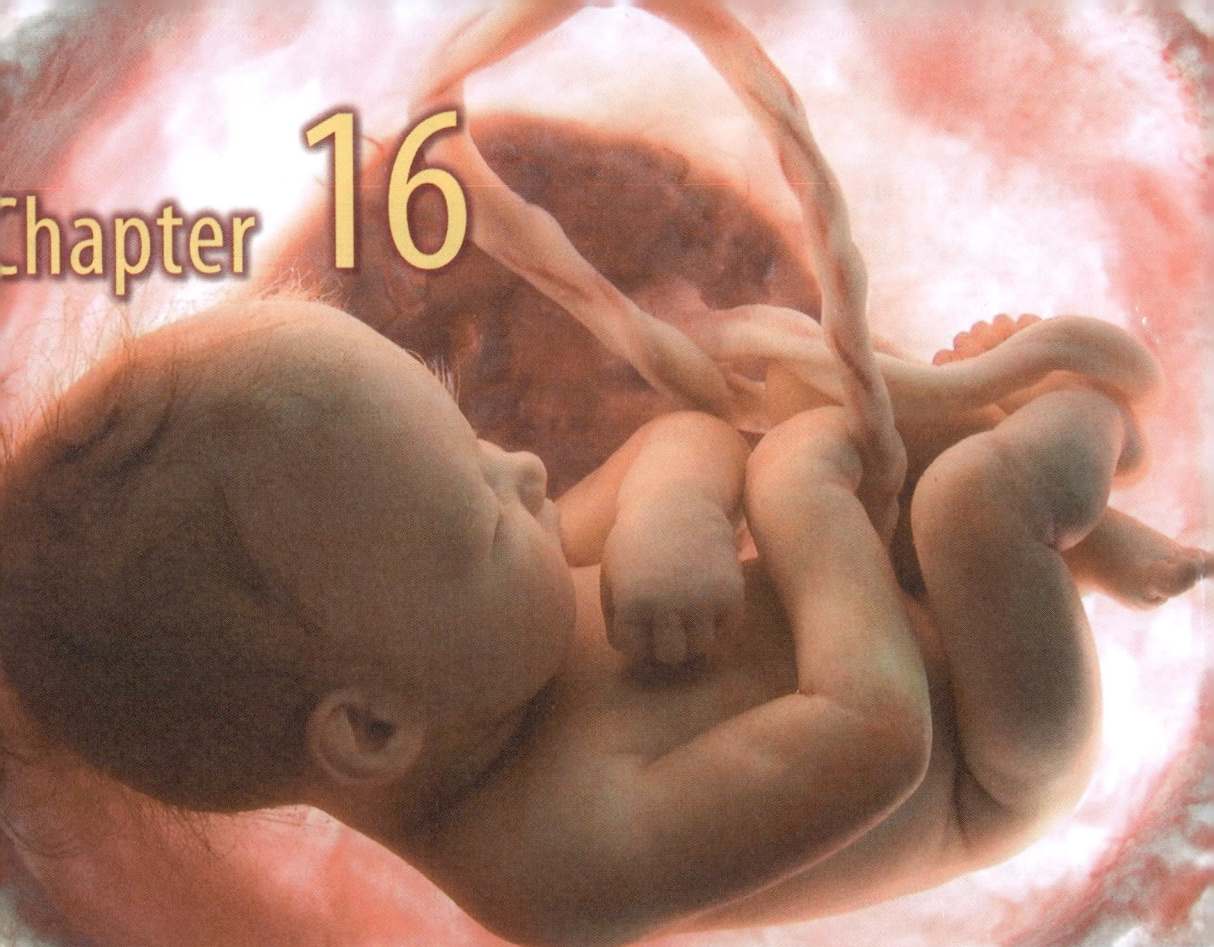

# Puberty

# INTRODUCTION

Puberty is the period during which adolescents reach sexual maturity and become capable of reproduction.

The time when puberty begins varies greatly among individuals; however, in girls puberty usually occurs in between the age of 10 and 14 years and in boys the age of puberty ranges from 12 to 16 years. Both genetic and environmental factors are involved in the timing of puberty. Body fat and/or body composition may play a role in regulating the onset of puberty. Puberty is associated with the development of secondary sex characteristics and rapid growth. Puberty may also be accompanied by emotional and mood changes. Table 1 enlists the stages of puberty in boys and girls.

**TABLE 1: Stages of puberty in boys and girls**

| Puberty | Boys | Girls |
|---------|------|-------|
| Stage one | **Prepubertal:** No sexual development | **Prepubertal:** No sexual development |
| Stage two | Testes enlarge, body odor | • Breast budding<br>• First pubic hair<br>• Body odor<br>• Height spurt |
| Stage three | • Penis enlarge<br>• Pubic hair starts growing<br>• Dermal ejaculation test | • Breasts enlarge<br>• Pubic hair darkens and becomes curlier<br>• Vaginal discharge |
| Stage four | • Continuous enlargement of penis and testis<br>• Penis and scrotal sac becomes darker in color<br>• Height spurt<br>• Male breast development | • Onset of menstruation<br>• Nipples are distinct from areola |
| Stage five | • Fully mature male<br>• Pubic hair extends to inner thighs<br>• Height increases abruptly then stops | • Fully mature female<br>• Pubic hair extends to inner thighs<br>• Height increases slowly then stops |

# DEVELOPMENT OF SEX ORGANS IN FEMALES

The physiology of puberty has been described in Figure 1.

## Breast Development

The first physical sign of puberty in girls is usually a firm, tender lump under the center of the areola of one or both breasts, occurring on average at about 10.5 years of age. This is referred to as thelarche. Tanner stage of breast development has been shown in Table 2.

## Pubic Hair

Pubic hair is often the second noticeable change in puberty, usually within a few months of thelarche. It is referred to as pubarche. The pubic hairs are usually visible first along the labia then around the whole pubic area. In about 15% of girls, the earliest pubic hair appears before breast development begins.

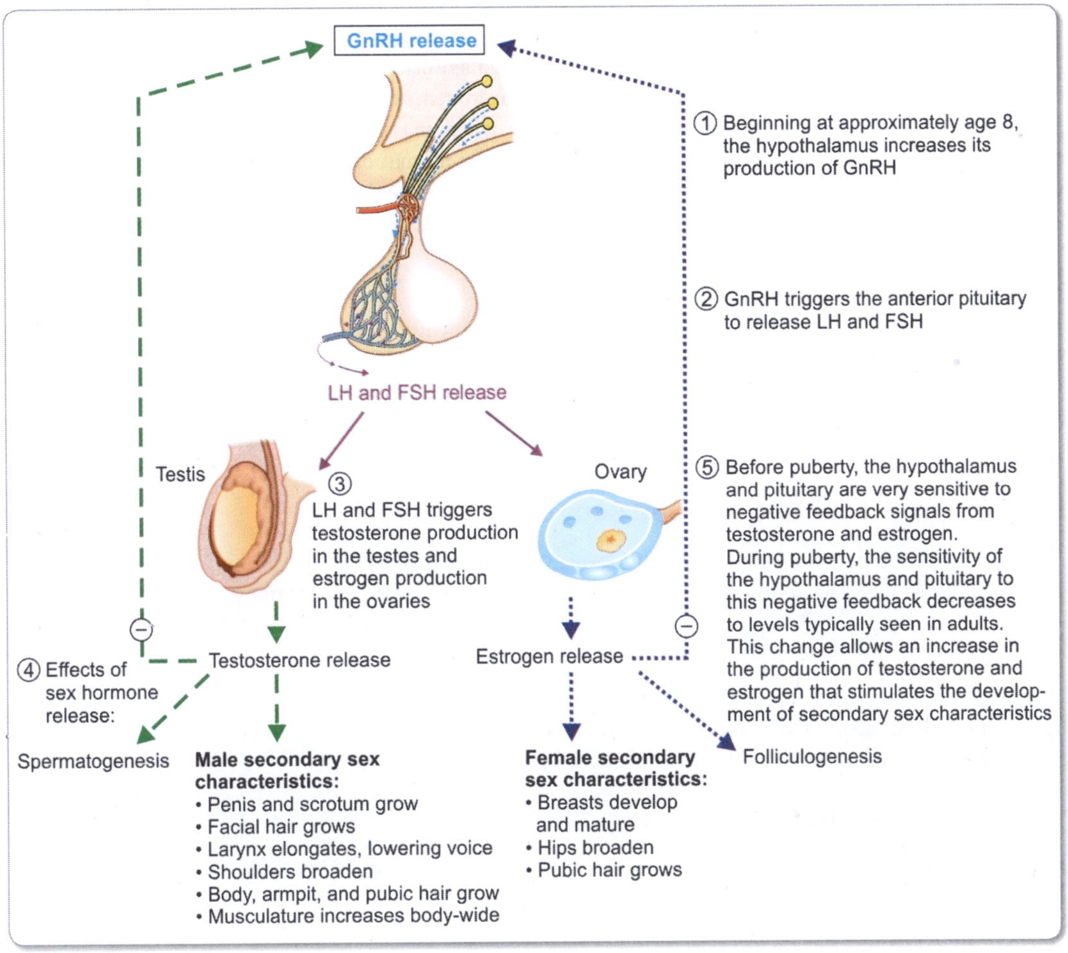

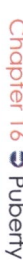

**GnRH release**

① Beginning at approximately age 8, the hypothalamus increases its production of GnRH

② GnRH triggers the anterior pituitary to release LH and FSH

**LH and FSH release**

Testis

Ovary

③ LH and FSH triggers testosterone production in the testes and estrogen production in the ovaries

⑤ Before puberty, the hypothalamus and pituitary are very sensitive to negative feedback signals from testosterone and estrogen. During puberty, the sensitivity of the hypothalamus and pituitary to this negative feedback decreases to levels typically seen in adults. This change allows an increase in the production of testosterone and estrogen that stimulates the development of secondary sex characteristics

Testosterone release

Estrogen release

④ Effects of sex hormone release:

Spermatogenesis

Folliculogenesis

**Male secondary sex characteristics:**
- Penis and scrotum grow
- Facial hair grows
- Larynx elongates, lowering voice
- Shoulders broaden
- Body, armpit, and pubic hair grow
- Musculature increases body-wide

**Female secondary sex characteristics:**
- Breasts develop and mature
- Hips broaden
- Pubic hair grows

**Fig. 1:** Physiology of puberty

*Abbreviations:* GnRH, gonadotropin releasing hormone; LH, luteinizing hormone; FSH, follicle stimulating hormone

**TABLE 2: Tanner stage of pubertal changes**

| Stage | Breast development | Pubic hair |
|---|---|---|
| 1 | **Prepubertal:** Papilla elevation only | **Prepubertal:** No pubic hair |
| 2 | **Breast bud:** Elevation of breast and papilla; enlargement of areola | Sparse, long, slightly pigmented hair on labia majora |
| 3 | Further enlargement of breast and areola; no separation of contour | Dark, coarse, curled hair, spreading sparsely over mons |
| 4 | Areola and papilla form secondary mound above level of breast | **Adult:** Type hair, abundant, limited to mons |
| 5 | Projection of papilla only, recession of areola to contour of breast | **Adult:** Type hair distribution to the medial thigh |

## Vagina, Uterus and Ovaries

Perineal skin keratinizes due to effect of estrogen increasing its resistance to infection. The mucosal surface of the vagina also changes in response to increasing levels of estrogen, becoming thicker and duller pink in color. Estrogen increases glycogen content in vaginal epithelium, which in future plays important part in maintaining vaginal pH. Whitish secretions (physiologic leukorrhea) are a normal effect of estrogen as well. In the two years, following thelarche, the uterus, ovaries and the follicles in the ovaries increase in size. Before puberty, uterine body to cervix ratio is 1:1, which increases to 2:1 or 3:1 after completion of pubertal period.

## Menstruation and Fertility

The first menstrual bleeding is referred to as menarche and typically, occurs about two years after thelarche. The average age of menarche is 12 years. The time between menstrual periods (menses) is not always regular in the first two years after menarche. A high proportion of girls with continued irregularity in the menstrual cycle several years from menarche will continue to have prolonged irregularity and anovulation, and are at higher risk for reduced fertility.

## Body Shape, Fat Distribution, and Body Composition

During this period, also in response to rising levels of estrogen, the lower half of the pelvis and thus, hips widen. Fat tissue increases in the areas of breasts, hips, buttocks, thighs, upper arms and pubis.

## Body Odor and Acne

Rising levels of androgen can change the fatty acid composition of perspiration, resulting in a more body odor. Another androgen effect is increased secretion of oil (sebum) from the skin. This change increases the susceptibility to acne, a skin condition that is characteristic of puberty.

## Visual and other Effects of Hormonal Changes

In girls, estradiol (the primary female sex hormone) causes thickening of lips and oral mucosa as well as further development of the vulva. Estradiol is also responsible for the increased production of pheomelanin, resulting in the characteristic red color of the lips, labia minora and sometimes labia majora. Estradiol together with other ovarian steroids also causes the darker coloration of the areola.

Testosterone will cause an enlargement of the clitoris and possibly has important effects on the growth and maturation of the vestibular bulbs, corpus cavernosum of the clitoris and urethral sponge.

## REVIEW OF MENSTRUAL CYCLE

The **menstrual cycle** is the regular natural change that occurs in the female reproductive system (specifically the uterus and ovaries) that makes pregnancy possible. The cycle is required for the production of oocytes, and for the preparation of the uterus for pregnancy (Fig. 2).

The first period usually begins between 12 and 13 years of age, a point in time known as menarche. Menstruation stops occurring after menopause which usually occurs between 45 and 55 years of age. Menstrual bleeding usually lasts around 2–7 days.

The menstrual cycle is governed by hormonal changes. Each cycle can be divided into different phases based on events in the ovary (ovarian cycle) or in the uterus (uterine cycle). The day count for menstrual cycle begins on the first day of menstruation when blood starts to come out of the vagina. In this section, the length of menstrual cycle has been assumed to be 28 days (which is the average among women).

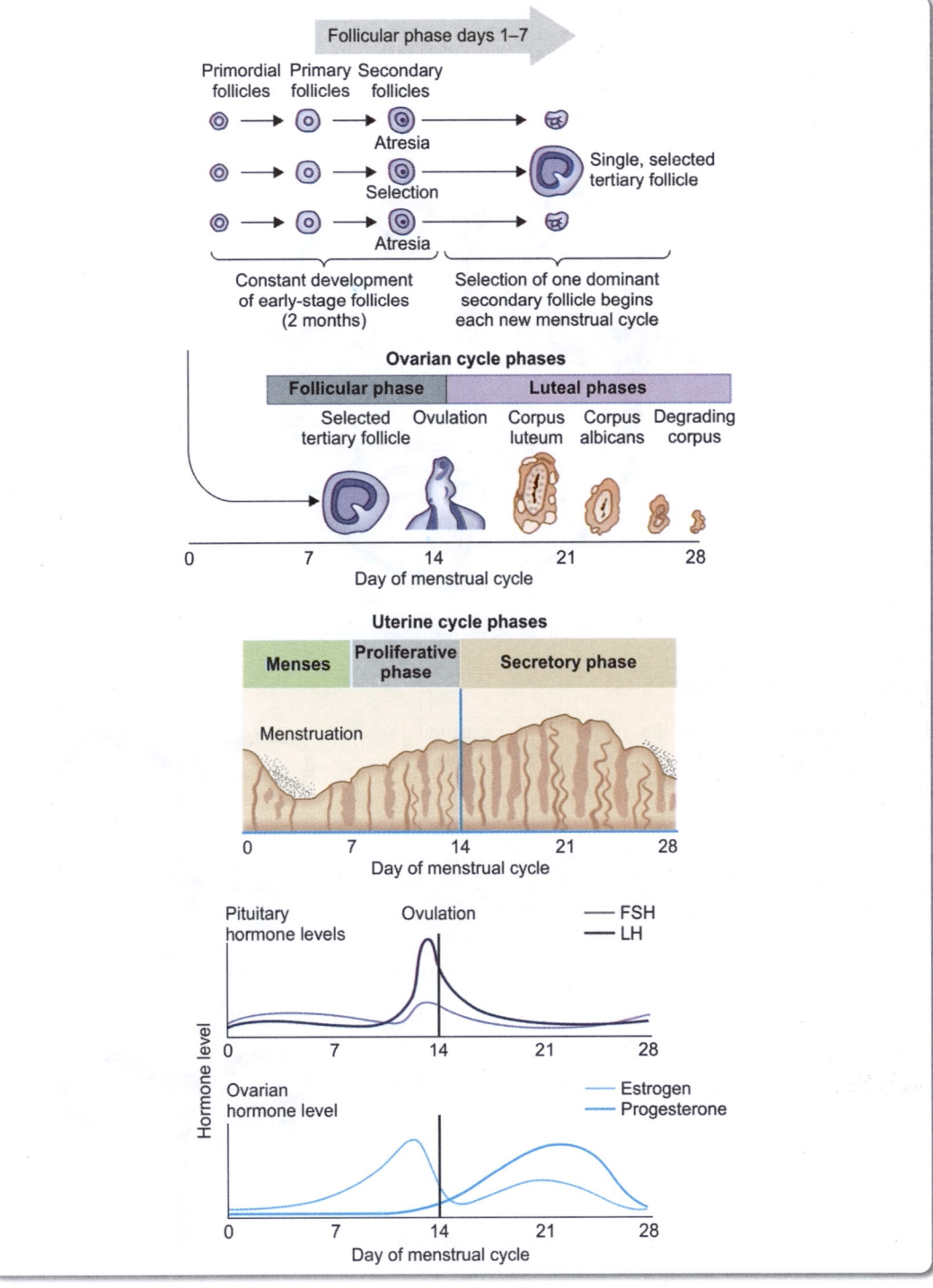

**Fig. 2:** Physiology of menstrual cycle

*Abbreviations:* FSH, follicle stimulating hormone; LH, luteinizing hormone

## Phases of Menstrual Cycle

**The entire duration of a menstrual cycle can be divided into four main phases:**

1. Menstrual phase (From day 1 to 5)
2. Follicular phase (From day 1 to 13)
3. Ovulation phase (Day 14)
4. Luteal phase (From day 15 to 28) (Fig. 3)

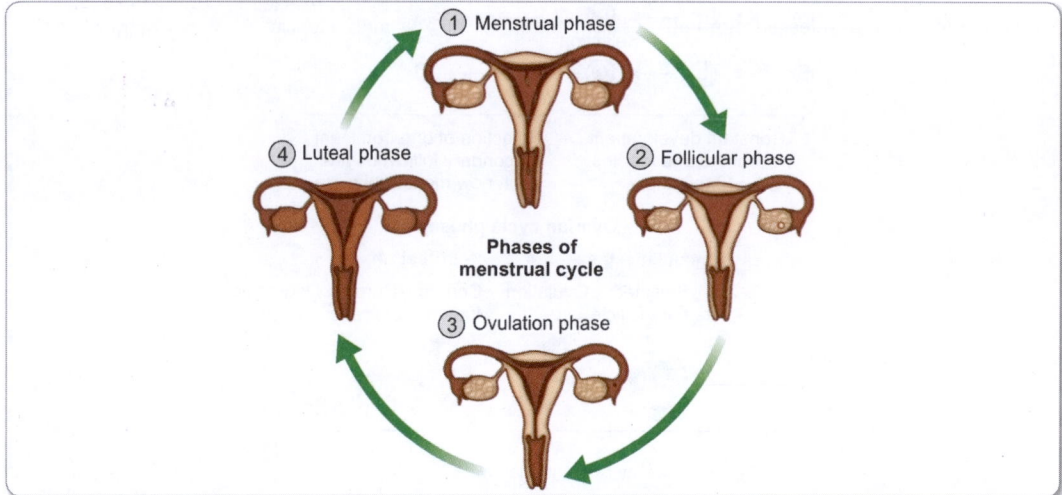

**Fig. 3:** Phases of menstrual cycle

### 1. Menstrual Phase (Day 1–5)

Menstrual phase begins on the first day of menstruation and lasts till the 5th day of the menstrual cycle (Fig. 4). The following events occur during this phase:

- The uterus sheds its inner lining of soft tissue and blood vessels which exits the body from the vagina in the form of menstrual fluid.
- Blood loss of 10–80 mL is considered normal.
- Person may experience abdominal cramps. These cramps are caused by the contraction of the uterine and the abdominal muscles to expel the menstrual fluid.

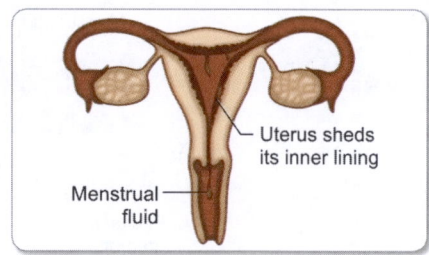

**Fig. 4:** Menstrual phase (day 1–5)

### 2. Follicular Phase (Day 1–13)

This phase also begins on the first day of menstruation, but it lasts till the 13th day of the menstrual cycle (Fig. 5). The following events occur during this phase:

- The pituitary gland secretes a hormone that stimulates the egg cells in the ovaries to grow.
- One of these egg cells begins to mature in a sac-like-structure called follicle. It takes 13 days for the egg cell to reach maturity.

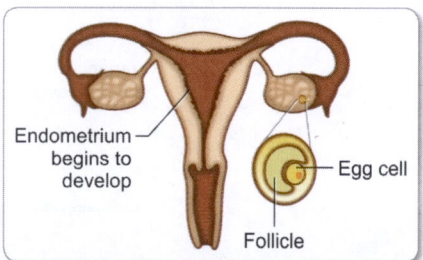

**Fig. 5:** Follicular phase (day 1–13)

- While the egg cell matures, its follicle secretes a hormone that stimulates the uterus to develop a lining of blood vessels and soft tissue called endometrium.

## 3. Ovulation Phase (Day 14)

On the 14th day of the cycle, the pituitary gland secretes a hormone that causes the ovary to release the matured egg cell (Fig. 6). The released egg cell is swept into the fallopian tube by the cilia of the fimbriae. Fimbriae are finger-like projections located at the end of the fallopian tube close to the ovaries and cilia are slender hair-like projections on each fimbria.

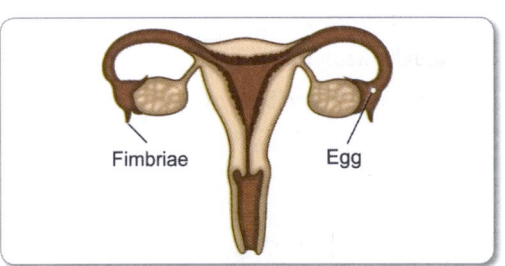

## 4. Luteal Phase (Day 15–28)

**Fig. 6:** Ovulation phase (Day 14)

This phase begins on the 15th day and lasts till the end of the cycle (Fig. 7). The following events occur during this phase:

- The egg cell released during the ovulation phase stays in the fallopian tube for 24 hours.
- If a sperm cell does not impregnate the egg cell within that time, the egg cell disintegrates.
- The hormone that causes the uterus to retain its endometrium gets used up by the end of the menstrual cycle. This causes the menstrual phase of the next cycle to begin.

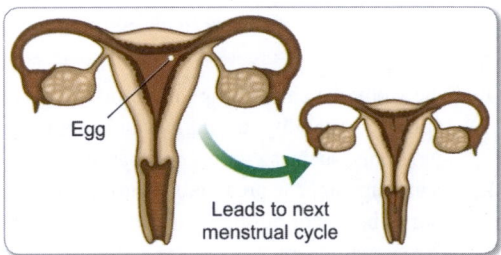

**Fig. 7:** Luteal phase (Day 15–28)

## PREMENSTRUAL SYNDROME

**Premenstrual syndrome (PMS)** refers to physical and emotional symptoms that occur one to two weeks before menstruation.

## Causes

The exact cause of premenstrual syndrome is unknown, but several factors may contribute to the condition:

- **Cyclic changes in hormones:** Signs and symptoms of premenstrual syndrome change with hormonal fluctuations and disappear with pregnancy and menopause.
- **Chemical changes in the brain:** Fluctuations of serotonin, a neurotransmitter that is thought to play a crucial role in mood states, could trigger PMS symptoms. Insufficient amounts of serotonin may contribute to premenstrual depression, as well as to fatigue, food cravings and sleep problems.
- **Depression:** Some women with severe premenstrual syndrome have undiagnosed depression, though depression alone does not cause all of the symptoms.

## Symptoms

The list of potential signs and symptoms for premenstrual syndrome is long, but most women only experience a few of these problems.

### Emotional and Behavioral Symptoms

- Tension or anxiety
- Depressed mood
- Crying spells
- Mood swings and irritability or anger
- Appetite changes and food cravings
- Insomnia (trouble falling sleep)
- Social withdrawal
- Poor concentration

### Physical Signs and Symptoms

- Joint or muscle pain
- Headache
- Fatigue
- Weight gain related to fluid retention
- Abdominal bloating
- Breast tenderness
- Acne flare-ups
- Constipation or diarrhea

## Diagnosis

There are no laboratory tests or unique physical findings to verify the diagnosis of PMS. The three key features are:

1. The woman's chief complaint is one or more of the emotional symptoms associated with PMS (most typically irritability, tension, or unhappiness). The woman does not have PMS if she only has physical symptoms, such as cramps or bloating.
2. Symptoms appear predictably during the luteal (premenstrual) phase, reduce or disappear predictably shortly before or during menstruation, and remain absent during the follicular (preovulatory) phase.
3. The symptoms must be severe enough to interfere with the woman's everyday life.

Mild PMS is common, and more severe symptoms would qualify as per-menstrual dysphoria disorder (PMDD).

## Treatment

Many things have been tried to ease the symptoms of PMS. No treatment works for every woman. Different treatments are required. Some treatment options include:

- Lifestyle changes
- Medications
- Alternative therapies

### Lifestyle Changes

A healthy lifestyle is the first step to manage PMS. For many women, lifestyle approaches are often enough to control symptoms to manage PMS:

- Drink plenty of fluids, like water or juice. Do not drink soft drinks, alcohol, or other beverages with caffeine. This will help reduce bloating, fluid retention, and other symptoms.
- Eat frequent, small meals. Do not go more than 3 hours between snacks. Avoid overeating.
- Eat a balanced diet. Include extra whole grains, vegetables, and fruit in your diet. Limit your intake of salt and sugar.
- Take nutritional supplements. Vitamin B6, calcium, and magnesium are commonly used. Tryptophan, which is found in dairy products, may also be helpful.
- Get regular aerobic exercise throughout the month. This helps in reducing the severity of PMS symptoms.
- Change sleep habits during night before taking drugs for insomnia.

## Medications

Commonly prescribed medications for premenstrual syndrome include:

- **Antidepressants:** Selective serotonin reuptake inhibitors (SSRIs)—which include fluoxetine (Prozac, Sarafem), paroxetine (Paxil, Pexeva), sertraline (Zoloft) and others—have been successful in reducing mood symptoms. These drugs are generally taken daily. But for some women with PMS, use of antidepressants may be limited to the two weeks before menstruation begins.
- **Nonsteroidal anti-inflammatory drugs (NSAIDs):** Taken before or at the onset of period, NSAIDs such as ibuprofen (Advil, Motrin IB and others) or naproxen (Aleve, Naprosyn and others) can ease cramping and breast discomfort.
- **Diuretics:** When exercise and limiting salt intake aren't enough to reduce the weight gain, swelling and bloating of PMS, taking diuretics can help the body shed excess fluid through kidneys. Spironolactone (aldactone) is a diuretic that can help ease some of the symptoms of PMS.
- **Hormonal contraceptives:** These prescription medications stop ovulation, which may bring relief from PMS symptoms.

## Alternative Therapies

Common complementary remedies used to soothe the symptoms of premenstrual syndrome are:

- **Calcium:** Consuming 1,200 mg in diet or with supplemental calcium daily, such as chewable calcium carbonate, may reduce the physical and psychological symptoms of PMS.
- **Magnesium:** Taking 360 mg of supplemental magnesium daily may help reduce fluid retention, breast tenderness and bloating in women with premenstrual syndrome.
- **Vitamin E:** This vitamin, taken in 400 IU daily may ease PMS symptoms by reducing the production of prostaglandins, hormone-like substances that cause cramps and breast tenderness.
- **Herbal remedies:** Some women report relief of PMS symptoms with the use of herbs, such as ginkgo, ginger, chaste berry and evening primrose oil.
- **Acupuncture:** A practitioner of acupuncture inserts sterilized stainless steel needles into the skin at specific points on the body. Some women experience symptoms of relief after acupuncture treatment.

# MENSTRUAL DISORDERS

There are a number of different menstrual disorders. Problems can range from heavy, painful periods to no periods at all. There are many variations in menstrual patterns, but in general women should be concerned when periods come fewer than 21 days or more than 3 months apart, or if they last for more than 10 days. Such events may indicate ovulation problems or other medical conditions.

## Dysmenorrhea (Painful Menstruation)

Dysmenorrhea is severe, frequent cramping during menstruation. Pain occurs in the lower abdomen but can spread to the lower back and thighs. Dysmenorrhea is usually referred to as primary or secondary.

- **Primary dysmenorrhea:** Primary dysmenorrhea is cramping pain caused by menstruation. The cramps occur from contractions in the uterus and are usually more severe during heavy bleeding.
- **Secondary dysmenorrhea:** Secondary dysmenorrhea is menstrual-related pain that accompanies another medical or physical condition, such as endometriosis or uterine fibroids.

## Causes of Dysmenorrhea (Painful Periods)

**Primary dysmenorrhea** is caused by prostaglandins, hormone-like substances that are produced in the uterus and cause the uterine muscle to contract. Prostaglandins also play a role in the heavy bleeding that causes dysmenorrhea.

**Secondary dysmenorrhea** can be caused by a number of medical conditions. Common causes of secondary dysmenorrhea include:

- **Endometriosis:** Endometriosis is a chronic and often progressive disease that develops when the tissue that lines the uterus (endometrium) grows onto other areas, such as the ovaries, bowels, or bladder. It often causes chronic pelvic pain (Fig. 8).
- **Uterine fibroid:** Fibroid are noncancerous growths that grow on the walls of the uterus. They can cause heavy bleeding during menstruation and cramping pain.
- **Other causes:** Pelvic inflammatory disease, ovarian cysts, and ectopic pregnancy. The intrauterine device (IUD) contraceptive can also cause secondary dysmenorrhea.

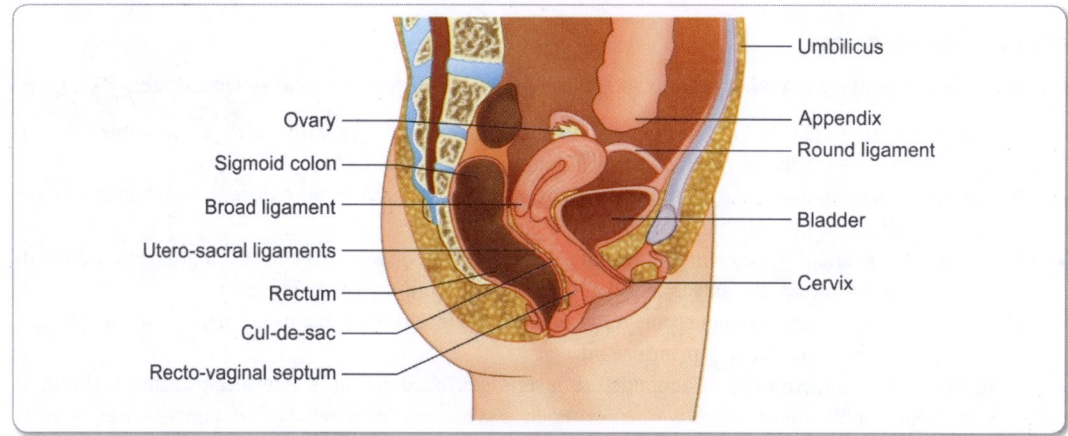

**Fig. 8:** Common sites for endometriosis

## Treatment

### Primary Dysmenorrhea

- Administer NSAIDs such as ibuprofen, naproxen, and acetylsalicylic acid (ASA).
- Oral contraceptives may also help reduce the severity of the symptoms. Implantable contraception and the Mirena IUD, which release low levels of the hormone progesterone, have also been found to be very helpful in decreasing pain.
- Nausea and vomiting may be relieved with an antiemetic medication.

### Secondary Dysmenorrhea

It varies with the underlying cause. Diagnostic laparoscopy, other hormonal treatments, or trial of transcutaneous electrical nerve stimulation (TENS) are potential next steps. Surgery can be done to remove fibroids or to widen the cervical canal if it is too narrow.

In addition to the above, other nonmedicinal treatments for the pain of dysmenorrhea include:

- Lying on back, supporting the knees with a pillow
- Holding a heating pad or hot water bottle on your abdomen or lower back
- Taking a warm bath
- Gently massaging your abdomen
- Doing mild exercises like stretching, walking, or biking—exercise may improve blood flow and reduce pelvic pain
- Getting plenty of rest and avoiding stressful situations as the menstruation approaches
- Yoga

## Menorrhagia (Heavy Bleeding)

Menorrhagia is menstrual flow that lasts longer and is heavier than normal. The bleeding occurs at regular intervals (during periods). It usually lasts for more than 7 days and women lose an excessive (more than 80 mL) amount of blood. Menorrhagia is often accompanied by dysmenorrhea because passing large clots can cause painful cramping.

**Menorrhagia is a type of abnormal uterine bleeding. Other types of abnormal bleeding are:**

- **Metrorrhagia** also called breakthrough bleeding, refers to bleeding that occurs at irregular intervals and with variable amounts. The bleeding occurs between periods or is unrelated to periods.
- **Menorrhagia** refers to heavy and prolonged bleeding that occurs at irregular intervals.
- **Menometrorrhagia** combines features of menorrhagia and metrorrhagia. The bleeding can occur at the time of menstruation (like menorrhagia) or in between periods (like metrorrhagia).
- **Dysfunctional uterine bleeding** (DUB) is a general term for abnormal uterine bleeding that usually refers to extra or excessive bleeding caused by hormonal problems, usually lack of ovulation (anovulation). DUB tends to occurs either when girls begin to menstruate or when women approach menopause, but it can occur at any time during a woman's reproductive life.
- **Other types of abnormal uterine bleeding** include bleeding after sex and bleeding after menopause.

### Causes

There are many causes for menorrhagia listed below:

- **Hormonal imbalances:** Imbalances in estrogen and progesterone levels can cause heavy bleeding. Hormonal imbalances are common around the time of menarche and menopause.
- **Ovulation problems:** If ovulation does not occur (anovulation), the body stops producing progesterone, which can cause heavy bleeding.
- **Uterine fibroids:** Uterine fibroids are a very common cause of heavy and prolonged bleeding (Fig. 9).
- **Uterine polyps:** Uterine polyps (small benign growths) and other structural problems or other abnormalities in the uterus may cause bleeding.
- **Endometriosis and adenomyosis:** Endometriosis, a condition in which the cells that line the uterus grow outside of the uterus in other areas, such as the ovaries, can cause heavy bleeding. Adenomyosis, a related condition where endometrial tissue develops within the muscle layers of the uterus, can also cause heavy bleeding and menstrual pain.

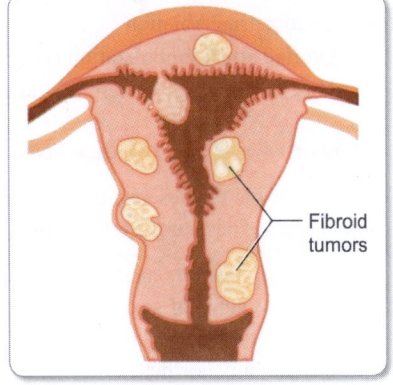

Fibroid tumors

**Fig. 9:** Uterine fibroid

- **Medications and contraceptives:** Certain drugs, including anticoagulants and anti-inflammatory medications, can cause heavy bleeding. Problems linked to some birth control methods, such as birth control pills or intrauterine devices (IUDs) can cause bleeding.
- **Bleeding disorders:** Bleeding disorders that stop blood from clotting can cause heavy menstrual bleeding. Most of these disorders have a genetic basis. Von Willebrand disease is the most common of these bleeding disorders.
- **Cancer:** Rarely, uterine, ovarian, and cervical cancer can cause excessive bleeding.
- **Infection:** Infection of the uterus or cervix can cause bleeding.
- **Pregnancy or miscarriage**
- **Other medical conditions:** Systemic lupus erythematosus, diabetes, pelvic inflammatory disorder, cirrhosis, and thyroid disorders can cause heavy bleeding.

### Treatment of Menorrhagia

#### Medications

*First line*

Intrauterine device with progesterone

*Second line*

- Tranexamic acid an antifibrinolytic agent
- NSAIDs
- Combined oral contraceptives pills to prevent proliferation of the endometrium

*Third line*

- Oral progestogen (e.g., norethisterone) to prevent proliferation of the endometrium
- Injected progestogen [depomedroxyprogesterone (DMPA)]

*Other options*

Gonadotropin-releasing hormone agonist.

#### Surgery

- Dilation and curettage (D&C)
- Endometrial Ablation
- Uterine artery embolization (UAE)
- Hysteroscopic myomectomy to remove fibroids

## Amenorrhea (Absence of Menstruation)

Amenorrhea is the absence of menstruation. There are two categories: *primary* amenorrhea and *secondary* amenorrhea. These terms refer to the time when menstruation stops.

- *Primary amenorrhea* occurs when a girl does not begin to menstruate by 16 years of age. Girls who show no signs of sexual development (breast development and pubic hair) by the age of 13 should be evaluated by a doctor. Any girl who does not have her period by 15 years of age should be evaluated for primary amenorrhea.
- *Secondary amenorrhea* occurs when periods that were previously regular, stop for at least 3 months.

# Oligomenorrhea (Light or Infrequent Menstruation)

Oligomenorrhea is a condition in which menstrual cycles are infrequent, greater than 35 days apart. It is very common in early adolescence and does not usually indicate a medical problem.

When girls first menstruate they often do not have regular cycles for several years. Even healthy cycles in adult women can vary by a few days from month to month. Periods may occur every 3 weeks in some women, and every 5 weeks in others. Flow also varies and can be heavy or light. Skipping a period and then having a heavy flow may occur; this is most likely due to missed ovulation rather than a miscarriage.

## *Causes*

Normal causes of skipped or irregular periods include pregnancy, breastfeeding, hormonal contraception, and perimenopause. Skipped periods are also common during adolescence, when it may take a while before ovulation occurs regularly. Consistently absent periods may be due to the following factors:

- **Delayed puberty:** A common cause of primary amenorrhea (absence of periods) is delayed puberty due to some genetic factors that delay physical development. Failure of ovarian development is the most common cause of primary amenorrhea.
- **Hormonal changes and puberty:** Oligomenorrhea (light or infrequent menstruation) is commonly experienced by girls who are just beginning to have their periods.
- **Weight loss and eating disorders:** Eating disorders are a common cause of amenorrhea in adolescent girls. Extreme weight loss and reduced fat stores lead to hormonal changes that include low thyroid levels (hypothyroidism) and elevated stress hormone levels (hypercortisolism). These changes produce a reduction in reproductive hormones.
- **Polycystic ovarian syndrome (PCOS):** PCOS is a condition in which the ovaries produce high amounts of androgens (male hormones), particularly testosterone. Amenorrhea or oligomenorrhea is quite common in women who have PCOS.
- **Endometriosis:** Endometriosis, and adenomyosis, can cause severe pelvic pain especially during menstruation. In endometriosis, cells from the tissue that lines the uterus grow in sites outside the uterus. In adenomyosis, these endometrial cells grow within and become attached to the muscular walls of the uterus.
- **Elevated prolactin levels (hyperprolactinemia):** Prolactin is a hormone produced in the pituitary gland that stimulates breast development and milk production in association with pregnancy. High levels of prolactin (hyperprolactinemia) in women who are not pregnant or nursing can reduce gonadotropin hormones and inhibit ovulation, thus causing amenorrhea.
- **Premature ovarian failure (POF):** POF is the early depletion of follicles before age 40. In most cases, it leads to premature menopause. POF is a significant cause of infertility.
- **Structural problems:** In some cases, structural problems or scarring in the uterus may prevent menstrual flow. Inborn genital tract abnormalities may also cause primary amenorrhea.
- **Stress:** Physical and emotional stress may block the release of luteinizing hormone, causing temporary amenorrhea.
- **Athletic training:** Amenorrhea or oligomenorrhea associated with vigorous activity may be related to stress and weight loss. Female athletes who use anabolic steroids will often have amenorrhea or oligomenorrhea.
- **Other medical conditions:** Epilepsy, thyroid problems, celiac sprue, metabolic syndrome, and Cushing's disease are associated with amenorrhea.

## Treatment

- In some women, nutritional deficiencies induced by dieting can cause amenorrhea. Such women should eat a properly balanced diet.
- In some women, excessive bodyweight can be the cause of amenorrhea. These women should restrict the amount of fat in their diet, and they should exercise moderately to maintain an ideal bodyweight.
- More than 8 hours of vigorous exercise a week may cause amenorrhea. A moderate exercise program may restore normal menstruation.
- In women with anorexia nervosa or excessive weight loss, normal menstrual cycles can often be restored by undergoing treatment to restore and maintain a healthy bodyweight.
- If amenorrhea is caused by emotional stress, finding ways to deal with stress and conflicts may help.
- Maintaining a healthy lifestyle by avoiding alcohol consumption and cigarette smoking is also helpful.

Some causes of amenorrhea can be managed by medical (drug) therapy. Examples include the following:

- **Dopamine agonists** such as Bromocriptine or pergolide (cabergoline), are effective in treating hyperprolactinemia. In most women, treatment with dopamine agonist's medications restores normal ovarian endocrine function and ovulation.
- **Hormone replacement therapy** consisting of an estrogen and a progestin can be used for women in whom estrogen deficiency remains because ovarian function cannot be restored.
- **Metformin (glucophage)** is a drug that has been successfully used in women with PCOD to induce ovulation.
- In some cases, **oral contraceptives** may be prescribed to restore the menstrual cycle and to provide estrogen replacement to women with amenorrhea who do not wish to become pregnant. Before administering oral contraceptives, withdrawal bleeding is induced with an injection of progesterone or oral administration of 5–10 mg of Medroxyprogesterone for 10 days.
- In case of anatomical abnormalities of the genital tract, surgery may be indicated.

## Cryptomenorrhea

**Cryptomenorrhea** also known as hematocolpos is a condition where menstruation occurs but is not visible due to an obstruction of the outflow tract. Specifically, the endometrium is shed, but a congenital obstruction such as a vaginal septum or on part of the hymen retains the menstrual flow.

The patient usually presents at the age of puberty when the commencement of menstruation blood gets collected in the vagina and gives rise to symptoms.

### Symptoms

Eugonadotropic primary amenorrhea and cyclical lower abdominal pain are the chief presenting complaints of hematocolpos. Patient may be brought in emergency urinary retention.

### Signs

- Abdominal examination: Swelling is felt on palpation.
- On vulval inspection: A tense, bulging, bluish membrane is seen, this finding varies according to the thickness of the obstructing membrane. It may be absent in patients with complete or partial vaginal agenesis.
- On rectal examination: A large bulging mass is felt.

## Investigations

It can be easily diagnosed on ultrasound, vagina is seen filled with blood and uterus is pushed upward. Associated hematosalpinx and hematometra may be seen.

## Complications

- Hematometra (collection of blood in the uterine cavity)
- Hematosalpinx (collection of blood in fallopian tubes)
- Endometriosis in long-standing cases
- In severe, untreated forms, infertility and urinary retention

## Treatment

A simple cruciate incision followed by excision of tags of hymen allows drainage of the retained menstrual blood. A thicker transverse vaginal septum can be treated with Z-plasty. A blind vagina will require a partial or complete vaginoplasty. Hematosalpinx may require laparotomy or laparoscopy for removal and reconstruction of affected tube. Infertility may require assisted reproductive techniques.

# Dysfunctional Uterine Bleeding

Dysfunctional uterine bleeding (DUB) is abnormal bleeding from the vagina that is due to changes in hormone levels.

## Causes

Dysfunctional uterine bleeding (DUB) most commonly occurs when the ovaries do not release an egg. Changes in hormone levels cause abnormal menstruation such as later or earlier and sometimes heavier than normal.

The cause can be psychological stress, weight (obesity, anorexia or a rapid change), exercise, endocrinopathy, neoplasm, drugs or it may be otherwise unknown.

## Signs and Symptoms

- Bleeding or spotting from the vagina between periods
- Periods that occur less than 28 days apart (more common) or more than 35 days apart
- Time between periods changes each month
- Heavier bleeding (such as passing large clots, needing to change protection during the night, soaking through a sanitary pad or tampon every hour for 2–3 hours in a row)
- Bleeding lasts for more days than normal or for more than 7 days

Other symptoms caused by changes in hormone levels may include:

- Excessive growth of body hair in a male pattern (Hirsutism)
- Hot flushes
- Mood swings
- Tenderness and dryness of the vagina

A woman may feel tired or have fatigue if she is losing too much blood over time. This is a symptom of anemia.

## Examination and Investigations

The health care provider will do a pelvic examination and may perform a Pap smear. Tests that may be done include:

- Complete blood count (CBC)
- Blood clotting profile
- Hormone tests
  - Follicle stimulating hormone (FSH)
  - Luteinizing hormone (LH)
  - Male hormone (androgen) levels
  - Prolactin
  - Progesterone
- Thyroid function tests
- Pap smear and culture to look for infection

Health care provider may recommend the following:

- Biopsy to look for infection, precancer, or cancer, or to help decide on hormone treatment
- Hysteroscopy, to look into the uterus through the vagina
- Transvaginal ultrasound to look for problems in the uterus or pelvis

## Possible Complications

- Infertility
- Severe anemia due to plenty of blood loss over time
- Increased risk for endometrial cancer

## Management

Management of dysfunctional uterine bleeding predominantly consists of reassurance, though mid-cycle estrogen and late-cycle progestin can be used for mid- and late-cycle bleeding respectively. Drug of choice is progesterone.

Nonspecific hormonal therapy such as combined high-dose estrogen and high-dose progestin can be given. Ormeloxifene is a nonhormonal medication that treats DUB but is only legally available in India.

The goal of therapy should be to arrest bleeding, replace lost iron to avoid anemia, and prevent future bleeding. A hysterectomy may be performed in some cases.

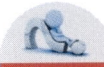

## ASSESS YOURSELF

### FREQUENTLY ASKED QUESTIONS IN EXAMS

1. Describe the development of female sex organs during puberty in detail.
2. Describe menstrual cycle along with diagram.
3. Enlist menstrual disorders. Explain in detail about dysmenorrhea.
4. Write short notes on:
   - Premenstrual syndrome
   - Dysfunctional uterine bleeding
   - Amenorrhea

### MULTIPLE CHOICE QUESTIONS

1. The first sign of puberty in girls is:
   a. Breast budding
   b. Growth spurt
   c. Menarche
   d. Pubic and axillary hair growth

2. The sequence of development of puberty in girls:
   a. Pubarche, thelarche, menarche
   b. Thelarche, pubarche menarche
   c. Menarche, thelarche, pubarche
   d. Pubarche, menarche, thelarche

3. Puberty occurs in girls between the age of:
   a. 10–14 years
   b. 10–12 years
   c. 14–16 years
   d. 8–12 years

4. Gonadal sex of the fetus is determined by:
   a. Secretion of testosterone
   b. Secretion of anti-Mullerian hormone
   c. Sex determining region on the Y chromosome
   d. Secretion of estrogen

5. Increased LH: FSH ratio is found in:
   a. Premature menopause
   b. Sheehan's syndrome
   c. Turner's syndrome
   d. Polycystic ovary syndrome

6. DES causes the following defects, except:
   a. Renal anomalies
   b. Parafimbrial cyst
   c. T-Shaped uterus
   d. Vaginal adenosis

7. Commonest cause of primary amenorrhea is:
   a. Genital tuberculosis
   b. Ovarian dysgenesis
   c. Müllerian duct anomalies
   d. Hypothyroidism

8. Menorrhagia means:
   a. Heavy bleeding
   b. Bleeding more than 7 days
   c. Bleeding with clots
   d. All of the above

9. Metrorrhagia means:
   a. Bleeding at irregular intervals
   b. Bleeding at regular interval
   c. Heavy bleeding
   d. Prolonged bleeding

10. Physical and emotional symptoms that occurs one to two weeks before menstruation is called:
    a. Premenstrual syndrome
    b. Dysfunctional uterine bleeding
    c. Menopausal symptoms
    d. None of the above

11. **Periods that were previously regular, and then stopped for at least 3 months indicate:**
    a. Secondary amenorrhea
    b. Primary amenorrhea
    c. Oligomenorrhea
    d. Dysmenorrhea

12. **Drug that has been successfully used in women with PCOD to induce ovulation:**
    a. Metformin
    b. Dopamine agonists
    c. Estrogen therapy
    d. All of the above

13. **Sexual infantilism is associated with:**
    a. Pituitary tumor
    b. Gonadal aplasia
    c. Dwarfism
    d. All of the above

14. **Gynecomastia is seen in:**
    a. Secondary syphilis
    b. Lepromatous leprosy
    c. HIV
    d. Klinefelter's syndrome

15. **When menstruation occurs but is not visible due to an obstruction of the outflow tract is called:**
    a. Cryptomenorrhea
    b. Dysmenorrhea
    c. Menorrhagia
    d. Amenorrhea

 **Answer Key**

| 1. a | 2. b | 3. a | 4. b | 5. d | 6. a | 7. b |
|------|------|------|------|------|------|------|
| 8. d | 9. a | 10. a | 11. a | 12. a | 13. d | 14. b & d |
| 15. a | | | | | | |

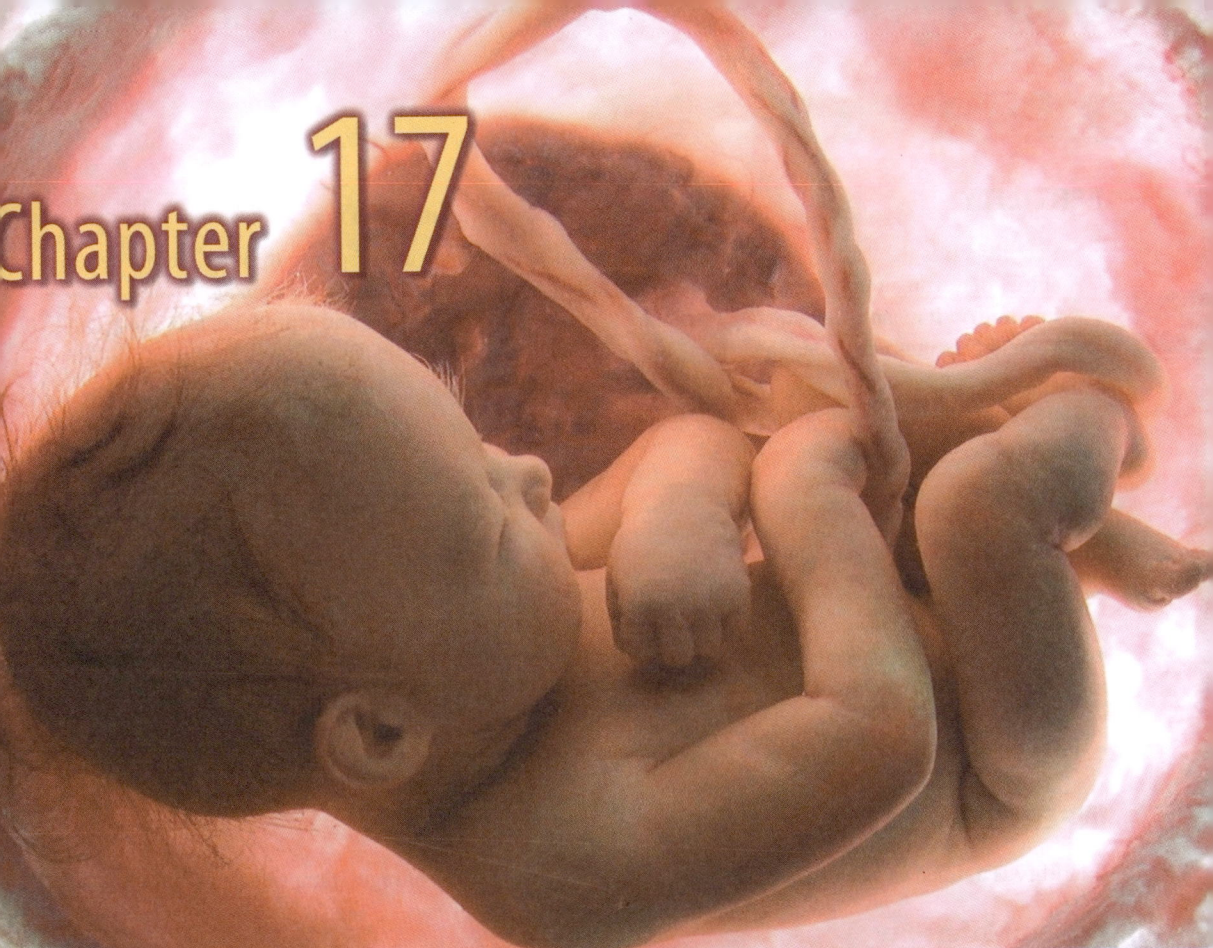

# Chapter 17

# Fertility and Infertility

## Learning Objectives

**Upon completing this chapter, the learner will be able to:**

➡ Define the terms fertility and infertility
➡ Describe the causes of male and female infertility
➡ Enumerate the investigations for infertility
➡ Explain the management of male and female infertility
➡ Understand the artificial reproductive techniques and their complications

## Chapter Outline

▲ Fertility
▲ Infertility

▲ Assisted Reproductive Technology

# FERTILITY

- **Fertility:** It is the "ability" of a man and a woman to reproduce an offspring. In other words, it is the ability of a woman to get pregnant and the ability of a man to make a woman pregnant.
- **Fecundity:** It means if a man and a woman utilize their fertility powers and reproduce, they are fecund. Fecundity is thus calculated in terms of the number of babies a couple has (Birth rate).

*Note that a man and woman might be fertile, i.e. capable of reproduction, but could not conceive (via protected sex, birth control pills, etc.) and hence would not be fecund. The other way round is not true for if a couple is fecund, they have to be fertile.*

## Factors Required for Fertility

- Healthy spermatozoa should be deposited high in the vagina at or near the cervix.
- Capacitation and acrosome reaction: Spermatozoa should undergo changes and acquire motility in cervical canal.
- **Motility:** Spermatozoa should ascend through the cervix into the uterine cavity and fallopian tubes.
- **Ovulation:** Ovum should reach the fimbriated end of the tube.
- Patent fallopian tube.
- Transportation of fertilized ovum to uterine cavity in 3–4 days.

# INFERTILITY

Infertility is defined as a failure to conceive within one or more years of regular unprotected coitus.

## Types of Infertility

- **Primary infertility:** Denotes couples who have never been able to conceive
- **Secondary infertility:** Indicates previous pregnancy but failure to conceive subsequently

## Causes of Infertility

- **Causes of male infertility** (Figs 1A to C)
  - *Endocrinal disorders*
    - Pituitary failure (tumor, radiation, surgery)
    - Hypothalamic dysfunction
    - Exogenous androgens
    - Hyperprolactinemia (drug, tumor)
    - Thyroid disorders
    - Adrenal hyperplasia
    - Gonadotropin deficiency
  - *Sexual dysfunction*
    - Retrograde ejaculation
    - Impotence
    - Decrease libido
  - *Anatomic disorders*
    - Congenital absence of vas deferens
    - Undescended testis

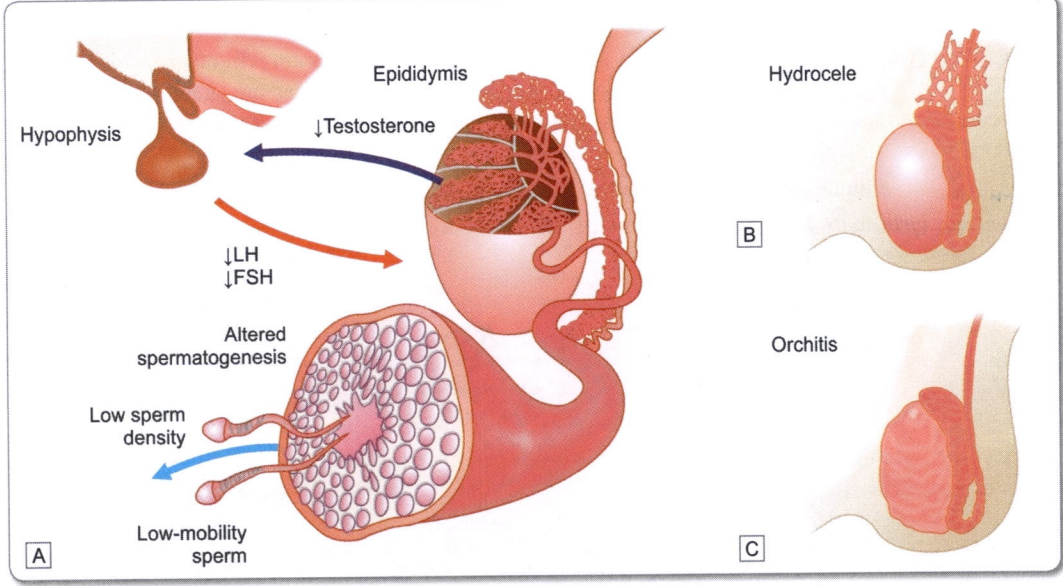

**Figs 1A to C:** Causes of male infertility

- ○ Hypospadias
- ○ Obstruction of vas deferens
- ○ Congenital abnormalities of ejaculatory system
- *Abnormal spermatogenesis*
  - ○ Chromosomal abnormalities
  - ○ Mumps orchitis, gonorrhea, tuberculosis
  - ○ Cryptorchidism
  - ○ Chemical or radiation exposure
- *Abnormal motility*
  - ○ Absent cilia
  - ○ Varicocele
  - ○ Antibody formation
- *Genetic factors*
  - ○ 47 XXY
  - ○ Y-chromosome deletions
  - ○ Single gene mutations
- *Toxins*
  - ○ Drugs
  - ○ Smoking
  - ○ Radiation
- *Surgery*
  - ○ Herniorrhaphy
  - ○ Vasectomy
  - ○ Bladder neck surgery

- **Causes of female infertility** (Fig. 2)
  - *Ovarian factors*
    - Central defects
      - Chronic hyperandrogenemic anovulation
      - Hyperprolactinemia (drugs, tumor, etc.)
      - Hypothalamic insufficiency
      - Pituitary insufficiency (trauma, tumor, congenital)

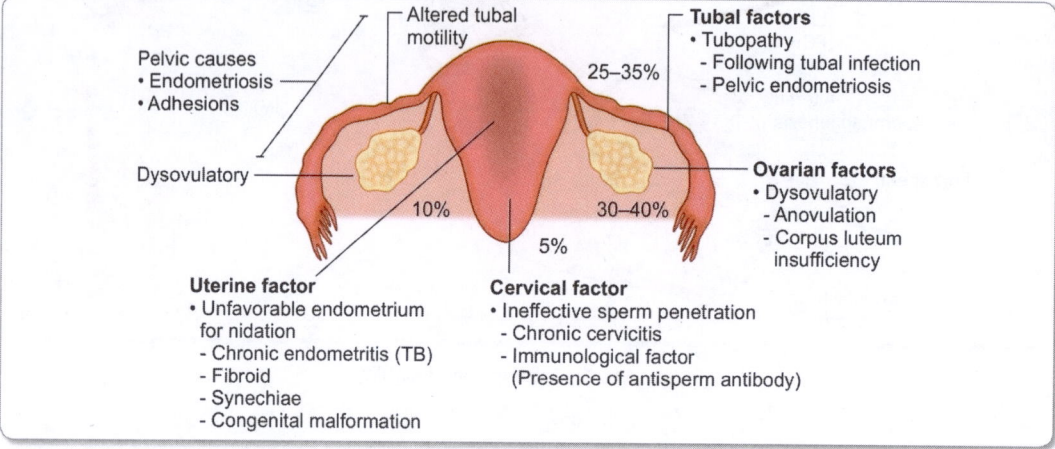

**Fig. 2:** Causes of female infertility

  - Peripheral defects
    - Gonadal dysgenesis
    - Premature ovarian failure
    - Ovarian tumor
    - Ovarian resistance
  - Metabolic disease
    - Thyroid disease
    - Liver disease
    - Renal disease
    - Obesity
    - Androgen excess, adrenal or neoplastic
  - *Tubal and peritoneal factors*
    - Peritubal adhesions
    - Endosalpingeal damage
    - Previous tubal surgery or sterilization
    - Salpingitis
    - Tubal or peritoneal endometriosis
    - Polyps within the lumen
    - Tubal spasm
  - *Uterine factors*
    - Uterine hyperplasia
    - Inadequate secretary endometrium

- o Fibroids
- o Endometritis
- o Uterine synechiae
- o Congenital malformations
- ■ *Cervical factors*
  - o Chronic cervicitis
  - o Presence of antisperm antibodies
  - o Congenital elongation of cervix
  - o Second degree uterine prolapse
  - o Acute retroversion of uterus
  - o Occlusion or cervical canal with polyp
  - o Pinhole os
  - o Scanty vaginal mucus
  - o Abnormal constituents in the mucus
- ■ *Vaginal factors*
  - o Atresia
  - o Septum
  - o Narrow introitus
- ■ *Pelvic factors*
  - o Infection
  - o Appendicitis
  - o Pelvic inflammatory disease
  - o Uterine adhesions
  - o Endometriosis
  - o Structural abnormalities
    - ♦ Diethylstilbestrol exposure
    - ♦ Failure of normal fusion of the reproductive tract
    - ♦ Myoma
- ■ *Combined factors*
  - o Age more than 35 years
  - o Infrequent intercourse during fertile period
  - o Apareunia and dyspareunia
  - o Anxiety and apprehension
  - o Use of lubricants during intercourse
  - o Immunological factors

## Investigations for Female Infertility

### *History Taking*

- **History:** Age, duration of marriage, sexual history, social habits, alcohol, smoking, etc.
- **Medical history:** Tuberculosis, sexually transmitted infections (STIs), pelvic inflammatory disease and diabetes.
- **Surgical history:** Abdominal or pelvic surgery that cause peritubal adhesions.
- **Menstrual history:** Duration of cycle, irregular/regular, amount of menstrual flow, any complication during menstruation.

- **Previous obstetric history:** In the case of secondary infertility, history of previous pregnancies, intervals, premature rupture of membranes or puerperal sepsis are taken.
- **Contraceptive practice:** Use of intrauterine contraceptive device (IUCD), oral pills, history of abortion can affect fertility pattern.
- **Sexual problems:** Dyspareunia and loss of libido.

## Examination

- **General examination**
  - Obesity
  - Too thin
  - Abnormal hairy growth
  - Underdevelopment of secondary sexual characteristics
- **Systemic examination**
  - Hypertension
  - Heart disease
  - Chronic renal lesions
  - Endocrinopathies
- **Gynecological examination:** To assess
  - Vaginal infection
  - Adequacy of hymenal opening
  - Length of cervix
  - Uterine size and shape
  - Presence of adnexal mass/nodules in the pouch of Douglas
  - Any cervical or vaginal discharge, lesion, etc.

## Diagnostic Tests

- **Basal body temperature:** Progesterone has a central thermogenic effect and elevates basal body temperature by an average of 0.8°C during the luteal phase.
- **Pelvic ultrasonography:** It gives evidence for ovulation. In the follicular phase, the developing follicles can be monitored to maturation and subsequent rupture.
- **Cervical mucus:** Within 48 hours of ovulation, cervical mucus changes under the influence of progesterone to become thicker, tacky and cellular, with loss of crystalline fern pattern on drying.
- **Hormone estimation**
  - Serum progesterone
  - Serum luteinizing hormone (LH)
  - Serum estradiol
  - Urinary LH
- **Endometrial biopsy:** To assess secretary changes are due to the action of progesterone on the estrogen - primed endometrium
  - **Laparoscopy examination** of recent corpus luteum or detection of the ovum from the aspirated peritoneal fluid to the pouch of Douglas is the direct evidence of ovulation
  - **Insufflation test (Rubin test)** to see the patency of fallopian tubes
  - **Hysterosalpingography** to detect the site of block in the tube, any abnormality in the uterus such as fibroid or synechiae
  - **Laparoscopic chromotubation** to detect pelvic inflammatory disease (PID), endometriosis and pelvic adhesions along with tubal patency.

## Investigations of Male Infertility

### History Taking and Examination

- **History:** Age, duration of marriage, history of previous marriage and proven fertility, if any are to be noted. Obtain sexual history, social habits, smoking and alcohol consumption habits.
- **Medical history:** STIs, mumps orchitis after puberty, diabetes, recurrent chest infection or bronchiectasis.
- **Surgical history:** Herniorrhaphy, operation on testes, etc.
- **Physical Examination:** To determine the general state of health.
- **Reproductive examination:** Includes inspection and palpation of the genitalia, testicular volume (measured by orchidometer), presence of varicocele should be elicited in the upright position.

### Investigations

- **Routine investigations** include urine and blood examination including postprandial sugar.
- **Semen analysis:** This should be the first step in investigation because if some gross abnormalities are detected, the couple should be counseled for the need of assisted reproductive technology (ART).
- **Hormonal testing** includes serum follicle stimulating hormone (FSH), LH, testosterone, prolactin and thyroid stimulating hormone (TSH).
- **Testicular biopsy** is done to differentiate primary testicular failure from obstruction as a cause of azoospermia or severe oligospermia.
- **Transrectal ultrasound** is done to visualize the seminal vesicles, prostate and ejaculatory ducts obstruction.
- **Vasogram** is a radiographic study done to evaluate the ejaculatory duct obstruction.
- **Postcoital test** is done to determine the number of active spermatozoa in the cervical mucus and length of sperm survival (in hours) after intercourse.
- **Sperm penetration assay:** These assays compare the ability of sperm to penetrate the zona-free hamster egg.
- **Sperm antibodies:** The immunobead test is mostly used and considered positive when only 20% or more of motile spermatozoa have immunobead binding.
- **Genetic testing:** Genetic abnormalities are relatively common causes of abnormal semen characteristic. Approximately 15% of azoospermic men and 5% of severe oligospermic men will have an abnormal karyotype.
- **Immunological tests:** Two types of antibodies that are detected: sperm agglutinating and sperm immobilizing.

## Management of Infertility

Management in fertility or subfertility would depend upon the cause, duration of marriage, age of the couple, environmental factors, etc.

### General Instructions

Instruct the couple regarding:

- **Weight optimization:** Overweight and underweight both affect the fertility. Therefore, achieving a normal body mass index (BMI) with appropriate diet and exercise regime is an important adjuvant for infertility management.
- **Environmental toxins:** Smoking and use of tobacco should be discouraged.

- **Stress management:** Instruct the couple to adopt different coping strategies to manage infertility- related stress, like yoga, meditation, listening music, and talk with friends/family members, etc.
- **Ideal intercourse frequency:** Instruct the couple to perform sexual intercourse during the period of ovulation.

- Use of at home "fertility monitor" and checking of vaginal mucus discharge to determine the optimal timing of intercourse may be most helpful.
- Do not use lubricants and douches.
- **Use of LH surge kit:** Use of kit can detect LH surge in urine by getting a deep blue color of dipstick. The test is performed between 12th and 16th day of regular cycle and timed intercourse over 24–36 hours after the color change reasonably succeeds to conception.
- Avoid the use of hormone by both partners as it affects fertility pattern.
- Provide psychological assurance to the infertile couple because they get more disturbed as the investigation progresses.

## *Management of Male Infertility*

- **General care**
  - Improve the health condition by adopting following measures:
    - Achieve a normal BMI with appropriate diet and exercise
    - Avoidance of alcohol and heavy smoking
    - Do not wear tight and synthetic undergarments
    - Avoidance of occupation that may elevate testicular temperature
  - Do not use medications that interfere with spermatogenesis such as
    - Cytotoxic drugs
    - Nitrofurantoin
    - Cimetidine
    - Anticonvulsant
    - Antidepressant
    - Beta blockers
- **Medications to treat specific causes:**
  - Dopamine antagonist (cabergoline) for hyperprolactinemia and altered testosterone level and to improve libido, potency and fertility
  - Human chorionic gonadotropin (hCG) hormone for hypogonadism
  - Gonadotropin releasing hormone (GnRH) therapy for hypogonadism
  - Antibiotic for genital tract infection
  - Clomiphene citrate to increase serum levels of FSH, LH and testosterone.
- **Special treatments for identified causes, like**
  - In vitro fertilization (IVF)
  - Intrauterine insemination (IUI)
  - Intracytoplasmic sperm injection (ICSI)
  - Artificial insemination with donor sperm
- **Surgical treatment**
  - If the testicular biopsy shows normal spermatogenesis, destruction of vas must be suspected. It is corrected by vasoepididymostomy or vasovasostomy.
  - Correction of hydrocele.
- **Impotency**
  - Psychosexual treatment.
  - Hyperprolactinemia needs further investigation and treatment.
  - **In case of erectile dysfunction:** Sildenafil (25–100 mg) or tadalafil (10–20 mg) is given.
  - Implanted devices, known as prostheses, can restore erection.

- **For ovulatory dysfunction**
  - Stimulation of ovulation
    - Clomiphene citrate
    - Letrozole
    - Human menopausal gonadotropin (hMG)
    - FSH
    - Insulin sensitizing agents
    - GnRH
  - *Correction of biochemical abnormality*
    - **Hyperinsulinemia:** Metformin
    - **Androgen excess:** Dexamethasone
    - **Prolactin raised:** Bromocriptine
  - *Substitution therapy*
    - **Hypothyroidism:** Thyroxin
    - **Diabetes mellitus:** Antidiabetic drugs
- **Surgery**
  - **For tubal adhesions:** Tubotubal anastomosis
  - **For polycystic ovarian disorder:** Laparoscopic ovarian drilling (LOD) or laser vaporization
  - **For tubal blockage:** Cannulation and balloon tuboplasty
  - **Fimbrial adhesion:** Fimbrioplasty
  - **For separation or division of division:** Adhesiolysis
  - **In case of complete tubal blockage:** Salpingostomy
  - **Ovarian/Adrenal tumor:** Surgical removal

## ASSISTED REPRODUCTIVE TECHNOLOGY

Assisted reproductive technology (ART) encompasses all methods used to achieve pregnancy by artificial or partially artificial means. It involves manipulation of gametes and embryos outside the body for the treatment of infertility. In ART, the process of intercourse is by passed either by IUI or fertilization of the oocytes in the laboratory environment as in IVF. Table 1 enlists the different ART techniques.

**TABLE 1: Different ART techniques**

| | |
|---|---|
| **IVF-ET** | *In vitro* fertilization and embryo transfer |
| **GIFT** | Gamete intrafallopian transfer |
| **ZIFT** | Zygote intrafallopian transfer |
| **POST** | Peritoneal oocyte and sperm transfer |
| **TET** | Tubal embryo transfer zone |
| **SUZI** | Subzonal insemination |
| **ICSI** | Intracytoplasmic sperm injection |
| **AH** | Assisted hatching |
| **IVM** | *In vitro* maturation of oocyte |
| **PGD** | Preimplantation genetic diagnosis |
| **Cryopreservation gestational surrogacy** | Embryo/oocyte/ovarian tissue/sperm |

## Sperm Retrieval Techniques

- **TESE:** Testicular sperm extraction
- **MESA:** Microsurgical epididymal sperm aspiration
- **PESA:** Percutaneous epididymal sperm aspiration

## In vitro Fertilization/Embryo Transfer

During IVF, mature oocytes from stimulated ovaries are retrieved transvaginally under ultrasonic guidance. Sperm and ova are then combined *in vitro* to prompt fertilization. If fertilization is successful, viable embryos are transferred transcervically into the endometrial cavity.

### Patient Selection

- Age <35 years
- Presence of ovarian reserve
- Husband → normal seminogram
- Couple must be screened negative for human immunodeficiency virus (HIV)/hepatitis
- Normal uterine cavity as evaluated by hysteroscopy/sonohysterography

### Indications of IVF

- Tubal disease or block
- Endometriosis
- Cervical hostility
- Unexplained infertility
- Ovarian failure

## Gamete Intrafallopian Transfer

It is similar to IVF but in this egg and sperm are placed via catheter through the fimbria and deposited directly into the fallopian tube via laparoscopy. **The prerequisite for GIFT procedure is to have normal uterine tubes** (Fig. 3).

### Indication

Same as IVF except the tubal factors.

## Zygote Intrafallopian Transfer

In this, eggs are removed from the women's ovaries and fertilized in the laboratory. The resulting zygote is then placed in the fallopian tube following one day *in vitro* fertilization through laparoscope (Fig. 4).

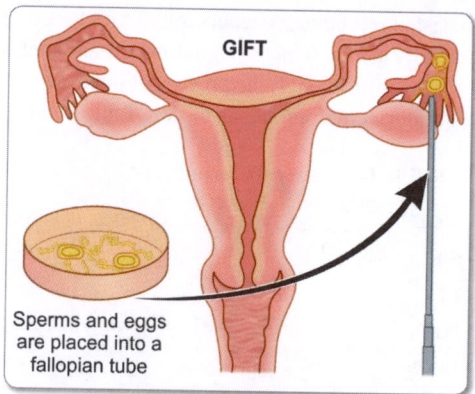

**Fig. 3:** Gamete intrafallopian transfer (GIFT)

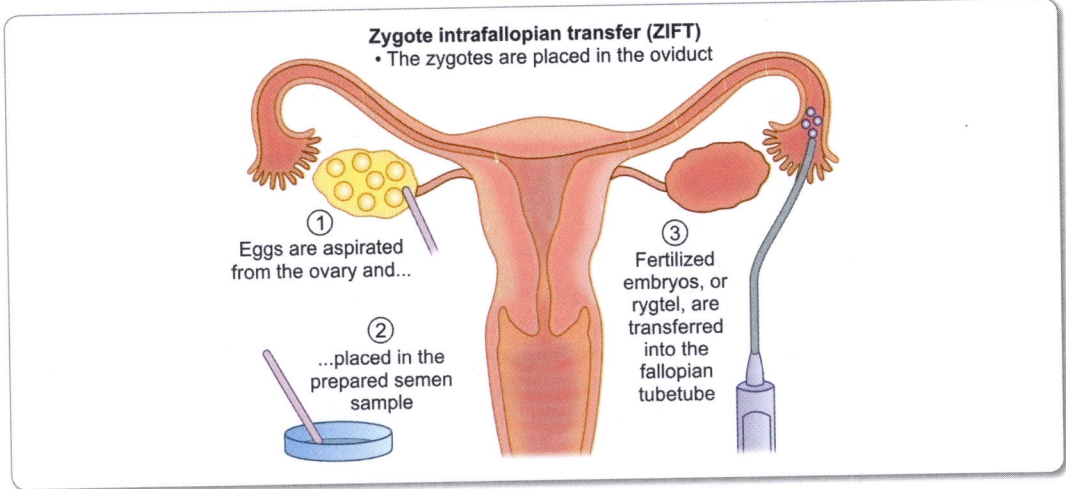

**Zygote intrafallopian transfer (ZIFT)**
• The zygotes are placed in the oviduct

① Eggs are aspirated from the ovary and...

② ...placed in the prepared semen sample

③ Fertilized embryos, or rygtel, are transferred into the fallopian tubetube

**Fig. 4:** Zygote intrafallopian transfer

### Indication and Prerequisite

Same as GIFT.

## Intracytoplasmic Sperm Injection

This procedure is done in case of male infertility where the sperm counts are very low or failed fertilization with previous IVF attempts.

In this procedure, single sperm is injected carefully into the center of an egg using a microneedle. Sperm is retrieved from the ejaculate or by testicular sperm extraction (TESE) or by microsurgical epididymal sperm aspiration (MESA) (Fig. 5).

### Indications

- Severe oligospermia
- Asthenospermia, teratospermia
- Presence of sperm antibodies
- Congenital absence of vas (bilateral)
- Obstruction of efferent duct
- Failure of fertilization in IVF

Clamp

Needle    Sperm    Egg cell (ovum)

**Fig. 5:** Intracytoplasmic sperm injection

## Embryo/Oocyte Donation

Egg donation is employed in the following circumstances:

- Infertility with ovarian failures or diminished ovarian reserve
- When offspring would be at risk for maternally genetic disease
  The oocytes are collected from sister, family members or friends. Oocyte donor, like the semen donor must be screened for infection and genetic disease. Successful implantation needs a perfect coordination of embryo and the endometrium. Estrogen therapy is started at the same time when the donor gets

cycle stimulation. Progesterone treatment in the recipient generally begins on the day the donor undergoes ovum retrieval. Generally, $D_3$ embryos are transferred on the fourth day of progesterone therapy.

## Preimplantation Genetic Diagnosis

In this technique 1 or 2 cell from a developing embryo is removed at 6–8 cell stage to screen for single gene defect and chromosomal disorders.

## Cryopreservation

- **Embryo cryopreservation:** In IVF, many eggs are retrieved to have ultimately one to three healthy embryos for transfer. This frequency leads to extra embryos. Successful freezing and thawing of embryo has been proved so that extra embryos can be freezed with cryopreservation which can be used in next cycle, without the need for ovarian stimulation and egg retrieval.
- **Cryopreservation of ovarian tissue:** Restoration of reproductive function of a woman undergoing chemotherapy or radiation therapy is possible these days with the help of cryobiology. Cryopreservation of ovarian tissue or auto transplantation may allow natural pregnancy later on. With this method, ovulation using exogenous gonadotropins can be achieved.
- **Oocyte cryopreservation:** It is an alternative method and done by freezing. Verification, using high concentration of cryoprotectant can solidify cells without ice formation. Human pregnancies and deliveries from vitrified mature oocytes have been recorded.

## Gestational Surrogacy

A woman without a functional uterus (developmental or hysterectomy) can have her genetic offspring with the help of ART. Embryos are transferred to the uterus of another woman who is willing to carry the pregnancy on behalf of the infertile couple.

## Causes of Failure of ART

- Less than optimal ovarian stimulation because of advanced maternal age and diminished ovarian reserve
- Poor fertilization
- Poor embryos quality because of advanced maternal age
- Poor technique of oocyte retrieval or embryo transfer
- Inadequate uterine receptivity

## Complications of ART

- Birth defect
- Increased rate of miscarriage
- Multiple pregnancy
- Ectopic pregnancy
- Increased changes of hydatidiform mole
- Increased rate of perinatal morbidity and mortality
- Chances of developing ovarian hyperstimulation syndrome
- Psychological stress/anxiety among couple

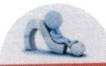

## ASSESS YOURSELF

### FREQUENTLY ASKED QUESTIONS IN EXAMS

1. **Define the following terms:**
   - a. Fertility
   - b. Infertility
   - c. Primary infertility
   - d. IVF
   - e. Surrogacy
2. **What are the causes of male and female infertility?**
3. **Describe the management of female infertility.**
4. **Enumerate artificial reproductive techniques and explain in detail about IVF and GIFT.**

### MULTIPLE CHOICE QUESTIONS

1. **When a woman has previous pregnancy but fails to conceive subsequently is called:**
   - a. Primary infertility
   - b. Secondary infertility
   - c. Subfertility
   - d. Sterility
2. **The cause of female infertility is:**
   - a. Hypothalamic insufficiency
   - b. Hyperprolactinemia
   - c. Tubal blockage
   - d. All of the above
3. **Most common indication for IVF is an abnormality in:**
   - a. Uterus
   - b. Fallopian tube
   - c. Anovulation
   - d. Azoospermia
4. **Time of ovulation is detected by:**
   - a. Urine LH
   - b. Urine FSH
   - c. Urine hCG
   - d. Serum Estradiol
5. **Sonosalpingography is done for:**
   - a. Measuring basal body temperature
   - b. To detect pregnancy
   - c. Testing tubal potency
   - d. Determining anovulatory cycle
6. **Drug used for ovulation induction is:**
   - a. Clomiphene citrate
   - b. Danazol
   - c. Cyproterone acetate
   - d. Tamoxifen
7. **The toxin that affects fertility in males:**
   - a. Smoking
   - b. Radiation
   - c. Drugs
   - d. All of the above
8. **The surgery in males that affects fertility:**
   - a. Herniorrhaphy
   - b. Vasectomy
   - c. Bladder neck surgery
   - d. All of the above
9. **Increased FSH level in azoospermic male indicates:**
   - a. Testicular atrophy
   - b. Hypothalamic failure
   - c. Cryptorchidism
   - d. Hypospadias

10. **Ferning pattern of drying cervical mucus suggests the action of:**
    a. Estrogen
    b. Progesterone
    c. Prolactin
    d. Prostaglandins

11. **Side effect of clomiphene citrate includes all except:**
    a. Multiple pregnancy
    b. Increased risk of ovarian cancer
    c. Abnormal vaginal uterine bleeding
    d. Teratogenic effect on offspring

12. **Basal body temperature elevates during the luteal phase by an average of:**
    a. 0.8°C
    b. 0.5°C
    c. 0.9°C
    d. 0.15°C

13. **PESA/MESA is helpful in:**
    a. Pretesticular azoospermia
    b. Testicular azoospermia
    c. Posttesticular azoospermia
    d. Asthenospermia

14. **In case of bilateral tubal blockage, the best treatment is:**
    a. Laparoscopy and hysteroscopy
    b. Hydrotubation
    c. IVF
    d. Tuboplasty

15. **Which is not ART technique?**
    a. GIFT
    b. ZIFT
    c. IVF and ET
    d. Artificial insemination

## Answer Key

| 1. b | 2. d | 3. b | 4. a | 5. c | 6. a | 7. d |
|------|------|------|------|------|------|------|
| 8. d | 9. a | 10. a | 11. d | 12. a | 13. c | 14. a |
| 15. d | | | | | | |

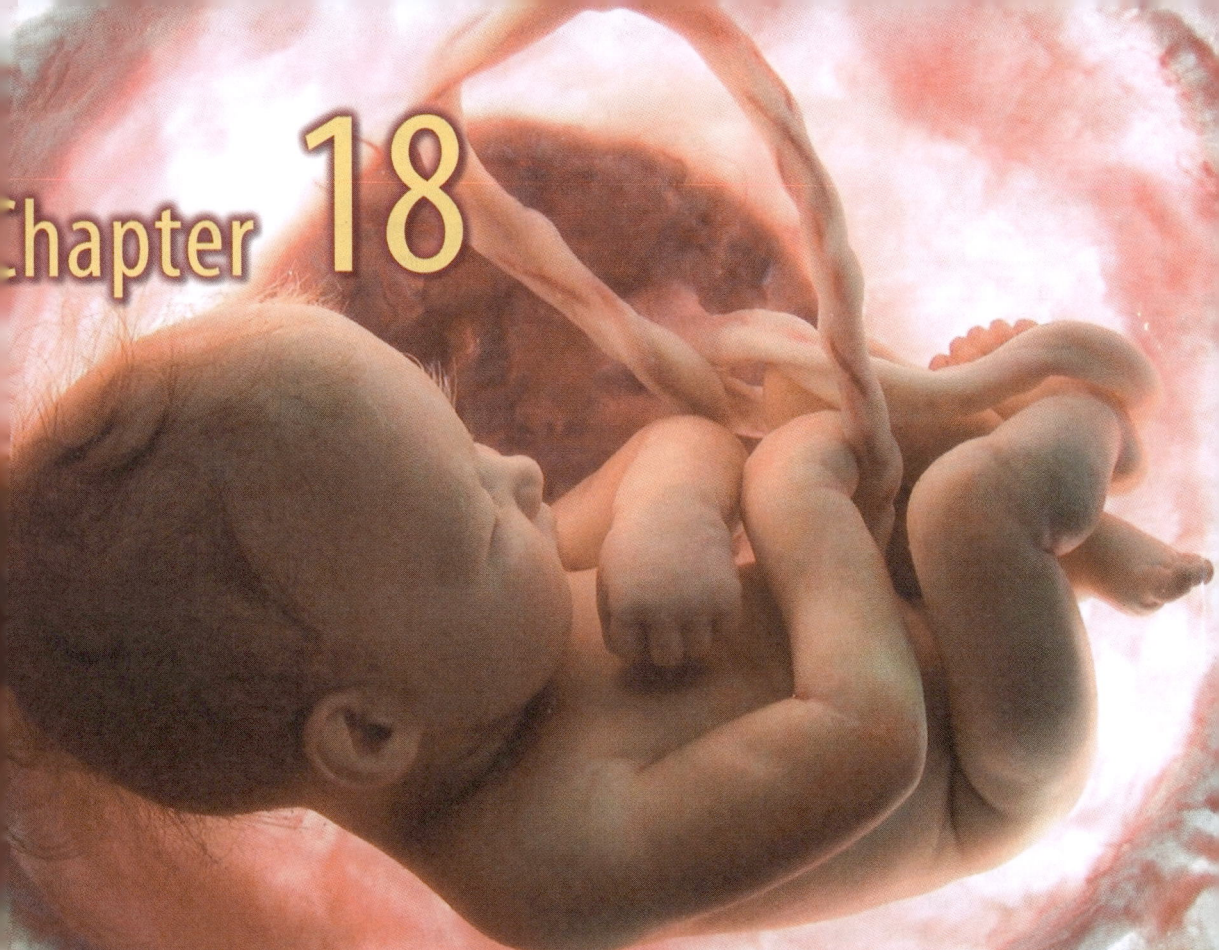

# Chapter 18

# Pelvic Infections

*Learning Objectives* ..............................................................

**Upon completing this chapter, the learner will be able to:**

➡ Understand vulvitis, its causes, signs and symptoms. Explain the preventive measures and treatment of vulvitis
➡ Define salpingitis, signs and symptoms and its treatment
➡ Discuss pelvis abscess in detail
➡ Describe pelvic inflammatory diseases, causes, signs and symptoms, and the treatment in detail
➡ Explain pelvic tuberculosis
➡ Enlist sexually transmitted diseases

# VULVAL INFECTIONS

## Vulvitis

Vulvitis is not a disease, but refers to the inflammation of the soft folds of skin on the outside of the female genitalia, the vulva.

### Causes

Vulvitis can be caused by many factors or irritants, including:

- The use of colored or perfumed toilet paper
- An allergic reaction to bubble bath or soap used to clean the genital area
- Use of vaginal sprays or douches
- Irritation by chlorinated swimming pool or hot tub water
- Allergic reaction to spermicidal cream/preparations
- Allergic reaction to sanitary napkins
- Wearing synthetic underwear or nylon pantyhose without a breathable cotton crotch
- Wearing a wet bathing suit for extended periods of time
- Bike or horseback riding
- Fungal or bacterial infections including scabies or pubic lice
- Herpes
- Skin conditions such as eczema or dermatitis

### Signs and Symptoms of Vulvitis

The symptoms of vulvitis can include:

- Extreme and constant itching
- A burning sensation in the vulvar area
- Vaginal discharge
- Small cracks on the skin of the vulva
- Redness and swelling on the vulva and labia (lips of the vagina)
- Blisters on the vulva
- Scaly, thick whitish patches on the vulva

### Investigations and Diagnosis

A pelvic examination often reveals redness and thickening and may reveal cracks or skin lesions on the vulva. If there is any vaginal discharge, a wet prep test may show that an infection is the cause.

## Complications

Itching of the vulva may be a sign of genital warts [human papilloma virus (HPV)], vulvar dystrophy, or precancerous or cancerous conditions of the vulva.

Sexually transmitted infections (STIs), which can cause vulvitis, may lead to other problems such as infertility. STIs should be treated appropriately.

## Prevention

- Daily cleansing with mild soap, adequate rinsing and thorough drying of the genital area can be helpful.
- Avoid using feminine hygiene sprays, fragrances, or powders in the genital area.
- Avoid wearing extremely tight-fitting pants or shorts, which may cause irritation by constantly rubbing against the skin and reducing air flow.
- Wear cotton underwear or cotton-crotch pantyhose. Avoid underwear made of silk or nylon, because these materials are not very absorbent and restrict air flow. This can increase sweating in the genital area, which can cause irritation and may provide a more welcoming environment for infectious organisms.
- Do not wear sweaty exercise clothing for prolonged periods.
- Infections that may spread by intimate or sexual contact may be prevented or reduced by avoiding sexual activities or using safer sexual behaviors.

## Treatment

- Stopping using any products that may cause irritation. Apply an over-the-counter cortisone ointment two or three times a day on the affected area for up to 1 week. If these methods do not relieve symptoms, consult with health care practitioner.
- Vaginal infections will be treated as appropriate. Cortisone ointment may be used to decrease vulval itching.
- If treatment does not work, biopsy of the skin of the vulva may be done to rule out vulvar dystrophy or vulvar dysplasia, a precancerous condition. A biopsy may also be necessary if any skin lesions are present.

## Bartholinitis

Bartholinitis is a disease characterized by the development of the inflammatory process in the Bartholin's gland.

## Causes

- A **body saturated in toxins,** which accumulate in different areas of the body, like in these glands.
- **Lack of feminine hygiene,** using tight clothing or synthetic fibers.
- **Excessive stress** could cause this inflammation.
- Frequent change of sexual partners, greatly increasing the risk of contracting diseases that are sexually transmitted.
- Due to scratching, rubbing, intertrigo of the genitalia.

### Signs and Symptoms

- Dark red **inflammation** in the area.
- According to the intensity of the infection and if a lump filled with a smelly fluid that has a strong and unpleasant odor.
- Strong pain and burning sensation.
- Pain and inflammation could increase if the woman stands or walks too much.
- Raised body temperature to 39°C.
- Weakness, chills, weakness.

### Prevention

- Observance of the rules of hygiene of external genital organs is of fundamental importance.
- Use of contraceptives during intercourse.
- Timely treatment of foci of chronic infection: urethritis, colpitis, caries, pyelonephritis, etc.
- Annual preventive visit to the gynecologist even in the absence of complaints.
- Avoiding wearing tight underwear, especially synthetic one.
- General strengthening of immunity: full sleep, proper nutrition, sufficiently active way of life, avoidance of hypothermia, etc.

### Treatment

- Treatment depends on the severity of symptoms. If there are no symptoms, no treatment may be needed.
- If a cyst is causing problems, drainage is recommended. The preferred method of drainage is the insertion of a Word catheter. The catheter stays in place for 2–4 weeks, draining the fluid and causing a normal gland opening to form, after which the catheter is removed. The catheters do not generally impede normal activity, but sexual intercourse is generally abstained from while the catheter is in place.
- Cysts may also be opened permanently, a procedure called Marsupialization, in which an opening to the gland is formed with stitches to hold the secretion channel open.
- If a cyst is infected, it may break open and start to heal on its own after 3–4 days. Nonprescription pain medication such as ibuprofen relieves pain, and a Sitz bath may increase comfort. Warm compresses can speed healing. If a Bartholin gland abscess comes back several times, the gland and duct can be surgically removed.

## VAGINAL INFECTIONS

### Vaginitis

Vaginitis refers to inflammation of the vagina that often occurs in combination with inflammation of the vulva, a condition known as vulvovaginitis. Vaginitis is often the result of an infection with yeast, bacteria, or *Trichomonas*, but it may also arise due to physical or chemical irritation of the area.

### Types and causes of Vaginitis

There are several types of vaginitis, depending on the cause. The most common are:

- **Atrophic vaginitis:** The endothelium, or lining of the vagina, gets thinner when estrogen levels decrease during the menopause, making it more prone to irritation and inflammation.
- **Bacterial vaginosis:** This results from an overgrowth of normal; bacteria in the vagina. Patients usually have low levels of normal vaginal bacteria called *lactobacilli*.

- **Trichomonas vaginalis:** Sometimes referred to as trich, it is caused by a sexually transmitted, single-celled protozoan parasite, *Trichomonas vaginalis*.
- **Candida albicans:** A yeast that causes a fungal infection, known as vaginal thrush.

## Risk Factors

Factors that increase the risk of developing vaginitis include:

- Hormonal changes, such as those associated with pregnancy, birth control pills or menopause
- Sexual activity
- Having a sexually transmitted infection (STI)
- Medications, such as antibiotics and steroids
- Use of spermicides for birth control
- Uncontrolled diabetes
- Use of hygiene products such as bubble bath, vaginal spray or vaginal deodorant
- Douching
- Wearing damp or tight fitting clothing
- Using an intrauterine device (IUD) for birth control

## Signs and Symptoms

A woman may have vaginal itching or burning and may notice a discharge. The discharge may be excessive in amount or abnormal in color (such as yellow, gray, or green).

The following symptoms may indicate the presence of infection:

- Irritation and/or itching of the genital area
- Inflammation (irritation, redness, and swelling caused by the presence of extra immune cells) of the labia majora, labia minora, or perineal area
- Vaginal discharge
- Foul vaginal odor
- Pain/irritation with sexual intercourse (dyspareunia)

## Diagnosis

The doctor will carry out a physical examination and ask about medical history. A sample of discharge may be taken to try to determine the cause of the inflammation.

The cause of vaginitis may be diagnosed by checking the appearance of the vaginal fluid, vaginal pH levels, the presence of volatile amines (the gas that causes a bad smell), and the microscopic detection of specific cells.

## Prevention

- Keep the area around your genitals clean and dry.
- Avoid irritating soaps and bath additives, vaginal sprays and douches.
- Change tampons and sanitary napkins frequently.
- Wear loose cotton underwear that does not trap moisture. Avoid nylon underwear.
- After swimming, quickly change wet bathing suit.

Because it is an STI and can be transmitted during sexual activity, the following measures are helpful to prevent this:

- Not having sex (abstinence).
- Having sex with only one uninfected partner.
- Consistently using male latex condoms during sexual intercourse, with or without a spermicide.

### Treatment

A variety of organisms and conditions can cause vaginitis, so treatment targets the specific cause:

- **Bacterial vaginosis:** In this condition administer metronidazole (Flagyl) tablets twice daily or metronidazole (MetroGel) gel or clindamycin (Cleocin) cream.
- **Yeast infections:** Yeast infections usually are treated with an over-the-counter antifungal cream or suppository, such as miconazole (Monistat 1), clotrimazole (Gyne-Lotrimin), butoconazole (Femstat 3) or tioconazole (Vagistat-1). Yeast infections may also be treated with a prescription oral antifungal medication, such as fluconazole (Diflucan).
- **Trichomoniasis:** Physician may prescribe metronidazole (Flagyl) or tinidazole (Tindamax) tablets.
- **Genitourinary syndrome of menopause (vaginal atrophy):** Estrogen in the form of vaginal creams, tablets or rings can effectively treat this condition.
- **Noninfectious vaginitis:** To treat this type of vaginitis, identify the source of the irritation and avoid it. Possible sources include new soap, laundry detergent, sanitary napkins or tampons.

## Trichomoniasis

Trichomoniasis is a sexually transmitted infection of the urogenital tract, is a common cause of **vaginitis** in women, while men with this infection can display symptoms of urethritis. Frothy, greenish vaginal discharge with a musty malodorous smell is characteristic.

### Causes

**Trichomonas vaginalis** is an anaerobic, flagellated protozoan parasite and the causative agent of trichomoniasis (Fig. 1). In women the infection can be found in the vagina and the urethra (tube where urine comes out). In men it can be found in the urethra. The infection is easily passed from one person to another through sexual contact.

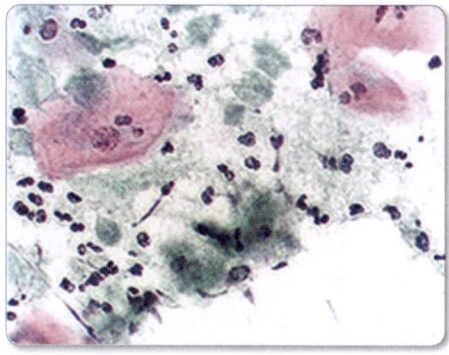

**Risk factors include:**
- History of other STIs
- Previous trichomoniasis infections
- Sex without a condom
- Multiple sexual partners

**Fig. 1:** Pap smear, showing infestation by *Trichomonas vaginalis*

### Signs and Symptoms

**In Women**

- Soreness, inflammation and itching in and around the vagina. This can cause discomfort when having sex.
- A change in vaginal discharge—there may be a small amount or a lot, and it may be thick or thin, or frothy and yellow. There is strong smell that may be unpleasant.
- Pain when passing urine.

**In Men**

- A discharge from the penis, which may be thin and whitish.
- Pain, or a burning sensation, when passing urine.
- Inflammation of the foreskin (this is uncommon).

## Diagnosis

A number of tests can diagnose trichomonas vaginalis, including:

- Examining samples of vaginal fluid (for women) or urethral discharge (for men) under a microscope
- Rapid antigen testing
- Transcription-mediated amplification
- Polymerase chain reaction testing

## Complications

- Preterm delivery.
- Low-birth-weight.
- Increased mortality as well as predisposing to human immunodeficiency virus (HIV) infection, acquired immunodeficiency syndrome (AIDS) and cervical cancer.
- *T. vaginalis* has also been reported in the urinary tract, fallopian tube and pelvis and can cause pneumonia, bronchitis and oral lesions.
- *Trichomonas vaginalis* infection in males has been found to cause asymptomatic urethritis and prostatitis. It may increase the risk of prostate cancer.

## Treatment

Trichomoniasis can be cured with antibiotics. Infection is treated and cured with metronidazole or Tinidazole. The center of disease control and prevention (CDC) recommends a onetime dose of 2 g of either metronidazole or tinidazole as the first-line treatment; the alternate treatment recommended is 500 mL of metronidazole, twice daily, for seven days if there is failure of the single-dose regimen. Do not drink any alcohol for the first 24 hours after taking metronidazole or the first 72 hours after taking tinidazole. It can cause severe nausea and vomiting. Avoid sexual contact for a week.

## Moniliasis/Candidal Vulvovaginitis

Moniliasis also known as **candidal vulvovaginitis** and **vaginal thrush**, is excessive growth of yeast in the vagina that results in irritation.

## Causes

Vaginal yeast infections are typically caused by the yeast species *Candida albicans*. **The causes of excessive** *Candida* **growth are not well understood,** but some predisposing factors have been identified:

- Pregnancy
- Uncontrolled diabetes mellitus
- Broad-spectrum antibiotics (occurs in 28–33%)
- Chemotherapy
- Vaginal foreign body
- Contraceptives may predispose to recurrent vaginal and vulval candidiasis

- Stress
- Lack of sleep
- Hormonal imbalance near menstrual cycle
- Weak immune system
- Poor eating habits including a lot of sugary foods

## Signs and Symptoms

### Signs

- Vulvar erythema, possible with fissuring
- Vulvar edema
- Satellite lesions
- Excoriation

### Symptoms

- Vaginal itching
- Swelling around the vagina
- Burning during urination or sex
- Pain during sex
- Soreness
- Redness
- Rashes
- Whitish gray and clumpy vaginal discharge is another telltale symptom. Sometime discharge looks like cottage cheese

## Investigations

- Routine vaginal swabs are not required.
- In suspected bacterial/resistant or complicated infection, take swabs from the anterior fornix or lateral vaginal wall and send for microscopy, culture and sensitivity.
- Take midstream specimen of urine (MSU) if symptoms could be due to urinary tract infection.

| Do's | Don'ts |
|---|---|
| • Eat a well-balanced diet. | • Wearing tight pants, pantyhose, tights, or leggings. |
| • Eat yogurt or take supplements with lactobacillus. | • Using feminine deodorant or scented tampons or pads. |
| • Wear natural fibers such as cotton, linen, or silk. | • Sitting around in wet clothing, especially bathing suits. |
| • Wash underwear in hot water. | • Sitting in hot tubs or taking frequent hot tub baths. |
| • Replace feminine products frequently. | • Douching. |

## Treatment

### Commence induction treatment

- Either three doses of fluconazole 150 mg (1 × 150 mg dose to be taken every 72 hours); or a topical imidazole treatment for 10–14 days according to response.
- A topical cream may be used in addition to the above for vulvar symptoms.

### Maintenance and further treatment

- Give a prescription for 'treatment as required' or prescribe a 6 months maintenance regimen.
- In either case, review the patient after 6 months.

- Possibilities for the maintenance regimen include:
  - 500 mg intravaginal clotrimazole once weekly.
  - 150 mg oral fluconazole once weekly
  - 50–100 mg oral itraconazole once daily.
- Zafirlukast 20 mg twice daily for six months may also induce remission. This may be an alternative for maintenance prophylaxis, particularly in atopic women.
- Cetirizine 10 mg daily for 6 months has also been shown to induce remission for women in whom fluconazole alone does not provide complete resolution of symptoms.

Approximately 90% of women will remain disease-free at 6 months and 40% at 1 year.

# INFECTIONS OF THE UTERUS, FALLOPIAN TUBES AND OVARIES

## Metritis

**Metritis** is inflammation of the wall of the uterus, whereas **endometritis** is inflammation of the functional lining of the uterus, called the endometrium The term pelvic inflammatory disease (PID) is often used for **metritis**.

### Causes

Endometritis is caused by an infection in the uterus. It can be due to chlamydia, gonorrhea, tuberculosis, or a mix of normal vaginal bacteria. It is more likely to occur after miscarriage or childbirth. It is also more common after a long labor or C-section.

The risk of endometritis is higher after having a pelvic procedure that is done through the cervix. Such procedures include:

- Dilation and curettage (D and C)
- Endometrial biopsy (EB)
- Hysteroscopy
- Placement of an intrauterine contraceptive device (IUCD)
- Endometritis can occur at the same time as other pelvic infections

### Signs and Symptoms

Endometritis typically causes the following symptoms:

- Abdominal swelling
- Abnormal vaginal bleeding
- Abnormal vaginal discharge
- Constipation
- Discomfort when having a bowel movement
- Fever
- General feeling of sickness
- Pain in the pelvis, lower abdominal area, rectal area

### Investigations

The health care provider will perform a physical exam with a pelvic examination. Uterus and cervix may be tender and the provider may not hear bowel sounds. Person may have cervical discharge.

The following tests may be performed:

- Cultures from the cervix for Chlamydia, gonorrhea, and other organisms
- Endometrial biopsy
- Erythrocyte sedimentation rate (ESR)
- Laparoscopy
- WBC
- Wet prep (microscopic examination of any discharge)

## Complications

- Infertility
- Pelvic peritonitis
- Collections of pus or abscesses in the pelvis or uterus
- Septicemia
- Septic shock

## Prevention

Endometritis is caused by STIs. To help prevent endometritis from STIs:

- Treat STIs early.
- Make sure sexual partners are treated in the case of an STI.
- Follow safer sex practices, such as using condoms.

*Women having a C-section may have antibiotics before the procedure to prevent infections.*

## Treatment

- **Antibiotic therapy:** The combination of clindamycin and gentamicin administered intravenously every 8 hours has been considered the criterion standard treatment. The combination of a second- or third-generation cephalosporin with metronidazole is another popular choice.
- Sexual partners may need to be treated if the condition is caused by a sexually transmitted infection (STI).
- Patient may need to be treated in the hospital if symptoms are severe or occur after childbirth.

Other treatments may involve:

- Intravenous fluid therapy
- Bed rest

## Salpingitis

If one or both the fallopian tubes are inflamed, then the condition is medically termed as salpingitis. The inflammation occurs due to infection, and often it has been noted that adjoining lymph node helps with mobility of infectious agent when one fallopian tube affected by infection and that extend to another fallopian tube.

## Causes

The infection usually has its origin in the vagina, and ascends to the fallopian tube from there. Because the infection can spread via the lymph vessels, infection in one fallopian tube usually leads to infection of the other.

## Risk Factors

- Endometrial biopsy
- Curettage
- Hysteroscopy

Another risks are the factors that alter the microenvironment in the vagina and cervix, allowing infecting organisms to proliferate and eventually ascend to the fallopian tube:

- Antibiotic treatment
- Ovulation
- Menstruation
- Sexually transmitted disease (STI)

Finally, sexual intercourse may facilitate the spread of disease from vagina to fallopian tube. Coital risk factors are:
- Uterine contractions
- Sperm, carrying organisms upwards.

## Types

**Salpingitis is of two types: Acute and chronic**

1. **Acute salpingitis:** In this type of salpingitis, the inner lining of the tube is stick together due to sticky fluid is discharged from the infection site. The fallopian tube gradually become reddened and inflamed and may attach with bowel wall.
2. **Chronic salpingitis:** The outbreak of the infection is sudden, but longer duration illness is associated. In this condition the infectious agent stayed in the fallopian tube for prolonged period and causes irritable inflammatory condition. Gradually the infection spread to the ovaries, as tubes become filled with pus and associated tissues are affected. This condition is termed as adhesion.

## Signs and Symptoms

The symptoms usually appear after a menstrual period. The most common are:

- Abnormal smell and color of vaginal discharge
- Pain during ovulation
- Pain during sexual intercourse
- Pain coming and going during periods
- Abdominal pain
- Lower back pain
- Fever
- Nausea and vomiting
- Bloating

## Investigations

- Pelvic examination
- Blood tests
- Vaginal or cervical swab
- Culture of the vaginal discharge

## Complications

- Infertility
- Increased risk of ectopic pregnancy due to damaged oviducts
- Infection of uterus and ovaries
- Infection of sexual partner
- Ovarian abscess
- Scarring of fallopian tubes

## Treatment

- Antibiotic therapy: Antibiotics are the common choice of treatment of salpingitis. For example, (doxycycline and lymecycline)
- Patients should abstain from sex during the treatment, otherwise the infection may persist.
- Both the sexual partners should be tested for STI.
- In serious cases where the antibiotics don't work and the infection persists, fallopian tubes, ovaries and/ or the uterus may need to be removed surgically

# Oophoritis

**Oophoritis** is an inflammation of the ovaries. It is often seen in combination with salpingitis (inflammation of the fallopian tubes). It may develop in response to infection.

## Causes

- Unprotected sexual intercourse
- Multiple sexual partners
- High-risk sexual behavior
- Immunosuppression
- Recent instrumentation of genital tract (endometrial biopsy, IUD placement)
- The partner is having STIs
- Douching also promotes the infection of the uterus and gradually spread to the fallopian tubes and ovaries.
- Infections of the cervix also lead to tubo-ovarian abscess formation

## Signs and Symptoms

In the initial stage the following symptoms are considered:

- The lower abdominal pain on both the sides, especially during menstrual cycle.
- Heavy vaginal bleeding during menstrual cycle
- Discomfort and pain during sexual intercourse
- Foul odor vaginal discharge
- Polyurea (frequent urination)
- Burning sensation during micturition
- Malaise
- During walking lower abdominal discomfort arises
- Pain extends up to the liver

In advanced stage, the following are the symptoms:

- Need to hospitalize the patient due to severe abdominal pain and tenderness
- Fever
- If tubo-ovarian abscess (TOA) become ruptured, then general peritonitis occurs

## Investigations

- **Complete blood count (CBC):** Elevation of the white blood cell count (WBC) to more than 10 K is a nonspecific indicator of infection. Early in the onset, however, the WBC may be normal.
- **Urinalysis:** To rule out cystitis.
- **Urine pregnancy test:** To rule out ectopic pregnancy.
- **Wet prep of cervical discharge:** Shows numerous WBCs and bacteria.
- **Cervical cultures for gonococcus (GC) and *Chlamydia:*** To rule out or diagnose and treat infection with these organisms (immediate results will not be available).
- Pelvic ultrasound may be needed if the physical exam does not allow for a thorough palpation of the adnexa.

## Treatment

### Medical Care

Outpatient treatment is appropriate for patients who are (1) Hemodynamically stable, (2) Reliable to return for follow-up care, (3) Immunocompetent, (4) Not pregnant, (5) Cannot tolerate oral medication due to nausea and vomiting, or (6) Have no evidence of a TOA.

Inpatient treatment is required for patients who (1) have already failed outpatient treatment, (2) are pregnant, (3) are infected with HIV, or (4) have evidence of a TOA.

The treatment method totally depends on patient's condition that how severe the infection and how much patient is affected.

- Initially patient is treated with antibiotic therapy to stop the microbial growth and also to kill the germs.
    - For symptomatic relief, application of hot pad at the lower abdomen. This may help to reduction of pain.
    - Warm bath is also recommended for 2–3 times a day for 10–15 minutes for reduction of the symptoms.
    - Avoidance of douching.
    - Avoidance of sexual activity till the infection becomes cure.

### Surgical Care

Oophoritis may be managed with surgery when medical treatment has shown no amelioration of symptoms after 48–72 hours. Surgical options may include laparoscopy with drainage of the abscess, removal of adnexa, and total abdominal hysterectomy-bilateral sagittal oophorectomy (TAH/BSO). Factors that influence the type of surgery used include the extent of the abscess, the degree of immunocompromised of the patient, and preservation of fertility for future child bearing potential. Interventional radiology can sometimes be used for drainage of abscesses in patients who are not surgical candidates.

## Cervical Erosion

Cervical erosion is a common condition where cells inside the cervical canal grow out and are found on the outer surface of the cervix. This condition is also called vaginal erosion or cervical ectropion. The outer part of the cervix is then left looking eroded, inflamed and infected. It can occur in pregnancy, young women and in menopause.

### Causes

- **Estrogen hormone changes**
- **Vaginal infections:** Some sexually transmitted infections (STIs), e.g., syphilis and herpes are also believed to lead to ulcerations in the cervix.
- **Trauma and inflammation:** For example, sexual intercourse, inserting speculum and other objects into the vagina is believed to be one of the causes of erosion.
- **Chemicals:** Include some contraceptive foams and creams, vaginal douches and even some bath soaps.

### Signs and Symptoms

- Vaginal discharge
- Bleeding after sex and between periods
- Pain
- Infertility

### Treatment

Cervical ectropion does not cause any problems in most women. Pain during and after sexual intercourse can also be a source of distress. These symptoms may require treatment. The general treatments available for cervical erosion are:

- **Cauterization:** Cauterization is used where there is much need to stop bleeding and spotting. The glandular cells are sealed off using this method to stop them from bleeding. Cauterization, also known as diathermy, uses electric current to cauterize the top layer of the bleeding cells.
- **Cryotherapy:** This is a freezing option that uses a cold treatment instead of electric current. Nitrogen oxide compound is used to destroy the bleeding cells and get rid of the symptoms such as bleeding and pain during intercourse.
- **Ablation treatment:** It is performed under local anesthesia. Ablation involves using a preheated probe (100°C) to destroy 3–4 mm of the epithelium.
- **In postpartum erosion:** Observation and re-examination are necessary for 3 months after labor.
- **Antibiotics for infections:** In the case of infections, which are likely to be common due to frequent bleeding in the cervical area, doctor may prescribe antibiotics. While antibiotics are not a direct treatment for cervical erosion, they may help control the infections.

## PELVIC ABSCESS

A pus-filled cavity in the pelvis due to infection. An abscess contains infected pus or fluid, and is walled off by inflammatory tissue.

### Causes

- A burst appendix
- A burst intestine
- A burst ovary
- Inflammatory bowel disease
- Infection in gallbladder, pancreas, ovary or other organs
- Pelvic infection
- Parasite infection

- Pelvic trauma
- Perforated ulcer disease
- Pelvic surgery
- Weakened immune system

## Signs and Symptoms

- Pelvic pain
- Pelvic tenderness
- Fever
- Increased urination frequency
- Diarrhea
- Painful urination
- Mucus in stool
- Malaise
- Anorexia
- Partial obstruction of small intestine
- Rectal mass on examination
- Vaginal mass on examination

## Investigations

- **CBC:** A high white blood cell count is a possible sign of an abscess of other infection.
- Ultrasound.
- Computed tomography (CT)/magnetic resonance imaging (MRI) scanning may be more effective at identifying the origin of the abscess.

## Management

- Arrange urgent admission to hospital.
- Management is usually by drainage of the abscess along with antibiotic treatment. Antibiotics used alone are occasionally effective for very early, small abscesses.
- Antibiotic choice is guided by the likely cause and local resistance patterns and guidelines, but usually needs to be broad-spectrum until the pathogens are determined.
- Procedures used for drainage of the abscess include:
  - Ultrasound-guided aspiration and drainage: Usually the abscess would be rectally drained in men, and in females it would be drained vaginally.
  - CT-guided aspiration and drainage. Percutaneous drainage often uses a trans-gluteal approach.
  - Endoscopic ultrasound-guided drainage.
  - Laparotomy or laparoscopy with drainage of abscess may be required in some cases.
- An abscess which is enlarging suprapubically needs draining urgently.
- In females, the abscess is more difficult to diagnose if coils of bowel lie between the abscess and the posterior fornix and it may have to be drained suprapubically.
- Abscess drainage with adjuvant thrombolytic treatment, such as tissue plasminogen activator (tPA), has been used to aid drainage.
- Definitive surgery may be required after initial drainage for some causes of pelvic abscess, such as appendectomy for abscesses due to appendicitis, or salpingo-oophorectomy for tubo-ovarian abscess.

# PELVIC INFLAMMATORY DISEASE

Pelvic inflammatory disease (PID) is an infection of the female upper genital tract, including the uterus, fallopian tubes and ovaries.

## Causes

Many types of bacteria can cause PID, but gonorrhea or chlamydia infections are the most common. These bacteria are usually acquired during unprotected sex, following childbirth, miscarriage or abortion.

## Risk Factors

- Being a sexually active woman younger than 25-year-old.
- Having multiple sexual partners.
- Being in a sexual relationship with a person who has more than one sex partner.
- Having sex without a condom.
- Douching regularly, which upsets the balance of good versus harmful bacteria in the vagina and might mask symptoms.
- Having a history of pelvic inflammatory disease or a sexually transmitted infection (STIs).

## Signs and Symptoms

- Pain in lower abdomen and pelvis.
- Heavy vaginal discharge with an unpleasant odor.
- Abnormal uterine bleeding, especially during or after intercourse, or between menstrual cycles.
- Pain during intercourse.
- Fever, sometimes with chills.
- Painful or difficult urination.
- Signs of shock, like fainting.
- Nausea and vomiting.

## Investigation

- Pelvic examination: To look for:
  - Bleeding from cervix
  - Fluid coming out of cervix
  - Pain when cervix is touched
  - Tenderness in uterus, tubes, or ovaries
- Lab tests to check for signs of infection:
  - Reactive protein (CRP)
  - Erythrocyte sedimentation rate (ESR)
  - WBC count
  Other tests include:
  - Vaginal or cervical Swab to check for gonorrhea, chlamydia, or other causes of PID.
  - Pelvic ultrasound or CT scan to see what else may be causing these symptoms. Appendicitis or pocket of infection around tubes and ovaries may cause similar symptoms.
  - Pregnancy tests.

## Complications

- Endometritis
- Salpingitis
- Tubo-ovarian abscess (TOA)
- Pelvic peritonitis
- Periappendicitis
- Perihepatitis

## Prevention

Regular testing for sexually-transmitted infections is encouraged for prevention. The risk of contracting pelvic inflammatory disease can be reduced by the following:

- Using barrier methods such as condoms.
- Seeking medical attention if person experiencing symptoms of PID.
- Using hormonal combined contraceptive pills also helps in reducing the chances of PID by thickening the cervical mucosal plug and hence preventing the ascent of causative organisms from the lower genital tract.
- Seeking medical attention after learning that a current or former sex partner has, or might have had a sexually-transmitted infection.
- Getting an STI history from current partner and strongly encouraging they be tested and treated before intercourse.
- Diligence in avoiding vaginal activity, particularly intercourse, after the end of a pregnancy (delivery, miscarriage, or abortion) or certain gynecological procedures, to ensure that the cervix closes.
- Reducing the number of sexual partners.
- Sexual monogamy that restricts sexual activities to two 'virgins' or partners remaining sexually exclusive with each other and having no outside sex partners.
- Abstinence.
- Get regular STI screening tests.
- Do not douche. Douching removes some of the normal bacteria in the vagina that protect the person from infection. Douching may also raise the risk for PID by helping bacteria travel to other areas, like uterus, ovaries, and fallopian tubes.
- Do not abuse alcohol or drugs. Drinking too much alcohol or using drugs increases risky behavior and may put the person at risk of sexual assault and possible exposure to STIs.

## Treatments

- **Antibiotics:** Typical regimens include cefoxitin or cefotetan plus doxycycline, and clindamycin plus gentamicin. An alternative parenteral regimen is ampicillin/sulbactam plus doxycycline.
- **Treatment for partner:** To prevent reinfection with an STI, sexual partner should be examined and treated. Infected partners might not have any noticeable symptoms.
- **Temporary abstinence:** Avoid sexual intercourse until treatment is completed and tests indicate that the infection has cleared in all partners.

# PELVIC TUBERCULOSIS

Pelvic tuberculosis is an infectious disease caused by the bacterium *Mycobacterium tuberculosis* (95%) or *Mycobacterium bovis* (5%). Pelvic tuberculosis is often a silent disease. It is common cause of infertility in developing countries and in Asia. It also creates an adnexal mass, ascites or both and thus can be difficult to distinguish from other PID causes.

The mode of spread is hematogenous or lymphatic and rarely from direct contiguity with an intra-abdominal organ or affected peritoneum. The fallopian tubes are the first and most commonly affected genitals organ followed by endometrium and ovaries.

## Signs and Symptoms

- Irregular menstrual periods
- Pain in the pelvic area
- Vaginal discharge which is heavy, continuous and stained with blood
- Bleeding from vagina after sex
- Severe pain while having sex
- Not able to conceive (infertility)
- Infertility

## Examination and Investigations

- **Hysterosalpingogram:** A hysterosalpingogram is an X-ray of the genital organs of a female. It is used to see tubal blocks. It also shows the peculiar lead pipe appearance of the fallopian tubes if the patient has tuberculous lesions in the tubes.
- **Endometrial biopsy:** A piece of the endometrial tissue is obtained in a laparoscopic procedure. Microscopic examination of the tissue might reveal tubercular bacteria.
- **Culture of menstrual blood:** A menstrual blood can be cultured to find out the presence of tubercular bacteria in the uterus.
- **Blood tests:** Blood tests show increased differential blood count and erythrocyte sedimentation rate.

## Treatment

- **Antibiotic therapy:** A course of antibiotics that lasts about 9 months to 1 year is prescribed. It is essential to complete the entire course in order to get rid of the tuberculosis completely. Although, the chances of recovering from infertility depend on the extent of the damage to the reproductive organs, like tubes and uterus.
- **IVF:** If the tuberculous process has not destroyed the endometrium, *in vitro* fertilization (IVF) can be done following successful anti-tubercular treatment (ATT). Blocked fallopian tubes is the most common cause of patient opting for IVF (*in vitro* fertilization).

# SEXUALLY TRANSMITTED DISEASES

(Already discussed in Chapter 8: Management of Complications during Pregnancy)

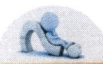

## ASSESS YOURSELF

### FREQUENTLY ASKED QUESTIONS IN EXAMS

1. Define vaginitis, its causes/signs and symptoms. Explain the preventive measures and treatment of vaginitis.
2. Explain in detail about pelvic inflammatory disease.
3. Define pelvic tuberculosis, its causes, signs and symptoms. Explain the management of pelvic tuberculosis.
4. Enlist sexually transmitted diseases.
5. Write short notes on:
   a. Oophiritis
   b. HIV/AIDS
   c. Syphilis

### MULTIPLE CHOICE QUESTIONS

1. A 32-year-old lady come to hospital with chief complaints of profuse vaginal discharge. The diagnosis of bacterial vaginosis is made upon all the following findings except:
   a. Absence of lactobacilli
   b. Abundance of gram variable coccobacilli
   c. Abundance of polymorph
   d. Absence of clue cells

2. Which of the following is the best drug of choice for treatment of bacterial vaginosis in pregnancy?
   a. Clindamycin
   b. Metronidazole
   c. Erythromycins
   d. Kanamycin

3. The cause of vulvitis is:
   a. Vaginal spray
   b. Bubble bath
   c. Synthetic underwear
   d. All of the above

4. Soreness inflammation and hatching of the vagina is the manifestation of:
   a. Salpingitis
   b. Trichomonas vaginalis
   c. Oophritis
   d. Metritis

5. Chlamydial infection is best treated by:
   a. Azithromycin + contact tracing
   b. Metronidazole
   c. Doxycycline + metronidazole
   d. Fluconazole + doxycycline

6. Which of the following is not STD?
   a. Echinococcus
   b. Candida
   c. Herpes
   d. Gonorrhea

7. Asymptomatic carrier of gonococcal infection in female is commonly seen in:
   a. Endocervix
   b. Vagina
   c. Urethra
   d. Fornix

8. Herpes simplex type II causes:
   a. Herpes labials
   b. Common in homosexual
   c. Carcinoma cervix
   d. All of the above

9. Which of the following does chlamydia trachomatis commonly cause:
   a. Malignancy
   b. Amenorrhea
   c. Postcoital bleeding
   d. Infertility

10. TB endometritis is caused by:
    a. Hematogenous spread
    b. Direct spread
    c. Lymphatic spread
    d. Retrograde spread

11. Most common cause of tubal block in India is:
    a. Gonorrhea
    b. Chlamydia
    c. Tuberculosis
    d. Bacterial vaginosis

12. The most common site of genital TB in women is:
    a. Tubes
    b. Uterus
    c. Cervix
    d. Vagina

13. The most common complication of pregnancy after complete treatment of genital tuberculosis is:
    a. Abortion
    b. Ectopic pregnancy
    c. Malpresentation
    d. IUD

14. The most sensitive method for detecting cervical chlamydia trachomatis infection is:
    a. Direct fluorescent antibody test
    b. Enzyme immunoassay
    c. PCR
    d. Culture on irradiated MC Conkey cells

15. Tuberculosis of female genital tract is most common in age group:
    a. Below 10 years
    b. 10–20 years
    c. 20–30 years
    d. Above 60 years

## Answer Key

| 1. c | 2. b | 3. d | 4. b | 5. a | 6. a | 7. a |
|------|------|------|------|------|------|------|
| 8. a | 9. d | 10. a | 11. c | 12. a | 13. b | 14. c |
| 15. c | | | | | | |

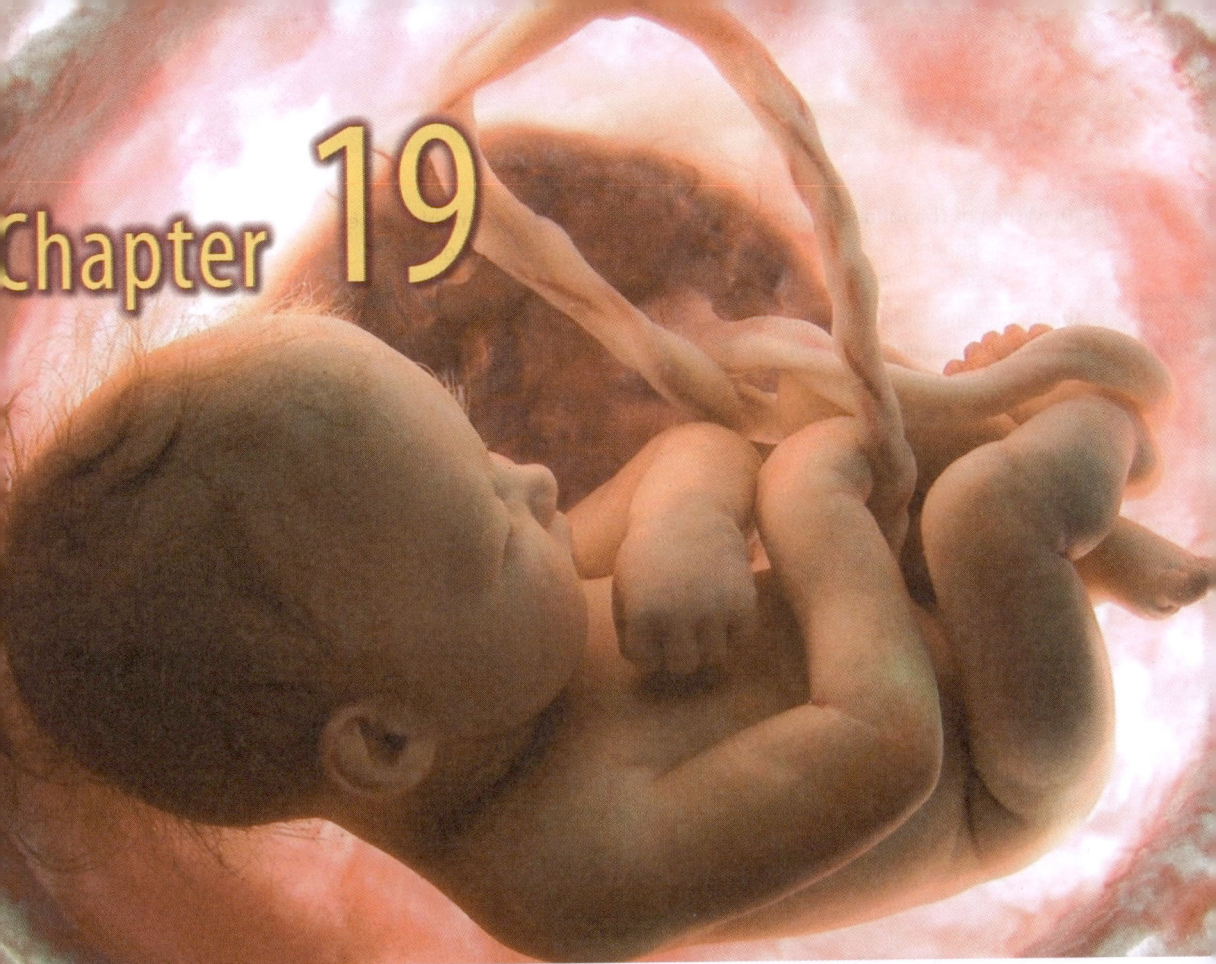

# Chapter 19

# Gynecological Disorders

# UTERUS

The uterus lies in the middle with bladder in the front and rectum behind. It can be described as anteverted with respect to vagina and anteflexed with respect to cervix.

- **Anteverted:** Rotated forward towards the anterior surface of the body.
- **Anteflexed:** Flexed towards the anterior surface of the body. Thus, it lies immediately posterosuperior to the bladder.

## Retroversion

**Retroversion** (Fig. 1) means when the organ or any body part is tilted backwards. A **retroverted** uterus (tilted uterus, tipped uterus) is a uterus that is tilted posteriorly. The uterus is bent backwards so that fundus points toward the sacrum and cervix toward the pubic symphysis.

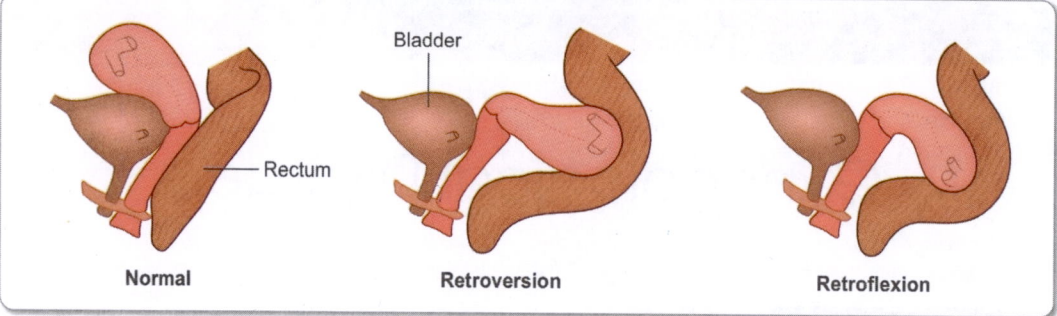

**Fig. 1:** Retroversion and retroflexion

## Retroflexion

**Retroflexion** (Fig. 1) means bending backwards upon itself. The uterus bends at an angle with the cervix, the position of which remains unchanged.

## Causes of Retroverted Uterus

In most cases, a retroverted uterus is genetic. Retroversion of the uterus may occur due to weakening of the pelvic ligaments at the time of menopause. Some cases are caused by pelvic surgery, pelvic adhesions, endometriosis, fibroids, pelvic inflammatory disease or childbirth.

## Signs and Symptoms

Generally, a retroverted uterus does not cause any problem. Problem may be due to associated disorder like endometriosis. A disorder like this could cause the following symptoms:

- Painful sexual intercourse
- Pain during menstruation (particularly if the retroversion is associated with endometriosis).

## Diagnosis

A retroverted uterus is usually diagnosed during a routine pelvic examination or with an internal ultrasound. A rectovaginal examination may be used to distinguish between a mass and a retroverted uterus.

## Prevention

There is no way to prevent the problem. Early treatment of uterine infections or endometriosis may reduce the chances of a change in the position of the uterus.

## Treatment

If a retroverted uterus is causing problems, treatment options can include:

- **Treatment for the underlying condition** such as hormone replacement therapy for endometriosis.
- **Exercises:** If movement of the uterus isn't hindered by endometriosis or fibroids, and if the doctor can manually reposition the uterus during the pelvic examination, exercises may help. However, in many cases, the uterus simply tips backwards again.
- **Pessary:** A small silicone or plastic device can be placed either temporarily or permanently to help prop the uterus into a forward lean. However, pessaries have been linked with increased risk of infection and inflammation. Another drawback is that sexual intercourse is still painful for the woman, and the pessary may cause discomfort for her partner too.
- **Surgery:** Using laparoscopic surgery techniques, the uterus can be repositioned so that it sits over the bladder. This operation is relatively straightforward and usually successful. In some cases, the surgical removal of the uterus (hysterectomy) may be considered.
- **Treatment options for incarcerated uterus** includes hospitalization, the insertion of a urinary catheter to empty the bladder, and a series of exercises (such as pelvic rocking) to help free the uterus.

## FISTULA

A fistula is an abnormal passage or hole that is formed between:

- Two organs in the body
- An organ and skin

   **A vaginal fistula is an** abnormal opening that connects vagina to another organ, such as bladder, colon or rectum that allows stool or urine to pass through vagina.
   **There are several types of vaginal fistulas:**

- **Vesicovaginal fistula:** Also called as bladder fistula, this opening occurs between vagina and urinary bladder (Fig. 2A).
- **Ureterovaginal fistula:** This type of fistula happens when the abnormal opening develops between vagina and ureters.

- **Urethrovaginal fistula:** In this type of fistula, also called a urethral fistula, the opening occurs between vagina and urethra.
- **Rectovaginal fistula:** In this type of fistula, the opening is between vagina and rectum (Fig. 2B).
- **Colovaginal fistula:** With a colovaginal fistula, the opening occurs between the vagina and colon.
- **Enterovaginal fistula:** In this type of fistula, the opening is between the small intestine and the vagina.

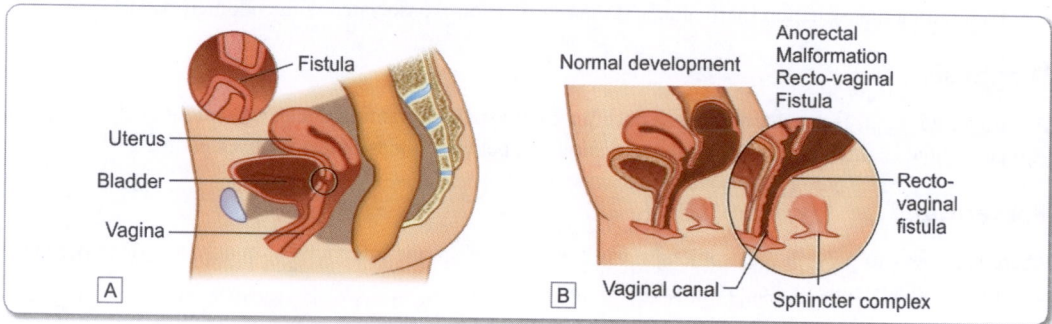

**Figs 2A and B:** **A.** Vesicovaginal fistula; **B.** Rectovaginal fistula

## Causes

- It is often caused by childbirth, when a prolonged labor presses the unborn child tightly against the pelvis, cutting off blood flow to the vesicovaginal wall. The affected tissue may necrotize, leaving a hole.
- Vaginal fistulas can also result from particularly violent cases of rape.
- It can also be associated with hysterectomy, cancer operations, radiation therapy and cone biopsy.
- A vaginal fistula sometimes happens after:
  - Surgery of the back wall of the vagina, the perineum, anus or rectum. Open hysterectomy is linked to most vesicovaginal tract fistulas.
  - Radiation treatment for pelvic cancer.
  - A period of inflammatory bowel disease (including Crohn's disease or diverticulitis).
  - A deep tear in the perineum or an infected episiotomy after childbirth.

## Symptoms

- In case of vesicovaginal fistula, fluid leaking or flowing out of vagina
- In rectovaginal, colovaginal, or enterovaginal fistula, foul-smelling discharge or gas coming from vagina
- Genital area may get infected or sore.

## Diagnosis

- History taking: E.g., any surgery, trauma, or disease that could cause a fistula.
- Physical examination: Doctor will use a speculum to look at the vaginal walls.
- **Other tests, such as:**
  - The use of dye in the vagina (and may be the bladder or rectum) to find all signs of leakage.
  - Urine analysis to check for infection.

- Blood test (complete blood count) to check for signs of infection in body.
- X-ray, endoscopy or magnetic resonance imaging (MRI) to get a clear look and check for all possible tissue damage.

## Complications

- Recurrent fistula formation
- Ureteric injury or obstruction
- Vaginal stenosis
- Reduced bladder capacity
- Irritative lower urinary tract symptoms

## Treatment

Depending on the cause of the fistula, in rare cases, observation and prolonged Foley's catheter drainage with bladder rest may be selected for trial of spontaneous healing. However, in most cases, surgical repair is necessary to repair vesicovaginal fistula.

Before surgery, doctor will see whether the tissue is healthy or needs to heal first.

- Administer medicine or wound care to heal the tissue before surgery.
- In case of inflammatory bowel disease, surgery should be avoided during a symptom flare.
- If there is a large rectovaginal fistula, colostomy will be created first to keep the fistula clear for the surgery. After the fistula repair heals, the colostomy is taken out.

## UTERINE PROLAPSE (PROCIDENTIA)

It is a condition that occurs when the **pelvic floor muscles** are no longer strong enough to support the **uterus.** As a result, the uterus **descends** toward or through the vagina.

### Types of Uterine Prolapse

Uterine prolapse can be categorized as incomplete or complete:

- **Incomplete uterine prolapse:** When an incomplete uterine prolapse occurs, the uterus is partially displaced into the vagina but does not protrude.
- **Complete uterine prolapse:** When a complete uterine prolapse occurs, there is a portion of the uterus protruding out of the vaginal opening.

**Prolapsed uterus (Fig. 3) can be described in the following stages:**

- **First degree:** The cervix descends downward into the vagina.
- **Second degree:** The cervix comes down to the opening of the vagina.
- **Third degree:** The cervix is outside the vagina.
- **Fourth degree:** The entire uterus is outside the vagina. This condition is also called procidentia. This is caused by weakness of all of the supporting ligaments.

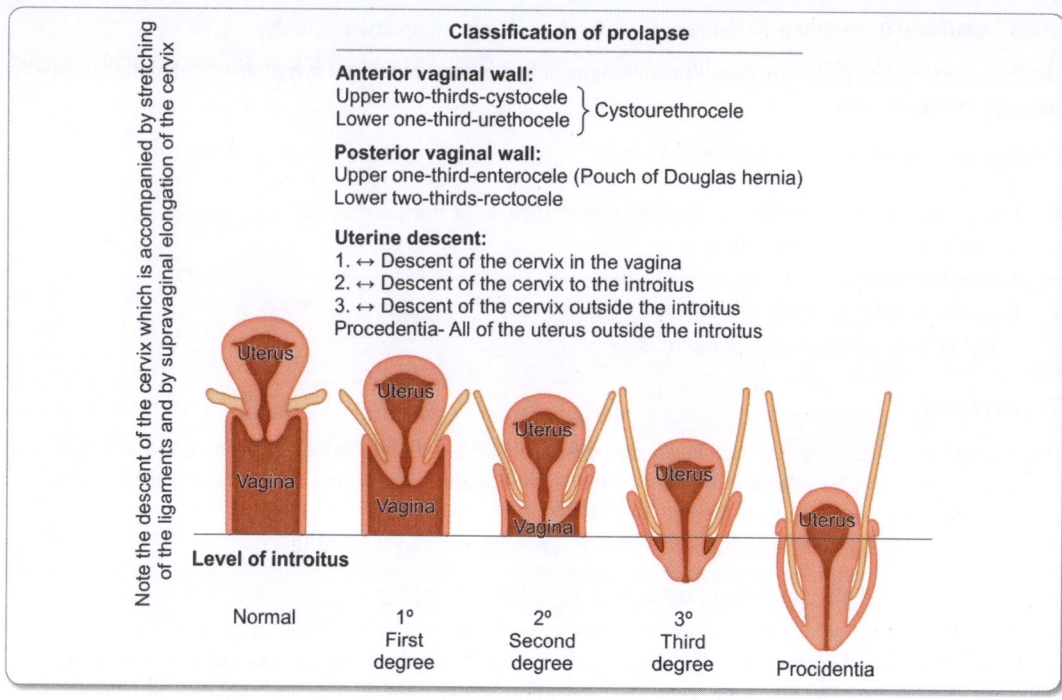

**Classification of prolapse**

**Anterior vaginal wall:**
Upper two-thirds-cystocele
Lower one-third-urethocele } Cystourethrocele

**Posterior vaginal wall:**
Upper one-third-enterocele (Pouch of Douglas hernia)
Lower two-thirds-rectocele

**Uterine descent:**
1. ↔ Descent of the cervix in the vagina
2. ↔ Descent of the cervix to the introitus
3. ↔ Descent of the cervix outside the introitus
Procedentia- All of the uterus outside the introitus

Note the descent of the cervix which is accompanied by stretching of the ligaments and by supravaginal elongation of the cervix

**Level of introitus**

Normal | 1° First degree | 2° Second degree | 3° Third degree | Procidentia

**Fig. 3:** Degrees of uterine prolapse

## Causes

Uterine prolapse results from the weakening of pelvic muscles and supportive tissues. Causes of weakened pelvic muscles and tissues include:

- Pregnancy
- Difficult labor and delivery or trauma during childbirth
- Delivery of a large baby
- Being overweight or obese
- Lower estrogen levels after menopause
- Chronic constipation or straining with bowel movements
- Chronic cough or bronchitis
- Repeated heavy lifting

## Risk Factors

**Factors that can increase the risk of uterine prolapse include:**

- One or more pregnancies and vaginal births
- Giving birth to a large baby
- Increasing age
- Obesity
- Prior pelvic surgery
- Chronic constipation or frequent straining during bowel movements
- Family history of weakness in connective tissue

## Signs and Symptoms

Mild uterine prolapse generally doesn't cause signs or symptoms. Signs and symptoms of moderate to severe uterine prolapse include:

- Sensation of heaviness or pulling in pelvis
- Tissue protruding from vagina
- Urinary problems, such as urine leakage (incontinence) or urine retention
- Trouble having a bowel movement
- Feeling of something coming out of vagina
- Sexual concerns, such as a sensation of looseness in the tone of vaginal tissue

## Complications

- **Cystocele:** A herniation (or bulging) of the upper front vaginal wall where a part of bladder bulges into the vagina, which may lead to urinary frequency, urgency, retention, and retention.
- **Enterocele:** The herniation of the upper vagina along with a segment of small intestine into the vagina. Standing leads to a pulling sensation and backache and is relieved when lying down.
- **Rectocele:** The protrusion forward of the back wall for the vagina, along with concomitant bulging forward of the rectum into the vagina. This may make bowel movements difficult to the point where the woman may need to push on the inside of the vagina to empty the rectum.

## Diagnosis

- The healthcare professional can diagnose uterine prolapse with a medical history and physical examination of the pelvis. The doctor may need to examine the patient in both standing and recumbent positions. She may be asked to cough or strain down to increase the intra-abdominal pressure.
- Specific conditions, such as urethral obstruction due to complete uterine prolapse, may need to be confirmed with an intravenous pyelogram (IVP) or a renal ultrasound. In an IVP, dye is injected into a vein. A series of X-rays is then taken to follow the dye through the urinary tract.
- Ultrasound may also be needed to rule out other pelvic problems. In this test, a probe is passed over the abdomen or inserted into the vagina to create images using sound waves.
- Other imaging tests such as MRI may be used to accurately image the pelvis.

## Prevention

- Repeated childbirth with short intervals cause UV prolapse.
- Woman should be advised to avoid pregnancies in quick succession.

### Labor

In case of uterine prolapse

- 1st stage
  - Avoid bearing down.
  - Breech or forceps delivery before full dilatation of cervix should not be attempted.
- 2nd stage
  - Avoid prolongation of this stage.
  - Perform episiotomy if tears or overstretching of perineum is feared.

- 3rd stage
  - Avoid Crede's method.
  - Episiotomy or tears should be carefully sutured.

## Puerperium

- Treat chronic cough and constipation.
- Avoid strenuous exercises and standing for prolonged time.

## Treatment

1.  **Exercises** (Figs 4A and B)

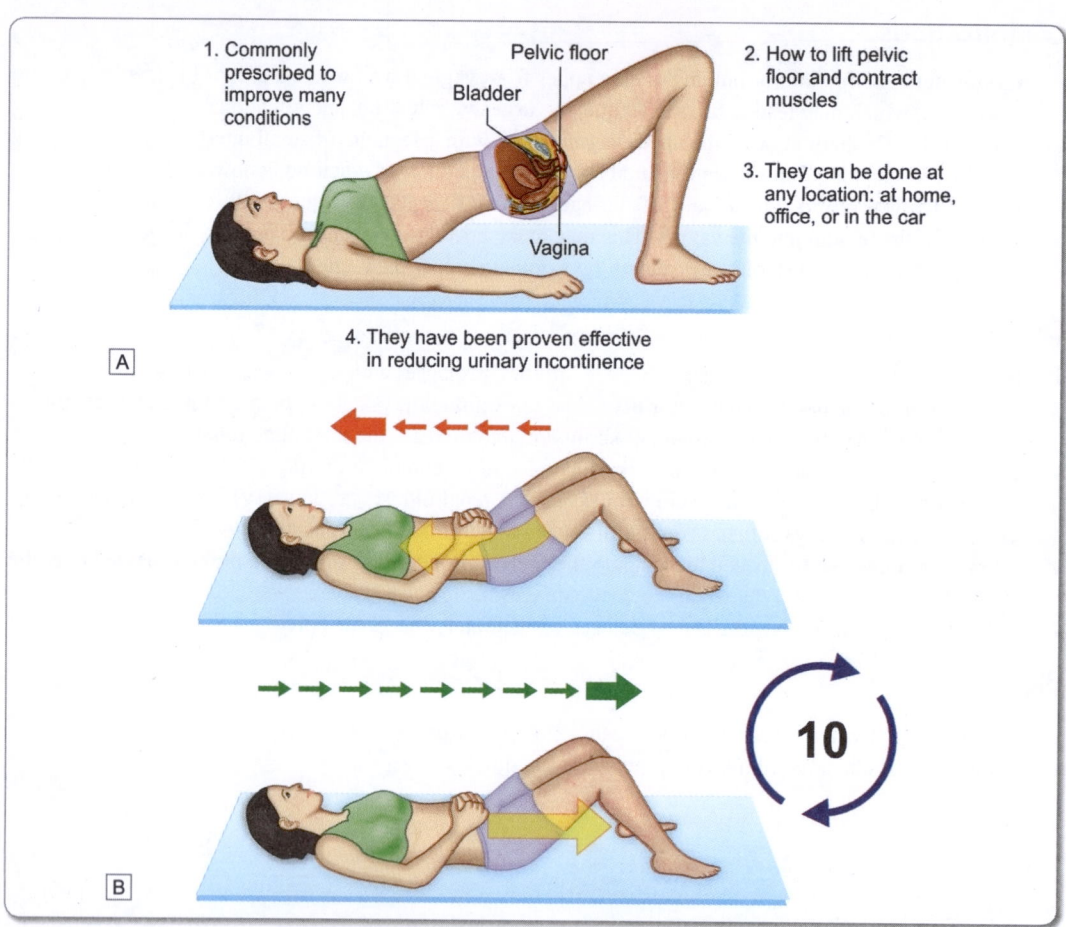

**Figs 4A and B:** Exercises for treatment of uterine prolapse

2.  **Nonsurgical treatment includes:**
    - Losing weight to take stress off pelvic structures.
    - Avoiding heavy lifting.

- Doing Kegel exercises, which are pelvic floor exercises that help strengthen the vaginal muscles
- Taking estrogen replacement therapy (ERT).
- Wearing a pessary, which is a device inserted into the vagina that fits under the cervix and helps push up and stabilize the uterus and cervix (Fig. 5).

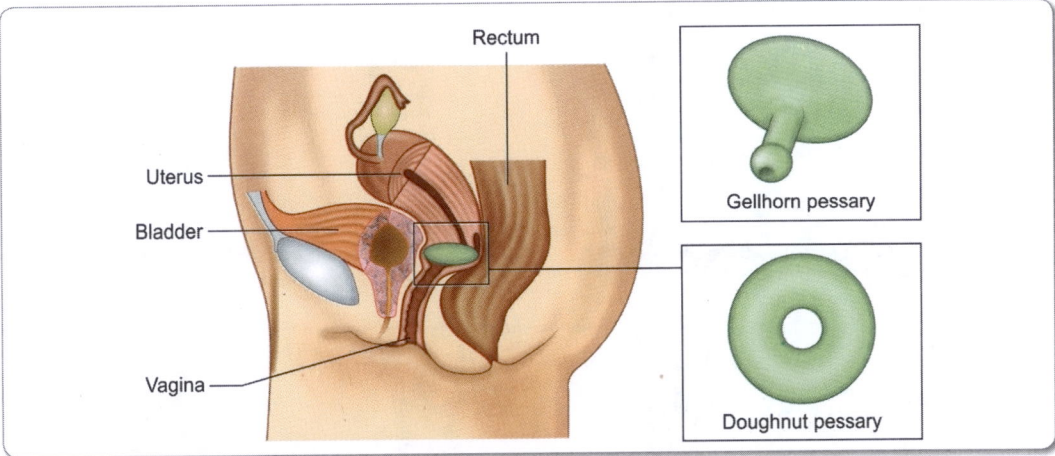

**Fig. 5:** Insertion of pessary

3. **Surgery:**
   - If uterine prolapse is severe, doctor might recommend surgery. Minimally invasive (laparoscopic) or vaginal surgery might be an option. Surgery can involve:
     - **Repair of weakened pelvic floor tissues:** This surgery is generally approached through the vagina but sometimes through the abdomen. The surgeon might graft person own tissue, donor tissue or a synthetic material onto weakened pelvic floor structures to support pelvic organs.
     - **Removal of uterus (hysterectomy):** Hysterectomy might be recommended if uterine prolapse is severe.

## UTERINE MALFORMATIONS

Uterine malformations (Fig. 6) are the result of an abnormal development of the Müllerian ducts during the woman's prenatal development of embryogenesis and they may affect fertility.

According to the classification of the **American Society for Reproductive Medicine**, some of the most common uterine malformations are:

- **Müllerian agenesis or absence of uterus:** This condition is not common and it is characterized by an absence of the Müllerian ducts, which form the uterus, during the prenatal development. Müllerian agenesis is the most serious of uterine malformations and it is frequently accompanied by problems in the development of the cervix and the vagina.
- **Unicornuate uterus:** Only one of the Müllerian ducts develops, therefore the uterus is half its normal size and the woman only has one fallopian tube.
- **Double or didelphys uterus:** Both Müllerian ducts develop but they do not fuse, so the woman has two uterine cavities, each with its own cervix and its own vagina. The woman may have two or more simultaneous pregnancies in both uteri, which have no communication between each other.

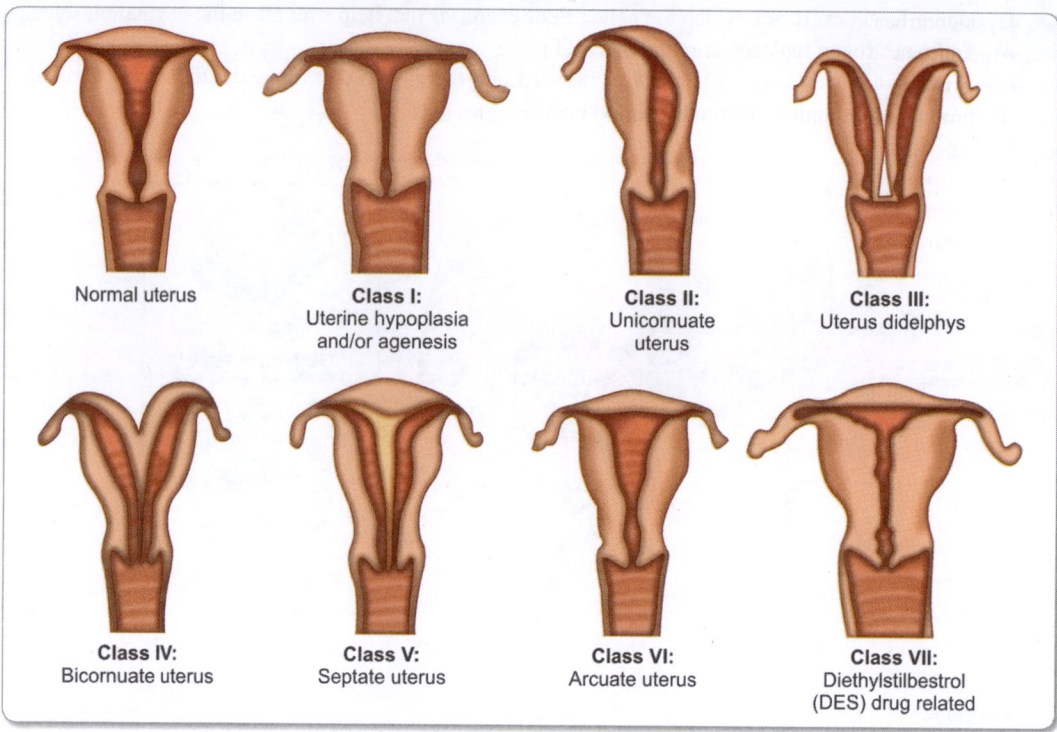

Normal uterus

Class I:
Uterine hypoplasia
and/or agenesis

Class II:
Unicornuate
uterus

Class III:
Uterus didelphys

Class IV:
Bicornuate uterus

Class V:
Septate uterus

Class VI:
Arcuate uterus

Class VII:
Diethylstilbestrol
(DES) drug related

**Fig. 6:** Uterine malformations

- **Bicornute uterus:** Due to an incomplete fusion of the Müllerian ducts, the uterus has a depression at the top, and because of this instead of the usual pear shape, it has the shape of a heart.
- **Septate uterus:** This is the most frequent uterine malformation, with a prevalence of over 50%. In this, the inside of the uterus is divided by a wall or septum that begins at the top of the uterine cavity and can extend to the cervix
- **Arcuate uterus:** It is variant of the septated uterus, in which the septum is much less pronounced. In general, women with an arcuate uterus have no fertility problems.
- **Diethylstilbestrol (DES) uterus:** This malformation is the least common and happens in daughters of women who took diethylstilbestrol during pregnancy. This synthetic estrogen was withdrawn from the market in 1975. However, it was widely used for about a decade to reduce the risk of abortion during the first three months of pregnancy.

## Risk Factors

Uterine malformations are associated with genetic and teratogenic factors. Using uncertified contraceptives (e.g., diethylstilbestrol), and any other substances with teratogenic potential, can be seen as problematic. Fetus is the most vulnerable in the period of 2–12 weeks.

## Signs and Symptoms

- Chronic pelvic pain
- Pain during intercourse (dyspareunia)

- Dysmenorrhea
- Amenorrhea
- Menorrhagia
- Abdominal inflammation especially during menstrual periods
- Endometritis
- Infertility
- Recurrent pregnancy loss
- Premature labor
- Low-birth-weight baby

## Diagnosis

A complete medical history and physical examination may lead us to suspect that a congenital uterine anomaly is present. However, imaging studies, such as a hysterosalpingogram (HSG) and ultrasound, or an MRI are required to visualize the uterus and confirm that a congenital uterine anomaly is present.

## Complications

- Infertility
- Endometriosis
- Hemometra
- Urinary tract anomalies
- Abortions
- Preterm deliveries
- Fetal malformations
- Malpresentation

## Treatment

Many women with uterine anomalies do not require treatment. If pain, miscarriage or infertility is an issue, a physician may recommend correcting the anomaly surgically. Most cases of uterine anomalies can be corrected through minimally invasive techniques, such as laparoscopy or hysteroscopy.

In the instance of a unicornuate uterus, an obstructed hemiuterus can be removed if the other side of the uterus is intact and functional. With a didelphic uterus, surgery is not usually recommended. A uterine septum can be resected in a simple out-patient procedure that combines laparoscopy and hysteroscopy. This procedure greatly decreases the rate of miscarriage for women with this anomaly.

Women who are at risk for preterm delivery or late pregnancy loss due to a uterine anomaly may need a stitch to be placed in the cervix (called a cervical cerclage) to prevent premature dilation.

# CYSTS

Cysts are abnormal, closed sac-like structures within a tissue that contain a liquid, gaseous, or semisolid substance. Cysts can occur anywhere in the body and can vary in size.

## Ovarian Cyst

An ovarian cyst is a fluid-filled sac within the ovary (Fig. 7).

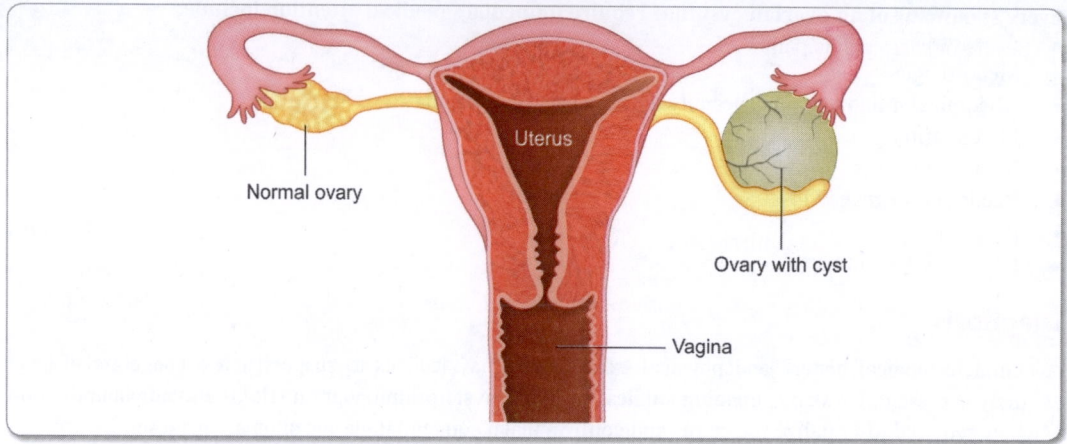

**Fig. 7:** Ovarian cysts

## Types of Ovarian Cysts

- **Functional ovarian cysts:** Cysts that develop as part of the menstrual cycle and are usually harmless and short-lived; these are the most common type of ovarian cyst
- **Pathological ovarian cysts:** Cysts that occur due to abnormal cell growth; these are much less common

## Risk Factors

- History of previous ovarian cysts
- Irregular menstrual cycles
- Infertility
- Polycystic ovarian syndrome
- Endometriosis
- Obesity
- Early menarche (11 years or younger)
- Hyperthyroidism
- Tamoxifen therapy for breast cancer

## Symptoms

Often ovarian cysts do not cause any symptoms. However, symptoms can appear as the cyst grows. Symptoms may include:

- Abdominal bloating or swelling
- Painful bowel movements
- Pelvic pain before or during the menstrual cycle
- Painful intercourse
- Pain in the lower back or thighs
- Breast tenderness
- Nausea and vomiting

**Severe symptoms of an ovarian cyst that require immediate medical attention include:**

- Severe or sharp pelvic pain
- Fever
- Faintness or dizziness
- Rapid breathing

## *Diagnosis*

- **Pelvic and transvaginal ultrasound:** Ovarian cysts are often detected during a pelvic examination. A pelvis ultrasound can allow the doctor to see the cyst with sound waves and help determine whether it comprises fluid, solid tissue, or a mixture of the two. In transvaginal ultrasound, doctor inserts a probe into the vagina in order to examine the uterus and ovaries.
- **Laparoscopic surgery:** During laparoscopic surgery, a doctor will make small incisions and pass a thin scope (laparoscope) through the abdomen. The laparoscope will allow the doctor to identify the cyst and possibly remove or perform biopsy of the cyst.
- **Serum CA-125 assay:** A cancer-antigen 125 (CA-125) blood test can help suggest if a cyst is due to ovarian cancer.
- **Hormone levels:** The doctor may order a pregnancy test and assess hormone levels. Blood tests can also be performed to test for other hormones that may cause polycystic ovarian syndrome.
- **Culdocentesis:** A fluid sample from the pelvis may be taken in order to rule out bleeding into the abdominal cavity. Culdocentesis is performed by inserting a needle through the vaginal wall behind the uterine cervix.
- **Imaging tools used to diagnose ovarian cysts include:**
    - Computed tomography (CT) scan
    - MRI
    - Ultrasound device

## *Treatment*

- **Birth control pills:** If there is occurrence of recurrent ovarian cysts, doctor can prescribe oral contraceptives to stop ovulation and prevent the development of new cysts. Oral contraceptives can also reduce the risk of ovarian cancer. The risk of ovarian cancer is higher in postmenopausal women.
- **Laparoscopy:** If cyst is small and results from an imaging test to rule out cancer, doctor can perform a laparoscopy to surgically remove the cyst. The procedure involves doctor making a tiny incision near navel and then inserting a small instrument into abdomen to remove the cyst.
- **Laparotomy:** In case of a large cyst, doctor can surgically remove the cyst through a large incision in abdomen, conduct an immediate biopsy and if they determine that the cyst is cancerous, hysterectomy to remove ovaries and uterus is performed.

## Bartholin's Cyst

A Bartholin's cyst is a fluid-filled swelling on one of the Bartholin's glands (Figs 8A and B). The Bartholin's glands are on each side of the opening of the vagina, on the lips of the labia. They secrete vaginal lubricating fluid. The fluid helps protect vaginal tissue during sexual intercourse.

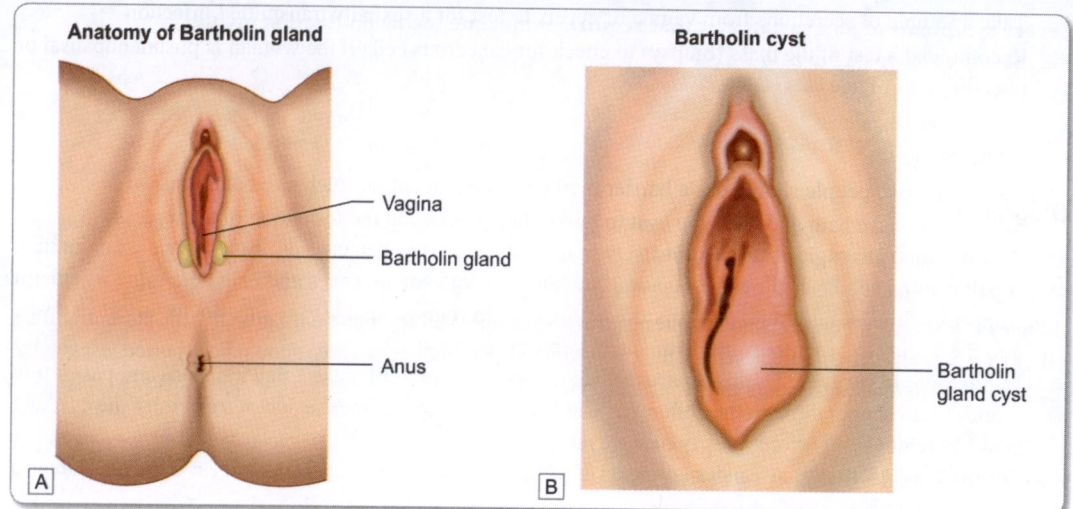

**Figs 8A and B:** Bartholin's cyst—symptoms, risk factors, treatment

## Causes

Cause of a Bartholin's cyst is a backup of fluid. Fluid may accumulate when the opening of the gland (duct) becomes obstructed, perhaps caused by infection or injury, irritation or an extra growth of skin.

In some instances, an infection can lead to the growth of a cyst. Bacteria that can infect a cyst include *Escherichia coli* and bacteria that cause gonorrhea or chlamydia.

**A woman is more likely to have a Bartholin's gland cyst when she is:**

- Young and sexually active
- Nulliparous woman
- Has just had one pregnancy

## Signs and Symptoms

Small Bartholin's cysts may not cause any symptoms. When symptoms occur, they usually include the following:

- A painless, small lump near the opening of the vagina
- Redness near opening of the vagina
- Swelling near the opening of the vagina
- Discomfort during sexual intercourse, walking, or sitting

If the cyst becomes infected, additional symptoms can develop. These include pus draining from the cyst, fever, and chills. When a cyst is infected, it is referred to as an abscess.

## Diagnosis

To diagnose a Bartholin's cyst, doctor may:

- Collect medical history
- Perform pelvic examination

- Take a sample of secretions from vagina or cervix to test for a sexually transmitted infection
- Recommend a test of the mass (biopsy) to check for cancerous cells if the woman is postmenopausal or over 40 years of age

## Prevention

- Sexually active people should use a barrier method of contraception, such as a condom.
- Sitting in a warm bath may help the cyst to burst, thus preventing the formation of an abscess.

## Treatment

If the cyst is small and presents no symptoms, the doctor may recommend no treatment—the patient will be asked to report any growth in the size of the cyst. Any lump in the vaginal area should be reported, especially if the patient has started the menopause.

### Medical Treatment

A doctor may perform a minor procedure where:

- A catheter is inserted into the cyst
- The catheter is inflated to fix it in place
- For 2–4 weeks, fluid is drained by the catheter, and a normal opening is formed

### Other Treatments

- **Marsupialization:** This involves cutting the cyst open and draining the fluid out. The edges of the skin are stitched open for the secretions to come through.
- **Carbon dioxide laser:** This can create an opening to help drain the cyst.
- **Needle aspiration:** A needle is used to drain the cyst. Sometimes, after draining the cyst, the cavity is filled with a 70% alcohol liquid solution for a few minutes before being drained out, to reduce the chances of infection.
- **Gland excision:** If the woman has many recurring cysts and does not respond well to any therapies, the doctor may recommend removing the Bartholin's gland.

## UTERINE FIBROID

Uterine fibroid is the most common benign (not cancerous) tumor of uterus. Fibroids are tumors of the smooth muscle found in the wall of the uterus. They can develop within the uterine wall itself or attach to it. They may grow as a single tumor or in clusters.

### Location and Classification

- **Subserosal fibroids** are located beneath the serosa (the lining membrane on the outside of the uterus). These often appear localized on the outside surface of the uterus or may be attached to the outside surface by a pedicle.
- **Submucosal fibroids** are located inside the uterine cavity beneath the inner lining of the uterus.
- **Intramural fibroids** are located within the muscular wall of the uterus.
- **Cervical fibroids** are located in the wall of the cervix (neck of the uterus). Rarely, fibroids are found in the supporting structures of the uterus that also contain smooth muscle tissue.

Figure 9 shows the classification of uterine fibroid.

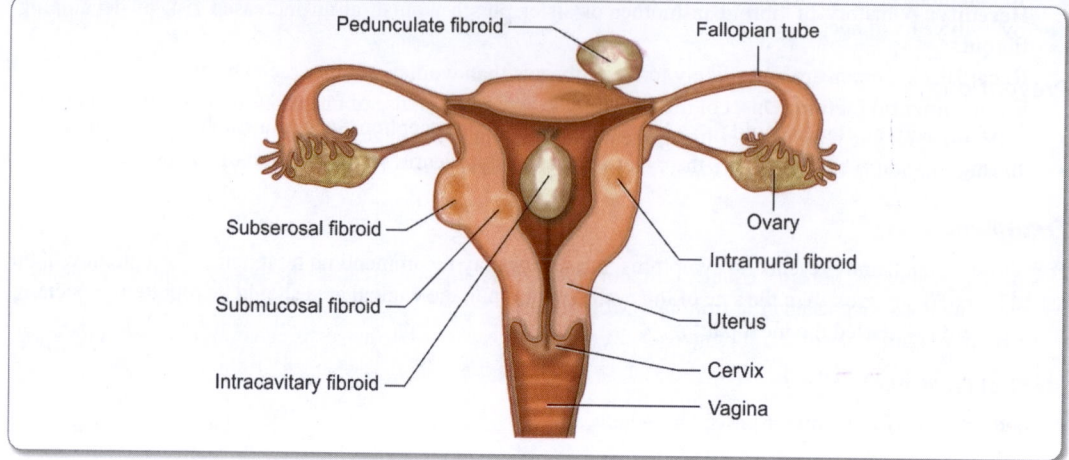

**Fig. 9:** Classification of uterine fibroid

## Signs and Symptoms

- Heavy menstrual bleeding (menorrhagia)
- Increased menstrual cramping
- Menstrual periods lasting more than a week
- Pelvic pressure or pain
- Frequent urination
- Difficulty emptying the bladder
- Constipation
- Backache or leg pain
- Pain during intercourse
- Swelling or enlargement of abdomen.

   **During pregnancy fibroid may also be the cause of:**

- Miscarriage
- Bleeding
- Premature labor
- Interference with the position of the fetus.

## Causes

- **Genetic changes:** Many fibroids contain changes in genes that differ from those in normal uterine muscle cells.
- **Hormones:** Estrogen and progesterone, two hormones that stimulate development of the uterine lining during each menstrual cycle in preparation for pregnancy, appear to promote the growth of fibroids.
- **Other growth factors:** Substances that help the body maintain tissues, such as insulin-like growth factor, may affect fibroid growth.

## Risk Factors

- **Heredity:** A history of fibroid in mother or sister puts a woman at an increased risk of developing fibroid.
- **Race:** Black women are more likely to have fibroids than women of other racial groups
- **Environmental factors:** Onset of menstruation at an early age; use of birth control; obesity; a vitamin D deficiency; having a diet higher in red meat and lower in green vegetables, fruit and dairy; and drinking alcohol, including beer, appear to increase the risk of developing fibroids.

## Complications

- Although uterine fibroids usually are not dangerous, they can cause discomfort and may lead to complications such as anemia from heavy blood loss.
- **Pregnancy and fibroids:** Submucosal fibroids may cause infertility or pregnancy loss. Fibroids may also increase the risk of certain pregnancy complications, such as placental abruption, fetal growth restriction and preterm delivery.

## Diagnosis

Fibroids are most often found during a routine pelvic examination. This, along with an abdominal examination, may indicate a firm, irregular pelvic mass to the physician. In addition to a complete medical history and physical and pelvic and/or abdominal examination, diagnostic procedures for uterine fibroids may include:

- **X-ray**
- **Transvaginal ultrasound**
- **Magnetic resonance imaging (MRI)**
- **Hysterosalpingography** (X-ray examination of the uterus and fallopian tubes that uses dye and is often performed to rule out tubal obstruction).
- **Hysteroscopy** (Visual examination of the canal of the cervix and the interior of the uterus using a viewing instrument [hysteroscope] inserted through the vagina).
- **Endometrial biopsy**
- **Blood test** (to check for iron-deficiency anemia if heavy bleeding is caused by the fibroid).

## Treatment

Since most fibroids stop growing or may even shrink as a woman approaches menopause, the healthcare provider may simply suggest "watchful waiting." With this approach, the healthcare provider monitors the woman's symptoms carefully to ensure that there are no significant changes or developments and that the fibroids are not growing.

In women whose fibroids are large or are causing significant symptoms, treatment may be necessary. Treatment will be determined by healthcare provider(s) based on:

- Patient overall health and medical history
- Extent of the disease
- Patient tolerance for specific medications, procedures, or therapies
- Expectations for the course of the disease
- Patient opinion or preference
- Patient desire for pregnancy

**In general, treatment for fibroids may include:**

- **Hysterectomy:** Hysterectomies involve the surgical removal of the entire uterus.
- **Conservative surgical therapy:** Conservative surgical therapy uses a procedure called a myomectomy. With this approach, doctor will remove the fibroid, but leave the uterus intact to enable a future pregnancy.
- **Gonadotropin-releasing hormone agonists (GnRH agonists):** This approach lowers levels of estrogen and triggers a "medical menopause". Sometimes GnRH agonists are used to shrink the fibroid, making surgical treatment easier.
- **Antihormonal agents:** Certain drugs oppose estrogen (such as progestin and Danazol), and appear effective in treating fibroids. Antiprogestins, which block the action of progesterone, are also sometimes used.
- **Uterine artery embolization (Fig. 10):** Also called uterine fibroid embolization, uterine artery embolization (UAE) is a newer minimally-invasive technique. The arteries supplying blood to the fibroids are identified, and then embolized (blocked off). The embolization cuts off the blood supply to the fibroids, thus shrinking them. Healthcare providers continue to evaluate the long-term implications of this procedure on fertility and re-growth of the fibroid tissue.
- **Myolysis:** In this laparoscopic procedure, radiofrequency energy, an electric current or laser destroys the fibroids and shrinks the blood vessels that feed them. A similar procedure called cryomyolysis freezes the fibroids.
- **Endometrial ablation:** This treatment, performed with a specialized instrument inserted into uterus, uses heat, microwave energy, hot water or electric current to destroy the lining of uterus, either ending menstruation or reducing your menstrual flow.

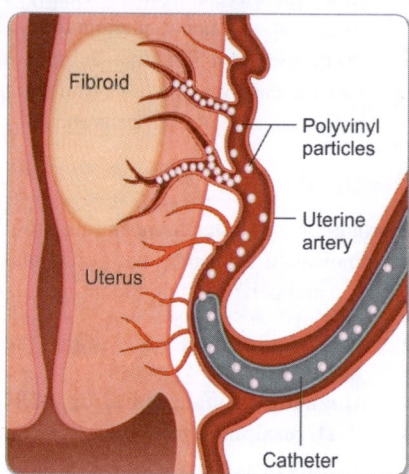

**Fig. 10:** Uterine artery embolization

- **Anti-inflammatory painkillers:** This type of drug is often effective for women who experience occasional pelvic pain or discomfort.

## ENDOMETRIAL POLYPS

Uterine polyps are growths attached to the inner wall of the uterus that extend into the uterine cavity (Fig. 11). Overgrowth of cells in the lining of the uterus (endometrium) leads to the formation of uterine polyps, also known as endometrial polyps. These polyps are usually noncancerous (benign), although some can be cancerous or can eventually turn into cancer (precancerous polyps).

### Causes

Hormonal factors appear to play a role. Uterine polyps are estrogen-sensitive, which means they grow in response to circulating estrogen.

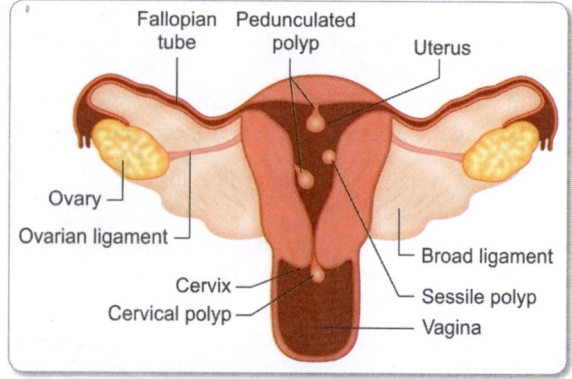

**Fig. 11:** Endometrial polyps

## Risk Factors

- Obesity
- High blood pressure
- History of cervical polyps
- Tamoxifen or hormone replacement therapy (HRT)

## Signs and Symptoms

- Irregular menstrual bleeding—for example, having frequent, unpredictable periods of variable length and heaviness
- Bleeding between menstrual periods
- Excessively heavy menstrual periods
- Vaginal bleeding after menopause
- Infertility
- Some women have only light bleeding or spotting; others are symptom-free

## Diagnosis

These tests may include the following:

- **Transvaginal ultrasound (TVS)**
- **Sonohysterography** is a related procedure that may be performed after the transvaginal ultrasound. A sterile fluid is introduced into the uterus through a thin tube called a catheter. The fluid causes the uterus to expand, providing a clearer image of any growths within the uterine cavity during the ultrasound procedure.
- **Hysteroscopy:** May be used to either diagnose or treat uterine polyps.
- **Endometrial biopsy**
- **Curettage:** It is done in an operating room. This procedure can both diagnose and treat polyps.

## Complications

Uterine polyps might be associated with infertility.

## Treatment

Treatment may not be necessary if the polyps do not cause any symptoms. However, polyps should be treated if they cause heavy bleeding during menstrual periods, or if they are suspected to be precancerous or cancerous. They should be removed if they cause problems during pregnancy, such as a miscarriage, or result in infertility in women who want to become pregnant. If a polyp is discovered after menopause, it should be removed.

- **Medications:** Drugs that help regulate the hormonal balance, such as progestins or gonadotropin-releasing hormone agonists, may be used as a temporary treatment. These medications help to relieve symptoms. However, the symptoms will usually return after the medications are stopped.
- **Hysteroscopy:** In this, the doctor will insert surgical instruments through the hysteroscope to remove any polyps that are found.
- **Curettage:** may be performed along with hysteroscopy. While using the hysteroscope to look at the interior of the uterus, the doctor uses a curette to scrape the lining and remove any polyps. The polyps

may be sent to a laboratory to determine whether they are benign or cancerous. This technique is effective for smaller polyps.

- Additional surgery may be necessary if a polyp cannot be removed using other methods, or if the polyps are cancerous. A hysterectomy may be necessary in cases where cancer cells are found in the uterine polyps.

# BENIGN AND MALIGNANT TUMORS OF THE REPRODUCTIVE TRACT

## Tumors of the Ovary

- Ovarian cancer is the fifth most common cancer in women all over the world. It is also the fifth leading cause of cancer death in women.
- Three cell types make up the normal ovary: The multipotential surface (coelomic) covering epithelium, the totipotential germ cells, and the multipotent sex cord/stromal cells. Each of these cell types gives rise to a variety of tumors.
- Neoplasms of the surface epithelial origin account for almost 90% of ovarian cancers.
- **Surface epithelial:** 65–70%
- **Stromal:** 15–20%
- **Germ cell tumors:** 5–10%
- **Metastatic tumors:** 5%
    - **Pathogenesis:** Several risk factors for epithelial ovarian cancers have been recognized.
        - Two of the most important are nulliparity and family history.
        - Prolonged use of oral contraceptives reduces the risk somewhat.
        - A majority of hereditary ovarian cancers seem to be caused by mutations in the BRCA1 and BRCA2 gene.

### Surface Epithelial Tumors

All types can be benign, borderline, or malignant.

### Serous Tumors

Serous tumors are the most common malignant ovarian tumors and account for 60% of all ovarian cancers. Grossly, may be small, but most are large, spherical to ovoid, cystic structures. Benign lesions are usually encountered between the age of 30 and 40 years, and malignant serous tumors are more commonly seen between 45 and 65 years of age (Figs 12A and B).

### Serous Cystadenoma

It is characterized by:

- Single layer of columnar ciliated epithelium is present
- Fine papillae

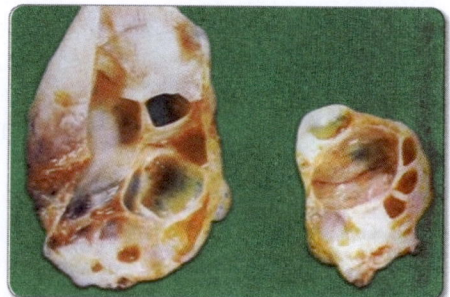

**Figs 12A and B:** Serous tumors

## Mucinous Tumors

- Mucinous tumors (Fig. 13) differ essentially from serous tumors in that the epithelium consists of mucin-secreting cells similar to those of the endocervical mucosa.
- Almost 10% of them are malignant, 10% are of low malignant potential and 80% are benign.
- The prognosis of mucinous tumors is better than for the serous counterpart, but the stage is the major determinant of treatment success.

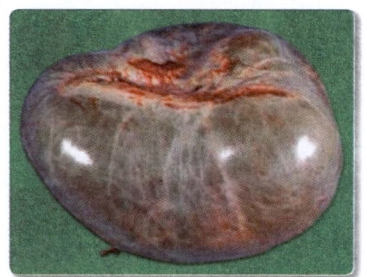

**Fig. 13:** Mucinous tumors

## Mucinous Cystadenoma-Borderline

Mucinous cystadenoma-borderline (Fig. 14) is characterized by:

- Papillary complexity
- Nuclear stratification and atypia
- No stromal invasion

## Endometrioid Tumors

- Endometrioid tumors (Fig. 15) may be solid or cystic, but sometimes they develop as a mass projecting from the wall of a cyst filled with chocolate-colored fluid.
- Microscopically, formation of tubular glands, similar to those of the endometrium.
- They are usually malignant tumors, although benign and borderline forms also exist.
- Approximately 15–30% of women with these ovarian tumors have a concomitant endometrial carcinoma.

## Granulosa Cell Tumor

- Granulosa cell tumor (Fig. 16) is a hormonally active tumor.
- It is the most common estrogenic ovarian neoplasm.
- The adult form occurs mainly in postmenopausal women, associated with endometrial hyperplasia and carcinoma.
- The juvenile type occurs in the first two decades and causes precocious sexual development.

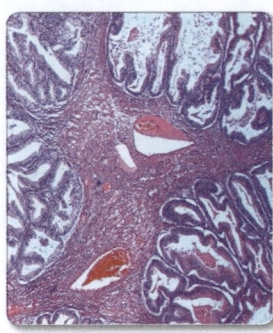

**Fig. 14:** Mucinous cystadenoma-borderline

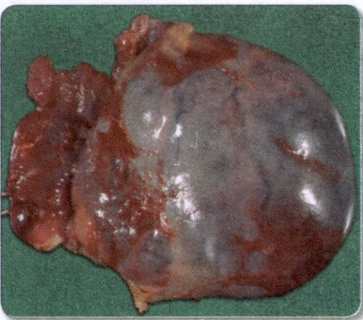

**Fig. 15:** Endometrioid tumors

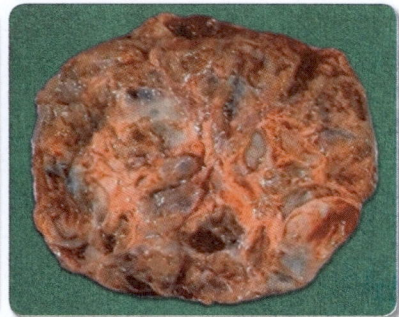

**Fig. 16:** Granulosa cell tumors

Chapter 19 ⊃ Gynecological Disorders

### Brenner's Tumor

- Brenner's tumor (Fig. 17) are uncommon, most are benign, solid, usually unilateral tumors, consisting of an abundant stroma containing nest of transitional-like epithelium resembling that of the urinary tract.
- Occasionally, the nests are cystic and are lined by columnar mucus-secreting cells.
- They are generally smoothly encapsulated.
- They may arise from the surface epithelium or from urogenital epithelium trapped within the germinal ridge.
- Rarely, they are formed as nodules within the wall of a mucinous.

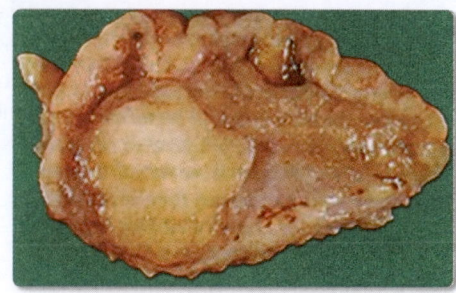

**Fig. 17:** Brenner's tumor

### Teratomas

- These are neoplasms of germ-cell origin and constitute 15–20% of ovarian tumors
- However, more than 90% of these are benign mature cystic teratomas. The immature malignant variant is rare.

### Benign (Mature) Cystic Teratomas

- Benign cystic teratomas (Fig. 18) are marked by differentiation of totipotent germ cells into mature tissues representing all three germ cell layers.
- Usually there are cysts lined by recognizable epidermis replete.
- On transection, they are often filled with sebaceous secretion and matted hair, when removed, reveal a hair-bearing epidermal lining. Sometimes teeth protrude from nodular projection.
- Occasionally, foci of bone and cartilage, nests of bronchial or gastrointestinal epithelium, and other recognizable lines of development are also present.
- Sometimes, they produce infertility for unknown reasons.

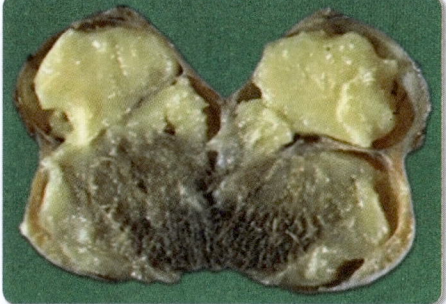

**Fig. 18:** Benign cystic teratomas

### Immature Malignant Teratomas

- Immature malignant teratomas (Fig. 19) are found early in life; the mean age is 18 years.
- They differ from benign teratomas as they are often bulky, and predominantly solid or near-solid on transection, and are punctuated by areas of necrosis.
- Uncommonly, one of the cystic foci may contain sebaceous secretion, hair, and other feature similar to those in the mature teratoma.
- Microscopically, the distinguishing feature is immature areas of differentiation toward cartilage, bone, muscle, nerve, and other structures.

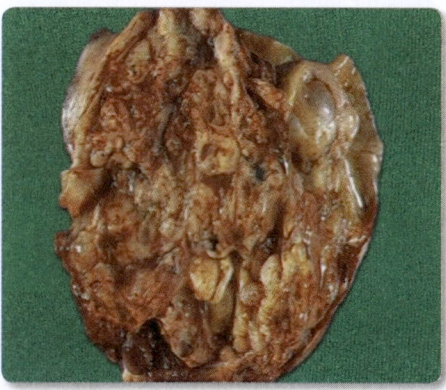

**Fig. 19:** Immature malignant teratomas

### Specialized Teratomas

- Struma ovarii is composed entirely of mature thyroid tissue that may hyperfunction and produce hyperthyroidism.
- They appear as small, solid, unilateral brown ovarian masses.
- Struma ovarii and carcinoid may be combined in the same ovary, One of these elements may become malignant.

## Uterine Tumors

### Endometrial Tumors

#### Endometrial Polyps

- These are sessile and usually hemispheric
- Histologically, they are composed of endometrium resembling the basalis, frequently with small muscular arteries
- More often they have cystic dilated glands, but some have normal endometrial architecture.
- They may occur at any age, but more commonly, they develop at the time of menopause.
- Clinical significance
  - Production of abnormal uterine bleeding.
  - Risk of giving rise to a cancer (rare).

#### Endometrial Carcinoma

It is the most frequent cancer occurring in the female genital tract.

- Appears most frequently between the ages of 55 and 65 years.
- There are two clinical settings in which endometrial carcinomas arise: in perimenopausal women with estrogen excess and in older women with endometrial atrophy. (*endometrioid* and *serous carcinoma* of the endometrium, respectively).
- Well-defined risk factors for endometrioid carcinoma: obesity, diabetes, hypertension and infertility
- These risk factors point to increased estrogen stimulation, and it is well recognized that prolonged estrogen replacement therapy and estrogen-secreting tumors increase the risk of this cancer.
- Marked leukorrhea and irregular bleeding are the first clinical indication of all endometrial carcinoma.
- With progression, uterus may be palpably enlarged, and in time, it becomes fixed to surrounding structures by extension of the cancer beyond the uterus.

### Myometrial Tumors

#### Leiomyoma

- Leiomyoma (Fig. 20) the most common benign tumor in females and are found in 30–50% of women during reproductive life. More frequent in blacks than in whites.
- They are often referred to as fibroids because they are firm.
- Estrogens and oral contraceptives stimulate their growth; conversely, they shrink postmenopausally.
- They may be entirely asymptomatic, discovered on routine pelvic examination. The most frequent manifestation, when present, is menorrhagia, with or without metrorrhagia. They may become palpable to the woman or may produce a dragging sensation.
- They rarely transform into sarcomas.

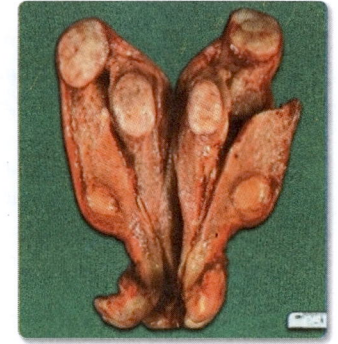

**Fig. 20:** Leiomyoma

### Leiomyosarcoma

- A uterine leiomyosarcoma (Fig. 21) is a rare malignant (cancerous) tumor that arises from the smooth muscle lining the walls of the uterus (myometrium).
- Smooth muscles react involuntarily in response to various stimuli For example, the myometrium stretches during pregnancy.
- Leiomyosarcoma is classified as a soft tissue sarcoma.

## Uterine Tube (Fallopian Tube) Tumors

Primary neoplasia of uterine tube includes the following:

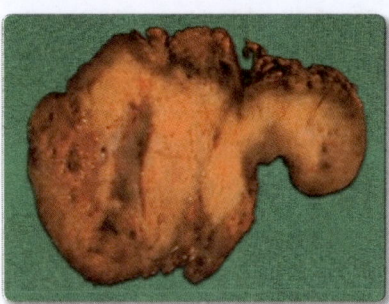

**Fig. 21:** Leiomyosarcoma

- Epithelial
  - Adenoma
  - Adenocarcinoma
- Mesenchymal
  - Leiomyoma
- Mixed tumors
  - Fibroadenoma
  - Adenomyoma
  - Metastatic granulosa cell tumor

### *Adenocarcinoma*

- Fallopian tube carcinoma is an uncommon tumor
- The etiology is unknown
- The typical presenting symptoms include abdominal pelvic pain or pressure and vaginal bleeding
- Primary adenocarcinoma with papillary features is the most common histologic type

### *Leiomyoma*

- Leiomyoma of the fallopian tube is extremely rare
- Most cases are asymptomatic and found incidentally at autopsy or unrelated operation
- These leiomyomas tend to be singular, small, and unilateral

## Tumors of the Cervix

- Cervical carcinoma is one of the major causes of cancer-related deaths in women, despite improvements in early diagnosis and treatment.
- Since introduction of the Papanicolaou (Pap) smear 50 years ago, the incidence of cervical cancer has decreased.
- The pap smear remains the most successful cancer screening test ever developed.
- Over the same period, the incidence precursor cervical intraepithelial neoplasia (CIN) has increased to more than 50,000 cases annually. It is important to know that nearly all invasive cervical squamous cell carcinoma arise from epithelial changes CIN.

### *Cervical Intraepithelial Neoplasia*

- Cytologic examination can detect cervical intraepithelial neoplasia (CIN) before the development of an overt cancer by many years. However, only a fraction of cases of CIN progress to invasive carcinoma.

- The peak incidence of CIN is about 30 years, whereas that of invasive carcinoma is about 45 years.
- Risk factors for the development of CIN and invasive carcinoma are:
  - Early age at first intercourse
  - Multiple sexual partners
  - Male partner with multiple previous sexual partners
  - Persistent infection by "High-risk" human papilloma virus (HPV)

## Invasive Carcinoma of the Cervix

- The most common cervical carcinoma are squamous cell carcinoma 75%, adenocarcinoma and adenosquamous carcinoma 20%, and small cell neuroendocrine carcinoma 5%.
- In some individual with aggressive intraepithelial changes, the time interval may be considerably shorter, whereas in other women CIN precursors may persist for life. The only reliable way to monitor the course of the disease is with careful follow-up and repeated biopsies.
- Symptoms include vaginal bleeding, leukorrhea, painful coitus, and dysuria.
- Detection of precursors by cytologic examination and their eradication by laser vaporization or cone biopsy is the most effective method of cancer prevention.
- Invasive carcinomas range from microscopic foci of early stromal invasion to grossly conspicuous tumors encircling the os. Tumors encircling the cervix and penetrate into the stroma produce a "barrel cervix", which can be identified by direct palpation.

# Tumors of Vulva

## Condylomas

Condylomas fall into two distinctive biologic forms:

- **Condylomata lata,** (*not commonly seen these days*), are flat, moist, minimally elevated lesions that occur in secondary *syphilis*
- **Condylomata accuminata,** (*more common*) may be papillary and distinctly elevated. They occur anywhere on the anogenital surface.

## High-grade Vulvar Intraepithelial Neoplasia and Carcinoma of the Vulva

- Carinoma of vulva represents about 3% of all genital tract cancers in women
- 90% of vulvar carcinomas are squamous cell carcinomas; and 90% of them are HPV related and most commonly by seen in relatively younger patients
- Non-HPV-related vulvar squamous cell carcinoma occurs in older women.

# Tumors of Vagina

- Vaginal tumors can be either intraepithelial neoplasia or squamous cell carcinoma
- Extremely uncommon, usually occurring in women older than age 60 years.
- Risk factors are similar to those for carcinoma of the cervix
- Associated with HPV infection in most cases.
- Vaginal clear cell adenocarcinoma, usually encountered in young women in their late teens whose mothers took diethylstilbestrol during pregnancy; overall risk is 1 per 1000 of those exposed in utero.
- Vaginal adenosis, are small glandular or microcystic inclusions appear in vaginal mucosa.

# PALLIATIVE CARE AND REHABILITATION

Palliative care is a term derived from Latin *palliare,* "to cloak". It refers to specialized medical care for people with serious illnesses. It is focused on providing people with relief from the symptoms, pain and stresses of a serious illness—whatever the prognosis. The goal is to improve quality of life for both the sick person and the family as they are the central system for care.

A World Health Organization (WHO) statement describes palliative care as "an approach that improves the quality of life of patients and their families facing the problems associated with life-threatening illness, through the prevention and relief of suffering by means of early identification and impeccable assessment and treatment of pain and other problems, physical, psychosocial and spiritual." More generally, however, the term "palliative care" may refer to any care that alleviates symptoms, whether or not there is hope of a cure by other means; thus, palliative treatments may be used to alleviate the side effects of curative treatments, such as relieving the nausea associated with chemotherapy.

## Palliative Care

- Provides relief from pain and other distressing symptoms
- Affirms life and regards dying as a normal process
- Intends neither to hasten or postpone death
- Integrates the psychological and spiritual aspects of patient care
- Offers a support system to help patients live as actively as possible until death
- Offers a support system to help the family cope during the patient's illness and in their own bereavement
- Uses a team approach to address the needs of patients and their families, including bereavement counseling, if indicated
- Will enhance quality of life and may also positively influence the course of illness
- Is applicable early in the course of illness, in conjunction with other therapies that are intended to prolong life, such as chemotherapy or radiation therapy, and includes those investigations needed to better understand and manage distressing clinical complications.

### Uses of Palliative Care

The term "palliative care" is increasingly used with regard to diseases other than cancer such as chronic, progressive pulmonary disorders, renal disease, chronic heart disease, human immunodeficiency virus (HIV)/acquired immunodeficiency syndrome (AIDS) and progressive neurological diseases. In addition, the rapidly growing field of pediatric palliative care has clearly shown the need for services geared specifically for children with serious illness.

Palliative care is given to people who have any serious illness and who have physical, psychological, social, or spiritual distress as a result of the treatment they are seeking or receiving. Palliative care increases comfort by lessening pain, controlling symptoms, and lessening stress for the patient and family, and should not be delayed when it is indicated. Evidence shows that end-of-life communication interventions decrease utilization (such as length of stay), particularly in the intensive care unit setting, and that palliative care interventions (mostly in the outpatient setting) are effective for improving patient and caregiver perceptions of care.

Palliative care is not reserved for people in end-of-life care and can improve quality of life, decrease depressive symptoms, and increase survival time. If palliative care is indicated for a person in an emergency department, then that care should begin in the emergency department immediately and with referral to additional palliative care services. Emergency care **physicians** often are the first medical professionals to open the discussion about palliative care and hospital **services** with people needing care and their families.

In some cases, medical specialty, professional organization recommend that sick people and physicians respond to an illness only with palliative care and not with a therapy directed at the disease. The following items are indications named by the American Society of Clinical Oncology as characteristics of a person who should receive palliative care but not any cancer-directed therapy.

- People who have a performance status limited ability to care for themselves
- People who have received no benefit from prior evidence-based treatments
- People who are ineligible to participate in any appropriate clinical trial
- The physician sees no strong evidence that treatment would be effective

## Rehabilitation

**Rehabilitation** describes specialized healthcare dedicated to improving, maintaining or restoring physical strength, cognition and mobility with maximized results. Typically, **rehabilitation** helps people gain greater independence after illness, injury or surgery.

It can also be described as the process of helping a person who has suffered an illness or injury restore lost skills and so regain maximum self-sufficiency. For example, rehabilitation work after a stroke may help the patient walk and speak clearly again.

**The purpose of rehabilitation** is to restore some or all of the patient's physical, sensory, and mental capabilities that were lost due to injury, illness, or disease. Rehabilitation includes assisting the patient to compensate for deficits that cannot be reversed medically.

Rehabilitation can take many forms but generally there are four ways that it can be delivered, i.e. physical therapy occupational therapy, respiratory therapy and speech therapy.

## Role of Nurse in Palliative Care and Rehabilitation

Nurses play a significant role in hospital/palliative care. In addition to the conventional nursing duties of observing and recording symptoms and treatments, they also provide emotional support to terminally ill patients and their families, through a series of roles.

- In rehabilitative care, nurses assist patients with temporary and long-term disabilities or chronic illnesses.
- They assist in adapting to their conditions, meeting their highest potential and living more independent lives.
- They commonly use holistic approaches to medical treatment to meet all needs of patients.
- They work with patients and family members to establish a treatment plan and establish short and long-term goals.
- They also prepare patients and caregivers for changes that occur in rehabilitative treatment.
- In palliative care, nurses work with other physicians and other medical professionals to diagnose, treat and provide care for individuals with terminal medical issues.
- They help patients and family deal with the condition by providing information, support, and access to counseling services.
- Palliative care nurses try to help patients receive the best possible medical treatment to alleviate their symptoms and pain to rest comfortably.
- They regularly meet with the family members and friends of patients to help provide coping strategies with the situation and discuss additional options for end-of-life care.

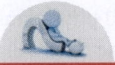

## FREQUENTLY ASKED QUESTIONS IN EXAMS

1. Define uterine prolapse. Explai.. degrees of uterine prolapse, its causes and signs and symptoms. Discuss the management of uterine prolapse.
2. Discuss uterine fibroids in detail.
3. Enlist the tumors of the reproductive tract. Discuss in detail the cervical cancer.
4. Write short notes on:
    a. Rectovaginal fistula
    b. Uterine polyps
    c. Vesicovaginal fistula

## MULTIPLE CHOICE QUESTIONS

1. Procidentia means:
    a. Fistulas
    b. Polyps
    c. Uterine prolapse
    d. Fibroids

2. When the cervix descends downwards into the vagina, the degree of uterine prolapse is:
    a. First degree
    b. Second degree
    c. Third degree
    d. Fourth degree

3. The herniation of the upper vagina along with a segment of small intestine into the vagina the condition is known as:
    a. Cystocele
    b. Enterocele
    c. Rectocele
    d. RVF

4. A 32-year-old lady came to hospital with chief complaints of sensation of heaviness in vagina, tissue protruding from vagina, urine retention, bowel problems, the gynecologist make the diagnosis of:
    a. Uterine prolapse
    b. Fistulas
    c. Cyst
    d. None of above

5. When two Müllerian ducts develop but they do not fuse, and the women has two uterine cavities each with its own cervix and its own vagina, this type of uterine malformation is known as:
    a. Unicornuate uterus
    b. Double uterus
    c. Bicornuate uterus
    d. Arcuate uterus

6. Which one of the following contraceptives leads to uterine malformations?
    a. IUD
    b. Oral contraceptive pills
    c. Diethylstilbestrol (DES)
    d. None of above

7. Abnormal fistulous tract extending between the bladder and the vagina that allows continuous involuntary discharge of urine into vaginal vault is called:
    a. VVF
    b. RVF
    c. CVF
    d. EVF

8. The cause of vesicovaginal fistula is:
    a. Infected episiotomy after childbirth
    b. Vaginal hysterectomy
    c. Radiation therapy for pelvic cancer
    d. All of the above

9. **Which hormone is responsible for the growth of uterine polyps:**
   a. Estrogen
   b. Progesterone
   c. LH
   d. FSH

10. **Fibroids cause all, except:**
    a. Menstrual irregularities
    b. Infertility
    c. Abdominal mass
    d. Amenorrhea

11. **Uterine fibroids are associated with:**
    a. PID
    b. Ovarian cancer
    c. Amenorrhea
    d. Endometriosis

12. **All drugs reduce the size of fibroids, except:**
    a. Danazol
    b. GnRH
    c. RU-486
    d. Estrogen

13. **Which of the following is the definitive treatment of adenomyosis?**
    a. LNG-Intrauterine device
    b. GnRH analog
    c. Danazol
    d. Hysterectomy

14. **True about cervical cancer is:**
    a. 90% associated with HPV
    b. Nulliparity
    c. OCP
    d. Immunocompromised patients

15. **Risk factor for cervical cancer is:**
    a. HPV
    b. Smoking
    c. Early sexual intercourse
    d. All of the above

16. **Earliest symptom of cervical cancer is:**
    a. Irregular vaginal bleeding
    b. Postcoital bleeding
    c. Foul smelling discharge
    d. Pain

17. **The most common cause of death in cervical cancer is:**
    a. Hemorrhage
    b. Uremia
    c. Infection
    d. Metastasis

18. **The most malignant endometrial carcinoma is:**
    a. Adenocarcinoma
    b. Adenoacanthoma
    c. Mixed adenosquamous
    d. Clear cell carcinoma

19. **Long-term tamoxifen therapy may cause:**
    a. Endometrial cancer
    b. Ovarian cancer
    c. Cervical cancer
    d. Vaginal cancer

20. **The most common germ cell tumor of the ovary is:**
    a. Choriocarcinoma
    b. Dysgerminoma
    c. Embryonal cell tumor
    d. Malignant teratoma

## 🔑 Answer Key

| 1. c | 2. a | 3. b | 4. a | 5. b | 6. c | 7. a |
|------|------|------|------|------|------|------|
| 8. d | 9. a | 10. d | 11. d | 12. d | 13. d | 14. a |
| 15. d | 16. a | 17. b | 18. d | 19. a | 20. b | |

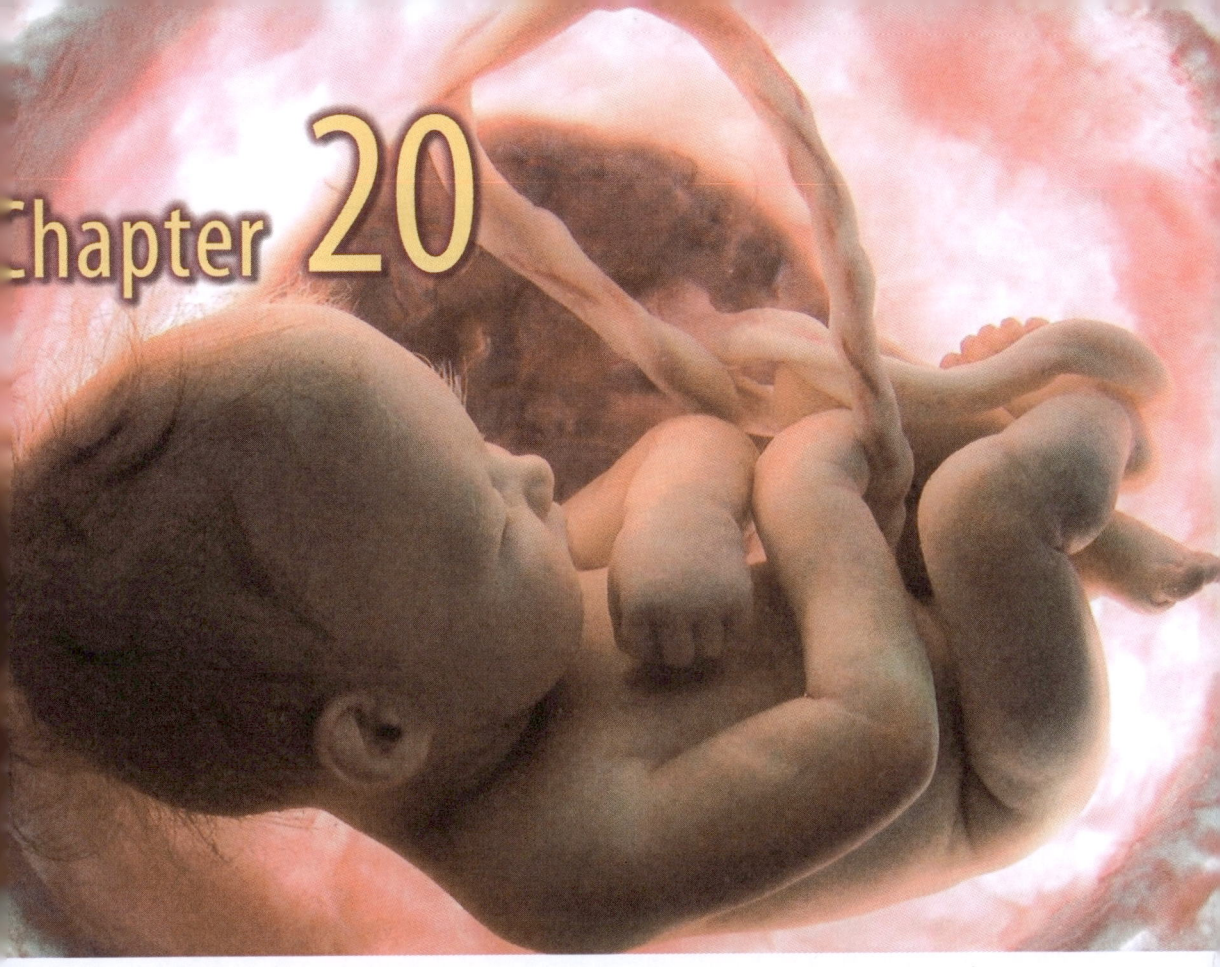

# Chapter 20

# Breast Disorders

## INTRODUCTION

Breast disorders may be noncancerous (benign) or cancerous (malignant). Most are noncancerous and not life threatening. Often, they do not require treatment. In contrast, breast cancer can mean loss of a breast or of life. Thus, for many women, breast cancer is their worst fear. However, potential problems can be detected early when women regularly examine their breasts themselves, are examined regularly by their doctor, and have mammograms as recommended. Early detection of breast cancer is essential to successful treatment. In this chapter, we will discuss the tumors of the breast.

A tumor is a mass of abnormal tissue. There are two types of breast tumors; those that are noncancerous, or 'benign', and those that are cancerous, which are malignant.

## BENIGN TUMORS

Benign tumors are noncancerous. A nonmalignant tumor can be serious if they are pressing a primary nerve, a main artery, or compresses any adjacent organs.

Benign breast conditions are very common and are encountered by most of the women. They are not life-threatening.

### Fibroadenoma

- A fibroadenoma (Fig. 1) is a very common benign breast condition. The most common symptom is a lump in the breast which usually moves when one touches it.
- Fibroadenomas often develop during puberty so are mostly found in young women, but they can occur in women of any age. Men can also get fibroadenomas, but this is very rare.
- A fibroadenoma is usually fell as a lump in the breast which has a rubbery texture, is smooth to the touch and moves easily under the skin.
- Fibroadenomas are usually painless, but sometimes they may feel tender or even painful, particularly just before a period.

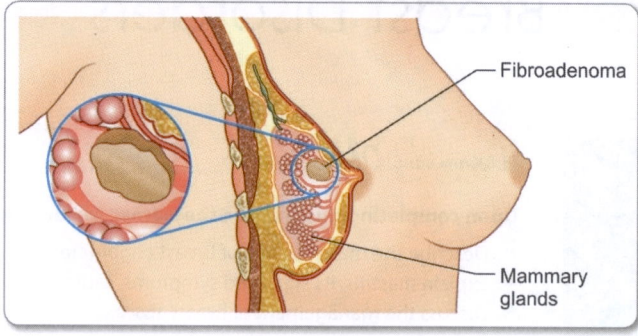

**Fig. 1:** Fibroadenoma

### Fibroadenosis

- Fibroadenosis also known by other names such as fibrocystic disease of breast or mammary dysplasia or chronic cystic mastitis.
- A biopsy of these lumps usually reveals fibrosis, adenosis, epitheliosis and cyst formation.

- It usually presents in the **reproductive age of a women—25–35 or 40 years.**
- The usual common presentation is as a breast lump or pain in the breast (mastalgia).
- The pain or lump may occur just before the menstrual periods and then disappear.

## Intraductal Papilloma

- Intraductal papillomas are benign, wart-like tumors that grow within the milk ducts of the breast.
- They are made up of gland tissue along with fibrous tissue and blood vessels (called fibrovascular tissue).
- **Solitary papillomas** (solitary intraductal papillomas) are single tumors that often grow in the large milk ducts near the nipple.
- They are a common cause of clear or bloody nipple discharge, especially when it comes from only one breast.
- They may be felt as a small lump behind or next to the nipple. Sometimes they cause pain.
- Papillomas may also be found in small ducts in areas of the breast farther from the nipple.
- In this case, there are often several growths and less likely to cause nipple discharge.

Figure 2A and B show intraductal papilloma.

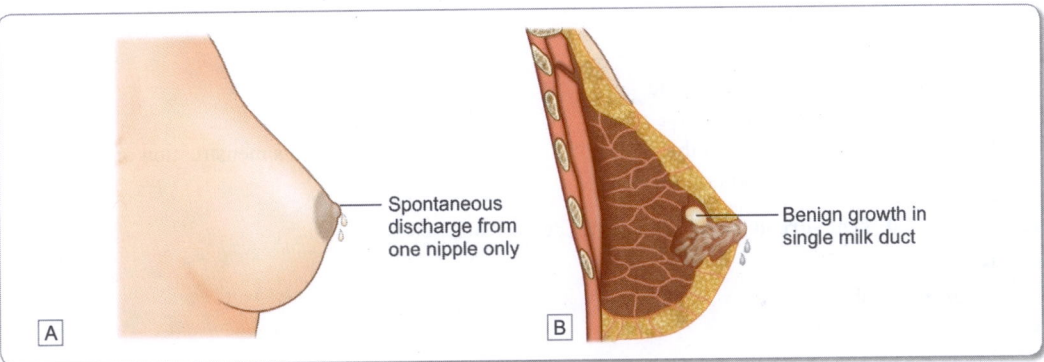

A — Spontaneous discharge from one nipple only

B — Benign growth in single milk duct

**Figs 2A and B:** Intraductal papilloma

## MALIGNANT BREAST CARCINOMA

It develops from breast tissue. Breast cancer usually starts off in the inner lining of milk ducts or the lobules that supply them with milk.

A breast cancer that originates in the lobules is known as lobular carcinoma, while one that develops from the ducts is called ductal carcinoma.

### Incidence

Breast cancer is the most common invasive cancer in females worldwide. It accounts for 16% of all female cancers and 22.9% invasive cancers in women. Approximately 18.2% all cancer deaths worldwide, including both males and females are from breast cancer.

### Risk Factors

- Early menarche
- Late menopause
- Nulliparity

- Obesity
- Late age of first birth (>35 years)
- Never breastfed
- Atypical lobular hyperplasia
- Nipple discharge other than milk
- High dose breast or chest irradiation
- High dietary fat intake
- Alcohol consumption
- Estrogen replacement therapy (ERT)
- Family history of cancer
- Carcinoma in the other breast
- Previous cancer of endometrium, ovary, colon
- Inherited mutations of BRCA 1 and BRCA 2 Genes

## Signs and Symptoms of Breast Cancer

- Lump in the breast
- Change in breast shape
- Dimpling of the skin
- Fluid/blood coming from the nipple
- Red scaly patch of the skin
- A pain in the armpits or breast that does not seem to be related to women's menstruation on period
- Pitting or redness of the skin of breast.

**In those with distant spread of the disease, there may be:**

- Bone pain
- Swollen lymph nodes
- Shortness of breath
- Yellow skin

Signs and symptoms of breast cancer are shown in Figure 3.

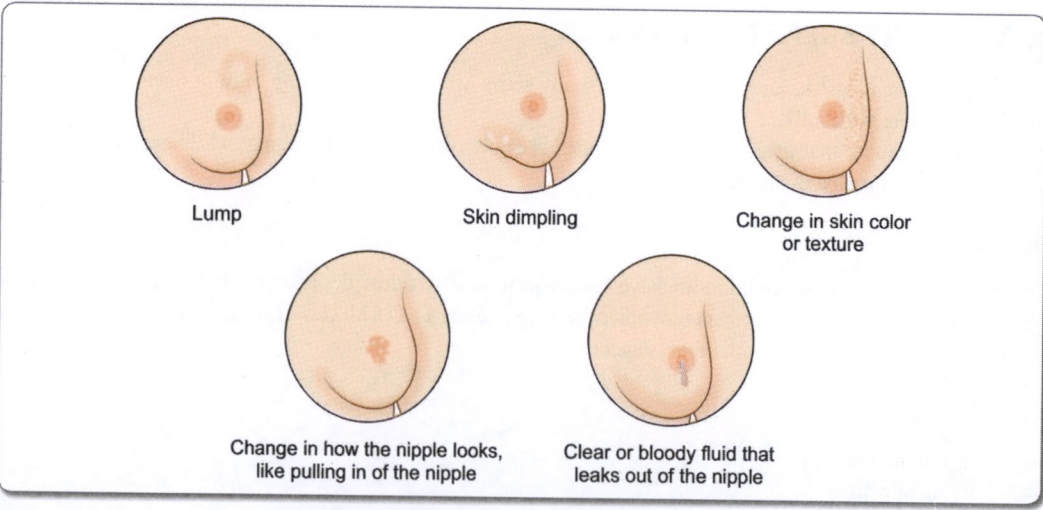

**Fig. 3:** Signs and symptoms of breast cancer

## Stages of Breast Cancer

Clinical staging is based on tumor, node, metastasis (TNM) system of the International Union Against Cancer. This classification considers tumor size, clinical assessment of axillary nodes and presence or absence of distant metastasis (Table 1).

**TABLE 1: Breast cancer surgical staging (TNM classification)**

| T | Stage | Stage grouping |
|---|---|---|
| $T_{1s}$ | *In situ* | O |
| $T_1$ | $\leq$2 cm | I |
| $T_2$ | >2 cm but $\leq$5 cm | IIA |
| $T_3$ | >5 cm | II A |
| $T_4$ | Involvement of skin or chest wall or inflammatory cancer | II B |
| **N** | **Stage** | |
| $N_0$ | No lymph node Involvement | III A |
| $N_1$ | 1–3 nodes | |
| $N_2$ | 4–9 nodes | |
| $N_3$ | $\geq$10 nodes | III B |
| **M** | **Stage** | |
| $M_0$ | No distant metastases | III C |
| $M_1$ | Distant metastases | IV |

## Diagnostic Evaluation

- **Mammography:** Mammography (Fig. 4) is the most reliable means of detecting breast cancer before a mass can be palpated in the breast.

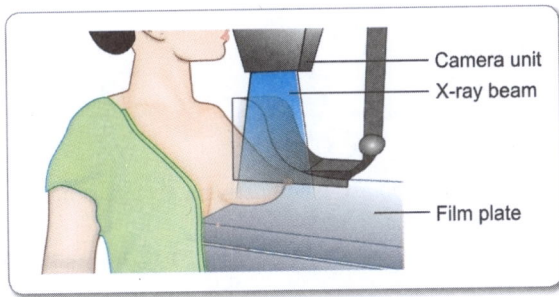

**Fig. 4:** Mammography

- **Biopsy technique:** Cytology
    - Fine needle biopsy and aspiration (Fig. 5)
    - Open biopsy
    - Image-guided localization biopsy

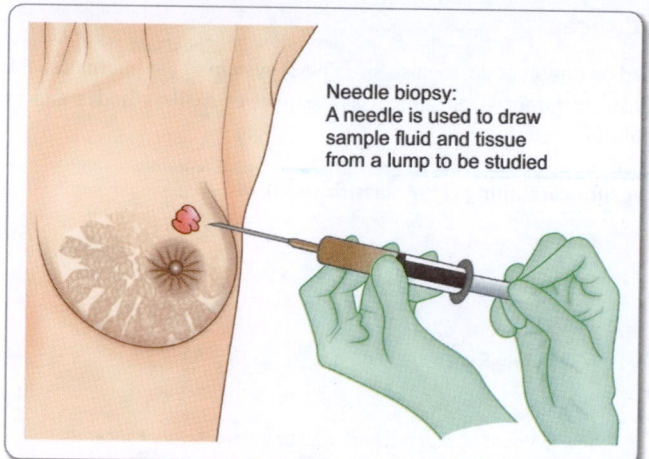

Needle biopsy:
A needle is used to draw sample fluid and tissue from a lump to be studied

**Fig. 5:** Needle biopsy

- **Laboratory finding:** A complete blood cell count, liver function test and β-human chorionic gonadotropin (hCG) in premenopausal patients to diagnosis pregnancy should be obtained as part of initial evaluation.
- **Radiographic findings:**
  - **Plain X-ray:** Posteroanterior and lateral chest X-ray may show pulmonary disease involvement and provides radiographic evaluation of the cardiac outline.
  - **Computed tomography (CT) scan of brain and liver** is only required for locally advanced disease.
  - **Magnetic resonance imaging (MRI)** is usually not used. In $T_0N_1$ patient may be helpful in better characterizing the soft tissues of the tumor.
  - **Radio nuclear scanning:** There is no role for this imaging in screening or in routine work-up of the patient. In evaluation of metastatic breast cancer, bone scans using Technetium-99m labeled phosphonates are important tools.

## Treatment of Breast Cancer

### Surgical Treatment

It includes:

- **Radical mastectomy:** In this entire breast, the underlying pectoralis muscles and contiguous axillary lymph nodes in continuity are removed.
- **Extended radical mastectomy:** In this internal mammary lymph node are also removed, but this did not enhance overall survival rate.
- **Modified radical mastectomy:** In this pectoralis major muscle is preserved. The breast is removed like radical mastectomy but axillary lymph node dissection and skin excision is not extensive (Fig. 6).
- **Total mastectomy:** In this entire breast, nipple and areolar complex is removed without resection of the underlying muscle or intentional excision of axillary lymph nodes. Low lying lymph node in upper outer portion of breast and low axilla are often excised. With this method, there is a higher risk of axillary recurrence (Fig. 7).

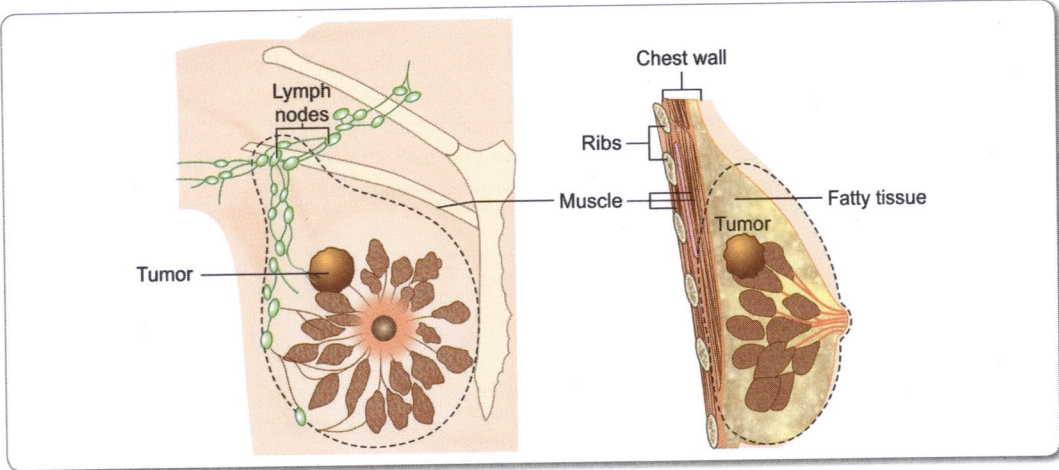

**Fig. 6:** Modified radical mastectomy

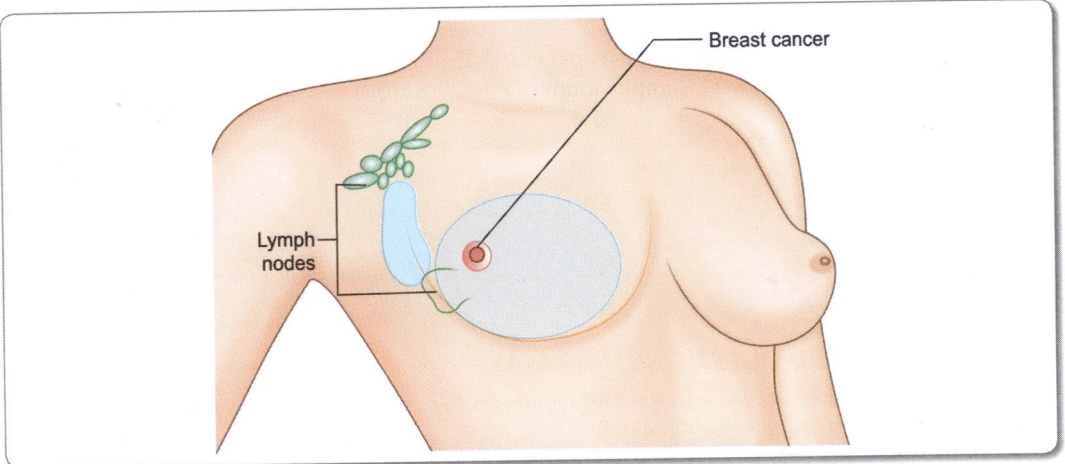

**Fig. 7:** Total mastectomy

## Breast Conservation Therapy (BCT) with or without Radiation Therapy

It involves a surgical procedure as lumpectomy: an excision of tumor mass with a negative surgical margin, an axillary evaluation and postoperative irradiation. Segmental mastectomy, partial mastectomy and quadrantectomy are also used in conjunction with radiation and are part of surgical component of BCT. BCT has gained increasing acceptance as a treatment option of stages I and II breast cancer.

## Radiotherapy

It is used when:

- Locally advanced cancer with distant metastasis in order to control ulceration, pain in breast and regional nodes.
- In treatment of certain bones or soft tissue metastasis to control pain or avoid pathologic fracture.

Chapter 20 ❂ Breast Disorders

### Hormonal Therapy

Tamoxifen is recommended as treatment of choice for hormonal therapy in premenopausal women with advanced breast cancer. In postmenopausal women, aromatase inhibitors and tamoxifen are the initial therapy of choice for metastatic breast cancer amenable to endocrine manipulation. Other agents are gonadotropin releasing hormones agonists as alternative to oophorectomy. Progestin, megestrol acetate and medroxyprogesterone acetate are alternative agents reserved mainly for cases resistant to tamoxifen.

### Chemotherapy

Cytotoxic drugs are indicated:

- If visceral metastasis present
- If hormonal treatment is unsuccessful
- If tumor is estrogen and progesterone receptor negative

### Bisphosphonate Therapy

It is recommended if bone metastasis is confirmed by plain X-ray, MRI/CT scans. It along with other palliative systemic treatment has been shown to reduce bony as well visceral metastasis. It is given intravenously every 3–4 weeks for 2 years or for the duration of other systemic treatment.

*Note:* **Mastitis, breast engorgement, breast abscess:** Already discussed in breast complications (Chapter 10: Management of Complications of Puerperium)

## ASSESS YOURSELF

### FREQUENTLY ASKED QUESTIONS IN EXAMS

1. **Define breast cancer, its causes, signs and symptoms. Explain the stages of breast cancer. Describe the treatment of breast cancer in detail.**
2. **Write short notes on:**
   a. Breast abscess
   b. Breast engorgement
   c. Mastitis

### MULTIPLE CHOICE QUESTIONS

1. **Noncancerous tumors also called:**
   a. Cystic tumor
   b. Polyp
   c. Benign tumor
   d. Malignant tumor
2. **Which is the form of benign tumor?**
   a. Fibroadenoma
   b. Fibroadenosis
   c. Duct papilloms
   d. All of the above
3. **Breast cancer is the form of:**
   a. Malignant tumor
   b. Benign tumor
   c. Fibroadenoma
   d. Cystic tumor

4. **Risk factors of breast cancer is:**
   a. Early menarche
   b. Family history of cancer
   c. Late menopause
   d. All of the above

5. **If the metastasis is *in situ*, the stage of cancer is:**
   a. Stage 0
   b. Stage I
   c. Stage II A
   d. Stage II B

6. **The definitive management to treat breast abscess is:**
   a. Antibiotic therapy
   b. Drainage of pus
   c. Hot fermentation
   d. Topical ointments

7. **In which of the following breast complications, breastfeeding at regular interval is necessary?**
   a. Breast abscess
   b. Breast engorgement
   c. Acute mastitis
   d. Retracted nipples

8. **The effective management of breast engorgement is:**
   a. Frequent suckling
   b. To support breast with binder/bra
   c. Manual expression of milk after each feed
   d. All of the above

9. **Treatment of choice for hormonal therapy in premenopausal women with advanced breast cancer is:**
   a. Methotrexate
   b. Tamoxifen
   c. Progestin
   d. Megestrol

10. **BCT means:**
    a. Breast cell tumors
    b. Breast conservation therapy
    c. Benign cancerous tumor
    d. Benign cell therapy

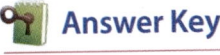 **Answer Key**

| 1. c | 2. d | 3. a | 4. d | 5. a | 6. b | 7. b |
|------|------|------|------|------|------|------|
| 8. d | 9. b | 10. b | | | | |

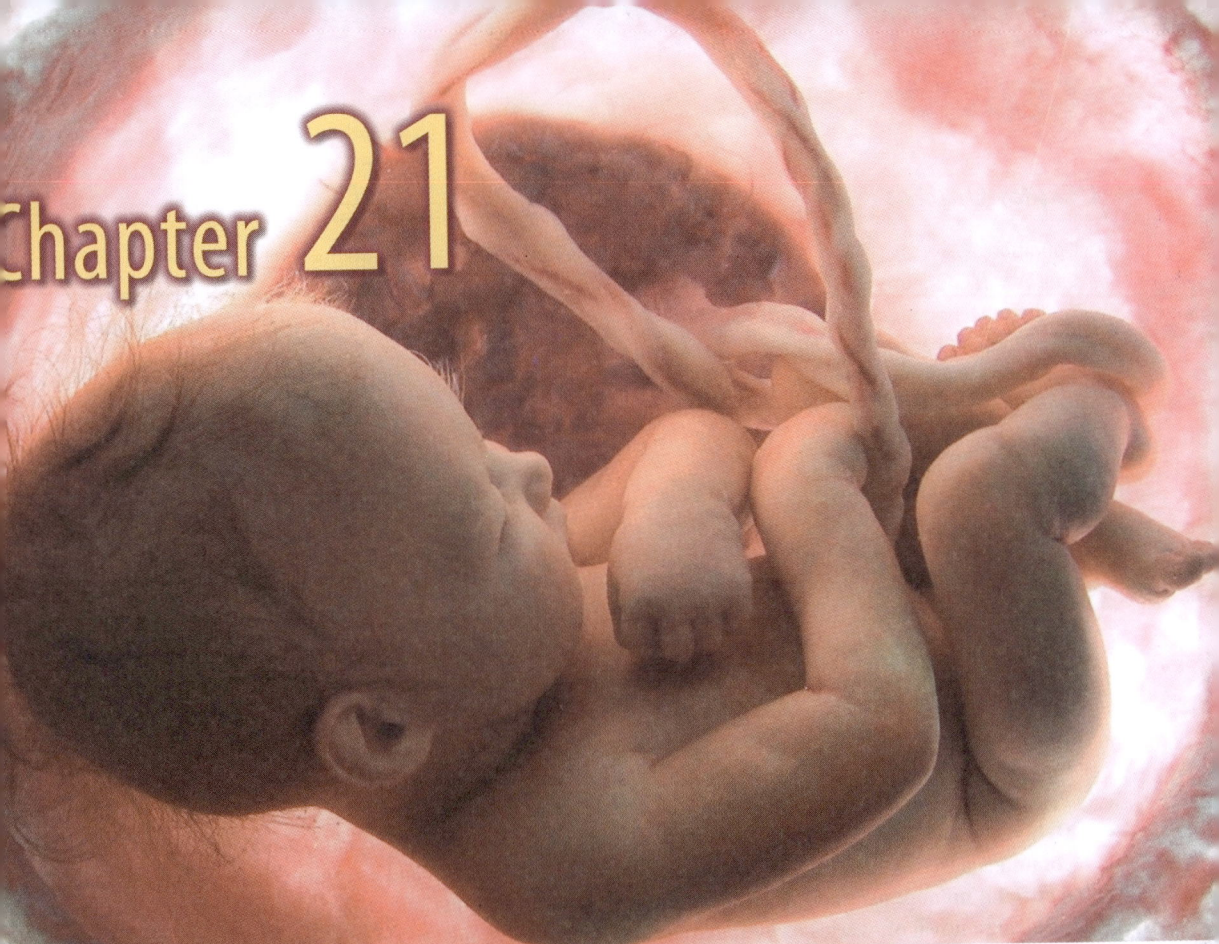

# Menopause

**Upon completing this chapter, the learner will be able to:**

- Define menopause and its signs and symptoms
- Describe the physiological changes due to menopause
- Discuss health education and counseling related to menopause
- Explain the role of hormonal replacement therapy in case of menopause
- Describe surgical menopause

## DEFINITIONS

- **Menopause:** The word "Menopause" literally means "end of monthly cycles". It means permanent cessation of menstruation at the end of reproductive life due to loss of ovarian follicular activity. It is the point of time when last final menstruation occurs. The clinical diagnosis is confirmed following stoppage of menstruation (amenorrhea) for twelve consecutive months without any other pathology (Fig. 1).
- **Climacteric:** It is the phase of aging process during which a woman passes from the reproductive to nonreproductive stage. This phase covers 5–10 years on either side of menopause.
- **Premenopause:** It is the part of the climacteric before menopause, when the menstrual cycle is likely to be irregular.
- **Postmenopause:** It is the phase of life that comes after the menopause.
- **Delayed menopause:** If the menopause fails to occur even beyond 55 years, it is called delayed. The common cause is constitutional, uterine fibroids, diabetes mellitus and estrogenic tumor of the ovary.
- **Artificial menopause:** Permanent cessation of ovarian function done by artificial means, for example, surgical removal of ovaries or by radiation is called artificial menopause.

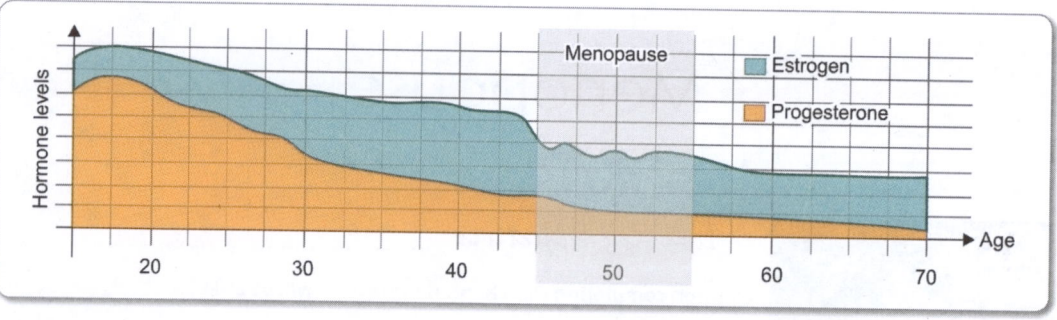

**Fig. 1:** Hormone levels in menopause

## CAUSES OF MENOPAUSE

- Menopause occurs as a result of exhaustion of eggs from ovarian follicles and consequent estrogen deprivation.
- Surgical removal of ovaries (surgical menopause).
- Ovarian failure from cancer therapy, such as chemotherapy or radiation treatments.

# TIMING OF MENOPAUSE

Menopause occurs at an average age of **45 years in India** and **51 years in west**. Genetic makeup, race and climate influence the age of menopause.

Premature menopause occurs before 35 years and delayed menopause occurs after 55 years. Delayed menopause is mainly due to some pelvic pathology (uterine fibroid) or in diabetes mellitus. Climacteric period gradually starts 2–3 years before and 2–5 years after menopause.

# PHYSIOLOGICAL CHANGES IN MENOPAUSE

- **General physical changes:**
  - Body weight decreases after 65 years
  - Skin becomes less elastic and wrinkles appear
  - Fat deposition in hip and thighs
  - Height diminishes after 65 years
  - Kyphosis develops due to spinal osteoporosis.
- **Bones:** Osteoporosis occurs due to postmenopausal estrogen insufficiency.
- **Hip:** Vertebral and forearm fractures become more common in women than men. Reduction of osteoblast and calcium loss in trabecular bone leads to reduction of bone mass.
- **Measurement of mineral density:** Bone mineral density (BMD) of bones is done. Dual energy X-ray absorptiometry (DEXA) is a good screening tool.
- **Cardiovascular:** Menstruating women get less ischemic coronary heart disease due to estradiol protection. The incidence rises and equals to that in men, (6–10 years after menopause).
- **Endocrinal:** Because of low negative estradiol feedback in postmenopausal women, follicle stimulating hormone (FSH) rises to 50 mIU/mL (50–150 mIU/mL).
  - Postmenopausal ovarian stroma produces androstenedione, which is converted to estrone in fatty tissue.
  - Progesterone secretion from ovary ceases due to failure of ovulation.
  - Testosterone (40% of total) is also secreted by ovarian stroma, thus serum testosterone levels do not appreciably fall.
  - Adrenal cortex secretes rest of androstenedione and testosterone.
  - Prolactin levels remain unchanged.
- **Genital effects:** In postmenopausal women progressive atrophy of genital organs with increased fibrosis occurs.
  - **Vagina:** Vaginal dryness occurs due to reduced estrogen level.
    - Vaginal pH increases, lactobacilli growth can be depressed and other bacteria tend to multiply and can lead to vaginitis.
    - Dyspareunia due to decrease in size of vaginal introitus and decreased lubrication during sexual stimulation.
  - **Ovary:** It is reduced to 5 cm, fibrotic, furrowed surface and follicles get exhausted.
  - **Fallopian tubes:** They show feature of atrophy. The muscle coat becomes thinner, the cilia disappear and the plicae become less prominent.
  - **Uterus:** Uterus becomes small and fibrotic. Endometrium atrophies, sometimes endometrial hyperplasia occurs due to estrogen effect. Cervix atrophies and flushes with vaginal vault. Vaginal epithelium atrophies with loss of rugosity.
  - **Vulva:** It gets atrophied with narrowing of vaginal orifice.

- **Bladder and urethra:** The epithelium becomes thin and is more prone to damage and infection. There may be dysuria, frequency, urge or even stress incontinence.
- **Loss of muscle tone:** It leads to pelvic relaxation, uterine descent and anatomic changes in the urethra and neck of the bladder. The pelvic cellular tissue becomes scanty and the ligaments supporting the uterus and vagina lose their tone. As such, preexisting weakness gets aggravated.
- **Breast:** Glandular tissue atrophies, breast becomes flabby and pendulous due to deposition of fat. Pubic and axillary hairs become sparse.
- **Sexual urge:** It increases at menopause due to rise in adrenal testosterone that declines after 65 years.
- **Psychological changes:** It includes feeling more emotionally labile, nervous or agitated with less control of their emotions, depressed mood or sometimes mood swings.

## SIGNS AND SYMPTOMS OF MENOPAUSE

**The three classical ways in which the menstrual period ceases are:**

1. Sudden cessation.
2. Gradual diminution in the amount of blood loss with each regular period until menstruation stops.
3. Gradual increase in the spacing of the periods until they cease for at least a period of 1 year.

The various signs and symptoms of menopause are enlisted in Figure 2.

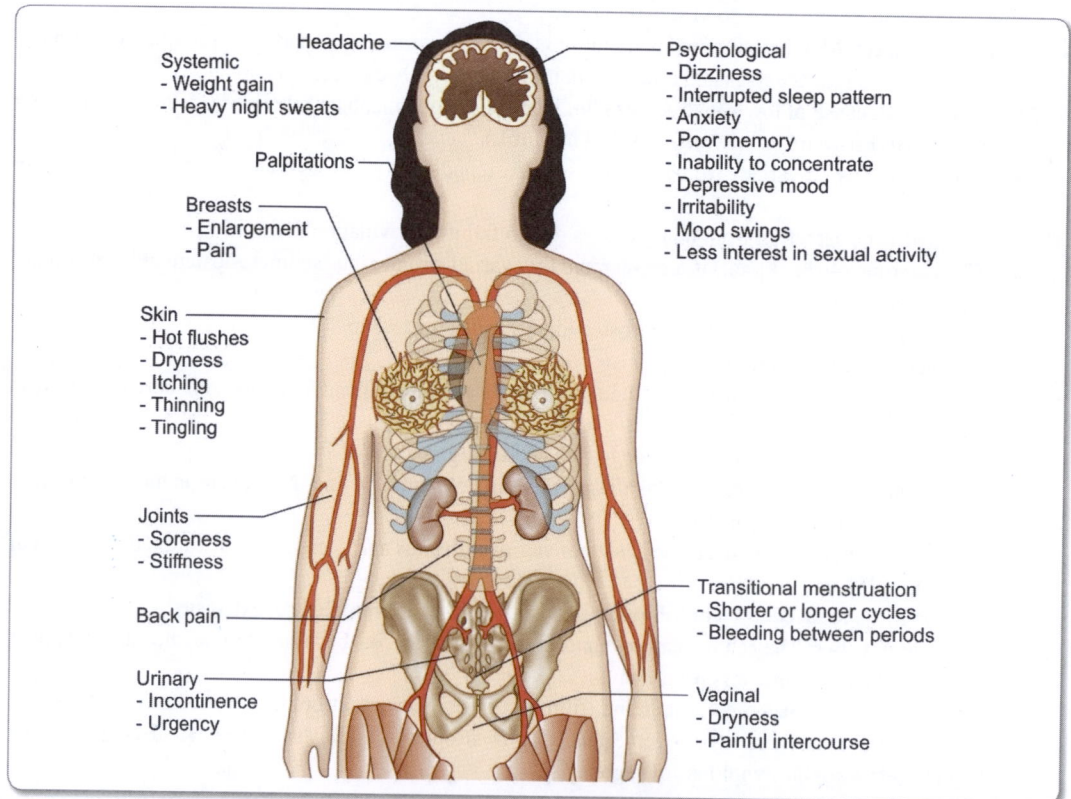

**Fig. 2:** Symptoms of menopause

## Other Symptoms

- Hot flushes
- Sweating
- Insomnia
- Headache
- Cancer phobia
- Irritability, depression
- Lack of concentration
- Neurological (paraesthesia → Sensations of pins and needles in the extremities)
- Urinary: Dysuria, stress incontinence and urge, recurrent infections
- Genital: Vaginal dryness, dyspareunia and loss of libido.

## Late Sequelae

**Menopausal women through the chronic estrogen deficiency are liable to develop:**

- Arthritis, osteoporosis and fracture
- Cardiovascular accident: Ischemic heart disease, myocardial infarction and atherosclerosis
- Stroke
- Skin changes (wrinkling of skin due to decreased collagen)
- Alzheimer's disease (due to estrogen deficiency)
- Colorectal cancer
- Tooth decay

# DIAGNOSIS OF MENOPAUSE

- History of various symptoms
- General examination: Includes blood pressure recording, palpation of the breast, weight and hirsutism
- Pelvic examination: Pap smear
- Blood examination, lipid profile, electrocardiogram (ECG)
- Mammography, pelvic ultrasound
- Bone density study. DEXA is a quick test with less radiation
- Estrogen levels and FSH decide the need of hormone replacement therapy (HRT)

# HORMONE REPLACEMENT THERAPY IN MENOPAUSE

Hormone replacement therapy is indicated in menopausal women to overcome the short-term and long-term consequences of estrogen deficiency.

## Indications of Hormonal Replacement Therapy

- Relief of menopausal symptoms
- Prevention of osteoporosis
- To maintain the quality of life in menopausal years

## Special Group of Women to whom HRT should be Prescribed

- Symptomatic women
- High risk cases for cardiovascular disease, osteoporosis, Alzheimer's syndrome and colonic cancer
- Following surgical oophorectomy in premenopausal women and premature menopause
- Gonadal dysgenesis
- Premature ovarian failure
- Those who demand HRT as prophylaxis

## Types of HRT

- Short-term HRT
- Long-term HRT

### Short-term HRT

It is for 6–12 months or more and can effectively relieve hot flushes (menopausal syndrome) within 3 months.

- **First line of drug:** It is estrone sulfate contained in conjugated equine estrogen—Tab. premarin 0.625 mg (28 tablets in a strip) is taken orally with water at bedtime continuously daily for 6 months or more following menopausal syndrome.
- Alternatively **lynoral (ethinyl estradiol)** 0.05 mg is taken daily continuously, like premarin for 6 months or more
- With intact uterus medroxyprogesterone acetate 5 mg is added for last 10 days every month along with estrogen
- In premenopausal menstruating women with hot flush, sleep disturbances. In this case, combined oral contraceptives (Mala D, ovral L) is also helpful.

### Long-term HRT

This is advocated for preventive health care in postmenopausal women. However, the risk of developing breast and endometrial carcinoma has not been yet solved on long-term HRT. **Estrogen is taken for 10 years or more to get *benefits*.**

#### Commonly used Drugs in Long-term HRT

- **Tablet premarin (only estrogen)** 0.625 mg is given to women without uterus. In women with uterus, premarin combined with medroxyprogesterone acetate 5 mg is taken continuously daily at bed time.

   While on premarin therapy if small withdrawal bleeding develops, patient is carefully followed when bleeding stops, brush cytology of endometrium can be done. In case of heavy bleeding, therapy is suspended. Endometrial curettage is done to exclude endometrial carcinoma.
- **Tablet tibolone** 2.5 mg is alternative therapy. It is 19-nortestosterone derivative steroid with estrogenic, Progestogenic and weekly androgenic property. One tablet is taken daily continuously like premarin. This has nonproliferative property in endometrium.
- Transdermal estradiol patches are not used in tropical countries since it causes skin irritation
- **Tablet calcium** 500 mg daily is given to patient who does not take adequate 2 glasses of milk or milk products.

# Contraindications to Estrogen Replacement Therapy

- **Absolute contraindications**
  - Estrogen dependent tumors
  - History of known or suspected pregnancy
  - Compromised liver function as in acute liver disease
  - Blood clotting disorders such as thrombophlebitis, myocardial infarction, etc.
  - Stroke
  - History of undiagnosed vaginal bleeding
  - Insulin dependent diabetes mellitus
- **Relative contraindications**
  - Hypertension
  - Endometriosis
  - Gallbladder disease

Table 1 gives the benefit-risk equation of long-term HRT.

**TABLE 1:** Benefit-risk equation of long-term HRT

| Benefit | Risk |
| --- | --- |
| Risk of coronary ischemic heart disease is reduced to 50% if estrogen is started within 1 year of menopause. | **Breast cancer:** Risk of developing breast cancer remains still unsolved. Long-term HRT shows potential risk of slight increase in breast cancer incidence although statistically insignificant. |
| Osteoporotic fractures can be prevented by prolonged HRT starting as above after menopause. | **Endometrial carcinoma:** Long-term HRT has been shown to cause endometrial hyperplasia, atypia and finally carcinoma. Use of progesterone can diminish estrogen receptors in endometrium thus in intact uterus progesterone is combined with estrogen as in short-term HRT. |
| Long-term HRT can improve vaginal and urethral atrophy. | **Venous thromboembolic disease** (VTE): It has been found to be increased with the use of combined oral estrogen and progestin. |
| Improvement of vasomotor symptoms (70–80%). | **Lipid metabolism:** Increased incidence of gallbladder disease has been observed following ERT due to rise in cholesterol (in bile). |
| Increase in bone mineral density (2–5%). | Dementia, Alzheimer's disease are increased. |
| Decreased risk in vertebral and hip fractures (25–50%). | |
| Reduction in colorectal cancer. | |

## Monitoring Prior to and during HRT

A base level parameter of the following and their subsequent checkups (at least annually) are mandatory:

- Physical examination including pelvic examination
- Blood pressure recording
- Breast examination and mammography
- Cervical cytology
- Pelvic ultrasound to measure endometrial thickness (normal <5 mm)

Any irregular bleeding should be investigated thoroughly (endometrial biopsy and hysteroscopy). Ideal serum level of estradiol should be 100 pg/mL during HRT therapy. Serum level of estradiol is useful to monitor the HRT therapy rather than that of serum FSH.

# HEALTH EDUCATION AND COUNSELING IN MENOPAUSE

**Counseling** is a method of communication. It is a way of working with people in which counselor tries to understand client's feelings and helps them to make decisions.

Counseling skills are useful when counselor talks to client or in our daily interaction. The communication skills will be discussed under two major headings:

1. Listening and learning skills
2. Building confidence and giving support

## Listening and Learning Skills

- Counseling place must be clean, calm and orderly. Greet the patient with a pleasant gesture. Accept her with dignity.
- Talk to her by name. Use proper soothing words.
- Maintain privacy and confidentiality of the client.
- Ask both open and closed ended question from the client to acquire proper information.
- Speak in a language which is easily understood by the client.
- Do not rush with questions; try to go with the pace of the client.
- Try not to interrupt the narration unnecessarily.
- Always be honest in your discussion.
- Try to be precise and to the point.

## Building Confidence and Giving Support

- Accept what the client thinks or feels.
- Recognize and praise what a client is doing right.
- Give practical help wherever possible.
- Give a little, relevant information.
- Use simple language.
- Make one or two suggestions, do not command.
- At the end, summarize what is so for discussed in the meeting.

Counseling the client should be based on current medical knowledge and keeping in mind the patient's best interests. In addition, we must give due respect to her own preference. Clear and simple communication fosters trust, facilitates access to services and improves quality of medical care.

Menopause is perceived by many as a loss of youth and it may be very disturbing experience for the woman. She is often depressed, anxious or irritable due to hormonal changes as well as due to psychosocial reasons. Good counseling sessions with the gynecologist can help these patients.

- Counseling of postmenopausal woman is important, health education, awareness about symptoms and their interpretation must be explained to the woman.
- Assurance of a good start of life and allaying various fears is important.
- A positive attitude of life is inculcated.
- Relaxation, massage, acupressure and Reiki help to reduce mental stress.

- Active participation of the patient in making changes in her lifestyle like:
  - **Contraceptives:** Advice on contraceptive is necessary. Until menopause is well established and amenorrhea has lasted for 12 months, couple is advised to use barriers method. Hormonal pills may not be safe because there is increased chances of thromboembolism. Progestogen pills or DEPOT injections may be alternative, but they cause irregular bleeding and depression.
  - **Exercise:** Instruct the patient for daily walk for 30 minutes and perform weight bearing exercises, (walking and aerobic) burns calories reliably and also prevent or delay osteoporosis.
  - **Diet:** Encourage the patient for a suitable natural diet with intake of fresh vegetables and fruits to avoid weight gain and stay healthy in menopausal years.
  - Smoking and alcohol intake is discouraged.
  - Talking with friend and family members, especially those who've gone through menopause.
  - **Stress reduction techniques:** Can be useful in reducing anxiety, depression and intensity of hot flushes, all common symptoms of menopause.
  - **Acupuncture:** Acupuncture points to treat the emotional and physical effects of menopause are located all over the body.
  - **Natural remedies:** There are many "herbal products" for sale that claims to help menopausal symptoms. Soy and Soy products have been used for alleviation of menopausal symptoms due to their high concentration of phytoestrogens.
  - **Aroma therapy** with essential oils of clary. Sage, lemon, jasmine, etc. help in overcoming emotional up and down.
  - **Bladder training** is a simple and effective treatment because in menopausal period there is stress incontinence.
  - **Sleep:** Taking 8-hour night and 2-hour nap a day is required.
  - **Hygiene:** Maintain personal hygiene; because of dry vagina, there are chances of genital tract infections also.
  - New creative hobbies are important in dealing with "Empty Nest Syndrome". She should be encouraged to use her time productively and pursue some hobby for which she may have been too busy in her younger days.

## SURGICAL MENOPAUSE

Surgical removal of both ovaries before the natural age of menopause is called surgical menopause (Figs 3A and B).

Surgical menopause is a type of induced menopause—menopause due to an unusual event. It is induced when the ovaries are surgically removed (by bilateral oophorectomy). Menopause can also be induced when the ovaries are gravely damaged by radiation, chemotherapy or other medications.

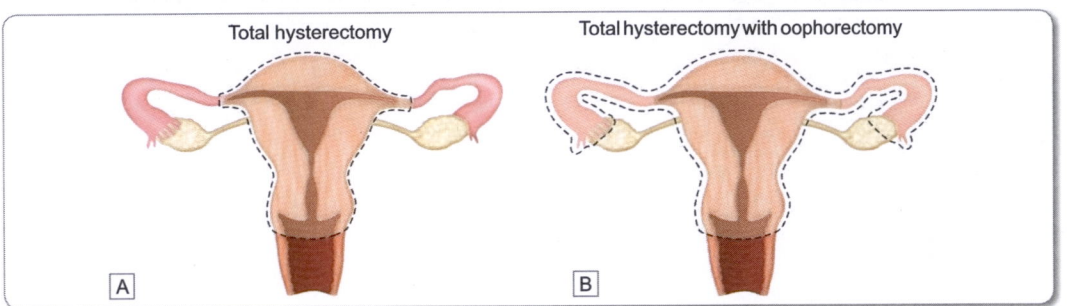

**Figs 3A and B:** Surgical menopause

Surgical removal of ovaries can be done at the time of hysterectomy or other pelvic surgery. The indications for surgical removal of ovaries either inherent ovarian disorders or done as preventive (prophylactic) measure. Weighing the risk and benefits for prophylactic oophorectomy and assessing the future risks associated with oophorectomy can be based on a growing number of scientific studies. If patient who has undergone hysterectomy and ovaries are left intact then patient have up to 50% chance of ovaries failing within 5 years of hysterectomy, this may be because the blood supply to the uterus has been cut off.

Radiation treatment following hysterectomy for cancer may also cause the ovaries to fail prematurely. Even after natural menopause the ovaries continue to produce a small amount of estrogen and more significant amount of testosterone up to 12 years. Therefore, there are indications that women having hysterectomy should have offered supplementation of testosterone and estrogen.

Compared with natural menopause, which is a gradual process, surgical menopause entails an abrupt withdrawal of estrogen, progesterone and androgens.

The sudden changes in hormones associated with surgical menopause are associated with more severe and prolonged menopausal symptoms. Long-term consequences of oophorectomy, particularly when it is performed before age 45 years, includes increased risk for emotional, cognitive and neurologic disease, as well as increased risk for cardiometabolic disorders and bone resorption. There is a survival benefit to retention of the ovaries up to age 65 years in women at low risk for ovarian cancer. Figure 4 enlists the HRT in surgical menopause.

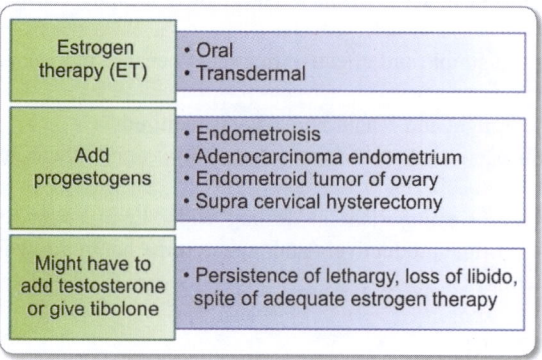

**Fig. 4:** HRT in surgical menopause

**Note:** (Physiological changes after menopause, Signs and symptoms and hormonal replacement therapy) →
    Similar to natural menopause, the only difference is given as follows →

*Women who undergo surgical menopause (bilateral oophorectomy) may benefit from testosterone replacement in addition to estrogen specially to improve libido. The place of testosterone in the treatment of over intact women with low libido requires further evaluation.*

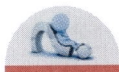

# ASSESS YOURSELF

## FREQUENTLY ASKED QUESTIONS IN EXAMS

1. Define menopause. Enlist the signs and symptoms of menopause. What are the physiological changes that occur during menopause?
2. As a midwife, how would you counsel postmenopausal women to alleviate menopausal symptoms?
3. Write short notes on:
   a. Surgical menopause
   b. Hormonal replacement therapy

## MULTIPLE CHOICE QUESTIONS

1. **HRT is used in all of the following except:**
   a. Vaginal atrophy
   b. Osteoporosis
   c. Flushing
   d. Coronary heart disease

2. **All of the following appear to decrease hot flushes in menopausal female, except:**
   a. Androgen
   b. Raloxifene
   c. Isoflavones
   d. Tibolone

3. **Estrogen administration in menopausal female increases:**
   a. Gonadotropin secretion
   b. LDL cholesterol
   c. Bone mass
   d. Muscle mass

4. **The investigation of choice in a 58-year-old postmenopausal female who has presented with postmenopausal bleeding is:**
   a. Pap smear
   b. Fractional curettage
   c. TVS
   d. CA-125

5. **Postmenopausal women who is overweight, hypertensive and diabetic, presents with bleeding per vagina. The most useful investigation in this period would be:**
   a. TVS
   b. Endometrial sampling
   c. Doppler ultrasound of pelvis
   d. CT scan of pelvis

6. **In case of surgical menopause, which hormone is prescribed in addition to estrogen specially to improve libido:**
   a. Testosterone
   b. hCG
   c. FSH
   d. Androgens

7. **Surgical removal of both ovaries before the natural age of menopause is called:**
   a. Artificial menopause
   b. Surgical menopause
   c. Post menopause
   d. Delayed menopause

8. **Average age of menopause for Indian women is:**
   a. 45 years
   b. 50 years
   c. 35 years
   d. 40 years

9. **Due to postmenopausal estrogen insufficiency, the bone effect is:**
   a. Osteoporosis
   b. Osteomalacia
   c. Fracture
   d. Osteoblastosis

10. Couple is advised to use barrier method, until menopause is well established and amenorrhea has lasted for how many months:
    a. 8 months
    b. 6 months
    c. 12 months
    d. 18 months

11. Which of the following product is rich in phytoestrogens that is helpful for alleviation of menopausal symptoms?
    a. Soy products
    b. Egg
    c. Green leafy vegetables
    d. Fruits

12. Which of the following is absolute contraindication for estrogen replacement therapy?
    a. Estrogen dependent tumors
    b. Stroke
    c. Diabetes type-1
    d. All of the above

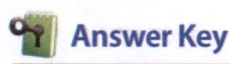
## Answer Key

| 1. d | 2. b | 3. c | 4. b | 5. b | 6. a | 7. b |
|------|------|------|------|------|------|------|
| 8. a | 9. a | 10. c | 11. a | 12. d | | |

# Appendices

## ANTENATAL EXAMINATION

**Definition:** It is systematic examination of the pregnant woman externally to know about the pregnant uterus and condition of fetus.

### Purposes

- To detect the high risk conditions of mother and fetus.
- To promote and maintain physical health.
- To ensure continued medical surveillance and prophylaxis.
- To obtain baseline information against which the subsequent changes are assessed and which are of importance in the determination of gestational age.
- To prevent, detect and treat any untoward complications at the earliest.
- To observe the signs of pregnancy.
- To detect any deviation from normal.
- To measure abdominal girth and fundal height.
- To assess abdominal muscle tone.
- To determine the possible location of fetal heart tones.
- To determine the fetal lie, presentation, position, variety (anterior/posterior) and engagement.
- To teach woman regarding importance of antenatal visits, diet, exercise, rest, prepare the mother for labor and sensitize about family planning.
- To clarify all her doubts associated with child-bearing and child rearing to reduce fear and anxiety.

### Articles

- **Examination of table/bed:** For the comfort of woman.
- **Soap:** To wash hands.
- **Thermometer:** To check temperature.
- **Blood pressure apparatus:** To note the blood pressure.
- **Watch:** To count pulse, respiration and fetal heart rate.
- **Measuring tape:** To measure abdominal girth.
- **Weighing machine:** To check the weight of mother.
- **Fetoscope:** To hear fetal heart sound.
- **Patient chart:** To record history, general and obstetrical assessment.

## Procedure

| Nursing action | Rationale |
| --- | --- |
| **Preprocedural steps:** | |
| • Arrange all the articles in the examination room and ensure about its adequate functioning. | • To save time. |
| • Approach the woman pleasantly. | • To establish rapport. |
| • Explain the procedure to the mother. | • To reduce anxiety. |
| • Collect complete history prior to examination, i.e. identification data of mother (name, age, address, religion, occupation, etc.), history of previous pregnancy, history of present pregnancy, medical history, family history. | • To know the woman completely. |
| • Make her comfortable while taking history. | • To gain her cooperation. |
| • Ask the woman to get her hemoglobin and urine tests done. | • For albumin and sugar test. |
| • Instruct the woman to empty the bladder after giving urine sample. | • To avoid discomfort during abdominal examination. |
| • Draw curtains around the bed. | • To maintain privacy. |
| **Intraprocedural steps:** | |
| • **General assessment:** Collect the data including appearance, gait, height, weight, blood pressure, pulse, respiration and temperature. | • To detect any abnormality. |
| • **Head to foot assessment:** Includes observation for following | |
| ▪ **Head:** Cleanliness, infection, pediculosis, etc. | |
| ▪ **Eye:** Signs of infection, jaundice, sclera and conjunctiva for pallor. | |
| ▪ **Ears:** Discharge, wax accumulation, hearing abnormality. | |
| ▪ **Nose:** Discharge, epistaxis. | |
| ▪ **Mouth:** Cheilosis, dental carries, gum swelling/bleeding, coated tongue, cracked lips. | |
| ▪ **Neck:** Shape, symmetry, lymph gland. | |
| ▪ **Breast examination:** Symmetry, shape, primary and secondary areola, tubercles, inverted/flat nipples and colostrum. | |
| ▪ **Upper extremities:** Check for any bone deformity. | |
| ▪ **Lower extremities:** Homan's sign, edema, bony deformity and varicose veins. | |
| ▪ **Bowel and bladder:** Constipation, incontinence. | |
| ▪ **Genital area:** Bleeding, discharge, infection, hemorrhoids and hygiene. | |

# Abdominal Examination

| Nursing action | Rationale |
|---|---|
| • Explain the woman what will be done and how she may cooperate during the procedure. | • Reduces anxiety and promotes relaxation during the procedure. |
| • Instruct the woman to empty her bladder. | • Avoids discomfort during palpation. |
| • Draw curtains around the bed. | • Provides privacy. |

| Inspection | |
|---|---|
| • Position the woman for examination (knees flexed) <br>    • Place a pillow under her head and shoulders <br>    • Have her arms by her sides <br>    • Expose her abdomen from below the breasts to the symphysis pubis. | • Promotes relaxation of abdominal muscles. <br><br> • Enables visualization of the whole abdomen. |
| • Inspect abdomen for the following: Scars, diastasis recti, hernia, linea nigra, striae gravidarum, contour of the abdomen, state of umbilicus and skin condition. | |
| • Determine the fundal height using the ulnar side of the palm <br> **12 weeks:** Level of symphysis pubis. <br> **16 weeks:** Midway between symphysis pubis and umbilicus. <br> **20 weeks:** 1–2 finger breadth below umbilicus. <br> **24 weeks:** Level of umbilicus. <br> **32 weeks:** Halfway between umbilicus and xiphoid process. <br> **36 weeks:** At level of xiphoid process. <br> **40 weeks:** 2–3 finger breadth below the xiphoid process if lightening occurs. | • In order to estimate if fetal growth corresponds to the gestational period. |

**Fig:** Fundal height at various weeks of gestation

*Contd...*

| Nursing action | Rationale |
|---|---|
| • Measure fundal height (see figure) using any one of the following methods:<br>　▪ **Using measuring tape:** Place zero line of the tape, measure on the upper border of the symphysis pubis and stretch the tape across the contour of the abdomen to the top of the fundus along the midline.<br>　▪ **Caliper method (pelvimeter):**<br>　　○ Place one tip of the caliper on the upper border of the symphysis pubis and the other tip at the top of the fundus. Both placements are in the midline.<br>　　○ Read the measurement on the centimeter scale located on the arc, close to the joint. The number of centimeters should be approximately equal to the weeks of gestation about 22–24 weeks after. | 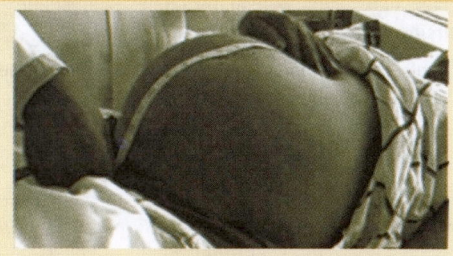<br>**Fig:** Measuring fundal height<br><br>• The number of centimeters measured should be approximately equal to the weeks of gestation after about 22–24 weeks.<br>• This method is more accurate. |
| • Measure the abdominal girth by encircling the woman's abdomen with a tape measure at the level of the umbilicus. (It is measured in inches). | • Normally the measurement is 2 inches (5 cm) less than the weeks of gestation.<br>E.g., 32 inches at 34 weeks' gestation. Measurements more than 100 cm (39.5 inches) are abnormal at any week of gestation. |
| • Instruct the woman to relax her abdominal muscles by bending her knees slightly and doing deep breathing. | • These steps reduce the stretching and tension of abdominal muscles. |
| • Be sure your hands are warm before beginning to palpate, rest your hand on the mother's abdomen lightly while giving explanation about the procedure. | • Cold hands may cause muscle contraction and discomfort. Resting hands on mother's abdomen would help her to become accustomed to your touch and dissipate muscle tightening. |
| • For the technique of palpation<br>　▪ Use the flat palmar surface of fingers and not finger tips. Keep fingers of hands together and apply smooth, deep pressure as firm as necessary to obtain accurate findings. | • These measures would aid in gathering greatest amount of information with least discomfort to the woman. |
| • **Perform the first maneuver (fundal palpation):**<br>　▪ Face the woman's head<br>　▪ Place your hands on the sides of the fundus and curve the fingers around the top of the uterus<br>　▪ Palpate for size, shape, consistency and mobility of the fetal part in the uterus. | • Round, hard, readily, movable part, ballotable between the fingers of both hands is indicative of head nonengagement.<br>• Irregular, bulkier, less firm and not well-defined or movable part is indicative of breech.<br>Neither of the above indicates transverse lie. |
| • **Do the second maneuver (lateral palpation):**<br>　▪ Continue to face the woman's head<br>　▪ Place your hands on both sides of the uterus about midway between the symphysis pubis and the fundus.<br>　▪ Apply pressure with one hand against the side of the uterus pushing the fetus to the other side and stabilizing it there.<br>　▪ Palpate the other side of the abdomen with the examining finger from the midline to the lateral side and from the fundus using smooth pressure and rotatory movements.<br>　▪ Repeat the procedure for examination of opposite side of the abdomen. | • A firm convex, continuously smooth and resistant mass extending from breech to neck is indicative of fetal back. Small knobby, irregular mass, which moves when, pressed or may kick or hit your examining hand is limbs of the fetus.<br><br>• Indicative of the fetal small parts all over the abdomen indicates posterior position. |

*Contd...*

| Nursing action | Rationale |
|---|---|
| • **Third maneuver (Pawlik's grip):**<br>  ■ Continue to face the woman's head make sure the woman has her knees flexed/bent.<br>  ■ Grasp the portion of the lower abdomen immediately above the symphysis pubis, if movable, it is indicative of an engaged head. It is done with one hand only. | • Avoids discomfort.<br><br>• If the fetal head is above the brim, it will be readily movable and ballotable. If not readily movable, it is indicative of an engaged head. |
| • **Fourth maneuver (pelvic palpation):**<br>  ■ Turn and face the woman's feet (make sure the woman's knees are bent).<br>  ■ Place your hands on the sides of the uterus, with the palm of your hands just below the level of umbilicus and your fingers directed towards the symphysis pubis<br>  ■ Press deeply with your fingertips into the lower abdomen and move them toward the pelvic inlet. | • Avoids pain with the maneuver. |
|   ■ The hand converge around the presenting part when head is not engaged.<br>  ■ The hands will diverge away from the presenting part and there will be no mobility if the presenting part is engaged or dipping. | • Cephalic prominence on the same side as the fetal small parts indicates vertex presentation with well flexed head. Cephalic prominence on the same side as the fetal back may be occiput in a face presentation with extended head prominences and are felt on both sides (brow presentation). |

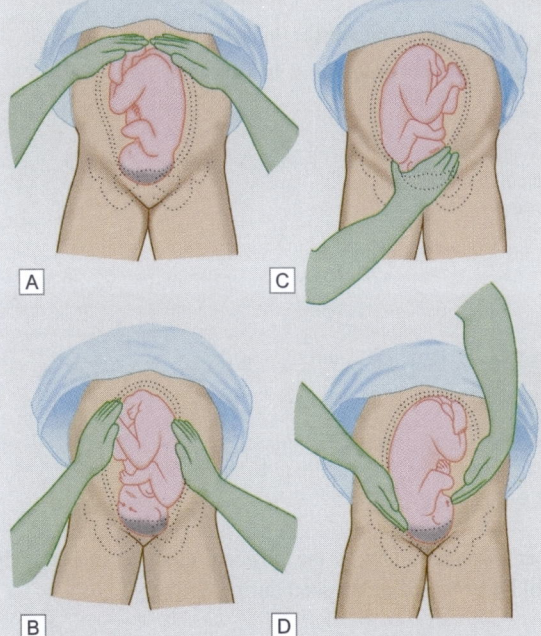

**Figs A to D:** Leopold's maneuvers. **A.** Fundal palpation; **B.** Lateral palpation; **C.** Pawlik's grip; **D.** Pelvic palpation

*Contd...*

| Nursing action | Rationale |
|---|---|
| **Auscultation** | |
| • Place fetoscope or stethoscope and over the convex portion of the fetus closest to the anterior uterine wall. Count fetal heart rate for 1 complete minute. | • Fetal heart sounds are heard over fetal back (scapula region) in vertex and breech presentation. Over chest in face presentation. |
| • Inform the mother of your findings. Make her comfortable. | |
| • Replace articles and wash hands | |
| • Record in the patient's chart the time, findings and remarks, if any | |

| Presentation and location of fetal heart sound | |
|---|---|

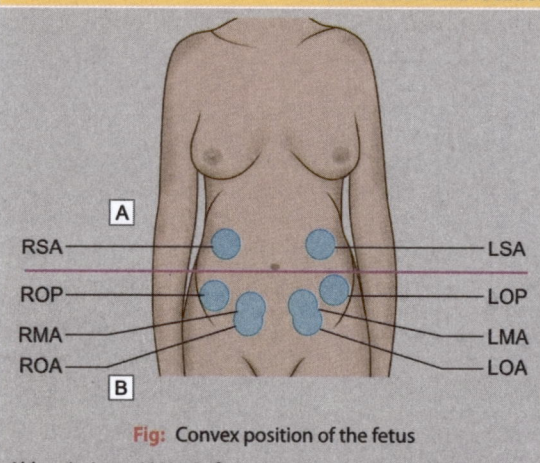

RSA
ROP
RMA
ROA

LSA
LOP
LMA
LOA

A

B

**Fig:** Convex position of the fetus

*Abbreviations:* LMA, Left mento-anterior; LOA, Left occiput anterior; LOP, Left occiput posterior; LSA, Left sacrum anterior; RMA, Right mento-anterior; ROA, Right occiput anterior; ROP, Right occiput posterior; RSA, Right sacrum anterior

• Location of the maximum intensity of the fetal heart rate

| Presentation | Location of FHR |
|---|---|
| Cephalic/vertex | Midway between umbilicus and level of anterior superior iliac spine |
| Breech | Level with or above umbilicus |
| Anterior | Close to the abdominal midline |
| Occiput transverse | In lateral abdominal area |
| Occiput posterior | In flank area |

## ANTENATAL EXERCISES

**Definition:** Systematic exercises to help the pregnant woman adapt to the physical changes in her body during pregnancy and to tone up the muscles that will be stretched or stressed during delivery.

### Purposes

• Keeping fit and healthy during pregnancy.
• To make body of the mother more prepared for the physical demands of labor, birth and puerperium.

## Advantages

- Reduction in aches and pains of pregnancy, e.g., backache and cramps.
- Improves posture and body awareness.
- Reduces constipation by accelerating movements in the intestine.
- Reduction in the minor ailments of pregnancy such as stiffness, tension, constipation and insomnia.
- Helps postnatal recovery.
- Improves ability to cope up with labor and childbirth.
- Helps to sleep better by relieving stress and anxiety that might make the mother restless at night.
- Exercise increases blood flow to the skin, and gives a healthy growth (glow).
- Mother receives an emotional lift from the release of internal hormones, like endorphins.
- Mother will feel more contented, as the release of tranquilizer hormones that follows exercise aids in relaxation.
- The energy level will be increased and mother will be better prepared for the labor.
- Mother will regain the shape more quickly after delivery.

## Articles

- Mat/Dari to do laying exercises comfortably.
- Chair to sit in a comfortable position

## Procedure

| Nursing action | Rationale |
|---|---|
| **Preprocedural steps:**<br>• Collect the articles necessary for the procedure.<br>• Explain the procedure to the patient.<br>• Ask the patient to empty her bowel and bladder.<br>• Make her wear comfortable loose clothes and well-fitted bra.<br>• Instruct the woman to take adequate fluid intake before and after the exercise.<br>• Educate the woman to start exercises slowly and rhythmically. | • To save time and energy.<br>• To win the confidence of the patient.<br>• Make the patient accustomed. |
| **Intraprocedural steps:**<br><br>**Exercise 1: Deep breathing exercise**<br>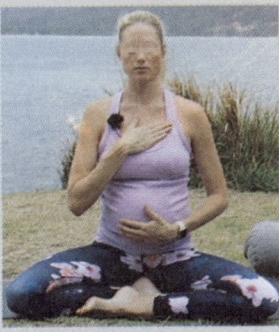<br>• Instruct the mother to assume comfortable sitting position. | • This exercise strengthens the diaphragmatic muscles and improves oxygenation of the blood.<br>• It is an effective pain reducing technique. |

*Contd...*

Appendices

| Nursing action | Rationale |
|---|---|
| • Breathe in deeply through nose.<br>• Sigh out through mouth.<br>• Repeat it five times (breathe in and out)<br>• Perform this exercise for six times a day | • This exercise aids oxygen supply to mother and fetus.<br>• It prevents hyperventilation.<br>• It relaxes the body and mind. |

**Exercise 2: Alternate nostril breathing**

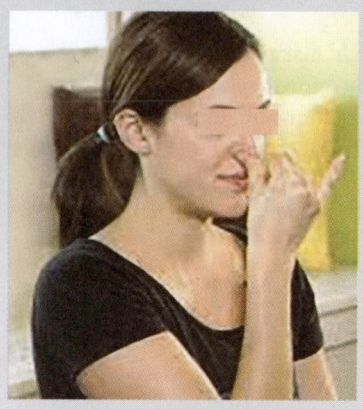

Instruct the mother to do the following steps:
- To start with, empty lungs completely.
- Close one nostril and take a deep breath through the other nostril.
- Try to fill lungs with as much air as possible.
- Hold the breath for few seconds.
- Breathe out through same nostril.
- Then repeat the same process with the other nostril closed.
- At one time 3–4 breaths are to be taken
- Do this exercise five times a day.

| **Exercise 3: Abdominal breathing**<br>• Instruct the mother to sit comfortably or kneel on all fours.<br>• Pull in the lower part of abdomen below the umbilicus while continuing to breathe normally.<br>• Hold the muscles in the drawn-in position for 10 seconds.<br>• Repeat up to 10 times. | • It strengthens the deep transverse abdominal muscles and also prevents backache. |

**Exercise 4: Pelvic tilting exercise**

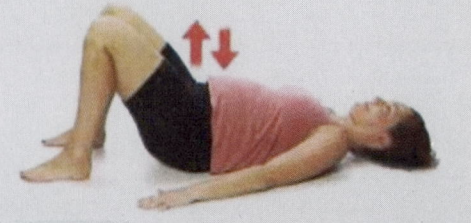

• It strengthens the pelvic floor and abdominal muscles that stretch during delivery.

*Contd...*

| Nursing action | Rationale |
|---|---|
| Teach the mother to do the following steps:<br>• Assume supine position, well supported with pillows, knees bent and feet flat.<br>• Place one hand under the back and other on top of the abdomen.<br>• Tighten the abdominal muscles and buttocks and press the surface of the back down on the underneath hand.<br>• Breathe normally, hold for 10 seconds and then relax<br>• Repeat up to 10 times. | |
| **Exercise 5: Tailor sit/Tailor stretching exercise**<br>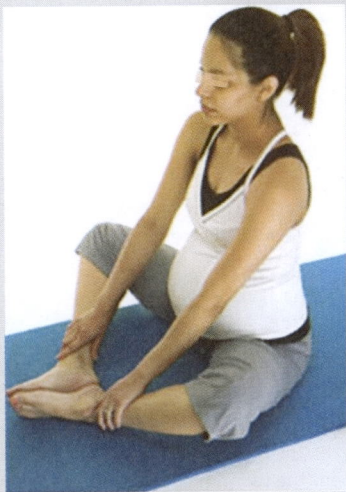<br>Instruct the mother to do the following steps:<br>• Sit with knees bent and place the soles of feet together.<br>• Pull feet closer to body.<br>• Place hands underneath knees.<br>• Inhale and press knees down against hands.<br>• While doing this, push hands against knees.<br>• Hold this pressure for a count of five. | • This exercise helps to strengthen the hip, thigh and pelvic floor muscles.<br>• Relieves lower back pain.<br>• Increases perineal circulation.<br><br><br>• To stretch the pelvic floor muscles. |
| **Exercise 6: Kegel exercise**<br>Instruct the woman to:<br>• Assume sitting/standing/half lie down position with legs slightly apart.<br>• Firmly tense or contract the muscles around the vagina as if to stop the flow of urine in midstream for 10 seconds then relax the muscles.<br>• Repeat up to 10 times<br>• One should aim to do 8–10 sets of 10 contractions each per day for maximum benefit. | |

Appendices

*Contd...*

| Nursing action | Rationale |
|---|---|
| **Exercise 7: Knee rolling exercise** | • This exercise helps to prevent backache and minimizes leg cramps. |

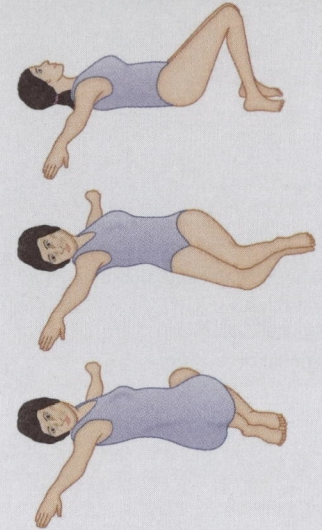

Tell the mother for the following steps:
• Lie on the back with knee bent and feet flat on the floor.
• Keep the shoulder down flat, lower both the knees slowly to the left, return them to center and then over to the right.
• Repeat in a rhythmical manner and gradually increase the range of movement.

| **Exercise 8: Hip up drawing exercise** | • It strengthens the calf muscles and relieves cramps |
|---|---|

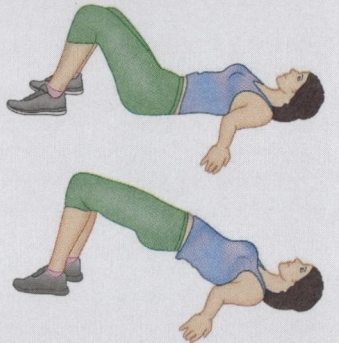

Ask mother to do the following procedure
• Lie on your back with bent knees and your feet in toward your hips.
• Press your palms into the floor alongside your body.
• Extend your right leg so that it is straight.
• Lift your hips up as high as you can.
• Hold this position for 30 seconds.

*Contd...*

| Nursing action | Rationale |
|---|---|
| **Exercise 9: Foot and leg exercise** | • It helps to improve circulation and reduces the occurrence of deep vein thrombosis. |

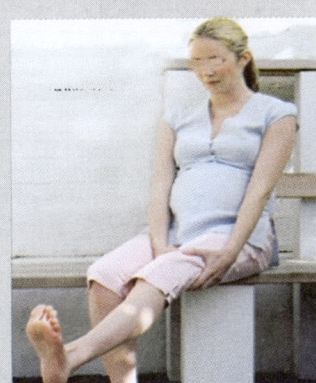

Instruct the mother to do the below procedure:
• Sit on the floor with the legs lie down or sit on a chair with the legs hanging down.
• Keep both knees and ankles relaxed.
• Now bend and stretch the ankles for 30–45 seconds, at least for 12 times.
• After this, make imaginary circles with your feet. Circle both feet at the ankles at least 20 times in each direction.
• Brace both knees for a count of four and then relax. Repeat 12 times.
• Bend and straighten knees.
• Perform this exercise before getting up from resting, last thing at night and several times a day.

**Exercise 10: Neck relaxer exercise**

• To relax body and mind.

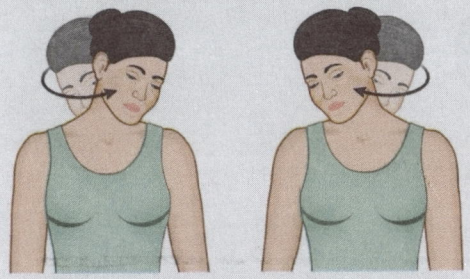

• Instruct the mother to assume comfortable sitting position.
• Close your eyes.
• Gently roll the head around, make a full circle and inhale while you do.
• Exhale and relax, letting the head drop forward comfortably.
• Repeat 4–5 times.
• Similarly, repeat this exercise in opposite direction.

*Contd...*

| Nursing action | Rationale |
|---|---|
| **Postprocedural steps:**<br>• Record time and details of exercise.<br>• Advice the mother to notify physician if any warning sign occurs as dizziness, blurred vision, heart palpitations, vaginal bleeding, lack of fetal movement, etc.<br>• Educate the mother regarding the benefits of exercises. | • To prevent complications.<br><br><br><br>• To motivate mother so that she should perform these exercises at home on regular basis during pregnancy. |

## Points to be Kept in Mind during Exercise

- Warm up and cool down at every exercise session.
- If woman feels faintness and dizziness, slow down or stop exercising.
- Drink plenty of fluids.
- Do not over heat the body as overheating of body is linked to some birth defects.
- Maintain good posture.
- Wear a well-fitted and supported brassiere.
- From midway throughout pregnancy, avoid exercising on the back as it places too much pressure on major veins and reduces $O_2$ supply to placenta and baby.

## Warning Signs to Stop Exercise

- Vaginal bleeding
- Dizziness or feeling pain
- Breathlessness
- Chest pain
- Headache
- Muscle weakness
- Calf pain/swelling
- Uterine contractions
- Decrease fetal movements
- Fluid leaking from vagina.

# URINE ANALYSIS

**Definition:** A urinalysis is an examination of urine. It is the process of analyzing urine scientifically, to detect abnormalities.

## Purposes

- To estimate the presence of glucose, albumin, pus cells in the urine.
- To help in diagnosis and treatment of a disease.

## Articles

- Spirit lamp
- Match box

- Test tube with test tube holder
- Test tube stand
- Benedict's solution and 2% acetic acid solution
- Dropper one for urine and second for reagents
- Kidney tray
- Specimen container
- One jar or bowl of water to rinse the dropper after use
- Clean, disposable gloves
- Reagent strips in container
- Litmus paper to check reaction of urine (activity/alkalinity)

## Procedure

### Testing Urine for Albumin

| Nursing action | Rationale |
| --- | --- |
| **Preprocedural steps:** | |
| • Explain the woman about the test to be done. | • To win the confidence of the patient. |
| • Provide container to the woman. | • For collecting urine |
| • Wear clean gloves. | • To maintain barrier nursing |
| • Collect urine specimen from patient. | • For urine analysis |
| **Intraprocedural steps:** | |
| • Take test tube and fill ¾ of it with urine | |
| • Fix the test tube holder on lower one-third of the test tube | • For proper fixing |
| • Check the reaction of urine, if found alkaline, add one drop of acetic acid and make it acidic | • If the urine is highly alkaline or acidic, it will give false reading |
| • Heat the upper third of urine over the spirit lamp and allow it to boil | • Prevent scalding |
| • Keep the mouth of the test tube away from your face | |
| • Observe the top heated column of the urine for a cloudy appearance. Clear urine indicates absence of albumin | • Confirms the presence of albumin |
| • If cloudy, add 5 drops of 2% acetic acid. A cloud may appear either due to phosphate or albumin | |
| • Add 2–3 drops of acetic acid into the test tube. If urine still remains cloudy, it indicates presence of albumin | |
|   Clear = nil | |
|   Trace = + | |
|   Cloudy = ++ | |
|   Thick cloudy = +++ | |
| If it becomes clear, it indicates the presence of phosphates. | |
| **Postprocedural steps:** | |
| • Discard the urine and rinse the test tube | • For next use |
| • Replace articles | • For further use |
| • Discard gloves and wash hands | • Prevent spread infection |
| • Record the procedure with date and time on patient chart | • Act as communication between the staff member |

*Contd...*

## Testing Urine for Sugar—Benedict's Solution Method

| Nursing action | Rationale |
|---|---|
| **Preprocedural steps:** | |
| • Explain about method of collecting a double voided specimen of urine | • It helps the patient to collect specimen in a correct manner |
| • Provide container for collecting urine | |
| • Wear gloves and collect urine specimen from patient | • To maintain barrier nursing |
| **Intraprocedural steps:** | |
| • Take test tube and fix in holder | |
| • Pour 5ml of benedict solution into the test tube | • Confirms the presence of sugar in the urine |
| • Light spirit lamp and heat benedict's solution for 2 minutes | • If color of the solution changes on heating, it means solution is not suitable for testing |
| • Keep the mouth of the test tube away from the face | • To avoid spillage of urine |
| • Add eight drops of urine using dropper, through the sides and allow it to boil for another few second | |
| • Put off the flame and allow it to cool | • Cooling completes color change when glucose is present in urine |
| • Watch for color change and compare with standard color code | • Normal urine does not contain sugar |
| ▪ Blue–nil | No sugar |
| ▪ Green liquid without deposit | +/1% sugar |
| ▪ Green liquid with yellow deposit | ++/2% sugar |
| ▪ Colorless liquid with orange deposit | ++++/3% sugar |
| ▪ Brick red | ++++/4% sugar |
| **Postprocedural steps:** | |
| • Discard the urine and rinse the test tube | • For further use |
| • Replace articles | |
| • Discard gloves | |
| • Wash hands | • To prevent infection |
| • Record the finding in patient's chart | • Acts as communication between staff members |

## Reagent Strip/Tape Method

| Nursing action | Rationale |
|---|---|
| **Preprocedural steps** (same as for benedict solution method) | |
| **Intraprocedural steps:** | |
| • Dip the portion of the strip with reagent in urine | • Color of the strip changes according to the amount of glucose present in urine |
| • Compare the color of the strip with color chart on the reagent strip container/separate chart (Fig.) | • Change in the color of the urine indicates presence of glucose in urine |

*Contd...*

| Nursing action | Rationale |
|---|---|
| 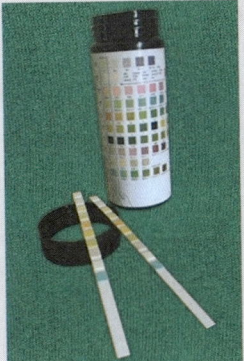<br>**Fig:** Urine strip test with color coding | |
| **Postprocedural steps:**<br>• Discard the urine and used strip<br>• Replace articles<br>• Discard gloves, wash hands<br>• Record the findings in patient's chart | • Acts as communication channel between staff members |

# PREGNANCY TEST (BY URINE SAMPLE)

**Definition:** A pregnancy test measures a hormone in the body called human chorionic gonadotropin (hCG). hCG is a hormone produced during pregnancy. It appears in the blood and urine of pregnant woman as early as 10 days after conception.

## Purpose

• To diagnose pregnancy.

## Articles

• Pregnancy test kit: It contains:
  ▪ Oval shape test card
  ▪ **Plastic dropper:** To be disposed of after the test
  ▪ Drying agent in a sachet—to keep the pouch moisture proof but is not required for the test
• Clean disposable gloves
• Urine sample
• Kidney tray

## Procedure

| Nursing action | Rationale |
|---|---|
| **Preprocedural steps:**<br>• Explain the woman about the test to be done<br>• Provide container to the woman<br>• Wear clean gloves<br>• Collect urine specimen from patient | • To win the confidence of the patient<br>• For collecting urine sample<br>• To maintain barrier nursing<br>• For urine analysis |
| **Intraprocedural steps:**<br>• Take out the preg-color card and place it on a flat surface<br>• Draw a little urine with a dropper and put just two drops in the circular test well that is usually marked "S"<br>• Do not spill urine on the reading strip<br>• Wait for 3–5 minutes (as per instruction of manufacturer's)<br><br>• Read the test result<br>  ▪ Look at the regions marked 'C' and 'T' on the test card. 'C' indicates a control. This band must always appear because this is the comparison band. 'T' indicates the test sample<br>  ▪ If only one pink/purple band appear, in the region marked 'C', it means the test is negative for pregnancy | • To maintain cleanliness during the procedure<br>• Read the result before stipulated time or waiting too long, can both lead to inaccurate readings |
|   ▪ If two pink/purple bands appear, one in the region marked 'C' and the other in the region marked 'T' it means that the test is positive for pregnancy<br>  ▪ In case no band appears, then the test is invalid. Repeat the test with a new pack after 72 hours<br>  ▪ If the line formed in region "T" is faint, this could be due to low levels of hCG hormone. In case of faint band, repeat the test with a new pack after 72 hours<br>**Postprocedural steps:**<br>• Discard the urine and preg color card<br>• Replace the articles<br>• Discard gloves and wash hands<br>• Record the finding on patient chart and also report the finding to patient and physician | <br><br><br><br><br><br>• For further use<br>• To control infection<br>• For further management |

## INTRANATAL ASSESSMENT

**Definition:** Intranatal assessment includes assessment of the mothers during labor and delivery.

## Purposes

- To assess the condition of the mother.
- To assess the condition of fetus.

- To avoid complication.
- To maintain partograph to monitor the progress of labor.
- To detect any complication at the earliest stage.

| Articles | Purposes |
|---|---|
| • Blood pressure apparatus<br>• Thermometer<br>• Stethoscope<br>• Watch<br>• Measuring tape<br>• Partograph chart | • To measure the blood pressure<br>• To note the temperature of the patient<br>• To hear fetal heart sound<br>• To note uterine contractions and fetal heart rate (FHR)<br>• To measure symphysis fundal height and abdominal girth<br>• To note the maternal and fetal data during labor |
| • Pen<br>• Gown, mask, cap, gloves<br>• Betadine solution<br>• Lubricating jelly<br>• Sterile tray for pervaginal examination contains:<br>  ▪ Sponge holder<br>  ▪ Cotton balls<br>  ▪ Gynecological pads<br><br>  ▪ Draw sheet | • To note the partograph<br>• To maintain barrier nursing<br>• For toileting the perineum<br>• To lubricate fingers before performing pervaginal examination<br>• For toileting the external genitalia and inner side of thighs<br><br>• To place on the mother's perineum after pervaginal examination<br>• To place below the mother perineum to provide a sterile field |

**Intranatal assessment includes:**

- Maternal assessment
- Fetal assessment
- Assessment of progress of labor

**Maternal assessment includes:**

| | |
|---|---|
| • Alert, oriented, gives response to command<br><br>• **Vital signs:** Temperature, pulse, respiration<br>• **Urinalysis:** Protein, ketones and glucose | • To assess condition of the mother with a hope she will participate well throughout the process of labor<br>• To detect any change in mother's condition<br>• To detect any complications such as increase in protein indicate preeclampsia; increase in glucose level indicate diabetes |

**Fetal assessment includes:**

| | |
|---|---|
| • Assessment of fetal size and position/ presentation<br>• Fetal heart rate<br>• Presence of blood or meconium in the liquor | • To diagnose whether the mother can undergo normal vaginal delivery or may need cesarean section<br>• To detect any fetal distress<br>• It indicates the possibility for the occurrence of fetal distress |

**Assessment of progress of labor includes:**

| | |
|---|---|
| • Descent of presenting part<br><br>• Dilatation and effacement of cervix<br><br><br>• Uterine contractions | • If the presenting part does not descend as duration of labor progress, it indicates cephalopelvic disproportion<br>• Full cervical<br>  **Dilatation:** 0–10 cm<br>  **Effacement:** 0–100%<br>• To note rate and rhythm of uterine contractions |

## Assessment as per Stages of Labor

### First Stage of Labor

- **History**
  - **Initial assessment:** Include a review of patient's antenatal care including confirmation of E.D.O.D from ultrasound and patient's verbal response.
  - **Focus history taking:** Include information regarding the frequency and time of onset of contraction, status of membrane (Intact, ruptured. If ruptured → when it happened, the color of amniotic fluid), the fetal movements, vaginal bleeding (present/absent)
- **Physical examination includes:**
  - Documenting maternal and fetal condition
  - Patient's vital sign
  - Head to toe examination
  - **Abdominal palpation:** To assess fetal lie, position, presentation
  - **Note the presence of peripheral edema:** Signs of preeclampsia
  - **Check for bladder distention:** It may impede progress of labor
- **Partograph:** To assess progress of labor.

## Partograph

**Definition:** Partograph (Fig. on page 652) is basically a graphic representation of the events of labor plotted against time in hours (by WHO).

**Components of partograph and its interpretation:**

- **Patient identification:** Includes patient's name, gravida, Para, hospital's name, consultant's name, period of gestation.
- **Time:** Recorded at hourly interval. Zero time for spontaneous labor is the time of admission in the labor ward and for induced labor, it is the time of induction.
- **Fetal heart rate:** Recorded every half hourly in 1st stage and every 15 minutes in 2nd stage or following rupture of membranes.

  > Normal fetal heart rate (FHR) is 110–150 beats/min measured by fetoscope or Doppler ultrasonic cardiography.

- **State of membranes and color of liquor:** If membranes are intact mark 'I', ruptured 'R'. If liquor is clear, mark 'C', if meconium stained, mark 'M'.
- **Cervical dilatation:**
  - **In latent phase:** Cervical dilatation up to 4 cm and rate of dilatation is 0.35 cm/hr.
  - **In active phase:** Starts with dilatation of 4 cm and ends till 8 cm. Rate of dilatation is 1.2–1.5 cm/hr.
  - **In transition phase:** Starts with dilatation of 8 cm and ends with 10 cm. Rate of critical dilatation is 1.5 cm/hr.

  **In cervicograph:** The alert line starts at 4 cm (WHO) of cervical dilatation and ends at 10 cm dilatation. The action line is drawn 4 hours to the right and parallel to the alert line.
  - In normal labor, cervical dilatation (cervicograph) should be either on the alert line or left to it.
  - When it falls on zone 2, it is abnormal and needs to be critically assessed.

- When it falls in zone 3, case should be reassessed by a senior person. Decision is to be made for termination of labor cesarean section/or for augmentation of labor [artificial rupture of membranes (ARM)/oxytocin].
- **Descent of presenting part:** Rate of descent of presenting part is less than 1 cm/hr in primi- and <2 cm/hr in multipara.
- **Uterine contractions:** The square in vertical columns are shaded according to duration and intensity. The contractions are weak (<20 sec), moderate (20–40 sec) and strong (>40 sec).
  - **During latent phase:** Contractions come at interval of 15–30 minutes and lasts for 30 seconds.
  - **In active phase:** Contractions come at interval of 3–5 minutes and lasts up to 60 seconds.
  - **In transition phase:** Contractions occur every 2–3 minutes lasting 60–90 seconds.
- **Drugs and fluids:** Concentration of oxytocin in the upper box and dose (mIU/min) in the lower box. Any drug (like diuretic, anticonvulsant, and antihypertensive, etc.) or fluids given during the time of labor are to be recorded carefully.
- **Blood pressure:** Recorded every 2 hourly and pulse at every 30 minutes.
- **Temperature:** Temperature is to be recorded every 4 hourly.
- **Urine analysis:** Check the urine volume and the presence of acetone bodies, proteins and glucose.

### Advantages of partograph

- A single sheet of paper can provide details of necessary information at a glance.
- No need to record labor events repeatedly.
- It can predict deviation from normal of labor.
- It reduces the incidence of prolonged labor and cesarean section rate.
- It saves time.
- Transfer of information becomes easy when labor status changes.
- Helpful to reduce maternal morbidity and mortality, perinatal morbidity and mortality rates.

### Second Stage of Labor

Continue to reassess the uterine contractions, fetal heart rate, progress of labor and plot the findings on the partograph.

### Third Stage of Labor

- Check vital signs of the mother so as to assess any deviation from normal
- Monitor baby's condition to detect earliest any sign of fetal distress
- Note the signs of separation of placenta
- Perform placental examination to check for its completeness
- Assess uterine condition. Immediately after delivery if no product is retained inside the uterine cavity— uterus feels hard, if product remains inside—uterus feels soft and boggy.

### Fourth Stage of Labor

- Monitor maternal vital signs every 15 minutes for 1 hour, then every 30 minutes for next 1 hour and then every 1 hourly, to monitor the condition of mother and identify any changes.
- Note fundal height, uterine tone and position—to assess whether uterus is contracting or relaxed.
- Assess the color, amount, odor of lochia—to check for any signs of PPH.

- If uterus is relaxed, massage it to make it hard because massaging the uterus can help to expel the blood clots.
- Assist and encourage the mother for breastfeeding as soon as possible.

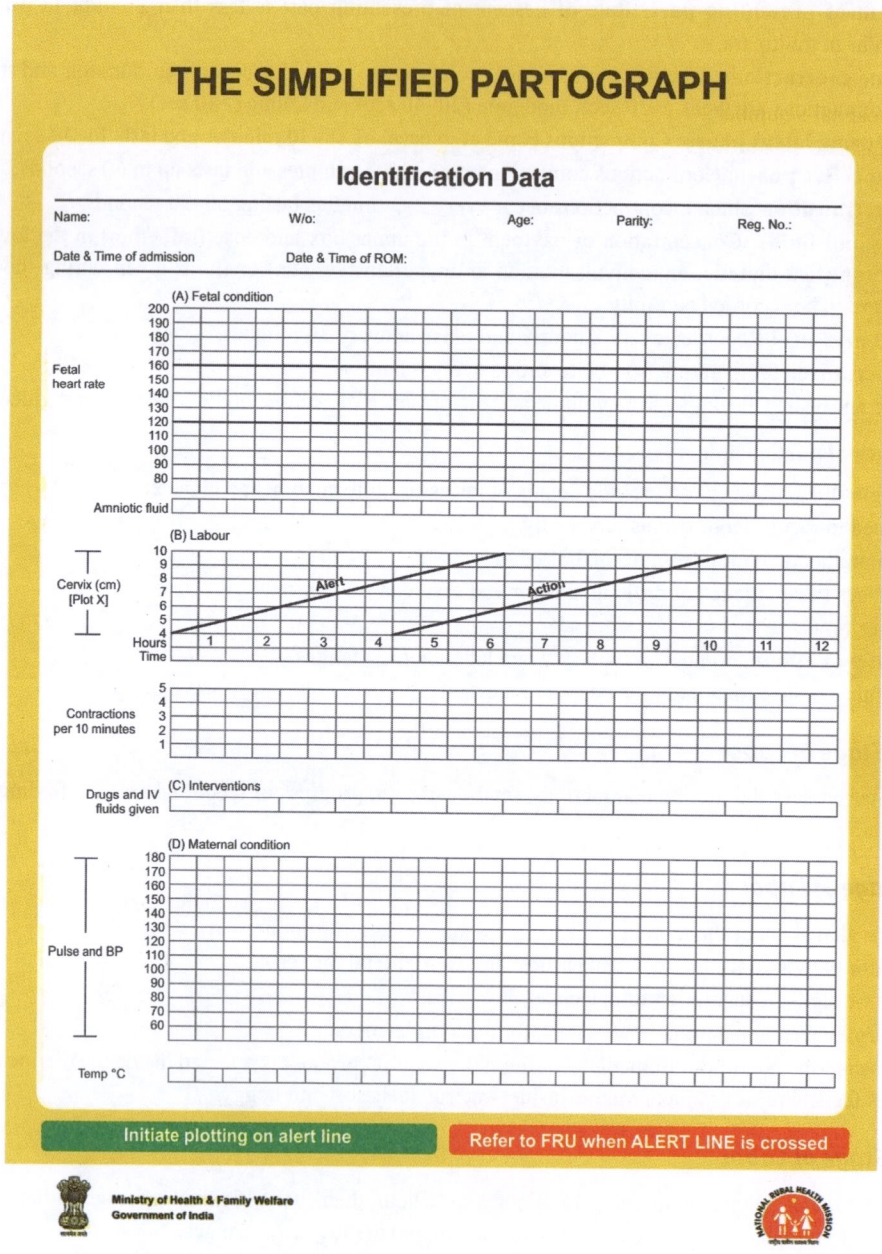

**Fig:** Partograph

## Intranatal Assessment Format

- **Identification data:**
  - Name
  - Age
  - Education
  - Hospital's number
  - Husband's name
  - Educational status of husband
  - Occupation of husband
  - Address
  - Family income
  - Date of admission
  - Reason for admission
- **Present obstetric history:**
  - Last menstrual period (LMP)
  - Expected date of delivery (EDD)
  - Period of gestation (POG)
  - GPLA
- **History:**
  - Trimester I
  - Trimester II
  - Trimester III
- **Past obstetrical history:**

| Sl. No. | Year | Nature of pregnancy | | | Nature of labor | Nature of puerperium | Condition of body | | | Remarks |
|---------|------|----------|---------|-----------|-----------------|---------------------|-------------------|-----|--------|---------|
|         |      | Abortion | Preterm | Full term |                 |                     | Alive/ stillbirth | Sex | Weight |         |
|         |      |          |         |           |                 |                     |                   |     |        |         |

- **Past medical/surgical history_____**
  - Personal history: Diet, sleep, habits, exercise, behavior _____
  - Family history, genetic disorder, joint/nuclear_____
- **Physical examination:**
  - Nourishment _____
  - Body built _____
  - Height _____
  - Weight _____
- **Vital sign:**
  - Temperature
  - Pulse
  - Respiration
  - Blood pressure

- **Head to toe examination:**
  - Face
  - Eyes
  - Mouth
  - Lips
  - Conjunctiva
  - Skin turgor
  - Warmth/cool
- **Abdominal examination:**
  - Size
  - Shape
  - **Skin condition:** Scars, diastasis recti, hernia, linea nigra, striae gravidarum, state of umbilicus _____
  - Contraction: Present/absent _____
  - **Fundal palpation:**
    **Inference:** Lie _____, presentation _____
    Position _____, attitude_____
  - **Lateral palpation:**
    Left side – Description _____
    Right side – Description _____
  - **Pelvic grip:** Presenting part engaged/nonengaged -------------
  - **Pawlick grip:** Presenting part: well-fixed/Mobile
  - **Auscultation:** FHR _____
- **Intranatal events:**
  - Time/date of onset of labor pain _____
  - Maternal general condition _____
  - **Condition of uterus:** Contracted/relaxed _____
  - **State of cervix:** Dilated/nondilated _____
  - Effacement of cervix (%) _____
  - Station of presenting part (+/–) _____
  - **Status of membrane:** (intact/ruptured) _____
  - **Color of liquor:** Clear/meconium stained _____
- Description of 3rd stage _____
  - **Description of 4th stage:** Condition of mother _____
  - Condition of baby _____

## PER VAGINAL EXAMINATION DURING LABOR

**Definition:** A vaginal examination in labor is a systematic examination to assess the status of vagina, vulva, cervix, membranes, liquor, presenting part and pelvis.

## Purposes

- **Vulva:** To assess for ulceration, condylomata, varices and any perineal scarring or rigidity.
- **Vagina:** To assess the presence or absence of following features.
  - Vaginal discharge
  - Full rectum
  - Vaginal stricture or septum
  - Presentation or prolapse of umbilical cord
- **Cervix:** To observe length, dilation and effacement
- **Membranes:** Whether membranes ruptured or intact
- **Liquor:** If membrane rupture, color of the liquor
- **Presenting part:** When palpating presenting part, four things that must be assessed:
  - What is the presenting part, e.g., head, breech or shoulder?
  - If head is presenting, what is the presentation, e.g., occiput, brow or face presentation?
  - What is the position of the present part in relation to mother's pelvis?
  - If presentation is occiput, vault or moulding is present?
- **Pelvis:** To assess the size of the pelvic inlet, the premonitory and retropubic area are palpated
  - To assess the size of mid pelvis, the curve of the sacrum, the sacrospinous ligaments and the ischial spines are palpated.
  - To assess the size of the pelvic outlet, the sub-pubic angle, inter-tuberous diameter and mobility of the coccyx are determined.

## Indications

- **At the onset of labor:** To assess presenting part and its position.
- **Progress of labor:** To assess dilatation, effacement of cervix and the station of the presenting part.
- **Following rupture of the membranes:** To exclude cord prolapse, color of the liquor.
- When any complication arises during labor.

## Equipment

- Artery clamp
- Sterile bowl
- Betadine solution
- Lubricating jelly
- Sterile cotton balls
- Sims' vaginal speculum
- Cap
- Gloves
- Plastic apron
- Mask
- Shoe cover
- Sterile drawsheet
- Sponge forceps
- Gynae pad

## Preliminaries/Points to be Kept in Mind

- Collect all the articles necessary for the procedure.
- Maintain aseptic technique during the procedure.
- Bladder should be empty.
- Explain procedure to the patient.
- Provide comfortable position to patient.
- Finger inserted per vagina should not be withdrawn until the required information has been obtained.
- Give perineal care before performing vaginal examination.
- It should be restricted or limited after membranes have ruptured.
- Avoid, vaginal examination in case of antepartum hemorrhage.

## Procedure

| Nursing action | Rationale |
|---|---|
| • Explain procedure to patient and also teach her how to relax during examination | • To promote compliance and for smooth performance of the procedure |
| • If bladder is full, ask the mother to void | • To avoid discomfort during procedure |
| • Draw curtains around the bed | • To maintain privacy |
| • Check the previous per vaginal finding, if any done | • Serves as baseline data |
| • Ask the woman to lie down in dorsal recumbent position with knees flexed at the edge of the examination table | • For good visualization |
| • Spread mackintosh with draw sheet | • To prevent soiling of the linen |
| • Do a surgical hand washing | • To maintain aseptic technique during the procedure |
| • Wear sterile gown and sterile gloves | • To prevent the spread of infection |
| • Observe the external genitalia for the following:<br>  ▪ Signs of varicosities, vulva/warts or scars<br>  ▪ Previous episiotomy scar or lacerations<br>  ▪ Discharge or bleeding per vagina<br>  ▪ Show<br>  ▪ **If membranes ruptured:** Color and odor of amniotic fluid | • External genitalia must be assessed before cleansing the vulva |
| • Clean the vulva and perineal area with betadine solution | |
| • Drape the perineal area with sterile perineal sheet | |
| • Dip the first two fingers of the right hand into the antiseptic cream | • Lubricate the fingers |
| • Holding the labia apart with thumb and index fingers of the left hand, insert the right hand gloved lubricated fingers into the vagina - palm side down and press downwards | |

*Contd...*

| Nursing action | Rationale |
|---|---|
| • With the finger inside, explore the vagina properly until required information is not attained but this must be kept in mind not to touch the clitoris and anus during examination. Note the following points: | • Repeated vaginal examination increases morbidity rate<br>• Touching clitoris causes discomfort<br>• Touching anus causes contamination |
| ▪ Condition of vulva (bulging, soft and stretchable)<br>▪ Feel on touch of vaginal walls<br>▪ Consistency of vaginal walls<br>▪ Scar from previous perineal wound, cystocele or rectocele | • Normal vagina is warm and moist with soft vaginal walls<br>• Hot, dry vagina, firm and rigid walls suggest obstructed labor |
| • Examine the cervix with the fingers in the vagina turned upwards; locate the cervical OS by sweeping the fingers from side to side; assess cervix for: | |
| ▪ Effacement: Taking up/shortening of the cervix (0–100%)<br>▪ Dilatation: Enlargement of internal OS indicates dilatation (0 – 10 cm) | • To assess the progress of labor |
| ▪ Position of cervix (central or lateral)<br>▪ Consistency (Soft, tense, tender, firm) | • Normally cervix is situated centrally<br>• Normal cervix is soft, elastic and well applied to the presenting part in normal labor |
| • Check the presence or absence of fore water | • Intact membranes, which become tense during contractions with well-fitting presenting part indicates fore water<br>• Protruding membranes are seen with ill-fitting presenting part<br>• Membranes will not be felt, if they ruptured early |
| • Assess the station of presenting part in relation to maternal ischial spines [minus (–) plus (+)] | • To assess the progress of labor |
| • Check the presentation, position of fetus and whether moulding takes place or not | • Presentation (vertex, breech face, brow)<br>• Position (anterior, posterior, lateral)<br>• Moulding overlapping of cranial bones (the parietal bones override the occipital bone in case of moulding |
| • At the completion of the examination withdraw fingers from vagina; take care to note the presence of any blood or amniotic fluid on the examining fingers | • To compare the current findings with the previous one |
| • Clean and dry the perineal area and buttocks | |
| • Provide sterile perineal pad, if leakage occurs | |
| • Remove gloves and wash hands | |
| • Remove gown and mask | |
| • Auscultate the fetal heart tones and record on the patient chart | • To assess the well-being of the fetus |

*Contd...*

| Nursing action | Rationale |
|---|---|
| • Shift the woman on bed and provide her left lateral position | |
| • Soiled cotton and gauze should be discarded in yellow bucket | • To prevent spread of infection (biomedical hazard) |
| • Wash all the articles used for the procedure and replace in the utility room | • For the further use |
| • Record the finding on the patient chart and report the progress of labor to the patient and physician | • Acts as communicator between the health professional and patient |

# SETTING TROLLEY AND CONDUCTION OF NORMAL VAGINAL DELIVERY

**Definition:** Conducting or managing normal vaginal delivery involves the hand maneuvers used to assist the baby's birth, delivery of the placenta and to provide immediate care to the newborn.

## Purposes

- To provide well prepared and safe environment to the mother during the time of labor.
- For the safe delivery (without trauma) to the mother and baby.
- To help the mother to go through the childbirth process without undue stress, injury and complications.
- To promote smooth and safe transition of newborn to the extra uterine life.
- To avoid complications.

## Articles

### For Mother

| A. Delivery table: For positioning the mother | |
|---|---|
| **B. Sterile delivery pack containing:** | |
| **Articles for cutting and suturing an episiotomy** | |
| • Episiotomy scissor—1 | • To give episiotomy cut |
| • Artery clamps—3 | • To clamp umbilical cord and for suturing |
| • Tissue forceps—2 | • To hold the soft tissues during episiotomy suturing |
| • Tooth thumb or plain thumb forceps | • To hold the soft tissues during episiotomy suturing |
| • Needle holder—1 | • To hold the needle while suturing |
| • Round body and cutting needle—1 | • To suture episiotomy wound |
| • Syringe 10 cc—1 | • For infiltration |
| • Catgut suture material | • For suturing |
| • Kocher's forceps—1 | • To clamp umbilical cord and for artificial rupture of membrane |
| • Sponge holding forceps—1 | • To hold cotton swabs |

*Contd...*

| | |
|---|---|
| • 1 Bowl with cotton swabs and gauze | • To clean perineum |
| • Kidney tray—1 | • To receive the placenta |
| • Sterile pad—1 | • To support the perineum during delivery of the head |
| • Infant tube feeding or Foley's catheter | • To catheterize the bladder |
| • Sterile pad—1 | • To apply on the perineum after delivery |

**Other articles**

**IV tray containing**

| | |
|---|---|
| • IV Set—1 | • For giving IV fluid |
| • IV cannula—1 | • For giving IV fluid |
| • Intravenous fluid | • Normal saline/ringer lactate |
| • Plaster | • To fix the cannula |

**C. Drugs**

| | |
|---|---|
| • Oxytocin, methergine | • To induce contraction |
| • Lignocaine (1%) | • For local anesthesia |

**D. Antiseptic solutions (Dettol/Savlon): For cleaning perineum**

**E. Personal protective equipment**

| | |
|---|---|
| • Shoe cover—1 pair | • To maintain asepsis and prevent cross infection |
| • Cap—1 | • To maintain asepsis and prevent cross infection |
| • Gown—1 | • To maintain asepsis and prevent cross infection |
| • Gloves—1 pair | • To maintain asepsis and prevent cross infection |
| • Plastic apron—1 | • To prevent soiling of staff's clothes |

## For Newborn

- Baby blanket or flannel cloth (2)—One to receive and dry the baby of excess secretions and another to wrap the baby.
- Neonatal resuscitation equipment checked and ready for use.
- Oxygen source with tubing.
- Suction apparatus and mucous extractor.
- Cord clamp.
- Bulb syringe for nasal and oropharyngeal suctioning of the baby.

## General Instructions

- Maintain strict aseptic technique.
- Make sure all the equipment used at the time of labor are in good working condition.
- Maintain partograph to assess the condition of the mother and fetus from time to time.
- Record and report if any deviation occur while maintaining partograph to avoid further complications.
- Give episiotomy at the peak of uterine contraction only.
- Instruct the mother to bear down along with uterine contractions and till full dilatation of cervix.

## Procedure

| Nursing action | Rationale |
|---|---|
| **Preprocedural steps:** | |
| • Provide local preparations as per agency policy (shaving the perineum) | • To prevent infection |
| • Administer enema | • To empty the bowel |
| • Provide hospital gown to the mother | • To prepare her for delivery |
| • Maintain partograph (cervical dilatation, effacement, maternal vital sign, fetal heart rate, uterine contraction, status of membranes, color of liquor, etc.) | • To assess the progress of labor |
| • Give liquid to the mother, avoid solid foods | • Emptying time of the stomach is delayed during labor and may cause regurgitation |
| • Instruct mother for relaxation techniques | • To promote relaxation and ensure more oxygen supply to fetus |
| • Explain the mother regarding deep breathing exercises and how to bear down at the time of labor | • To get cooperation from the mother |
| **Intraprocedural steps:** | |
| • Once the head of the baby is visible at the introitus and bulging of the perineum take place, immediately shift the mother to the delivery room | |
| • Place the woman in dorsal position with knees bent at the lower end of the delivery table | • To ensure proper positioning for delivery |
| • Perform surgical hand washing | • To prevent spread of infection |
| • Wear sterile gown, mask and gloves | • To maintain barrier nursing |
| • Open the delivery pack, arrange all the articles and pour cleansing solution in the bowl | • For convenience and timely use |
| • Drape the mother's perineum and delivery area | • Obtain a sterile field for delivery |
| • Clean the perineum in the following manner using one cotton ball separately for each stroke<br> ▪ Mons pubis in zigzag manner from level of clitoris upwards<br> ▪ Clitoris to fourchette one downward stroke<br> ▪ Labia minora farther side first then nearest side<br> ▪ Labia majora farther side first them nearest side<br> ▪ Thighs in long strokes away from the perineum<br> ▪ Anus in one circular stroke | • Proper cleansing makes the perineum free from microorganism |
| • **Delivery of the head:**<br> ▪ As the head becomes visible at the introitus, place the pads of your fingertips on the portion of the vertex at vaginal introitus<br> ▪ Use other hand to support the perineum<br> ▪ Encourage the mother to bear down during uterine contractions<br> ▪ Infiltrate the perineum in facing manner at right lateral if episiotomy is required | • Giving pressure against the fetal head will keep it well flexed<br><br>• To prevent perineal tear<br>• To facilitate descent of the head<br><br>• To desensitize the perineal area before episiotomy |

*Contd...*

| Nursing action | Rationale |
|---|---|
| • When the suboccipital is placed under the symphysis pubis and the perineum is fully stretched, bulges out and threatens to tear—give episiotomy | • The ideal time to give episiotomy and to cut short second stage of labor |
| • Slow delivery of the head in between contractions is to be regulated. This is done when suboccipital frontal diameter emerges out | • To prevent intracranial damage to baby and laceration to perineum |
| • Immediately following delivery of the head, the mucus and blood in the mouth and pharynx are to be wiped with sterile gauze piece held on a little finger | • To clear the airway |
| • Sweep the fingers in both directions to feel for the umbilical cord | • To detect the presence of nuchal cord, which prevents descent of the fetus and delivery of the body |
| • If cord is loose around the neck, slip it over the baby's head as the baby is being born. But if it is sufficiently tight it is cut in between with the help of Kocher's forceps (1 inch apart) | • To prevent strangulation of the neck by the cord |
| • **Delivery of the shoulders:** | |
|   • Wait for a contraction and watch for restitution and external rotation of head | • Allows time for shoulders to rotate to the anteroposterior diameter of the outlet |
|   • When the shoulders reach the anteroposterior diameter of the pelvic outlet, proceed to deliver one shoulder at a time in the following manner: | |
|     o Place hands on each side of the head over the ears and apply downward traction to deliver the anterior shoulder | • Avoid overstretching of the perineum |
|     o Give methergin (0.2 mg) intramuscularly, following delivery of anterior shoulder to escape over the posterior vaginal wall | |
| • **Delivery of the trunk** | |
|   • Place the fore finger of each hand under the axillae and deliver the trunk gently by lateral flexion | |
|   • Record the time of birth | • Important life event |
|   • Place two clamps on the cord about 8–10 cm away from umbilicus and cut it while covering it with gauze | • Covering the cord will prevent the delivery field becoming bloody |
|   • Place the baby on mother's abdomen until the delivery of placenta. (If baby's Apgar score is normal) | • To promote bonding between mother and baby |
| **After delivery** | |
| • Place one hand over the fundus | • To feel the contraction of the uterus |
| • Continue to monitor the mother as she progresses to the third stage of labor | • To detect any change in mother's condition |
| • Watch for signs of placental separation (e.g., lengthening of cord, gush of bleeding, round firm fundus, descending of placenta into the vagina) | • Forceful pulling of placenta causes breakage of cord from placenta and as a result placenta is retained inside uterine cavity |
| • When the placenta is expelled out through the birth canal, grasp it in cupped hands, twist the placenta round and round with gentle traction | • For the intact stripping of the membranes |
| • Examine the placenta | • For its completeness |
| • Explore the genital tract | • For any laceration and any retained bits of placenta |

*Contd...*

| Nursing action | Rationale |
|---|---|
| • Massage the uterus | • To make it contract for expulsion of retained bits of membranes |
| • Suture the episiotomy in the following sequence with catgut 'O' suture (from inside outside) | • For proper approximation of episiotomy wound |
| ▪ 1st – Mucosa in continuous manner | |
| ▪ 2nd – Muscle in interrupted manner | |
| ▪ 3rd – Skin in figure of 8 manner or mattress sutures | |
| • Clean the vulva and surrounding area with antiseptic solution | |
| • Place perineal pad | |
| **Postprocedural steps** | |
| • Provide comfortable position to the mother | • To promote relaxation |
| • Remove gloves, gown, mask and wash the hands | • To prevent spread of infection |
| • Clean and replace the article | • For further use |
| • Record the delivery process, condition of the mother, baby on patient's chart | |

# PLACENTAL EXAMINATION

**Definition:** A thorough inspection and examination of the placenta and membranes, soon after expulsion for its completeness and normalcy.

Normally, the human placenta is:

- Discord, because of its shape.
- Hemochorial, because of the direct contact of the chorion with the maternal blood.
- Deciduate, because of the connection between the mother and fetus through umbilical cord.

## Purposes

- To assess whether the placenta is in normal size (15–20 cm in diameter), shape (discoid) and weight (1/6 of the fetal weight; 500–700 g).
- To detect any abnormalities such as additional lobes, missing cotyledons (normally 15–20), infarction, etc.
- To make sure that entire membrane and placenta have been expelled out.
- To assess the length of cord (30–100 cm, 50 cm average), site of insertion of cord (at center of placenta).
- To prevent postpartum hemorrhage and infection.

## Equipment

| Articles | Purposes |
|---|---|
| **A clean tray containing:** | |
| • Gloves and apron | • To protect yourself from infection and contamination |
| • Mackintosh | • To protect the table from soiling |
| • Pin | • To measure the thickness of placenta |
| • Measuring tape | • To measure the length of cord |
| • Cotton thread | • To measure the diameter of placenta and length of the cord |
| • Cotton swab | • To spread the membranes |
| • Kidney tray/paper bag | • To discard waste |
| • Weighing machine | • To measure weight of placenta |
| • Plastic bin (yellow) | • To discard the placenta |

## Procedure

| Nursing action | Rationale |
|---|---|
| • Wash hands | • To prevent cross infection |
| • Wear gloves and apron | • To protect yourself from infection and contamination |
| • Take placenta in a tray and wash it under running water in washbasin | • To remove blood clots and for clear visualization of placenta |
| **Examination of the membranes** | |
| • Using gloved hand, hold the placenta by the cord allowing the membranes to hang (twisting the cord twice around the fingers will provide a firm grip) | • For easy visualization |
| • Identify the hole through which the baby was delivered | • If membranes are intact, a single round hole can be identified clearly. |
| • Put hand inside the hole and spread out fingers to view the membranes and blood vessels | • The position of cord insertion and the course of blood vessels can be noted in this position |
| • Remove hand from inside the membranes and keep the placenta on a flat surface and examine both placental surfaces under membrane | |
| • With the cotton swab try to separate the amnion and chorion | • For clear visualization |
| • The amnion should be peeled from the chorion right up to the insertion of the umbilical cord in the fetal surface. And chorion is up to the margin of the placenta | • To check abnormalities |
| • Check the presence of any extra hole in the membrane | • To check abnormalities |
| • Examine the amnion and chorion for its completeness and presence of abnormal vessels and lobe. Amnion is smooth and shining but chorion is dull, rough and shaggy. | • To check abnormalities |
| **Examination of the placenta** | |
| • Invert the placenta, expose the maternal surface and remove if any clots present | • For clear visualization |
| • Put the placenta on flat surface | |
| • Check the diameter of the placenta with thread or measuring tape | |
| • Put pin in the center and margin of placenta. | • To check thickness of placenta |

*Contd...*

| | |
|---|---|
| • Examine the maternal surface by spreading it in the palms of both hands | • To assess for any missing part |
| • Then put the placenta on a flat surface, place the cotyledons in close approximation (any broken fragments must be replaced before accurate assessment is made). Ensure that no parts of placenta or membranes are left inside the uterus | • To prevent retention of bits of membranes inside the uterine cavity and hence prevent the occurrence of postpartum hemorrhage |
| • Check the presence of abnormalities such as infarctions, calcification or succenturiate lobes | |
| • Examine the fetal surface for numbers of lobes, color, appearance, insertion of cord and distribution of blood vessels | • To check any abnormality |

**Examination of cord**

| | |
|---|---|
| • Check for the presence of true and false knot | • To check any abnormality |
| • Measure the length of the cord by holding it extended against a graduated surface/side of the measuring scale. (The length of the cord on the baby may be added to get total length if possible) | • Average cord length is 50 cm |
| • Inspect the cut end of umbilical cord presence of three umbilical vessels | • Two arteries and one umbilical vein. Absence of an artery may be associated with renal abnormalities |

**Weighing the placenta**

| | |
|---|---|
| • Spread the plastic paper on the weighing machine | • To prevent it from soiling |
| • Weigh the placenta by placing it on the weighing scale | • Normally placental weight is 1/6 of fetal weight (500–700 g) |

**After care of articles and mother**

| | |
|---|---|
| • Place the placenta in yellow bin and send it for incineration | • For proper biomedical waste management |
| • Clean the area used for examination of the placenta and membranes, the weighing scale and bowl | |
| • Discard all waste | |
| • Remove the gloves and wash hands | |
| • Record the findings regarding placental examination on patient's chart and if any abnormality found report to physician | • Acts as a communication between staff members |

9

## PERFORMING AND SUTURING EPISIOTOMY

### Episiotomy

It is surgically planned incision given on the perineum during second stage of labor to enlarge the vaginal introitus, to facilitate safe and easy delivery of the fetus.

## Objectives

- To enlarge the size of vaginal orifice.
- To prevent perineal tear (if given on time).
- To reduce stress and strain on fetal head.
- To cut-short second stage of labor.
- To maintain the integrity of pelvic floor.

## Indications

- Large fetus more than 4 kg.
- Preterm or small for gestational age baby in order to minimize the risk of intracranial hemorrhage.
- Presence of rigid perineum.
- Face to pubis delivery, breech delivery or shoulder dystocia.
- Fetal distress, to make the delivery fast.
- When large laceration seems inevitable.
- In case of operative delivery like forceps/ventouse.
- Previous history of pelvic floor repair, perineal reconstructive surgery.

## Types (Fig)

Four types of episiotomy are:

- **Mediolateral:** Incision is given downward and outwards from the midpoint of fourchette. The cut may be given either towards right or left side and about 2.5 cm.
- **Median/midline:** The incision is given from the center of fourchette and extends posteriorly. The cut is 2.5 cm in length.
- **Lateral:** Incision starts from about 1 cm away from the center of fourchette and extends laterally.
- **J-shaped:** The incision starts from center of fourchette and is directed posteriorly about 1.5 cm and then points towards downward and outwards along 5 or 7 o'clock.

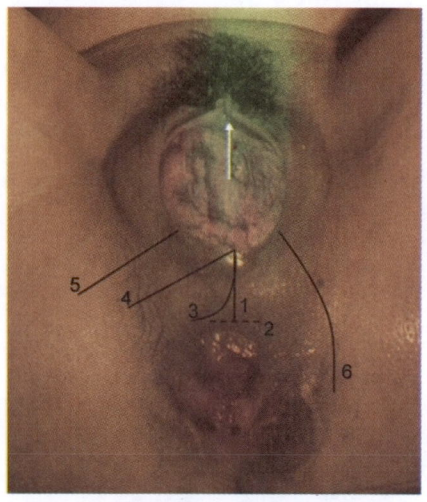

**Fig:** Types of episiotomy.
*Pointers:* 1: Median episiotomy; 2: Modified median episiotomy; 3: 'J'-shaped episiotomy; 4: Mediolateral episiotomy; 5: Lateral episiotomy; 6: Radical lateral (Schuchardt incision)

## Articles

| Articles | Purposes |
| --- | --- |
| • Episiotomy scissor | • For giving episiotomy |
| • Draping sheets | • To minimize exposure and prevent infection |
| • Xylocaine (1%) | • For local infiltration |
| • 10 mL disposable syringe with 21 gauge needle | • For local infiltration |
| • Gauge pieces | • To apply betadine on episiotomy wounds |

*Contd...*

| Articles | Purposes |
|---|---|
| • Cotton swabs | • To clean the perineum |
| • Antiseptic solution: Savlon, betadine | • For toileting of vagina |
| • Sterile gloves | • To prevent infection |
| • Suture material | • Chromic catgut 'O' for suturing episiotomy |
| • Sponge/Tampon | • To soak the bleeding |
| • Tooth thumb forceps | • To hold the edges of episiotomy while suturing |
| • Round body needle | • For suturing mucosal and muscle layers |
| • Cutting body needle | • For suturing skin |
| • Needle holder | • To hold the needle while suturing |

## Procedure

| Nursing action | Rationale |
|---|---|
| **Preprocedural steps:**<br>• **Preparation of mother**<br>  ■ Physical preparation:<br>    ○ Shave the perineum as per the hospital policy during first stage of labor<br>    ○ Provide lithotomy or dorsal position with thigh flexed and separated<br>    ○ Drape the mother<br>  ■ Psychological preparation:<br>    ○ Explain the procedure to the mother<br>    ○ Encourage and reassure during the procedure<br>  ■ Preparation of the environment:<br>    ○ Arrange for good source of light<br>    ○ Maintain privacy<br>    ○ Maintain sterile field | • To prevent infection and for clear visualization of vaginal orifice during birth process<br>• Gives clear visualization<br><br>• To maintain privacy<br>• To win the confidence<br><br><br>• To avoid unnecessary hurry |
| **Intraprocedural steps:**<br>• Clean the perineum thoroughly with antiseptic lotion and drape properly<br>• Infiltrate the perineum using 10 mL of local anesthetic (1% lignocaine). Wait for 3–5 minutes for the anesthetic to act<br>• Place index and middle fingers in the vagina with palmer side down; separate them slightly and exert outward pressure on perineal body and predict the length of the incision, accordingly | • To prevent infection<br><br>• To reduce pain during incision<br><br>• To provide protection to the presenting part in two ways:<br> (i) The fingers are against the presenting part and are thick enough so that scissors, if properly placed will not hurt the baby<br> (ii) The outward pressure flattens the perineal body a bit more, making it easier to incise using a single cut |
| • Place the blades of scissors in a straight up and down position, so that one blade is against the skin of the perineal body with the point where the blades cross at the middle of posterior fourchette. | |

*Contd...*

| Nursing action | Rationale |
|---|---|
| • Adjust the length of the blades of the scissors on the perineal body and predict the length of the incision, accordingly | • The length of the incision should be adequate to deliver the fetal head |
|   ▪ If mediolateral incision is given, cut is given downward and outward and from the midpoint of fourchette | |
|   ▪ If median/midline episiotomy is given, the incision is given from the center of fourchette and extends posteriorly | |
|   ▪ Apply pressure with a gauge piece (4", 4") | • To control bleeding |
| • After the conduction of delivery, assist/perform episiotomy suturing | |
| • Wipe the incisional area with sterile antiseptic cotton swabs | • To prevent the spread of infection |
| • Focus light on the perineal area | • For clear visualization of the perineum. |
| • Pack the vagina with vaginal plug | • Continuous bleeding may obscure the place of suturing |
| • **Vaginal mucosa** is sutured first. Identify the apex of mucosa and the first bite/suture is taken 0.5–1 cm above the apex. Continuous suture is used to repair vaginal mucosa from the above downwards till the fourchette is reached | |
| • Repair the **perineal muscle** by interrupted sutures, include the deeper tissue to enclose dead space from above downwards till the fourchette is reached | |
| • **Perineal** skin is opposed by mattress suture or figure of eight | |
| **Postprocedural steps:** | |
| • Remove the vaginal pack which was inserted during suturing | |
| • Rectal examination is made in order to ensure that no sutures have penetrated the rectal mucosa | • To prevent fistula formation |
| • Clean the perineum and apply perineal pad | |
| • Straighten patient's legs and assist her to supine position with legs crossed | • To make patient comfortable and reduce the chances of bleeding |
| • Clean all the instruments used for delivery and for episiotomy | • For further use |
| • Record in the labor record, the time of episiotomy, type of episiotomy, suturing carried out and the patient reaction. | • Acts as communication between staff members. |

## After Procedure Care

- **Dressing:** The wound is to be dressed each time following urination and defecation, to keep the area clean and dry. The dressing is done by swabbing with cotton swab soaked in antiseptic solution by antiseptic powder or ointment
    - Check for any bleeding or formation of hematoma
    - Check vital signs
    - Check for any tear or laceration
- **Comfort:** To relieve pain in the area, the following can be done:
    - Sitz bath with potassium permanganate
    - Application of infrared light
    - Ice application
- **Removal of stitches:** Catgut suture are absorbed by itself. If nonabsorbable material, like silk or nylon is used, remove the stitches on 6th day.

# 10

# EPISIOTOMY CARE

**Definition:** Cleaning the patient's external genitalia, sutures and surrounding skin using antiseptic solution.

## Purposes

- To clean the perineum
- To inspect the perineal region for redness, edema, ecchymosis, discharge, approximation (REEDA)
- To reduce the occurrence of infection in the perineal region
- To provide soothing effect
- To relieve pain
- To relieve inflammation
- To promote healing
- To stimulate circulation
- To reduce body odor and improve self-image
- To promote the sense of well being
- To observe the lochia

## Points to be Kept in Mind

- Maintain privacy during the procedure.
- Always clean from more clean area to less clean area.
- Use correct concentration of antiseptic solution.
- Collect specimen of discharge if required before cleaning the area.

## Articles

- **A clean tray containing:**
  Antiseptic solution 2% Dettol or Savlon (2 mL Savlon/Dettol in 100 mL of water)

## Normal Saline in a Bottle

- Cheatle forceps
- Sterile sanitary pad
- Kidney trays
- Sterile gloves
- Mackintosh with sheet/towel
- **Sterile tray continuing**
  - Artery forceps—1
  - Dissecting forceps—1
  - Cotton bolls
  - Gauze pieces
  - Sterile gallipot/bowl → to pour antiseptic solution
  - Sterile towel to wipe hands of after surgical
  - Scrub—draw sheet

## Other Articles

- Bedpan
- Screen
- Plastic apron
- Mask
- Infrared lamp

## Procedure

| Nursing action | Rationale |
|---|---|
| **Preprocedural steps:** | |
| • Collect all the articles at the bedside of patient | • To save time and energy |
| • Explain the procedure to the patient | • To win the cooperation |
| • Ask the patient to empty her bowel and bladder | • To ensure cleanliness and reduce the number of microorganism in perineal area |
| • Spread curtain/screen around the bed | • To maintain privacy |
| • Provide dorsal recumbent position | • To facilitate better viewing and provide comfort |
| • Ask the mother to remove undergarments and sanitary pad | • For better visualization |
| • Spread mackintosh under patient's hips along with newspaper lining | • To prevent soiling of linen |
| • Observe lochia (color, odor, consistency) | • To detect any abnormality |
| • Discard the pad in yellow bin | • As per biomedical waste management protocol |
| **Intraprocedural steps:** | |
| • Keep bedpan under the buttocks of the patient | • To collect the normal saline/sterile water that is poured due to excessive sticky lochial discharge |
| • Pour warm water/normal saline on the perineal area | • To remove excessive clots/discharge |
| • Remove bedpan | |
| • Wash hands with soap | • To maintain barrier nursing |
| • Open the sterile tray, arrange articles with cheatle forceps and pour antiseptic solution in the sterile gallipot in tray | |
| • Wear gloves | |
| • Drape the area using diamond draping method | |
| • Separate the vestibule using two gauge pieces with nondominant hand and clean the vestibule starting from clitoris to fourchette | |
| • Inside of labia minora downward, farther side first, then nearer side | |
| • Take off the nondominant hand | |
| • Labia majora downward, father side first then nearer side | |
| • Discard the used artery forceps | |
| • Take one gauze piece, dip in Savlon/normal saline, squeeze it properly | |
| • Roll it over the episiotomy suture line from inside to outside without lifting your hand. Do not use cotton balls for this purpose | • To clean the area uniformly and to facilitate drainage, if any |

*Contd...*

| Nursing action | Rationale |
|---|---|
| • Repeat it until episiotomy wound becomes clean<br>• Assess the episiotomy wound healing using REEDA scale<br>• Remove the gloves and discard them<br>• Adjust the position of infrared lamp so that it shines on the perineum at the distance of 45–50 cm | • To assess the status of wound healing<br><br>• To prevent cross infection<br>• Infrared lamp promotes episiotomy wound healing |
| • Provide the infrared lamp therapy with infrared lamp of 230 volts that emits infrared rays at a distance of 45–50 cm for 10–15 minutes<br>• Place sanitary pad from front to back. Do not shift position of the pad once applied<br>• Dress the patient appropriately and make the patient comfortable; and leave the unit clean<br>**Postprocedural steps:**<br>• Discard the waste in the right biomedical waste bin (yellow color code bin)<br>• Wash the articles, dry these and replace in the utility room<br>• Remove gloves and wash hands<br>• Record the findings of the REEDA scale on the patient's chart<br>• Report to physician if REEDA scale shows abnormal findings | <br><br>• Avoid chances of contamination<br><br>• Promotes confidence and self-esteem<br><br><br>• For maintaining proper biomedical waste management<br><br>• For further use<br><br>• To prevent cross infection<br>• Acts as communication channel |

## PERINEAL CARE

**Definition:** Cleaning the perineum, external genitalia and surrounding area using antiseptic solution to prevent infection prior, during and after delivery and after any vaginal surgery is known as perineal care.

Or

It is an antiseptic irrigation or sponging of the perineum during a specific period following delivery or operation on the reproductive system, urinary meatus or anus.

### Purposes

- To clean the perineum before any surgery or delivery
- To inspect the perineal region for redness, edema, ecchymosis, discharge, approximation (REEDA)
- To reduce the occurrence of infection in the perineal region
- To provide soothing effect
- To relieve pain
- To relieve inflammation

- To promote healing
- To stimulate circulation
- To reduce body odor and improve self-image
- To promote the sense of well-being
- To observe the lochia

## Points to be Kept in Mind

- Maintain privacy during the procedure.
- Always clean from more clean area to less clean area.
- Use correct concentration of antiseptic solution.
- Collect specimen of discharge if required before cleaning the area

## Articles

- **A clean tray containing:**
  - Antiseptic solution 2% Dettol or Savlon (2 mL Savlon/Dettol in 100 mL of water)
  - Normal saline in a bottle
  - Cheatle forceps
  - Sterile sanitary pad
  - Kidney trays
  - Sterile gloves
  - Mackintosh with sheet/towel
- **Sterile tray containing:**
  - Artery forceps—1
  - Dissecting forceps—1
  - Cotton balls
  - Gauze pieces
  - Sterile gallipot/bowl → to pour antiseptic solution
  - Sterile towel to wipe hands after surgical scrub
  - Draw sheet
- **Other articles:**
  - Bedpan
  - Screen
  - Plastic apron
  - Mask
  - Infrared lamp

## Procedure

| Nursing action | Rationale |
|---|---|
| **Preprocedural steps:** | |
| • Collect all the articles at the bedside of patient | • To save time and energy |
| • Explain the procedure to the patient | • To win the cooperation |
| • Ask the patient to empty her bowel and bladder | • To ensure cleanliness and reduce the number of |
| • Spread curtain/screen around the bed | microorganisms in perineal area |
| • Provide dorsal recumbent position | • To maintain privacy |

*Contd...*

| Nursing action | Rationale |
|---|---|
| • Ask the mother to remove undergarments and sanitary pad | • To facilitate better viewing and provide comfort |
| | • For better visualization |
| • Spread mackintosh under patient's hips along with newspaper lining | • To prevent soiling of linen |
| • Observe lochia (color, odor, consistency) | • To detect any abnormality |
| • Discard the pad in yellow bin | • As per biomedical waste management protocol |
| **Intraprocedural steps:** | |
| • Keep bedpan under the buttocks of the patient | • To collect the normal saline/sterile water that is poured due to excessive sticky lochial discharge |
| • Pour warm water/normal saline on the perineal area | • To remove excessive clots/discharge |
| • Remove bedpan | |
| • Wash hands with soap | • To maintain barrier nursing |
| • Open the sterile tray, arrange articles with cheatle forceps and pour antiseptic solution in the sterile gallipot in tray | |
| • Wear gloves | |
| • Drape the area using diamond draping method | |
| • Take the cotton swabs with artery forceps, dip in the Savlon and squeeze excess lotion with dissecting forceps into the kidney tray | • To prevent contamination |
| ▪ Clean the mons pubis in a C-shape stroke in one stroke and in the same manner from other side | |
| ▪ Clean the farther side of the labia majora with one swab in one down ward stroke. Repeat cleaning the nearer side of the labia majora with another swab | |
| ▪ Using the thumb and index finger of nondominant hand, separate the labia majora | |
| ▪ Clean the farther side of the labia minora with one swab in one downward stroke. Repeat on the nearer side of the labia minora using another swab | |
| ▪ Clean the vestibule starting from vestibule to vagina with one swab in one downward stroke and from vagina to fourchette using another swab in one downward stroke | |
| ▪ Wipe all traces of antiseptic away with sterile normal saline swabs in the same manner as described above using thumb/artery forceps | • Because antiseptic solution may cause irritation |
| ▪ Place sanitary pad from front to back. Do not shift position of the pad once it is applied. | |
| ▪ Help the mother to wear undergarment (panty) | • To absorb the discharge |
| **Postprocedural steps:** | |
| • Make the patient comfortable and leave the unit clean | • For maintaining proper biomedical waste management |
| • Discard the waste in the right biomedical waste bin (yellow color code bin) | • For further use |

*Contd...*

| Nursing action | Rationale |
|---|---|
| • Wash the articles, dry these and replace in the utility room | • To prevent cross infection |
| • Remove gloves and wash the hand | • Acts as communication channel between health professionals |
| • Record the findings on the patient's chart | |
| • Report to physician if any abnormality is found | • For further management |

# BREAST CARE

**Definition:** Breast care is a procedure to clean and prepare the breast tissue, nipple and supporting tissue during pregnancy and lactation for the breastfeeding.

## Purposes

- To clean the breast.
- To prevent infection and inflammation.
- To detect any abnormality like breast engorgement, breast abscess, mastitis, etc.
- To prevent breast complications.
- To prepare the mother for breastfeeding.
- To stimulate milk ejection.
- To prevent cracked and sore nipples during lactation.
- To provide comfort to the mother.

## Articles

- Jug with hot water
- Jug with cold water
- Basin
- Bowl to pour
- Wet swabs
- Hand sanitizer
- Soap
- Kidney tray
- Bowl with lid
- Mackintosh with draw sheet
- Towel

## Procedure

| Nursing action | Rational |
|---|---|
| **Preprocedural steps:** | |
| • Collect and assemble all the articles required for the procedure near the bedside of mother | • Saves time and energy |
| • Explain the procedure to the mother | • To win the cooperation of the mother |
| • Ask the mother to empty the bladder and bowel | • To be relaxed during the procedure |
| • Spread curtains/screen around the bed | • To provide privacy |
| • Give comfortable position to the mother (lying/sitting) | • To provide comfort to the patient |
| • Spread the mackintosh with towel over the top of mother (sitting position) or under back (lying down) | • To prevent soiling of linen |
| • Pour hot and cold water in a basin and make sure temperature of the water should be checked by the mother | • To avoid discomfort |
| • Wash hands | • To prevent cross infection |
| • Stand on the right side of the patient | • To carry out the procedure easily |
| **Intraprocedural steps:** | |
| • Expose both breasts first and check the symmetry | • To find out abnormality |
| • Expose the farthest breast covering the near one | |
| • Inspect the breast for size, inverted/cracked/retracted nipples or sign and symptom of infection | • To find out abnormality |
| • Place kidney tray under breast | • To collect waste water |
| • Pour lukewarm water with a bowl on breast | • To make the breast soft and promote circulation |
| • Lubricate hands and breast with soap | |
| • Apply soap on your hands and apply on the breast | • To clean the breast |
| • Do not apply soap on nipples | |
| • Follow the below discussed steps | |
| **1. Rolling** | |
| ▪ Start at the top of the breast. Move fingers in a circular motion on one spot on the skin | • To detect any abnormality |
| ▪ Press firmly into the chest wall. Give special attention while massaging over hard areas | |
| ▪ After few seconds, move the fingers to the next area on the breast | |
| ▪ Spiral around the breast towards the areola using this massage | |
| ▪ The motion is similar to that used in breast examination | |
| **2. Stroking** | |
| ▪ Start from the top of breast towards the nipple with a light tickle-like stroke | • Provide relaxation and stimulate milk ejaculation reflex |
| ▪ Continue this stroking motion from chest wall to nipple around whole breast nipple for 2–3 minutes | |

*Contd...*

| Nursing action | Rational |
|---|---|
| **3. Shaking** | |
| ▪ Support the breast with one hand and shake with other hand for 2–3 minutes | • Gravity will help the milk eject |
| Or | |
| Shake the breast while leaning forward | |
| ▪ Remove the soap thoroughly with water | • To clean the breast |
| ▪ Dry the breast with clean towel | |
| ▪ Clean nipple with clean swab gauze piece | |
| **4. Expressing the milk** | |
| • **Position:** | |
| ▪ Position the thumb and first two fingers about I"–1.5" behind the nipple | • The place of milk reservoir |
| ▪ Place the thumb pad above the nipple and the finger part below the nipple forming the letter "C" with the hand | |
| ▪ Note the fingers are positioned so that milk reservoirs lie beneath them | |
| ▪ Avoid cupping the breast | |
| • **Push:** | |
| ▪ Push straight into the chest wall | |
| ▪ Avoid spreading the fingers apart | |
| ▪ For large breast, first lift and then push into the chest wall | |
| • **Roll:** | |
| ▪ Roll thumb and fingers forwards at the same time | • To drain the reservoirs |
| ▪ The rolling motion of the thumb and the fingers compresses and empties the milk reservoirs without hurting sensitive breast tissue | |
| • **Repeat rhythmically:** | |
| ▪ Repeat rhythmically | |
| ▪ Position, push, roll; position, push, roll | |
| **Rotate** the thumb and finger position to express the milk from the other reservoirs. Use both hands on each breast | |
| **Avoid these motions:** | |
| • Avoid squeezing the breast | • This can cause bruising |
| • Avoid pulling out the nipple and breast | • This can cause tissue damage |
| • Avoid sliding on the breast | • This causes skin burns |
| *Steps on second breast are same as given above.* | |
| **Postprocedural steps:** | |
| • Provide comfortable position to the patient | • For further use |
| • Wash articles and replace in the utility room | • To prevent cross infection |
| • Wash hand | • For further management |
| • Record the findings on the patient's chart | |
| • Report if any abnormality is found, to the physician | |

# 13

# POSTNATAL ASSESSMENT

**Definition:** Postnatal period is a post delivery period when the maternal system returns to a prepregnant state. This is a 6-week period, which is divided into three phases:

  i. **Immediate:** 24 hours after delivery
 ii. **Early:** Up to 7 days
iii. **Late:** Up to 6 weeks

## Purposes

- To assess the normal physiological changes in maternal body during the postnatal period.
- To assess the normal psychological changes in the immediate postnatal period.
- To assess the involution of reproductive organs.
- To assess the mother for potential medical problems after delivery.
- To teach the postnatal mother regarding care of herself and baby.

## Articles

| Articles | Purposes |
|---|---|
| • Hand washing articles<br>  ▪ Soap<br>  ▪ Soap dish<br>  ▪ Towel | • To prevent the spread of infection |
| • Gloves, gown, mask | • To maintain barrier nursing during the procedure |
| • Draw sheet and mackintosh | • To prevent soiling of the linen |
| • Weighing machine | • To note the weight of the mother |
| • Measuring tape | • To measure fundal height |
| • Screen | • To provide privacy to mother |
| • TPR tray | • To check the vital sign of mother |
| • Treatment chart | • To record the finding |
| • Perineal care tray | • To provide perineal care for the proper assessment of episiotomy wound and also to note the color, odor, amount of lochia |

## Procedure

| Nursing action | Rationale |
|---|---|
| **Preprocedural steps:**<br>• Collect all the articles required for the procedure and keep the articles on the right side of the patient bed | • To avoid unnecessary wastage of time |
| • Greet the mother | • It opens the channel for communication |

*Contd...*

| Nursing action | Rationale |
|---|---|
| • Explain the procedure to the mother<br>• Ask the mother to empty the bladder<br>• Provide comfortable position to the mother<br>• Spread screen around patient's bed<br>• Wash hands | • To win the confidence of the mother<br>• For correct estimation of fundal height<br>• To provide comfort to the patient<br>• To provide privacy to the mother<br>• To prevent spread of infection |
| **Intraprocedural steps:**<br>• History taking<br>  ▪ **Biodata:** Name, age, education, occupation<br>  ▪ Chief complaints<br>  ▪ Present pregnancy history<br>    ○ Para<br>    ○ Gravida<br>    ○ EDOD<br>    ○ Any other problem (specify)<br>  ▪ Family history<br>    ○ Support person<br>    ○ No of children<br>    ○ Any history of genetic disorder<br>  ▪ Delivery history<br>    ○ Duration of labor<br>    ○ Any problem faced during labor<br>    ○ Position of fetus<br>    ○ Date and time of delivery<br>    ○ Types of delivery | • To provide treatment/care accordingly.<br>• A quick review of pregnancy history is useful for further planning<br><br><br><br><br><br><br><br>• With this information, the activity level required from mother will be known and accordingly instructions can be given.<br><br>• This information will help to plan postnatal procedures such as episiotomy care, etc. |
|   ▪ Neonatal data<br>    ○ Sex of baby<br>    ○ Weight of the baby<br>    ○ Difficulty faced during birth process<br>    ○ Any congenital abnormality<br>    ○ Breastfeeding<br>  ▪ Postpartum data<br>    ○ Activity level after delivery<br>    ○ General health<br>    ○ Characteristics of lochia<br>    ○ Problems during postpartum period (physiological/psychological) | • This information helps to plan care for the newborn<br><br><br><br><br>• This information is helpful in assessment of the mother's present condition and planning of her care and health education to be imparted to her and the family |
| **Physical examination** | |
| **A. General physical examination**<br>  ▪ General appearance<br>    ○ Gestures of pain and her facial expressions<br>    ○ Face: Edematous<br>    ○ Hair: Combed, – Yes/No<br>    ○ Dressed up neatly – Yes/No<br>    ○ Well oriented: Yes/No<br>  ▪ Vital signs<br>    ○ Temperature: 100.4°F – normal after delivery<br>    ○ If >100.4°F – Check for following possible infection like laceration, sutures, breast, lochia | • Helps in detecting any deviation from normal physiological changes |

*Contd...*

| Nursing action | Rationale |
|---|---|
| ○ Pulse: Varies from 70 to 80/min. Pulse more than 100/min should be investigated for fever and shock.<br>○ Respiration: Observe the respiration whether it is normal or abnormal (i.e., labored, shallow or fast breathing).<br>○ Blood pressure: Remains unchanged after delivery. If history of HTN, preeclampsia, eclampsia – check BP every hour during early postpartum period. | |
| **B. Head to foot examination**<br>• **Head:** Infection, clean lines, pediculosis, etc.<br>• **Eyes:** Sclera/conjunctiva for pallor, signs of infection and jaundice<br>• **Ears:** Hearing abnormality, discharge, accumulation of wax<br>• **Nose:** Discharge, DNS, epistaxis<br>• **Mouth:** Cracked lips, cheilosis, dental caries, gum swelling or bleeding, coated tongue | • To detect any complication in the immediate postnatal period |
| • **Neck:** Symmetry, shape, lymph adenopathy<br>• **Breast exam:** Symmetry, shape, primary and secondary areola, tubercles, inverted or flat nipples and colostrum<br>• **Upper extremities:** Check for bony extremities, capillary refill<br>• **Lower extremities:** Homan's sign, edema, bony deformity, varicose vein<br>• **Bowel and bladder:** Constipation, incontinence<br>• **Genital area:** Bleeding, discharge, infection, hemorrhoids and hygiene | |
| **C. Postnatal assessment**<br>The acronym BUBBLEHE is commonly used to remember the necessary components of the postnatal assessment. It is as follows:<br>B – Breast<br>U – Uterus<br>B – Bowel<br>B – Bladder<br>L – Lochia<br>E – Episiotomy<br>H – Homan's sign<br>E – Emotions | • Provides a guide for the thorough assessment in postnatal period |
| **Breast**<br>• **Inspection:** Inspect the breast for its color, shape, contour, abnormal discharge from the nipples<br>• **Palpation**<br>  ▪ Gently palpate each breast<br>  ▪ Check for any tenderness, firm ness and fullness | • To rule out any abnormality and help in detecting breast complication that will create difficulty in breastfeeding |

*Contd...*

| Nursing action | Rationale |
|---|---|
| **Abdominal breathing:**<br><br>▪ Instruct the woman to sit comfortably<br>▪ Instruct her to inhale through nose, keep the ribcage as stationary as possible and allow the abdomen to expand and then contract the abdominal muscles as she exhales slowly through the mouth<br>▪ Instruct her to place one hand on the chest and one on the abdomen when inhaling. The hand on the abdomen should rise and the hand on the chest should remain stationary<br>▪ Repeat for five times | |
| **Head lift**<br><br>▪ This exercise can be started within few days after childbirth<br>▪ Instruct the mother to lie in supine position with knees bent and arms out-stretched at her side<br>▪ Instruct her to inhale deeply at first and then exhale while lifting the head slowly, to hold the position for a few seconds and relax | • This exercise strengthens the abdominal muscles |
| **Head and shoulder raising:**<br><br>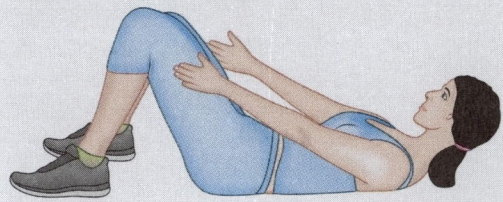<br><br>On 2$^{nd}$ postpartum day, instruct the mother to:<br>▪ Lie flat without pillow and raise head until the chin touches the chest<br>▪ On 3$^{rd}$ postpartum day, raise both head and shoulders off the bed and lower them slowly<br>▪ Repeat for 10 times | • It strengthens the abdominal and diaphragmatic muscles |
| **Leg raising:**<br><br>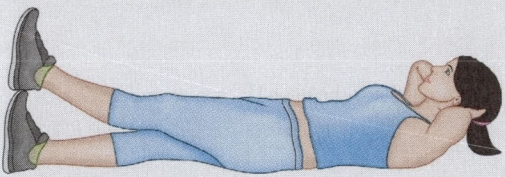<br><br>▪ Instruct the mother to start this exercise on 7th postpartum day<br>▪ Instruct her to lie flat on the floor with no pillows under the head, point toes and slowly raise one leg, keeping the knee straight | • This exercise strengthens the abdominal muscles and helps in involutions of reproductive organs |

*Contd...*

| Nursing action | Rationale |
|---|---|
| ▪ Lower the leg slowly<br>▪ Gradually, increase the frequency to ten times with each leg | |
| • **Knee and leg rolling** | • This exercise will strengthen the oblique abdominal muscles |

| Nursing action | Rationale |
|---|---|
| ▪ Instruct the mother to lie on the bed/floor with knee bent and feet flat on floor<br>▪ Keep the shoulders and feet stationary and roll the knees to side to touch one side of the bed first and then other<br>▪ Repeat it five times<br>▪ Later, as flexibility increases, the exercise can be varied by the rolling of one knee only (the mother rolls her left knee to touch the right side of the bed, returns to center and rolls the right knee to touch the left side of the bed | |
| • **Pelvic tilting/rocking**<br>(same as in antenatal exercises) | |
| • **Hip hitching**<br>▪ Instruct the mother to lie on her back with one knee bent and other knee straight<br>▪ Slide the heel of the straight leg downwards, thus lengthening the leg<br>▪ Shorten the same leg by drawing the hip up toward the ribs on the same side<br>▪ Repeat up to 10 times keeping the abdomen pulled in<br>▪ Change to the opposite side and repeat | • It strengthens the deep transverse muscles which are the main support for the spine and thus prevents backache problem in the future |

*Contd...*

| Nursing action | Rationale |
|---|---|
| • **Abdominal tightening**<br>   ▪ Instruct the woman to sit comfortably or kneel on all fours<br>   ▪ Breathe in and out, then pull the lower part of the abdomen below the umbilicus while continuing to breathe normally<br>   ▪ Hold for 10 seconds<br>   ▪ Repeat up to 10 times | • It strengthens the abdominal muscles and helps in involution of uterus after delivery |
| **2. Circulatory exercises**<br>   Foot and leg exercise<br>   (same as in antenatal exercise)<br>**3. Pelvic floor exercises**<br>   Kegel exercise<br>   (same as in antenatal exercise)<br>**4. Chest exercises**<br><br>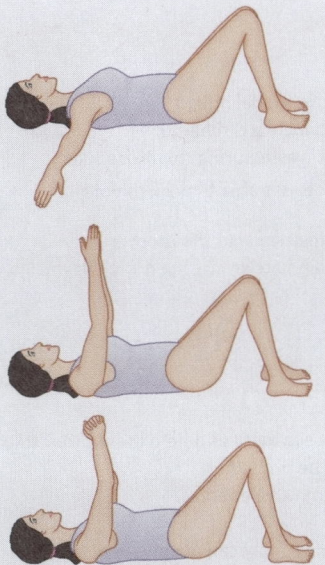<br><br>   ▪ Instruct the mother to lie flat on the floor mat with arms extended straight out to the side, bring both hands together above the chest, while keeping the arms straight, hold for a few seconds and return to the starting position<br>   ▪ Repeat the exercise five times initially and follow the advice of the health care provider for increasing the number of repetitions<br>   ▪ Instruct the mother to bend her elbows, clasp her hands together above her chest, and press her hands together for a few seconds<br>   ▪ Repeat up to five times | • To strengthen the diaphragmatic muscles |

**Postprocedural steps** (same as in antenatal exercise)

# MEASURING INVOLUTION OF UTERUS

**Definition:** Involution is a process by which the reproductive organs return to their prepregnant state both anatomically and physiologically (almost 6 weeks).

## Purposes

- To estimate the rate of involution.
- To assess the general condition during puerperium.
- To rule out complications.

## Articles

| Articles | Purposes |
|---|---|
| • **A tray containing:** | |
| ▪ Inch-tape | • To measure fundal height |
| ▪ Sanitary pad | • To absorb lochial discharge |
| ▪ Kidney tray | • To collect waste during the procedure |
| • Bedpan | • If mother is not able to walk to void |
| • Draping sheet | |
| • Screen | • To provide privacy to the mother |
| • Gloves | • To maintain barrier nursing during vaginal pad check-up |

## Procedure

| Nursing action | Rationale |
|---|---|
| **Preprocedural steps:** | |
| • Explain the procedural to the patient | • To reduce anxiety and help the mother to cooperate during the procedure |
| • Collect all the articles needed for the procedure in a tray and place it near the bed side locker | • Saves time and energy |
| • Ask her to void before the procedure and if mother is not able to walk, provide bedpan | • Full bladder may cause upward displacement of uterus |
| • Spread the curtains/screen around the bed | • To provide privacy to the patient |
| **Intraprocedural steps:** | |
| • Position the mother flat in bed with the head comfortable on a pillow; if it is uncomfortable the woman may flex her legs | • Flat position prevents false assessment of fundal height |
| • Drape the patient, exposing only the lower abdomen | • Enhances easy assessment |
| • Determine the uterine firmness | |
| ▪ Rub your palms to warm up | • To prevent chillness to abdomen |
| ▪ Gently place one hand on the lower segment of the uterus and keep the other hand on the lateral side of the fundus | • It provides support to the uterus |

*Contd...*

| Nursing action | Rationale |
|---|---|
| <ul><li>Check for engorgement of breast, i.e. tender, painful and heavy</li><li>**Check the nipples:** Inverted, erected, cracked, bleeding, bruises and presence of colostrum and milk.</li></ul>**Abdomen:**<ul><li>Provide supine position to the woman.</li><li>Place a pillow under her head and upper shoulders</li><li>Have her arms by her sides</li><li>Expose her abdomen from below the breast to the symphysis pubis</li><ul><li>Note the shape of abdomen, linea nigra, striae gravidarum and previous surgical scars</li><li>If cesarean delivery, check the incision site for healing or for infection</li><li>Note the involution of uterus by using following steps:</li><ul><li>Instruct the woman to empty her bladder</li><li>Uterus is to be centralized and with a measuring tape, the fundal height is measured above the symphysis pubis</li><li>Following delivery, the fundus lies about 13.5 cm above the symphysis pubis</li><li>During first 24 hours, the level remains constant, there after there is steady decrease in height by 1.25 cm in 24 hours, so that at the end of 2nd week uterus becomes the pelvic organ</li></ul><li>Note for subinvolution of uterus, which occurs when the uterus is not completely contracted and retracted</li><li>Palpate the uterus to note its consistency normally after delivery, if there is no product of conception remains inside the uterine cavity, uterus feel firm and hard. If uterus is soft and boggy, it means contraction are inadequate and blood continues to flow</li></ul></ul>**Bladder**<ul><li>Inspect and palpate the bladder simultaneously while checking the height of fundus</li><li>Teach the mother about:</li><ul><li>Perineal care</li><li>Always wipe from front to back after voiding and defecating</li><li>Frequent emptying of bladder</li><li>Early ambulation</li></ul><li>Measure the first three voiding, it should be at least 150 cc. Frequent small voiding with or without pain and burning may indicate infection or retention</li></ul> | <ul><li>To provide comfort to the woman</li></ul><br><br><br><br><br><br><br><br><br><br><br><br><br><br><br><br><br><br><br><br><br><br>• Subinvolution of uterus causes postpartum hemorrhage<br><br><br>• To rule out the atonicity of the uterus in the immediate postpartum period<br><br><br><br><br><br>• To help the uterus to contract and retract properly and prevent the atonicity of the uterus |

*Contd...*

| Nursing action | Rationale |
|---|---|
| **Bowel** | |
| • Ask the patient regarding daily bowel movement, she must not become constipated | • To prevent constipation |
| • If the bowel of postnatal mother is not emptied till 2nd postpartum day, start mild laxative | |
| • Auscultate for bowel movement | |
| • Encourage mother to drink extra fluid | |
| • Have mother select fruits and vegetables from her menu | |
| • Increase fiber and fluid intake | |
| • Encourage early ambulation | |
| **Genital area:** | |
| • Assess the perineal area for any redness, edema, tenderness | • For better visualization |
| • Inspect the episiotomy thoroughly using flashlight | |
| • Use the acronym REEDA to guide assessment | |
|   R – Redness | |
|   E – Edema | |
|   E – Ecchymosis | |
|   D – Discharge | |
|   A – Approximation of suture line | |
| • Note the color, composition, odor, amount of lochial discharge | |
| • Normal characteristic of lochia | |
|   ▪ **Odor:** Peculiar, offensive, fishy smell | • If offensive, it indicates infection |
|   ▪ **Reaction:** Alkaline | |
|   ▪ Color | |
|   ▪ Lochia rubra (1–4 days), red | |
|   ▪ Lochia serosa (5–9 days), yellow, pink, pale brownish | • Persistence of red color beyond normal limit signifies subinvolution or retained bits of placenta |
|   ▪ Lochia alba (10–15 days), pale white | |
|   ▪ Composition | |
|     ○ **Lochia rubra:** Blood, shreds of fetal membranes and decidua, vernix caseosa, lanugo, meconium | |
|     ○ **Lochia serosa:** RBC, leucocytes, wound exudate, mucus from cervix | |
|     ○ **Lochia alba:** Plenty of decidual cells, leucocytes, mucus, fatty and granular epithelial cells | |
|   ▪ **Amount:** Average amount for first 5–6 days is estimated 250 mL | • Scanty or excessive indicates infection |
| **Rectal area:** | |
| • Check the rectal area for hemorrhoids | • To relieve pain |
| • Encourage the mother to take sitz bath and local analgesics as prescribed by physician | • Help in detection of infection |

*Contd...*

| Nursing action | Rationale |
|---|---|
| **Homan's sign:**<br>• Provide supine position to the mother<br>• Press down gently on the patient's knee (legs extended flat on bed)<br>• Ask the mother to dorsiflex her feet<br>• If mother feels pain or tenderness in the calf muscles, it indicates thrombophlebitis<br>• Examine the lower extremities for the presence of redness, pain and edema, it indicates deep vein thrombosis | • Provides a sign for detection of DVT |
| **Emotional status:**<br>• Assess the emotional state of the mother to diagnose postpartum blues, postpartum depression, postpartum psychosis | • To detect any psychological complication in the postnatal period |
| **Postprocedural steps:**<br>• Provide comfortable position to the patient<br>• Wash all the articles used during the procedure and replace in the utility room<br>• Remove gloves, wash hand<br>• Record the finding on the patient chart and report to physician if any abnormality found<br>• Inform the mother about time and date of next visit. | • To provide comfort to the mother<br><br>• To prevent cross infection<br>• Acts as communication channel between the health professionals<br>• To provide continuity of care |

## POSTNATAL EXERCISES

**Definition:** A series of physical exercises that are performed by the postnatal mother to bring about optimal functioning of all systems and prevent complications.

### Purposes

- To educate about correct posture and body mechanics.
- To prevent genital prolapse.
- To prevent stress incontinence of urine.
- To improve muscle tone, especially perineal and abdominal muscle that are stretched during pregnancy and labor.
- To minimize the risk of deep vein thrombosis (DVT).
- Reduction in aches and pains after delivery, e.g., backache and cramps.
- Improves posture and body awareness.
- Reduces constipation by accelerating movements in the intestine.
- Helps postnatal recovery.
- Helps to sleep better by relieving stress and anxiety that might make the mother restless at night.

- Exercise increases blood flow to the skin, and gives a healthy growth (glow).
- Mother will receive an emotional lift from the release of internal hormones like endorphins.
- Mother will feel more contented, as the release of tranquilizer hormones that follows exercise aids relaxation.
- Mother will regain the shape more quickly after delivery.

## Articles

- Mat/Dari to do laying exercises comfortably
- Chair to sit in a comfortable position

## Points to be Taken Care

- Warm up and cool down at every exercise session.
- If woman feels faintness and dizziness, slow down or stop exercising.
- Drink plenty of fluids.
- Do not over heat the body as overheating of body has been linked to some birth defects.
- Maintain good posture.
- Wear a well-fitted and supported brassiere.
- From midway throughout pregnancy, avoid exercising on the back as it places too much pressure on major veins and reduces $O_2$ supply to placenta and baby.

## Warning Sign to Stop Exercise

- Vaginal bleeding
- Dizziness or feeling pain
- Breathlessness
- Chest pain
- Headache
- Muscle weakness
- Calf pain/swelling
- Uterine contractions
- Decreased fetal movements
- Fluid leaking from vagina

## Procedure

| Nursing action | Rationale |
|---|---|
| **Preprocedural steps:** (Same as for antenatal exercise) **Intraprocedural steps:** **Exercise 1: Abdominal exercises** | • It strengthens the diaphragmatic muscles and improves oxygenation of the blood |

*Contd...*

| Nursing action | Rationale |
|---|---|
| • **Abdominal breathing:**<br>  ▪ Instruct the woman to sit comfortably<br>  ▪ Instruct her to inhale through nose, keep the ribcage as stationary as possible and allow the abdomen to expand and then contract the abdominal muscles as she exhales slowly through the mouth<br>  ▪ Instruct her to place one hand on the chest and one on the abdomen when inhaling. The hand on the abdomen should rise and the hand on the chest should remain stationary<br>  ▪ Repeat for five times | |
| • **Head lift**<br>  ▪ This exercise can be started within few days after childbirth<br>  ▪ Instruct the mother to lie in supine position with knees bent and arms out-stretched at her side<br>  ▪ Instruct her to inhale deeply at first and then exhale while lifting the head slowly, to hold the position for a few seconds and relax | • This exercise strengthens the abdominal muscles |
| • **Head and shoulder raising:**<br>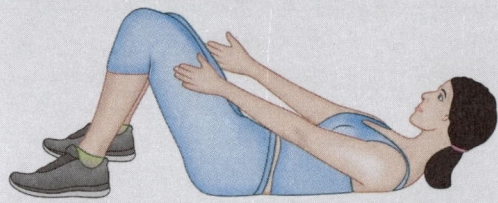<br>On 2nd postpartum day, instruct the mother to:<br>  ▪ Lie flat without pillow and raise head until the chin touches the chest<br>  ▪ On 3rd postpartum day, raise both head and shoulders off the bed and lower them slowly<br>  ▪ Repeat for 10 times | • It strengthens the abdominal and diaphragmatic muscles |
| • **Leg raising:**<br>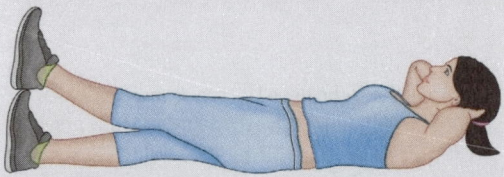<br>  ▪ Instruct the mother to start this exercise on 7th postpartum day<br>  ▪ Instruct her to lie flat on the floor with no pillows under the head, point toes and slowly raise one leg, keeping the knee straight | • This exercise strengthens the abdominal muscles and helps in involutions of reproductive organs |

*Contd...*

| Nursing action | Rationale |
|---|---|
| <ul><li>Lower the leg slowly</li><li>Gradually, increase the frequency to ten times with each leg</li></ul> <br> • **Knee and leg rolling** <br><br> <br><br> <ul><li>Instruct the mother to lie on the bed/floor with knee bent and feet flat on floor</li><li>Keep the shoulders and feet stationary and roll the knees to side to touch one side of the bed first and then other</li><li>Repeat it five times</li><li>Later, as flexibility increases, the exercise can be varied by the rolling of one knee only (the mother rolls her left knee to touch the right side of the bed, returns to center and rolls the right knee to touch the left side of the bed</li></ul> | • This exercise will strengthen the oblique abdominal muscles |
| • **Pelvic tilting/rocking** <br> (same as in antenatal exercises) | |
| • **Hip hitching** <br> <ul><li>Instruct the mother to lie on her back with one knee bent and other knee straight</li><li>Slide the heel of the straight leg downwards, thus lengthening the leg</li><li>Shorten the same leg by drawing the hip up toward the ribs on the same side</li><li>Repeat up to 10 times keeping the abdomen pulled in</li><li>Change to the opposite side and repeat</li></ul> | • It strengthens the deep transverse muscles which are the main support for the spine and thus prevents backache problem in the future |

*Contd...*

| Nursing action | Rationale |
|---|---|
| • **Abdominal tightening**<br>  ▪ Instruct the woman to sit comfortably or kneel on all fours<br>  ▪ Breathe in and out, then pull the lower part of the abdomen below the umbilicus while continuing to breathe normally<br>  ▪ Hold for 10 seconds<br>  ▪ Repeat up to 10 times | • It strengthens the abdominal muscles and helps in involution of uterus after delivery |
| **2. Circulatory exercises**<br>  Foot and leg exercise<br>  (same as in antenatal exercise)<br>**3. Pelvic floor exercises**<br>  Kegel exercise<br>  (same as in antenatal exercise)<br>**4. Chest exercises**<br>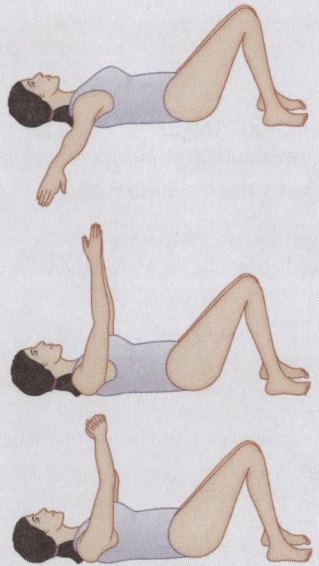<br>  ▪ Instruct the mother to lie flat on the floor mat with arms extended straight out to the side, bring both hands together above the chest, while keeping the arms straight, hold for a few seconds and return to the starting position<br>  ▪ Repeat the exercise five times initially and follow the advice of the health care provider for increasing the number of repetitions<br>  ▪ Instruct the mother to bend her elbows, clasp her hands together above her chest, and press her hands together for a few seconds<br>  ▪ Repeat up to five times | • To strengthen the diaphragmatic muscles |

**Postprocedural steps** (same as in antenatal exercise)

# MEASURING INVOLUTION OF UTERUS

**Definition:** Involution is a process by which the reproductive organs return to their prepregnant state both anatomically and physiologically (almost 6 weeks).

## Purposes

- To estimate the rate of involution.
- To assess the general condition during puerperium.
- To rule out complications.

## Articles

| Articles | Purposes |
|---|---|
| **A tray containing:** | |
| ▪ Inch-tape | • To measure fundal height |
| ▪ Sanitary pad | • To absorb lochial discharge |
| ▪ Kidney tray | • To collect waste during the procedure |
| • Bedpan | • If mother is not able to walk to void |
| • Draping sheet | |
| • Screen | • To provide privacy to the mother |
| • Gloves | • To maintain barrier nursing during vaginal pad check-up |

## Procedure

| Nursing action | Rationale |
|---|---|
| **Preprocedural steps:** | |
| • Explain the procedural to the patient | • To reduce anxiety and help the mother to cooperate during the procedure |
| • Collect all the articles needed for the procedure in a tray and place it near the bed side locker | • Saves time and energy |
| • Ask her to void before the procedure and if mother is not able to walk, provide bedpan | • Full bladder may cause upward displacement of uterus |
| • Spread the curtains/screen around the bed | • To provide privacy to the patient |
| **Intraprocedural steps:** | |
| • Position the mother flat in bed with the head comfortable on a pillow; if it is uncomfortable the woman may flex her legs | • Flat position prevents false assessment of fundal height |
| • Drape the patient, exposing only the lower abdomen | • Enhances easy assessment |
| • Determine the uterine firmness | |
| ▪ Rub your palms to warm up | • To prevent chillness to abdomen |
| ▪ Gently place one hand on the lower segment of the uterus and keep the other hand on the lateral side of the fundus | • It provides support to the uterus |

*Contd...*

| Nursing action | Rationale |
|---|---|
| <ul><li>Palpate the abdomen until the top of the fundus is located</li><li>Note whether fundus is firm and hard or soft/boggy</li><li>If fundus is soft/boggy, massage it, until it becomes firm</li></ul><ul><li>Determine the height of fundus</li><li>Measure the height of the top where the fundus is felt in finger breadth</li><li>With the help of inch-tape, measure from the level of fundus to the upper border of symphysis pubis</li></ul> | <ul><li>A firm fundus indicates that muscles are contracted and bleeding will not occur</li><li>Massaging helps to remove the blood clot from uterine cavity</li></ul><ul><li>Finger breadth measurement should correspond to the number of days after delivery</li></ul> |

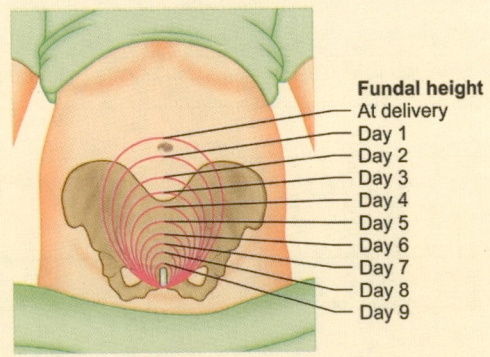

**Fundal height**
- At delivery
- Day 1
- Day 2
- Day 3
- Day 4
- Day 5
- Day 6
- Day 7
- Day 8
- Day 9

**Fig:** Involution of uterus

- On 1st day - fundus is felt 10–12 cm above symphysis pubis
- From 2nd-11th day – fundus descends at rate of ½ inch, 1 finger breadth (1.25 cm) per 24 hour
- On 11th day—uterus sinks below the level of symphysis pubis and becomes a pelvic organ
- Bleeding and odor assessed for infection

| Nursing action | Rationale |
|---|---|
| <ul><li>Wear gloves</li><li>Check perineal pad for color, presence of clots and odor of lochia</li><li>Offer perineal pad if needed</li></ul>**Postprocedural steps:**<ul><li>Wash the articles and replace in the utility room</li><li>Remove gloves and wash hands</li><li>Record the fundal height in patient chart</li></ul> | <ul><li>To maintain hygiene and prevent infection</li></ul><ul><li>For next time use</li><li>To prevent spread of infection</li><li>Documentation helps in obtaining a clear picture about involution of uterus</li></ul> |

## ARTERY FORCEPS

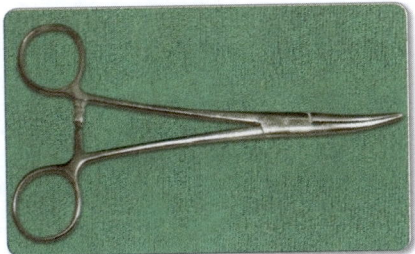

### Purposes

- To clamp bleeding vessels during hemorrhage.
- To grasp tissue at the time of operation.
- To hold stay sutures.

## ALLIS' FORCEPS

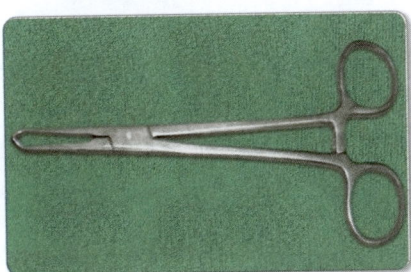

### Purposes

To grasp tough structures, like rectus sheath or fascia in operations, like tubectomy, lower segment cesarean section, abdominal hysterectomy.

## BABCOCK'S FORCEPS

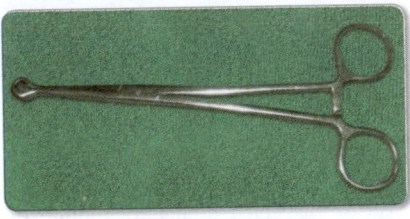

### Purpose

To grasp tubular structures, like Fallopian tube in tubectomy (modified pomeroy operation), ureter, appendix, etc. because tip of the instrument is atraumatic as there is no sharp tooth.

## PUNCH BIOPSY FORCEPS

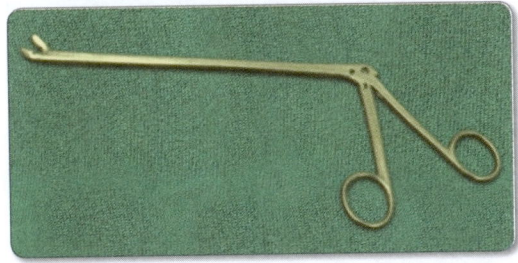

### Purpose

To take biopsy from the cervix.

## NEEDLE HOLDER

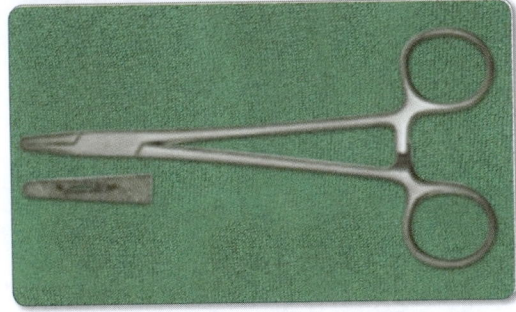

### Purposes

- This instrument is used for **grasping needle at the time of suturing.**
- The inner surface of tip has serrations and a small grove for firm grasp of the curved needle.
- The box joint is placed very close to tip to give adequate pressure because of the lever effect.

## MAYO SCISSORS

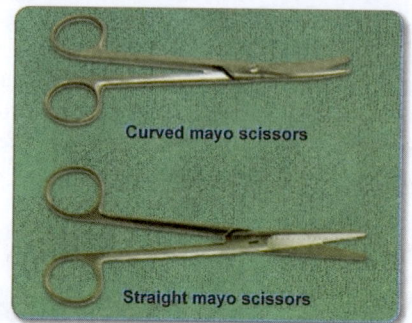

Curved mayo scissors

Straight mayo scissors

### Purposes

- To cut the umbilical cord.
- To make episiotomy.
- To cut suture materials as in cesarean section.

## EPISIOTOMY SCISSORS/ PERINEORRHAPHY

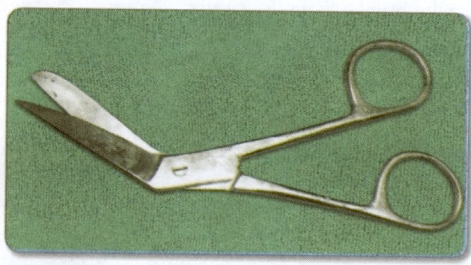

### Purpose

To give episiotomy cut during the time of labor.

## AYRE'S SPATULA

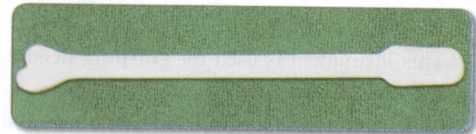

### Purposes

- To take Pap smear for screening carcinoma of cervix.

- To take cells from lateral vagina for knowing the hormonal status.

## UTERINE CURETTAGE

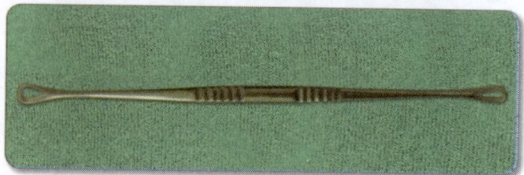

### Purposes

- It may be sharp at both ends or sharp at one end and blunt at the other.
- In D+E operation, the curettage is done by blunt curette as the uterine wall is very soft.
- It is used in incomplete abortion for D+C.
- It can also be used in D+C operation one week following evacuation of hydatidiform mole.

## CUSCO'S BIVALVE SELF-RETAINING VAGINAL SPECULUM

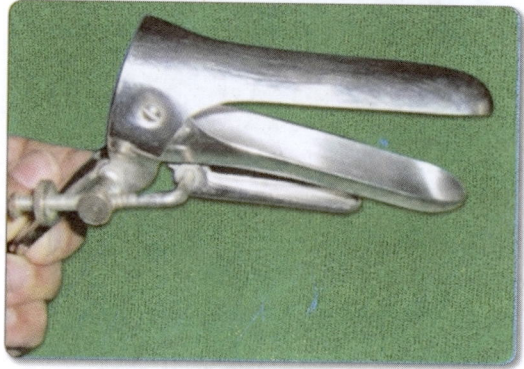

### Purposes

- To visualize the cervix and vaginal fornices for any local cause (polyp, ectopy) of APH.
- For taking Pap smear.
- Used during Cu-T insertion and removal.
- To detect leakage of liquor from cervical Os in case of suspected premature rupture of membranes (PROM).

## DOYEN'S RETRACTOR

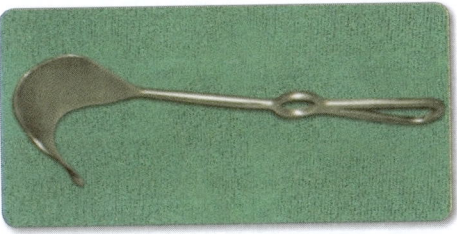

### Purpose

It is used for retracting bladder and abdominal wall during abdominal operations like lower segment cesarean section (LSCS), abdominal hysterectomy, laparotomy.

## DISSECTING FORCEPS (TOOTHED AND NONTOOTHED)

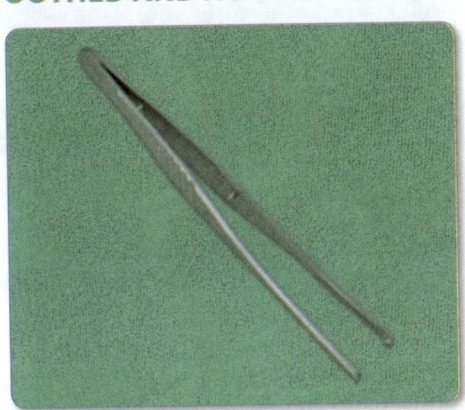

**Toothed**

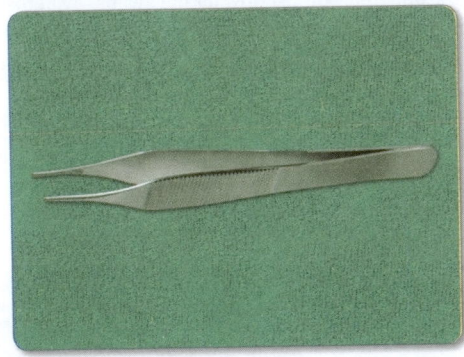

**Nontoothed**

### Purpose

To hold tough structures, like rectus sheath, cut margins of vaginal flaps pelvic floor repair (PFR) of the skin margins during suturing.

## GREEN ARMY TAGE FORCEPS

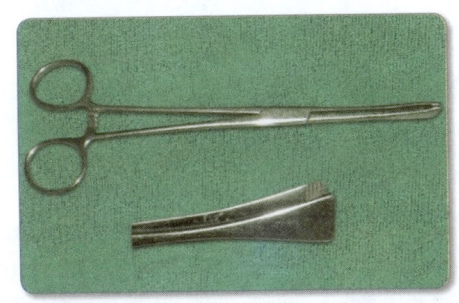

### Purposes

- This forceps is used as a **hemostat in cesarean operation**. As the tips are broad, wide area can be compressed.
- In LSCS, the cut uterine edges bleed, this forceps is applied to the two angles and lower and upper edge of the incision.
- The common indicators for LSCS are fetal distress in first stage, chronic pelvic disease (CPD), abnormal presentations like transverse lie, brow, breech in primi, previous two scars on the uterus.

## HEGAR'S DILATOR/DAS'S DILATOR

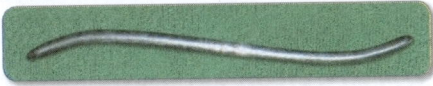

## HAWKIN-AMBLER DILATOR

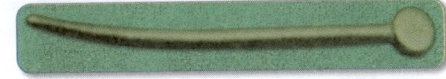

### Purposes

- It is a long rod-like instrument with gentle curve and tapering tip.

- It is used for dilatation of the cervix in procedures like D&C, D&E, Fothergills operation, hysteroscopy, cervical stenosis, primary dysmenorrhea.
- It can cause perforation if too much force is used. Very large dilatation can cause cervical incompetence.

## KOCHER'S FORCEPS (CLAMP)

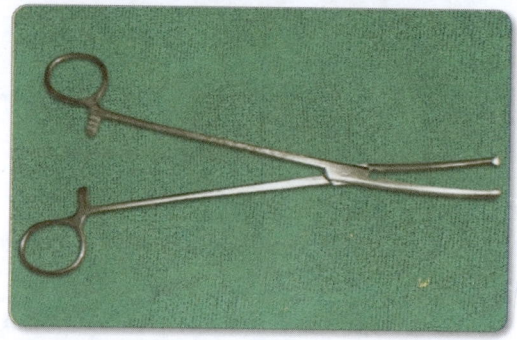

## Purposes

- This instrument is used for holding Fallopian tube in hysterectomy.
- The tips of the blades have teeth so that the tissue does not slip.
- The blades can either be straight or curved. This instrument is used in hysterectomy to clamp fallopian tube which are then transfixed.
- It is also used for salpingectomy in ectopic or oophorectomy in ovarian mass. This can also be used for clamping umbilical cord of newborn at the time of delivery or for artificial low rupture of membranes (ARM).

## OVUM HOLDING FORCEPS

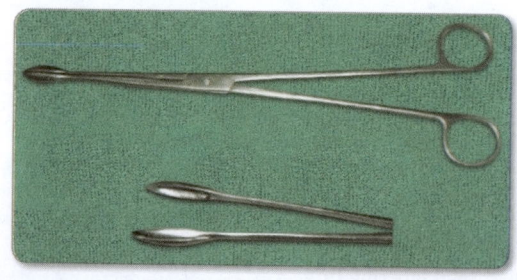

## Purposes

- This instrument is used for **removing the products of conception in inevitable, incomplete abortion and in MTP operations.**
- The tip of this instrument is rounded cup-like to avoid perforation and to hold large tissue.
- This instrument has no catch. This is to avoid perforation of wall.

## SIMS' SPECULUM

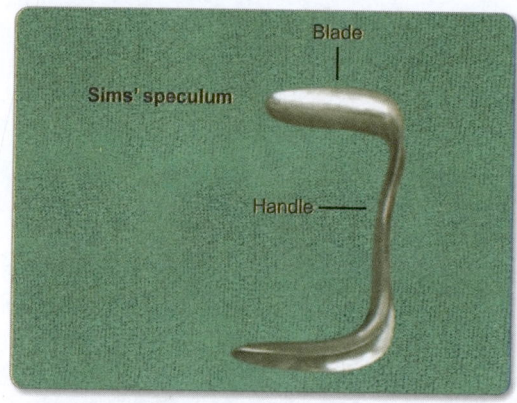

## Purposes

- Sims' speculum is used for inspection of vagina and cervix in the OPD. It retracts posterior vaginal wall.
- For complete visualization, anterior vaginal wall retractor must be used.
- **Used in gyne OPD for following procedures:** Taking pap smear, insertion and removal of Copper-T, colposcopy, taking swabs, hysterosalpingography (HSG).
- **Used in gyne operations:** D&C, cervix biopsy, vaginal hysterectomy, Fothergills, repair of vesicovaginal fistula, hysteroscopy.

## SIMS' ANTERIOR VAGINAL WALL RETRACTOR

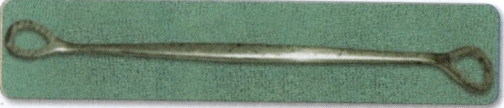

## Purposes

- This instrument is **used with Sims' speculum.** It is a long instrument with blunt loops at both the ends making an angle for easy **visualization of cervix and vagina**, especially useful in case of **cystocele.**
- **Used in obstetrics:**
  - For inspection (bluish discoloration in early pregnancy, local cause for threatened abortion, local cause in antepartum hemorrhage [APH]).
  - First trimester MTP by suction curettage.
  - In second trimester MTP by ethacredyl lactate os tightening or cervical encerclage.
  - Removal of os tightening stitch at the onset of labor or at 38 weeks.
- Inspection for suspected rupture of membranes.
- After forceps delivery to trace for cervical tears.
- **Advantage:**
  - **Wide area for inspection. Instrumentation is easy.**
- **Disadvantages:**
  - **Needs assistant (Not self-retaining)**
  - **Must bring patient to edge of the table.**

## SPONGE HOLDER/SPONGE HOLDING FORCEPS

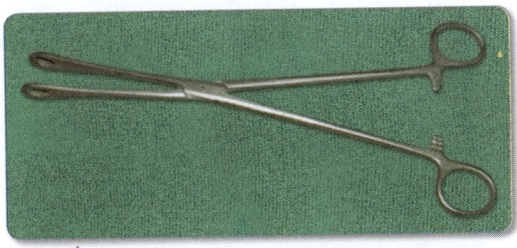

## Purposes

- This instrument is used for **holding sponge or a gauze piece** for painting the area before operation.
- This is also used for **grasping the cervix in obstetrics** in os tightening operation.
- Second trimester MTP (to hold the cervix before insertion of Foley's catheter).

- In exploring cervix, after forceps delivery (three sponge holding forceps are used). In LSCS, this can be used instead of green armytage for clamping the bleeding edges of uterine incision).

## SUCTION CURETTE

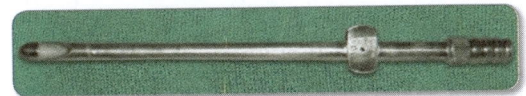

## Purposes

- This instrument is used for **first trimester MTP, suction of vesicular mole.**
- It is numbered as per outer diameter.
- **The size of the cannula selected is equal to number of weeks of pregnancy.**
- The tip is blunt (to prevent perforation) and below the tip are two sharp openings **for suction and curetting** the cavity.
- Usually, suction force of 60 mm Hg is applied. Rotational to and fro movements are done to empty the cavity.
- Grating sensation and gripping of the cannula indicates the procedure is complete.

## SHIRODKAR'S CERCLAGE NEEDLE

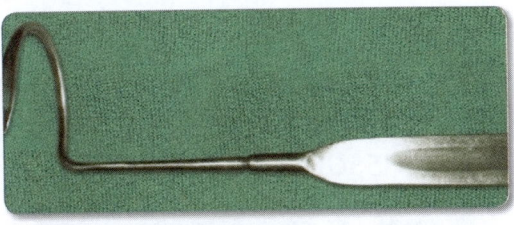

## Purposes

- This is specially designed needle for **putting stitch around the cervix.**
- The needle is inserted around the cervix through the opening made in vagina.
- The suture material (Mersilene tape) is threaded on the eye present at the tip and withdrawn.
- Another needle with curvature in reverse direction is used for other side.
- The knot is placed once the vagina is closed.

## SURGICAL BLADES/SCALPEL

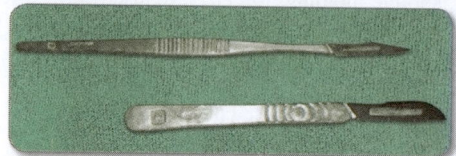

### Purpose

To give surgical cut during the time of operation.

## UTERINE SOUND

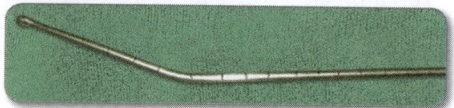

### Purposes

- It is a long instrument with blunt tip (to avoid perforation).
- About 5 cm from the tip it is bent to make angle of 30°.
- It has marking on it for measurements.
- The angle helps to negotiate **curvature of the uterus** (anteflexion).
- It is used for measuring **uterocervical length, length of the cervix**, to feel for any pathology inside the cavity like fibroid (submucus, polyp) Congenital anomalies like septa or bicornuate UT adhesions. To feel for the misplaced intrauterine contraceptive device (IUCD).

## LANES TISSUE FORCEPS

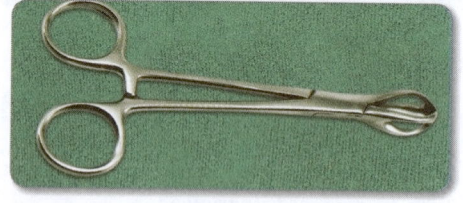

### Purposes

- To hold parietal wall (bulk of tough tissues) for retraction during abdominal operations with transverse incision.

- To hold the polyp or fibroid in polypectomy or myomectomy operations.
- To hold the towel during draping.

## UTERINE HOLDING FORCEPS

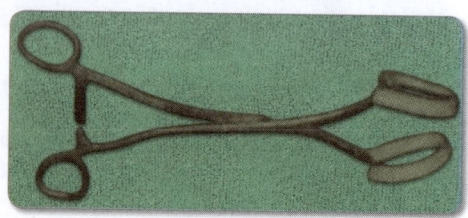

### Purpose

To fix and steady uterus when conservative surgery is done on the adnexae.

## BLADDER SOUND

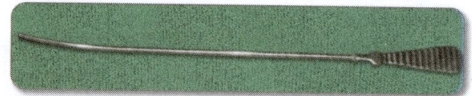

### Purposes

- It is a long instrument with gentle curve (not angled like uterine sound) and has no markings on it.
- It is used to define **extension of bladder cystocele and vaginal hysterectomy.**

## TROCAR AND CANNULA

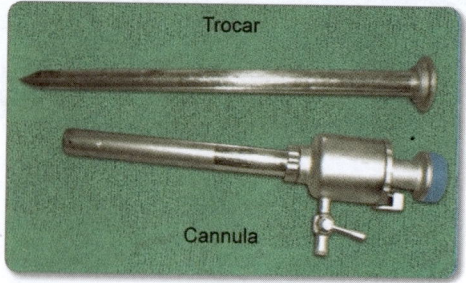

Trocar

Cannula

### Purposes

- Trocar is put into the cannula and then inserted into abdominal cavity for laparoscopy.

- It is also called port (port of entry to telescope and other instruments). It is numbered as per outer diameter.
- About 10 mm is used for operative telescope, 7 mm is used for band applicator for tubal ligation, 5 mm is used for other hard instruments like grasper, etc.
- A reducer sleeve is available to use large size port for small instrument.
- It has a trumpet valve to prevent gas leak. On one side there is opening for connecting it to gas ($CO_2$ or air).

## SINGLE-TOOTHED VULSELLUM

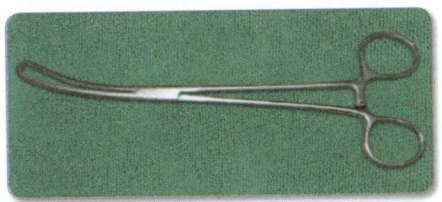

### Purposes

- To hold the cervix after opening the vault of vagina and to give traction while the remaining vault is being cut in total abdominal hysterectomy.
- To hold new cervical stump after amputation of the cervix and Fothergill's operation.
- To hold the cervical stumps left after subtotal hysterectomy.
- Sometimes to hold anterior lips of multiparous cervix in operation of D+C.

## TENACULUM

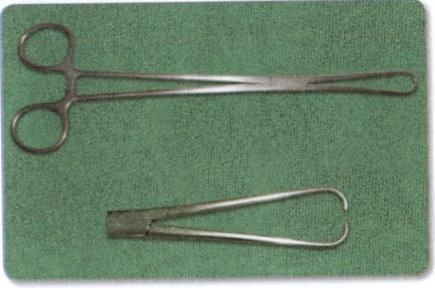

### Purposes

- This instrument is a straight instrument and has only single bite for grasping the cervix.
- It is used for **hysterosalpingography, hysteroscopy, laparoscopic chromopertubation.**

## EXTRACTOR (VENTOUSE)—SILASTIC CUP

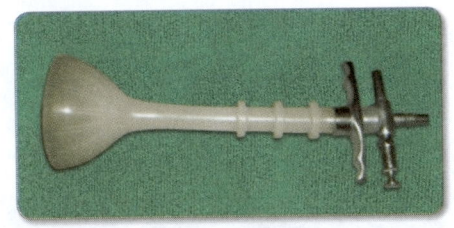

## EXTRACTOR (VENTOUSE)—METALLIC CUP

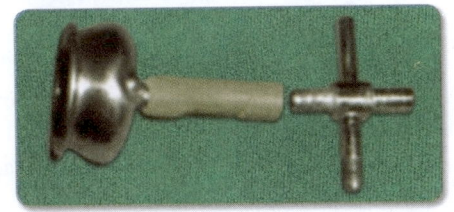

### Purposes

- **Alternative to forceps delivery.**
- Causes less trauma to mother and fetus. Prerequisites almost same. Available in two forms: Metal cup and silastic cup.
- Can be used when rotation is not complete.
- Produces artificial caput called chignon. Not to be used in pre term delivery.

## PINARD'S FETAL STETHOSCOPE

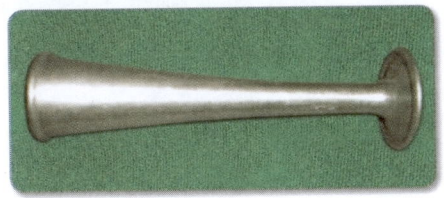

## Purposes

- This is used for **auscultation of fetal heart**. The tapering rim is applied to ear and the other side to mother's abdomen.
- With other instruments available for auscultation of fetal heart, this is now **rarely used**.

## TOWEL CLIP

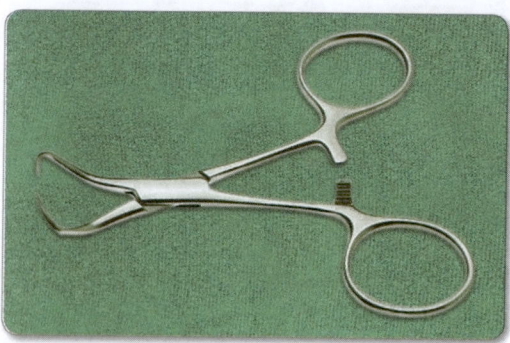

## Purposes

- It is used in draping the operative area-abdominal or vagina.
- The towels or sheets are fixed to the skin and each other with these clips.

## UMBILICAL CORD CLAMP

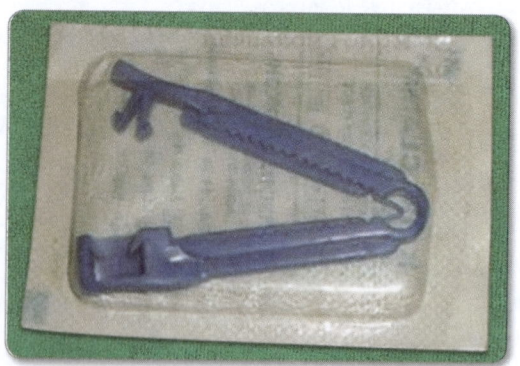

## Purpose

To clamp the umbilical cord of the newborn.

## UMBILICAL CORD CUTTING SCISSORS

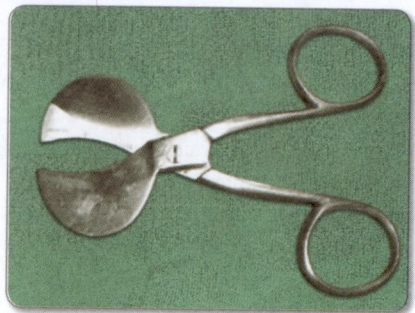

## Purpose

To cut the umbilical cord at the time of birth of the baby so as to separate the baby from the mother.

## FOLEY'S CATHETER

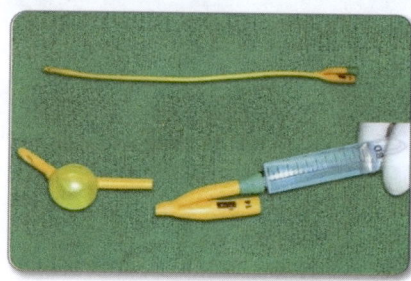

## Purposes

- This is a self-retaining catheter most commonly used for **drainage of the urinary bladder** after surgery.
- It is used in operations, like abdominal vaginal hysterectomy, Wertheim's hysterectomy, repair of vesicovaginal fistula.
- It is also used for diagnosis of incompetent cervix and for sonosalpingography.
- It has a bulb below the tip. This can be inflated by normal saline. It has two channels. One for inflating bulb and has a valve. The other channel is for drainage of urine to which urobag is attached. Number 14 or 16 are used in adult. Number 8 for sonosalpingography.

## PAIN CATHETER/FEMALE RUBBER CATHETER

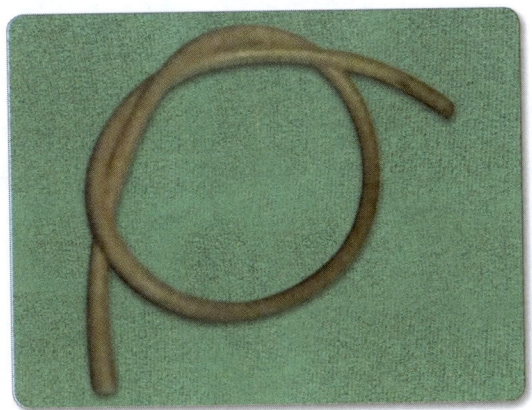

### Purposes

- To empty the bladder in retention of urine.
- To use as a tourniquet in myomectomy operation as alternative clamp.

# Index

Refer *'f'* for figure and *'t'* for table, respectively